MW01109975

Arthur Grove, Jr MD
Mass. Eye & Ear Infirmary
Boston

TUMORS of the EYE

I am most grateful to the Eye Cancer Foundation

for subsidizing the color section of this book.

A.B.R.

TUMORS
of the EYE

THIRD EDITION

ALGERNON B. REESE

M.D., D.Sc. (Hon.), M.D. (Hon.), LL.D. (Hon.), Department of Ophthalmology,
The Columbia-Presbyterian Medical Center, New York, New York

Medical Department
Harper & Row, Publishers
Hagerstown, Maryland
New York, San Francisco, London

DRUG DOSAGE

The authors and publisher have exerted every effort to ensure that drug selection and dosage set forth in this text are in accord with current recommendations and practice at the time of publication. However, in view of ongoing research, changes in government regulations, and the constant flow of information relating to drug therapy and drug reactions, the reader is urged to check the package insert for each drug for any change in indications and dosage and for added warnings and precautions. This is particularly important when the recommended agent is a new and/or infrequently employed drug.

TEXT AND COVER DESIGNED BY MARIA S. KARKUCINSKI

COMPOSITION BY AMERICAN BOOK–STRATFORD PRESS
PRINTING BY PEARL PRESSMAN, LIBERTY, PHILADELPHIA

76 77 78 79 80 81 10 9 8 7 6 5 4 3 2 1

Tumors of the Eye, Third Edition. Copyright © 1976 by Harper & Row, Publishers, Inc. All rights reserved. No part of this book may be used or reproduced in any manner whatsoever without written permission except in the case of brief quotations embodied in critical articles and reviews. Printed in the United States of America. For information address Medical Department, Harper & Row, Publishers, Inc., 2350 Virginia Avenue, Hagerstown, Maryland 21740
Library of Congress Cataloging in Publication Data
Reese, Algernon B.
  Tumors of the eye, Third Edition.
  Includes bibliographies and index.
  1. Eye—Tumors. I. Title.
RC280.E9R43   1976   616.9'92'84   76-17288
ISBN 0-06-142241-X

CONTENTS

CONTRIBUTORS

D. JACKSON COLEMAN, M.D.

pp. 332–342

Assistant Professor of Clinical Ophthalmology,
Department of Ophthalmology, Columbia University
College of Physicians and Surgeons, New York, New York

ROBERT M. ELLSWORTH, M.D.

pp. 343–350

Associate Professor of Clinical Ophthalmology,
Department of Ophthalmology, Columbia University
College of Physicians and Surgeons, New York, New York

RAMON L. FONT, M.D.

pp. 351–366

Assistant Chief, Ophthalmic Pathology Division, Armed
Forces Institute of Pathology; Clinical Professor of
Pathology and Ophthalmology, Departments of
Pathology and Ophthalmology, Georgetown University
Medical Center, Washington, D.C.

J. DONALD M. GASS, M.D.

pp. 367–372

Professor of Ophthalmology, Department of Ophthalmology,
University of Miami School of Medicine, Miami, Florida

IRA SNOW JONES, M.D.

pp. 238–241

Clinical Professor, Department of Ophthalmology,
Columbia University College of Physicians and
Surgeons, New York, New York

F. DAVID KITCHIN, M.D., F.R.C.P.

pp. 125–131

Associate Professor of Clinical Medicine, Department of
Medicine, Columbia University College of Physicians
and Surgeons, New York, New York

PATRICIA TRETTER, M.D.

pp. 373–377

Associate Professor of Clinical Radiology, Department of
Radiology, Columbia-Presbyterian Medical Center,
New York, New York

STEPHEN L. TROKEL, M.D.

pp. 378–384

Associate Ophthalmologist, Department of
Ophthalmology, Columbia University Medical Center,
Edward S. Harkness Eye Institute; Assistant Professor of
Clinical Ophthalmology, Department of Ophthalmology,
Columbia University College of Physicians and
Surgeons, New York, New York

PREFACE

Instead of joining the rocking chair brigade at my time of life I have chosen, like the sea squid, to leave in my wake a blast of black ink. The result is the third edition of Tumors of the Eye.

Like the two previous editions, it gives an overall view of all tumors and tumor-like lesions which directly or indirectly affect the eye, including descriptions of various types of lesions that must be included in the differential diagnosis. Special emphasis is placed upon the clinical and practical aspects of tumors encountered in the practice of ophthalmology.

In preparing this new edition, I have had the benefit of over ten additional years of experience in a consulting practice weighted toward tumors of the eye and adnexa, and I have attempted to keep abreast of new concepts and techniques. In virtually all the cases reported from the Edward S. Harkness Eye Institute, the diagnoses were made or confirmed here at the Algernon B. Reese Laboratory of Ophthalmic Pathology.

For those wishing to study types of eye tumors in depth, the references at the end of each chapter reflect contributions, new and old, to our specialty.

Since new growths are thought to develop in any tissue capable of cell division, it is surprising that to my knowledge no tumors have been reported arising from the epithelium of the lens. However, Mann* was able to induce a malignant lesion of the mouse lens if it was given a blood supply. The assumption was that the lens epithelium in man fails to develop neoplasms because of its avascularity, and not because of any inherent intracellular immunity.

The aim of this volume, based largely on my own clinical experience, observations and records, as well as a review of the literature, is to guide and aid the ophthalmologist and the ophthalmology resident in the detection, identification, and therapy of tumors of the eye. It is hoped that the coverage is sufficiently comprehensive to be of value to general pathologists and oncologists as well. In order to make room for new material it has been necessary to omit many references, as well as some figures and text that appeared in the first and second editions of this book; they may be consulted by readers seeking a fuller historical background.

* Mann J: Induction of an experimental tumour of the lens. Br J Cancer 1:63–67, 1947

ACKNOWLEDGMENTS

I am deeply grateful to a number of friends and colleagues for their help in the preparation of this edition. Eight recognized experts in different areas of ophthalmology have contributed sections on advances and current concepts in their particular fields of interest, broadening the scope of this work. Dr. Gordon M. Bruce has given me the benefit of his clinical experience and felicitous phrasing. Dr. Michael M. Mund undertook the important task of keying into the text the précis of new references and suggested that others be added. Dr. Lorenz E. Zimmerman promptly answered requests for advice and for pictorial material from the Armed Forces Institute of Pathology. Dr. Frederick A. Jakobiec and Dr. Nathan Lane clarified a number of areas in pathology. I am also indebted to Dr. Arnold W. Forrest, Dr. David H. Abramson and Dr. Philip E. Duffy for reviewing certain sections and making suggestions. Harper & Row, my publishers, have cooperated throughout the long period of preparation. They have earned my deep gratitude for recommending Elma T. Wadsworth, who has lent good cheer along with her considerable editorial skills to this endeavor. I am indebted to my secretary, Rita B. Dolan, whose efficiency and careful attention to detail have lightened this task.

COLOR ILLUSTRATIONS

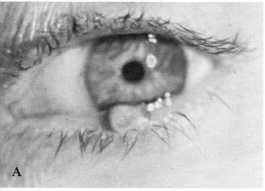

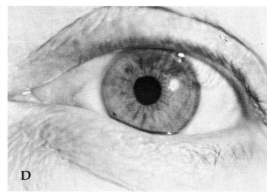

FIG. 1–1. Carcinomas of the lid. **A.** Squamous-cell. **B.** Basal-cell. **C.** Pigmented basal-cell before excision. **D.** After the lesser resection (see Fig. 1–12). (See p. 39.)

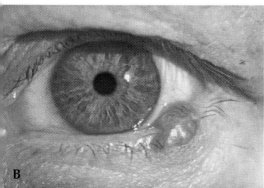

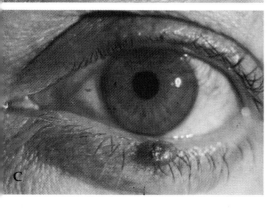

FIG. 1–2. Basal-cell carcinoma of the inner canthus and adjacent areas of both lids. (See p. 39.)

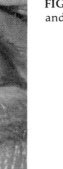

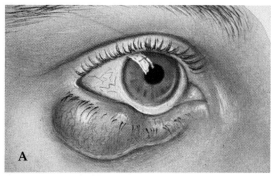

A

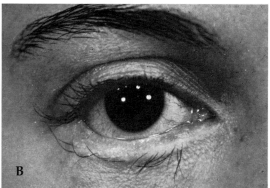

B

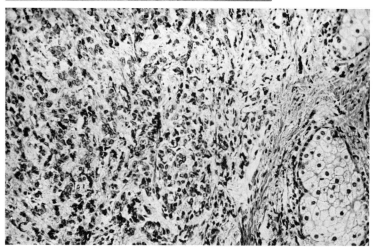

C

FIG. 1–7. Meibomian gland carcinoma of the lid. A tumor of the lower lid in a 20-year-old girl had grown slowly for four years. **A.** Clinically, the inflammatory element bears some resemblance to a diffuse chalazion. **B.** Appearance of the eye after a Hughes operation and cilia graft. **C.** Some meibomian gland tissue is seen at right in section studied microscopically. (See p. 41.) (Courtesy of J. H. Dunnington and W. Hughes.)

FIG. 1–18. Diffuse basal-squamous epithelioma of the lids and orbit. Extension of the tumor into the orbit has caused some degree of exophthalmos and limited motion of the eyeball. The lids are markedly indurated. Some inflammatory reaction, particularly in the upper lid, is characteristic of such extensive growths. (See p. 52.)

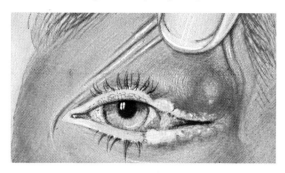

FIG. 1–19. Squamous-cell epithelioma of the bulbar conjunctiva at the limbus. (See p. 53.)

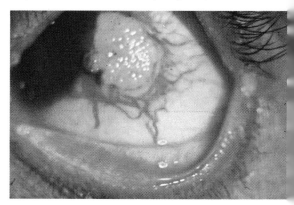

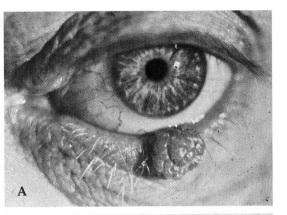

A

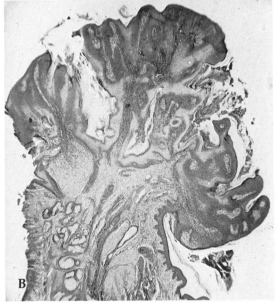

B

FIG. 1–23. Papilloma of the left lower lid. **A.** Clinical appearance. **B.** Section of the excised lesion. (See p. 55.)

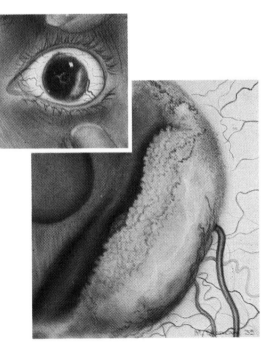

FIG. 1–24. Pigmented papilloma of the limbus and cornea of the left eye. The tumor, extending from 1 to 6 o'clock in a 50-year-old black woman, before beta radiation. The tumor regressed completely. Inset shows eye with residual scarring on the cornea over the tumor site. There was no recurrence after 12 years. (See p. 55.)

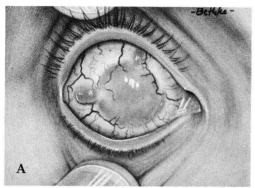

FIG. 1–25. Intraepithelial epithelioma of the cornea and limbus. A. The right eye of a 62-year-old man harbored three fleshy masses at the limbus, and the cornea was covered by uneven, elevated opaque tissue. B. Section shows abrupt transition from normal to tumor tissue, and a chronic inflammatory reaction in and under the epithelium. (See p. 56.)

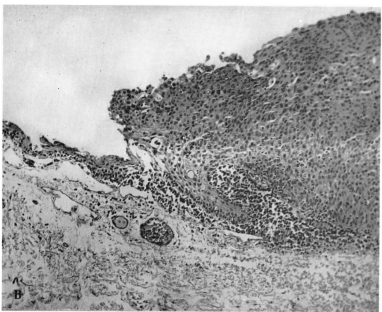

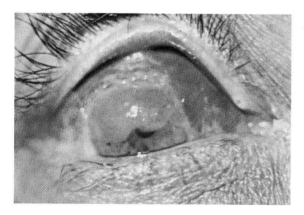

FIG. 1–26. Intraepithelial epithelioma of the cornea and bulbar conjunctiva. The pannus on the right cornea in a 46-year-old woman with active bilateral trachoma became thicker and more dense over a two-year period; the bulbar conjunctiva in the limbal area was thickened and indurated. The diagnosis was established when the epithelium was excised. (See p. 56.) (Courtesy of J. S. McGavic.[40])

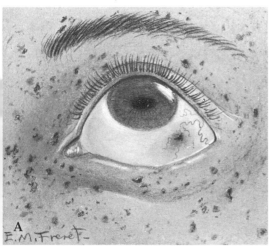
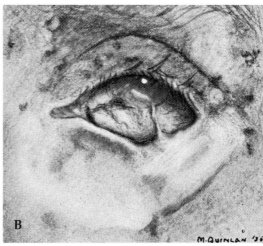

FIG. 1-28. Xeroderma pigmentosum. **A.** The left eye of a patient with early xeroderma pigmentosum. The lower lid shows some atrophy and loss of cilia. **B.** Within 15 years the atrophy is marked; there is symblepharon, congestion of the eyeball, and exposure keratitis of the cornea. (See p. 58).

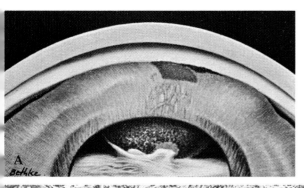

FIG. 2–14. Adenocarcinoma of the ciliary body. **A.** Examination by gonioscope shows the tumor mass through the pupillary area, its contact with a cataractous lens, and its extension to the anterior surface of the iris which is pushed forward. **B.** Structure of the tumor at a site where it extends through the periphery of the iris. (See p. 73.) (Courtesy of J. A. C. Wadsworth.[62])

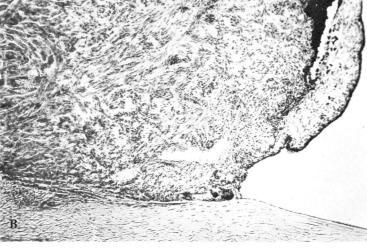

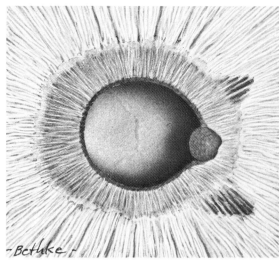

FIG. 2–19. Adenoma of the pigment epithelium of the iris. Lesion noted during a routine eye examination in a 60-year-old woman proved to be a globular pigmented tumor at the temporal pupillary margin, with a nodular mulberrylike surface. Some of the tumor is visible through interstices of the adjacent stroma. (See p. 77.) (Courtesy of F. Bracken.)

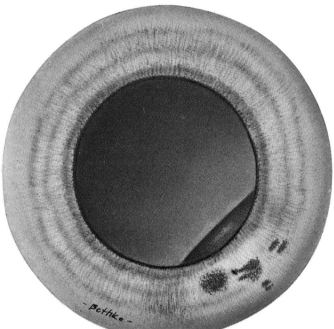

FIG. 2–30. Intraepithelial cyst of the iris with pigment changes in the overlying stroma. The iris stroma corresponding to the site of the cyst bulges forward, occluding the angle. Pigmentation in the stroma is due to migration of the pigmented epithelial cells. (See p. 86.)

FIG. 3–16. Exophytum type of retinoblastoma. The tumor has caused a complete funnel-shaped detachment of the retina. White calcium foci are seen above and below. (See p. 102.)

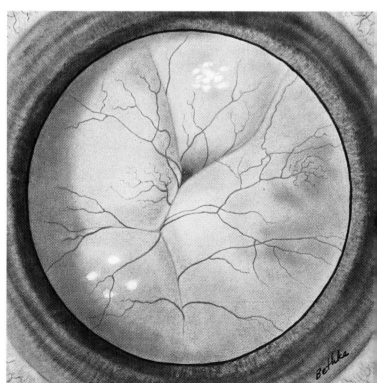

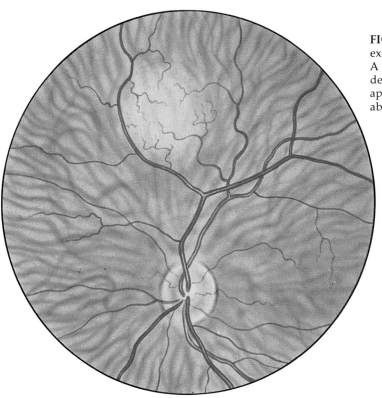

FIG. 3–17. Early intraretinal or exophytum type of retinoblastoma. A very slightly elevated, poorly demarcated, light-colored tumor of approximately 1 dd can be seen above the disc. (See p. 102.)

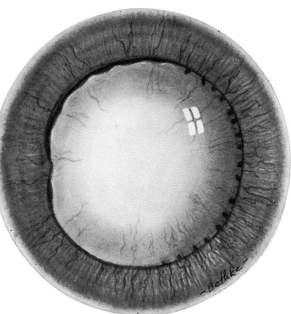

FIG. 3–24. Persistent hyperplastic primary vitreous. Behind the lens is a pinkish opaque tissue in which blood vessels tend to course radially. This tissue is densest in its yellow center. The equator of the lens is visible inside the dilated pupil. Ciliary processes are seen temporally. Blood vessels are present in the iris. (See p. 109.)

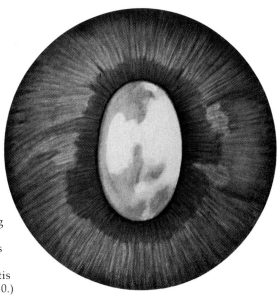

FIG. 3–27. Metastatic retinitis following a case of measles. A normal eye became painful and red during an attack of measles. A yellowish-white opaque inflammatory exudate in the vitreous obscured details of the fundus. The iris was atrophic and transmitted light freely. The clinical diagnosis of metastatic retinitis was confirmed by microscopic examination. (See p. 110.)

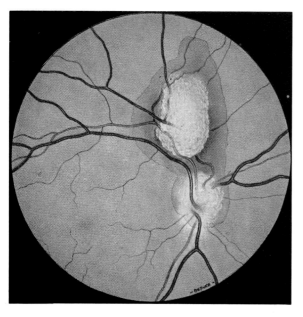

FIG. 4–8. Retinal and disc tumors in a case of tuberous sclerosis. The fundus shows a typical tumor of the optic nerve and retina. A mass of waxy translucent bodies presenting a nodular mulberrylike surface rises 4 diopters from the disc. A similar lesion elevated 6 diopters is seen in the retina above; lesions in the fellow eye were of the same type except that the retinal tumor was located beneath the inferior nasal vessels. (See p. 144.)

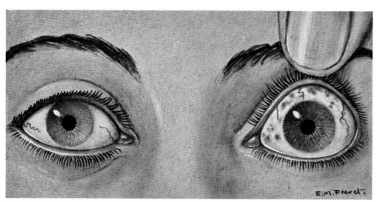

FIG. 7–2. Congenital ocular melanocytosis. The sclera of the left eye shows mottled pigmentation. Both the iris and fundus are darker than in the fellow eye. (See p. 183.)

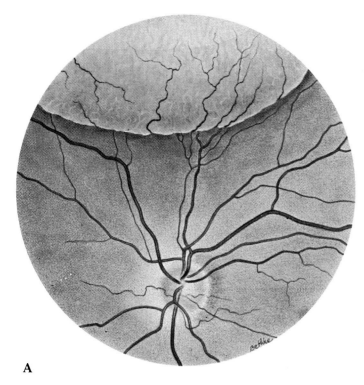

FIG. 7–13. Hourglass malignant melanoma of the choroid. **A.** Clinical appearance. **B.** Extension of tumor through sclera seen in enucleated eye. **C.** Microscopic appearance: (*a*) extension of tumor through emissary and (*b*) long ciliary nerve. (See p. 189.) (Courtesy of J. H. Dunnington.)

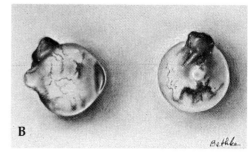

B

A

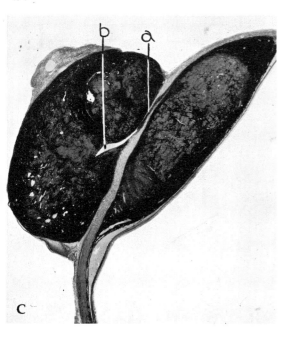

Fig. 7–13 *(continued)*

C

FIG. 7–23. Benign melanoma of the choroid immediately above the fovea. White dots over the surface represent excrescences of the lamina vitrea (drusen). The patient had no symptoms referable to the lesion, and no field defect was elicited. (See p. 198.)

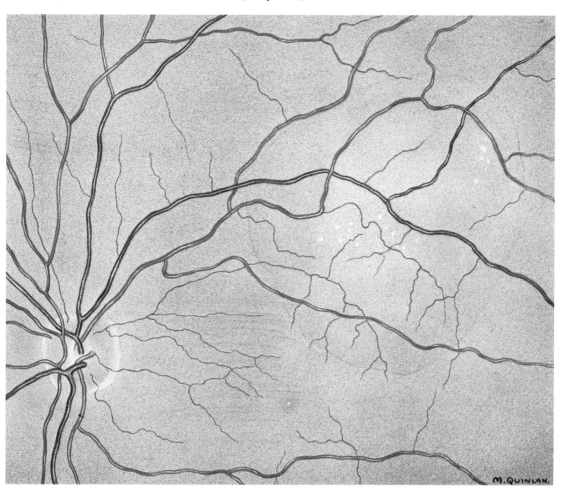

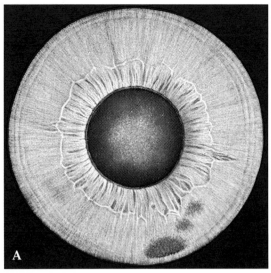

FIG. 7–28. Multiple foci of melanomas. **A.** The iris of an eye harboring a malignant melanoma of the choroid had three benign melanomas; there were none in the fellow iris. **B, C.** Sections of this eye, each showing a benign melanoma. (See p. 203.)

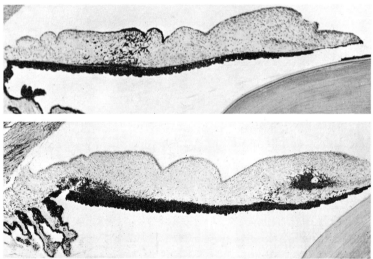

FIG. 7–35. Extension of malignant melanoma through the retina. **A.** The tumor has grown through the lamina vitrea and invaded the retina. **B.** Clinical appearance. (Courtesy of J. P. Macnie.) **C.** Malignant melanoma of the choroid in the macular area. The central well-demarcated mottled portion with hemorrhage has extended through the lamina vitrea, and the surrounding gray portion of the tumor has remained in the choroid. Tension lines of the retina are seen along the nasal margin. (See p. 209.)

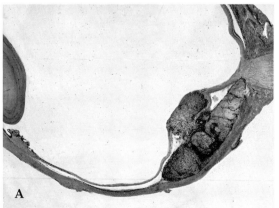

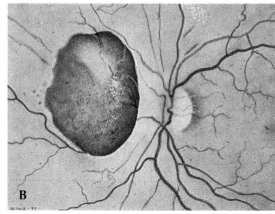

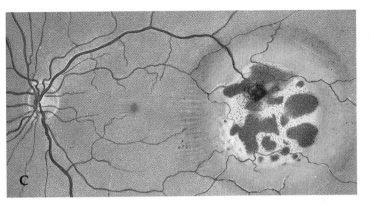

C

Fig. 7–35 *(continued)*

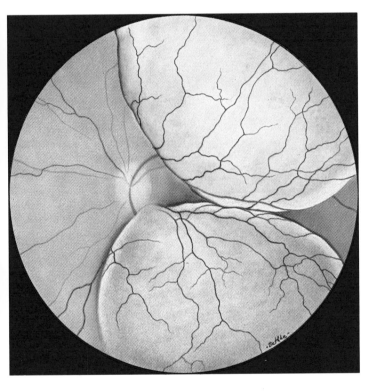

FIG. 7–36. Fundus of an eye with malignant choroidal melanoma showing a solid detachment of the retina above and a serous detachment below. The diagnosis was verified microscopically. (See p. 211.)

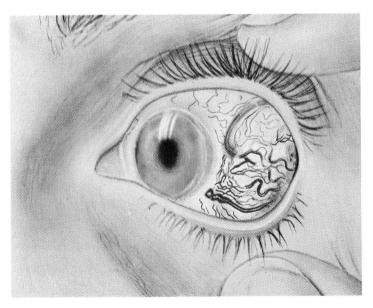

FIG. 7–39. Extraocular extension of a malignant choroidal melanoma. (See p. 212.)

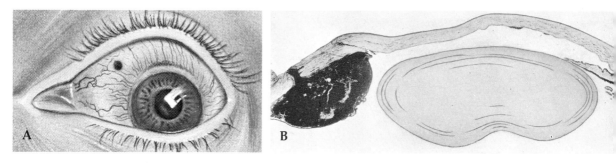

FIG. 7–40. Extension of a malignant melanoma of the ciliary body through an emissary of the anterior ciliary artery. **A.** This extension was the first sign of the tumor. The ciliary body tumor was not seen; the diagnosis was established by a biopsy of the extraocular nodule. **B.** Microscopic section of the eye. There were tumor seeds in the opposite angle. (See p. 212.)

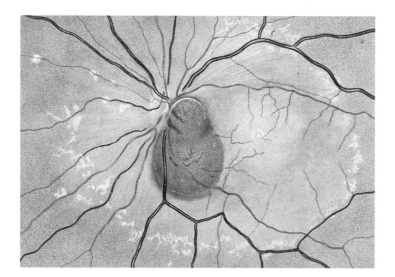

FIG. 7–42. Clinical appearance of a juxtapapillary malignant melanoma of the choroid. The tumor extends around the lamina vitrea into the disc and protrudes as a red globular mass. (See p. 212.) (Courtesy of R. Castroviejo.)

FIG. 7–43. Early malignant melanoma of the choroid. **A.** Viewed by direct ophthalmoscopy, a grayish-white lesion above the macula, suspected of being a melanoma, shows some edema or flat detachment. **B.** Scatter illumination reveals a dark, sharply demarcated mass with characteristic luminosity of the overlying retinal vessels. (See p. 213.)

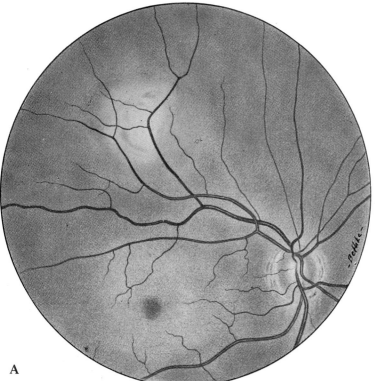

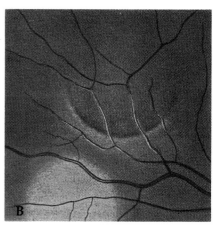

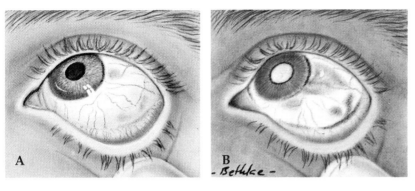

FIG. 7–44. Detection of the extent of pigmented conjunctival lesions by ultraviolet light. **A.** An eye from which a precancerous melanosis of the bulbar conjunctiva had been excised shows recurrence of two faint areas of melanosis, by ordinary light. **B.** The same eye seen by ultraviolet light. (See p. 216.)

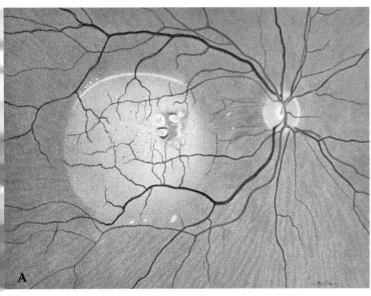

FIG. 7–47. Disciform degeneration in the macular region simulating a new growth. **A.** The elevated, dark lesion shows an area of mottled pigmentation and a number of punctate hemorrhages. (Courtesy of R. L. Pfeiffer.) **B.** Microscopic section from an eye with similar disciform degeneration. Between the retina over the site of the fovea (*a*) and the lamina vitrea (*b*) is a large plaque of fibrous tissue (*c*) containing bone (*d*). The fibrous tissue resulted principally from metaplastic proliferation of the pigment epithelium. (See p. 219.)

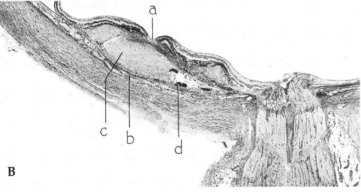

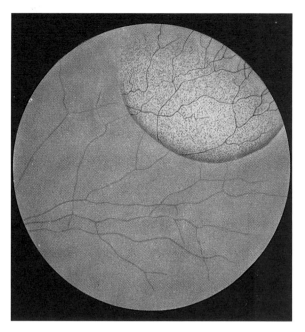

FIG. 7–51. Retinoschisis simulating a new growth. (See p. 221.)

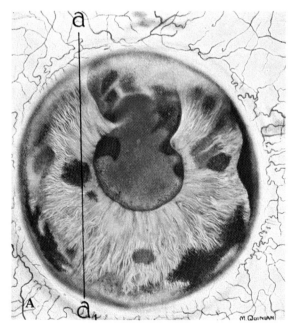

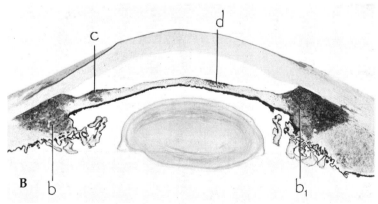

FIG. 7–53. Ring-type malignant melanoma of the ciliary body. **A.** Extensive, diffuse implantation growths cover the surface of the iris. The patient had secondary glaucoma, treated by an iridectomy. The line (*a* to *a₁*) indicates the site of the microscopic section in **B,** below. **B.** In the anterior sector of this eye, the tumor of the ciliary body (*b* to *b₁*) extends over the surface of the iris and into the stroma (*c*). An implantation growth is seen at *d*. (See p. 224.) (Courtesy of J. H. Dunnington.)

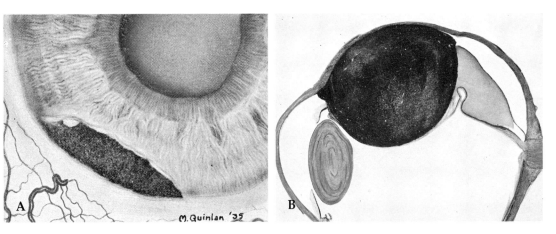

FIG. 7–55. Malignant melanoma of the ciliary body. **A.** Tumor projects into the anterior chamber; over the tumor site the anterior ciliary arteries are dilated. **B.** Microscopic section shows a serous detachment of the retina posterior to the tumor. (See p. 224.) (Courtesy of J. P. Macnie.)

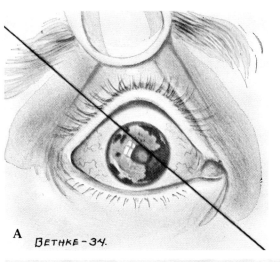

FIG. 7–60. Diffuse ring melanoma of the iris. **A.** This flat tumor was noted in a 62-year-old woman with secondary glaucoma. The diagonal line indicates the site of section shown in **B,** below. **B.** Anterior section under low power shows tumor cells in the angle at *a* and an implantation growh at *b.* (See p. 229.)

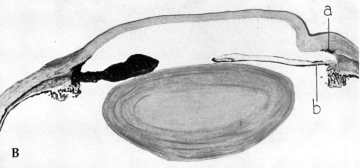

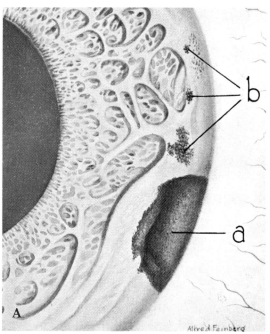

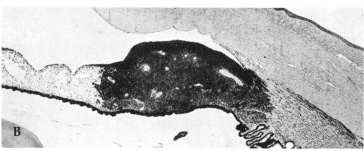

FIG. 7–62. Multiple origins of melanoma of the iris. A. The malignant melanoma at *a* arose from a benign melanoma which had shown no active growth during eight years of observation. The three microscopically identified iris freckles at *b* appeared successively with active growth of the malignant tumor. They do not represent implantation growths. B. Microscopic section. (See p. 230.)

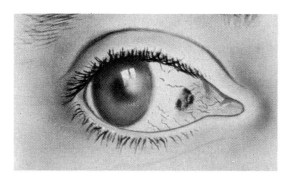

FIG. 7–77. Nevus of the conjunctiva. A typical elevated, pigmented, sharply demarcated nevus of the bulbar conjunctiva. (See p. 244.)

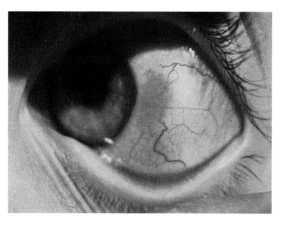

FIG. 7–80. Nonpigmented nevus of the conjunctiva. This slightly elevated lesion has a nutrient vessel and appears salmon-colored. (See p. 245.)

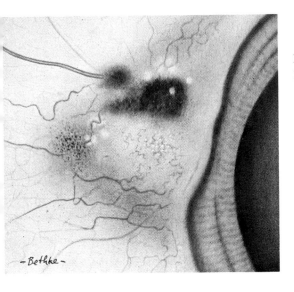

FIG. 7–81. Flat nevus of the bulbar conjunctiva extending partially onto the cornea. (See p. 245.)

FIG. 7–84. Nonpigmented nevus of the limbus. Because of its multiple conjunctival cysts (inset), this tumor is sometimes referred to as gelatinous nevus. (See p. 247.) (Courtesy of J. H. Dunnington.)

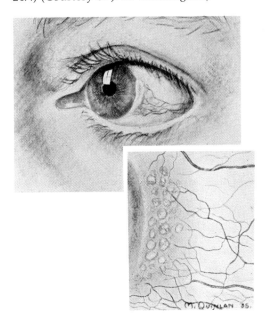

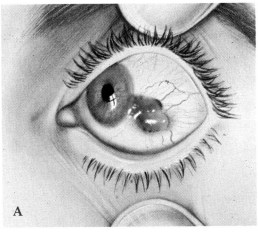

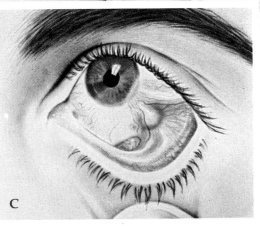

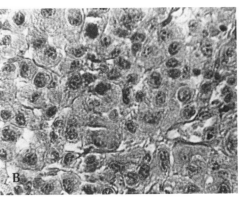

FIG. 7–89. Malignant melanoma of the conjunctiva arising from a congenital nevus. A 29-year-old man had had a pigment spot on the bulbar conjunctiva as long as he could remember. It was diagnosed as a congenital nevus when he entered the army at age 24. When the patient was 27 the lesion began to grow and become more elevated, leading to excision two years later. A. The lesion before surgery, supplied by dilated nutrient vessels. B. Malignant cells seen in section from the excised tumor. The cell border of the protoplasm is well demarcated. The nuclei vary in size and there is a tendency toward multinucleated cells. C. Recurrence three months after excision. (See p. 250.)

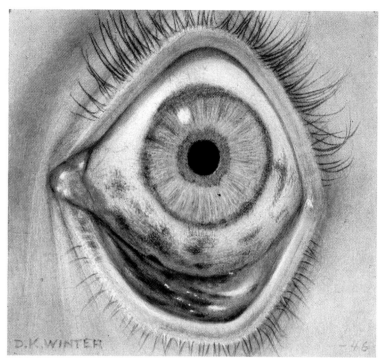

FIG. 7–94. Cancerous melanosis developing from precancerous melanosis. A 27-year-old woman noted a small pigmented area on the conjunctiva of the left eye near the inner canthus. At age 35 it began to enlarge, slowly at first, but rapidly after age 38. At age 45, immediately before exenteration of the eye, a diffuse, nonelevated, granular pigmentation involved the palpebral and bulbar conjunctiva, the caruncle, the semilunar fold, and the lid margin. (See p. 252.)

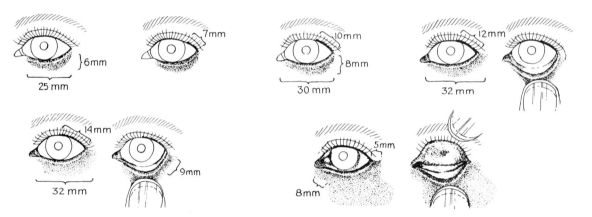

FIG. 7–96. Development of cancerous melanosis from precancerous melanosis. A 23-year-old man noted a pigmented pinpoint-sized spot along the left lower lid, and by the time he was 35, it had reached pinhead size. Thereafter it enlarged more rapidly, and a biopsy when he was 40 revealed precancerous melanosis. The drawings show changes with the passing years. *Top row:* Appearance at ages 41, 42, 43, and 46. *Bottom row:* Appearance at ages 46½ and 50. Despite the steady progression to a malignant state, the patient refused exenteration.

Color pictures show the cancerous melanosis at age 50. Pigmentation of **(A)** both lids and the bulbar conjunctiva; **(B)** the lower palpebral conjunctiva, fornix, and bulbar conjunctiva (lower lid retracted); **(C)** the upper and lower lids and the upper palpebral conjunctiva (upper lid retracted); and **(D)** the upper and lower lids, bulbar conjunctiva, caruncle, and semilunar fold (lower lid retracted). The tumor did not appear to be elevated except perhaps slightly in the lower fornix. (See p. 253.)

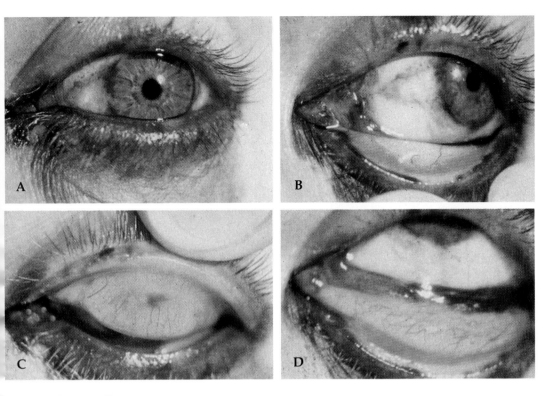

Fig. 7–96 *(continued)*

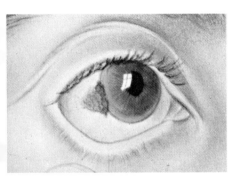

FIG. 7–97. Precancerous melanosis with spontaneous regression. This rather extensive lesion in a 55-year-old woman had developed over an 11-year period from a hemorrhage the size of a pinhead on the right eye. At age 51 a nonelevated pigmented lesion of the bulbar conjunctiva temporally, adjacent to the limbus, measured 7 x 7 mm and encroached 1 mm on the cornea. It then began to regress without treatment. Two years later the fine granular pigmentation had disappeared spontaneously, but within the next year it was observed with the slit-lamp at and around the site of the former lesion. (See p. 254.)

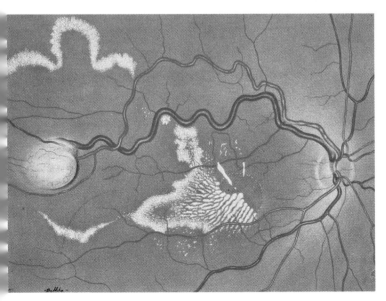

FIG. 8–8. Angiomatosis retinae (von Hippel's disease). The fundus in a 29-year-old man showed a globular angioma temporal to the macula and connected with the disc by a dilated artery and vein. Hard white deposits (residual edema) are seen in the retina around the tumor and in the macular area. (See p. 267.)

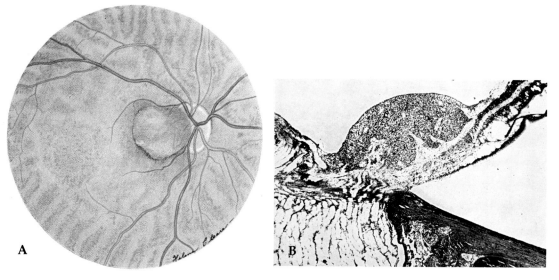

FIG. 8–9. Angiomatosis of the disc (von Hippel's disease). **A.** The tumor extended toward the macula which showed recent edema that led to rapid deterioration of vision. **B.** Section of the tumor confirms its classification in the angiomatosis retinae group. (See p. 267.) (Courtesy of B. F. Souders.[66])

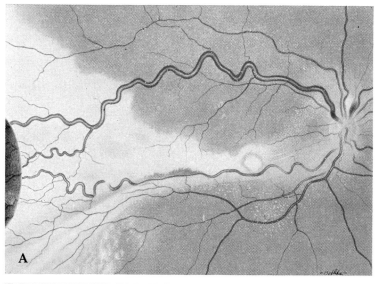

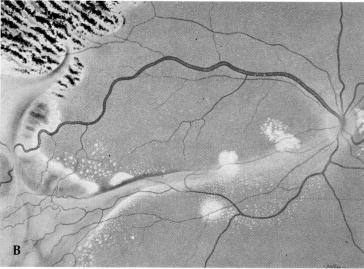

FIG. 8–11. Angiomatosis retinae (von Hippel's disease) treated by diathermy. **A.** Both afferent and efferent vessels in the fundus are markedly distended. The tumor is surrounded by fibrous tissue and hard, white, retinal deposits. **B.** Three months after diathermy treatment the horizontal vessels are appreciably smaller; scar tissue is visible over the site of the angioma and pigment changes above it. The patient showed no progression of the disease during the next 14 years. (See p. 268.)

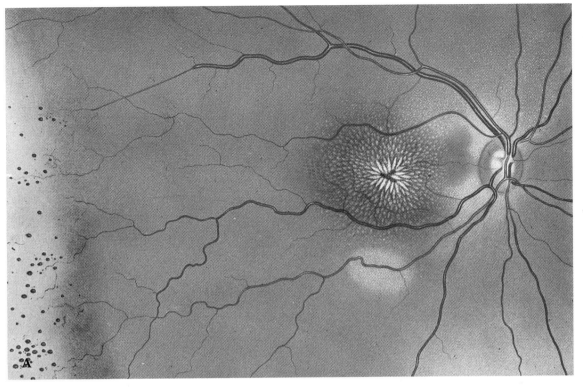

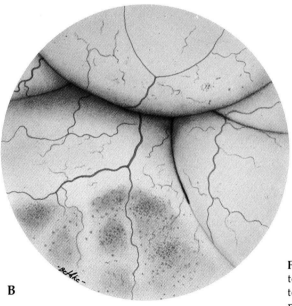

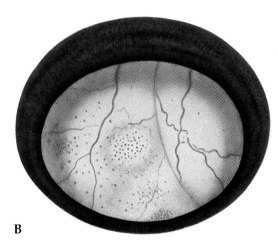

B

B

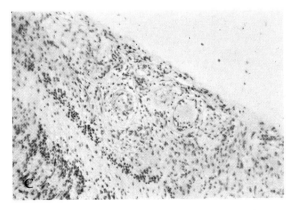

FIG. 8–13. Retinal telangiectasis which progressed to Coats's disease. **A.** Fundus of the right eye shows telangiectatic blood vessels temporally in the white retina, and white residual edema in the macula. **B.** One year later the telangiectatic blood vessels and some hemorrhage can be seen over the bullous detachment. **C.** Section from the lesion shows large vascular channels whose walls are either thickened to varying degrees or occluded by the red homogeneous PAS-positive material in the vessel walls (periodic acid stain). **D.** Section of the same retinal lesion stained with hematoxylin and eosin shows less specificity than the PAS. (Courtesy of Arthur Unsworth.) **E.** High-power view of retinal blood vessels in a case of Coats's disease. David Cogan and Toichiro Kuwabara prepared the retina by their trypsin digestion technique. The thick-walled vessels, consistent with those found in Coats's disease, showed a marked increase in PAS-positive material. (See p. 270.)

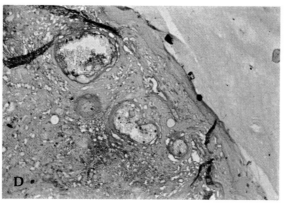
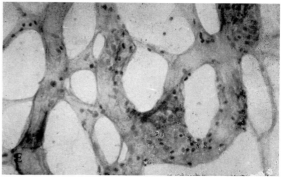

Fig. 8–13 *(continued)*

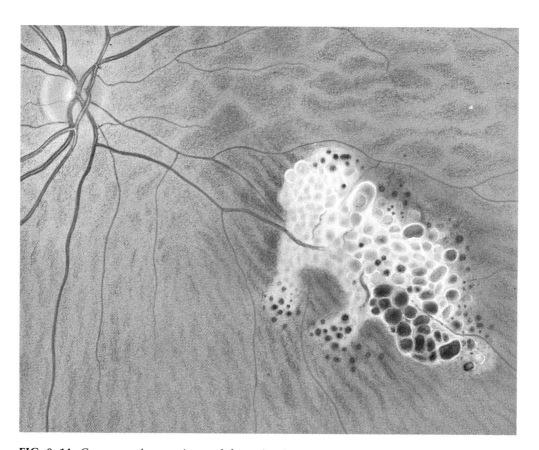

FIG. 8–14. Cavernous hemangioma of the retina in an 11½-year-old girl. (See p. 272.)

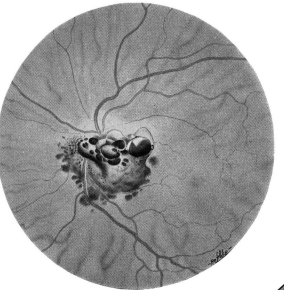

FIG. 8–18. Cavernous hemangioma (arteriovenous aneurysm of the disc and adjacent retina). The lesion was discovered during a routine eye examination of a 14-year-old boy with 20/20 vision. Subsequently there were several hemorrhages into the vitreous which cleared, leaving the vision normal. The lesion has not changed essentially for 30 years. (See p. 276.) (Courtesy of J. H. Dunnington and J. A. C. Wadsworth.)

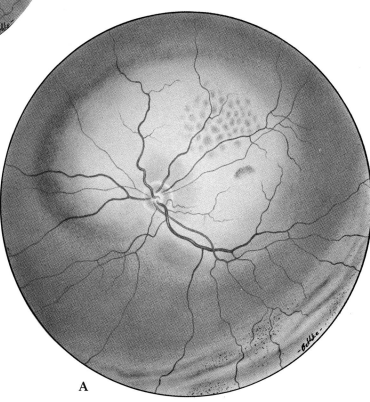

A

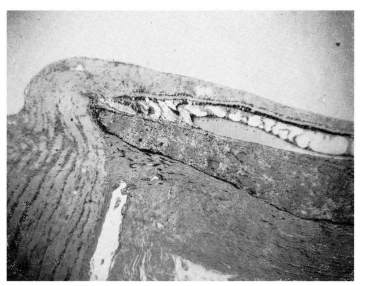

FIG. 8–19. Hemangioma of the choroid. **A.** Three years after the appearance of macular edema in a 39-year-old woman, the condition had definitely progressed, with a serous detachment seen below. The overlying retina appeared honeycombed, and the tumor area transmitted light by retroillumination. The eye was enucleated. **B.** Section in the region of the optic disc. Many cystic spaces in this external plexiform layer of the overlying retina confirm the diagnosis of a choroidal hemangioma. (See p. 277.)

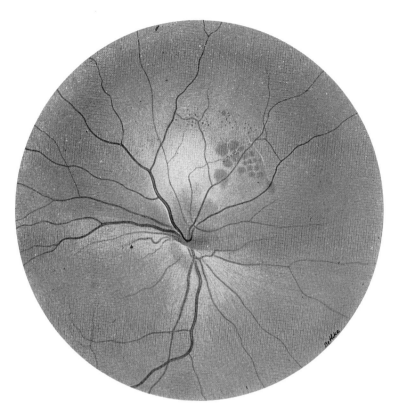

FIG. 8–22. Hemangioma of the choroid diagnosed clinically and confirmed microscopically. Over the upper half of the fundus of the right eye in a 31-year-old pregnant woman the retina was elevated and honeycombed in the central part. She had complained of blurred vision, and examination showed 20/200 vision, compared with 20/20 in the fellow eye. The lesion transmitted light by retroillumination. A serous detachment was found in the lower part of the fundus, and dustlike opacities in the vitreous. Vision in the affected eye worsened with two succeeding pregnancies; four years after the first examination the findings were complete detachment of the retina and secondary glaucoma. Numerous blood vessels in the iris and newly formed vessels over the retinal surface led to much bleeding at the time of enucleation. (See p. 278.)

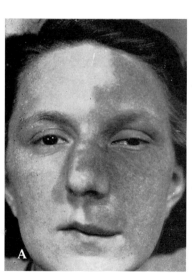

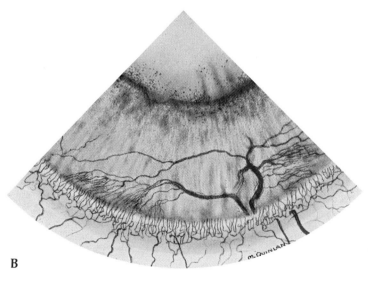

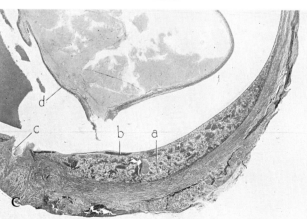

FIG. 8–23. Sturge-Weber syndrome. A. Unilateral facial hemangioma in a 20-year-old girl. B. Drawing shows angiomatous area in the left iris. C. Section of this eye, enucleated because of absolute glaucoma, showed a choroida hemangioma (a), with an epichoroidal membrane (b), glaucomatous cupping of the disc (c), and partial detachment of the retina (d). (See p. 279.) (Courtesy of L. Guy)

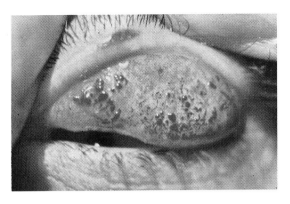

FIG. 8–25. Diffuse hemangioma of the palpebral conjunctiva. (See p. 282.)

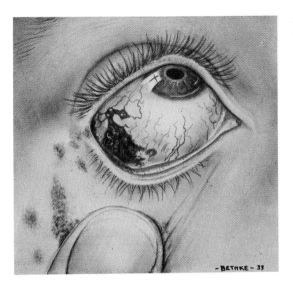

FIG. 8–26. Hemangioma of the conjunctiva and the adjacent skin. (See p. 282.)

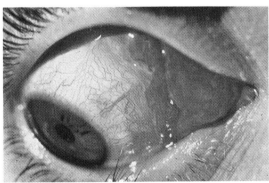

FIG. 8–27. Hemangioma of the conjunctiva near the inner canthus. (See p. 282.)

FIG. 8–31. Hemangioma of the right lids, orbit, brow, and scalp. **A.** Before treatment with sodium morrhuate injections and applications of carbon dioxide snow. **B.** Six years after treatment the lesion shows regression. The levator function is unimpaired. (See p. 285.)

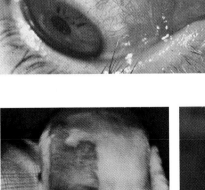
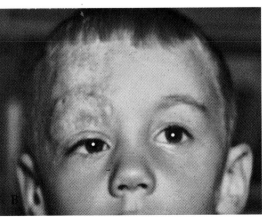

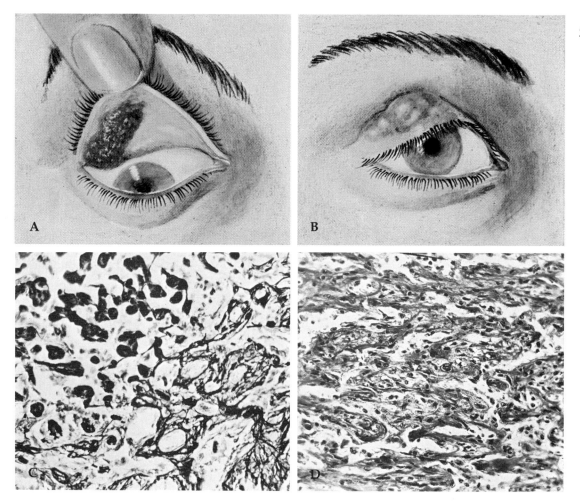

FIG. 8–38. Recurrent malignant hemangioendothelioma. A. This tumor of the right upper lid, which involved the bulbar conjunctiva, recurred after each of nine excisions. B. View from the skin surface. C. Intraluminal growth of the endothelium is clearly seen in section stained with silver for reticulin. D. Section stained with hematoxylin and eosin. (See p. 290.) (Courtesy of A. P. Stout.[68])

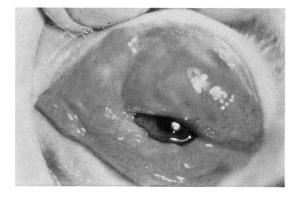

FIG. 8–40. Lymphangioma of the palpebral conjunctiva. (See p. 291.)

FIG. 8–43. Lymphangioma of the right orbit and face. (See p. 292.)

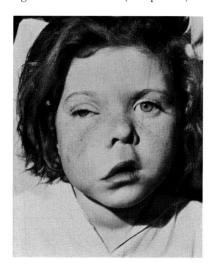

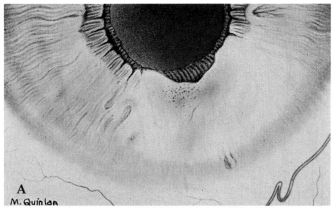

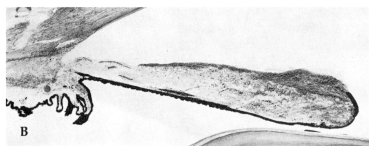

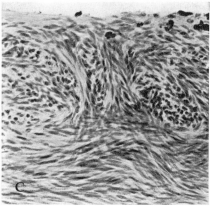

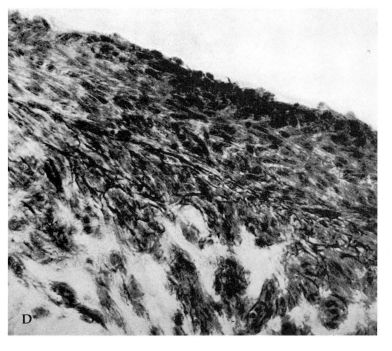

FIG. 9–1. Leiomyoma of the iris. **A.** Diffuse flat lesion with some ectropion uveae is seen clinically.**B.** The tumor occupies the pupillary third of the iris and extends along its surface. **C.** Interlacing bands of tissue and a tendency toward palisading of the nuclei. **D.** Myoglial fibrils are revealed by the gold impregnation stain. (See p. 298.) (Courtesy of A. D. Frost.[8])

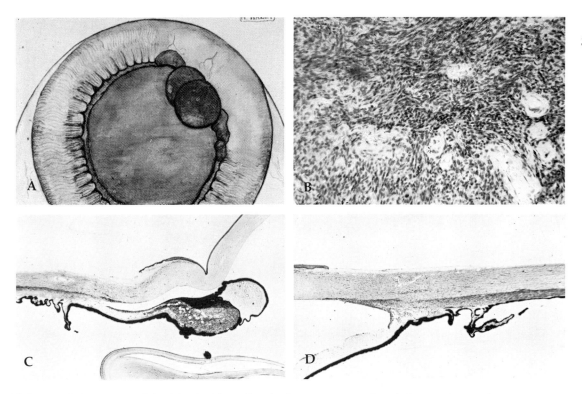

FIG. 9–2. Leiomyoma of the iris. **A.** Clinically, the lesion appears flat, diffuse and vascularized, with cysts and some ectropion uveae at the pupillary margin. **B.** Myoglial fibrils are demonstrated by the gold chloride and Masson trichrome stains. Reactions to the van Gieson phosphotogunstic acid and the Wilder stains were consistent with leiomyoma. **C.** The tumor extends along the anterior surface of the iris, and a large cyst is seen. **D.** The opposite angle shows some tumor extension which caused glaucoma. (See p. 299.)

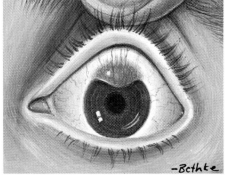

FIG. 11–13. Fibroxanthoma (Hand-Schüller-Christian disease). **A.** A fleshy lesion 8 × 7 mm straddled the limbus in a 16-year-old boy. **B.** Papular skin lesions scattered over the body were noted in profusion in the axilla. During the next four years the condition exacerbated; new lesions of the cornea, limbus, and conjunctiva were treated by excision and radiation. **C.** At the sites of residual scar the corneal stroma became thin but not ectatic (see slit lamp inset at right). After 13 years of treatment the eye remained quiet; vision was 20/30 in each eye with contact lenses. (See p. 326.)

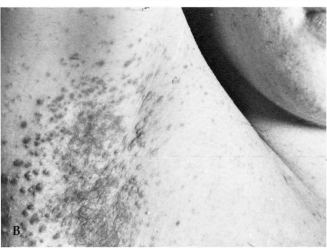

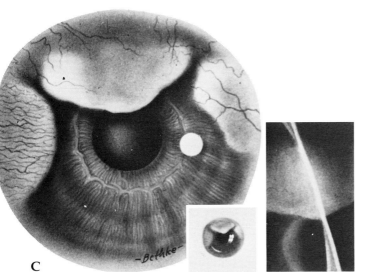

C

Fig. 11–13 *(continued)*

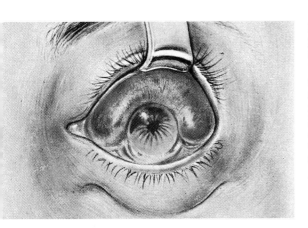

FIG. 13–1. Lymphatic leukemia. Exophthalmos and protrusion of the bulbar conjunctiva led a 69-year-old man to seek medical advice. The markedly congested bulbar conjunctiva protruded like a sausage concentric to the limbus. The thick, indurated lids appeared to be pushed outward by uniform infiltration of the tumor in and posterior to the lids. A tissue biopsy from under the bulbar conjunctiva revealed a solid mass of lymphocytes. The patient's white cell count was 160,000 with 94% small lymphocytes. (See p. 388.) (A. B. Reese and L. Guy.[51])

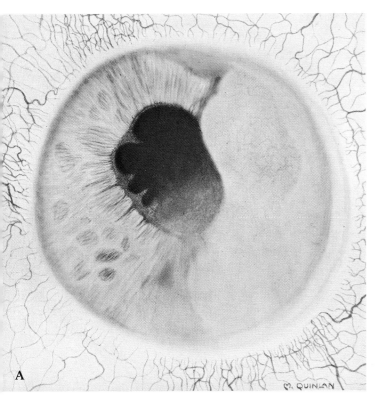

A

FIG. 13–3. Malignant lymphoma (lymphocytic-cell type) of the iris. **A.** Tumor tissue fills the temporal half of the anterior chamber and in the periphery touches the posterior surface of the cornea. **B.** Low-power magnification shows that infiltration is confined to the iris. **C.** High-power view shows structure of the tumor. (See p. 389.)

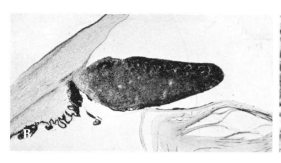
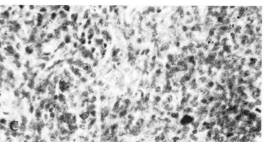

Fig. 13–3 *(continued)*

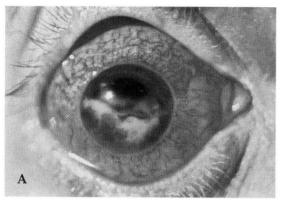

FIG. 13–4. Malignant lymphoma (reticulum-cell type) of the iris. **A.** Tumor tissue fills the lower half of the anterior chamber and rests against the posterior surface of the cornea. Yellowish-white purulent material covering the surface of the tumor trickles down between it and the cornea. **B.** Microscopic section shows involvement of the iris, ciliary body, and anterior choroid. The fact that the tumor is partially necrotic seems to account for the inflammatory reaction. Inset shows the cytology. (See p. 389.)

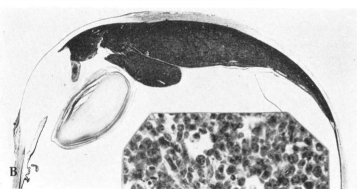

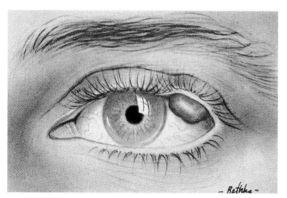

FIG. 13–5. Hodgkin's disease. The enlarged lacrimal gland protrudes below the upper lid. (See p. 390.)

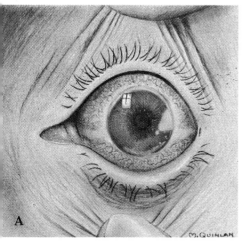
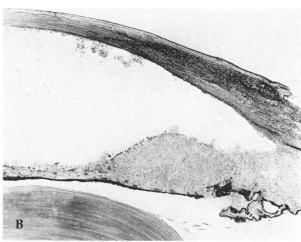

FIG. 16–1. Metastatic carcinoma of the iris simulating iridocyclitis with secondary glaucoma. The primary site in the stomach was discovered only at autopsy. **A.** Grayish mass is seen in the anterior chamber temporally. There was marked acute iridocyclitis with corneal deposits and hypopyon. **B.** Microscopic section showing the neoplastic metastasis in the iris. The partially necrotic tumor had provoked a marked inflammatory reaction, with deposits of inflammatory cells on the cornea. (See p. 425.)

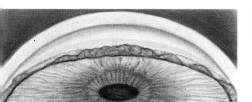

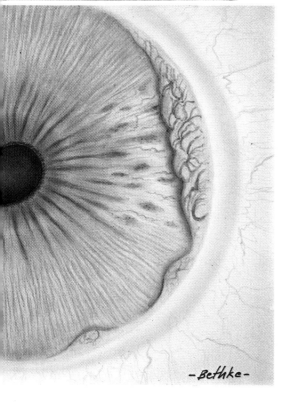

FIG. 16–3. Metastatic ring carcinoma at the angle, from a primary site in the breast. (See p. 425.)

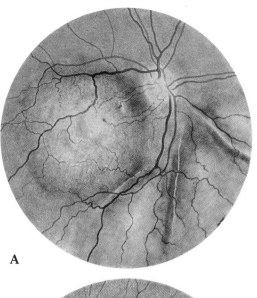

A

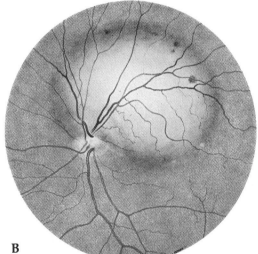

B

FIG. 16–5. Metastatic carcinoma of the choroid of both eyes from a primary site in the thyroid gland. The eye manifestations were noted before the primary site was known. **A.** In the right fundus the tumor is in the macula; there is a serous detachment of the retina below. **B.** In the left fundus, the localized and elevated tumor lies above the disc. It is light in color with a slightly mottled surface. **C.** Section of the right eye shows the localized elevated tumor in the macular area and the serous detachment. (See p. 426.)

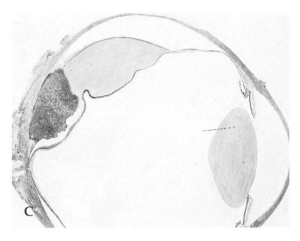

C

FIG. 16–7. Metastatic carcinoma of the orbit from a primary site in the breast. Necrosis of the tumor has resulted in a marked inflammatory reaction. Exophthalmos is present. (See p. 427.)

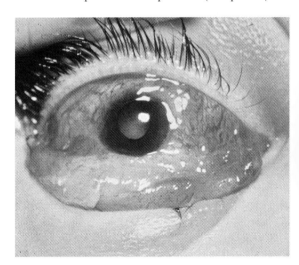

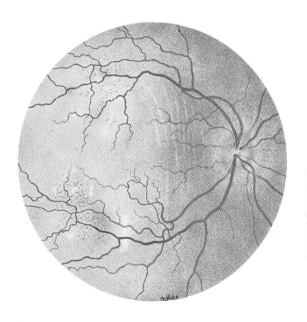

FIG. 16–6. Metastatic carcinoma of the choroid from a primary site in the breast. The tumor, in the macular region, is flat, light in color, with some mottling over the surface. Concentric striae between the tumor and the disc represent tension folds of the internal limiting membrane of the retina. (See p. 427.)

TUMORS
of the EYE

1

EPITHELIAL TUMORS
OF THE LID,
CONJUNCTIVA, CORNEA,
AND LACRIMAL SAC

Many different tumors affect the lids because of the combination there of skin, mucous membrane, and various glandular structures. As a group these tumors are relatively benign in that they do not usually metastasize. Their overt nature often makes possible early successful treatment by surgery or radiation.

CARCINOMAS AND ADNEXAL TUMORS OF THE LID

Eyelid carcinomas are the same histologically and clinically as other facial varieties. However, they have a predilection for the lid margin where excision necessitates plastic repair, and irradiation may produce complications. These lesions are potentially destructive because when uncontrolled they may invade the orbit or contiguous bone and sinuses, resulting in fatality. Even a small basal-cell epithelioma of the skin of the lid may reach the orbit, producing exophthalmos and in one case even a superior orbital fissure syndrome.[14]

INCIDENCE AND CLASSIFICATION

Although most facial carcinomas develop on the nose, the eyelid is a close second. The order of frequency is lower lid, inner canthus, upper lid, and outer canthus.

Epithelial tumors of the lid, the lid margin, and the lacrimal caruncle are classified as follows:

1. Basal-cell type
   a. Adnexal tumors of hair follicles, sweat glands, and sebaceous (meibomian) glands
   b. Basal-cell carcinomas
2. Squamous-cell type
   a. Intraepithelial tumors (Bowen's disease)
   b. Squamous-cell (epidermoid) carcinomas

The adnexal tumors and the basal-cell carcinomas are essentially the same but in various stages of differentiation. The most highly differentiated types—the so-called folliculo-mas[33,52] of hair follicles, the adenomas of sebaceous glands, and the syringocystadenomas of sweat glands—are benign hamartomas. As they become less differentiated, they are frequently referred to as epitheliomas (trichoepitheliomas, sebaceous epitheliomas, and cylindromas) and, when their identification is lost, as basal-cell carcinomas.

Basal-cell carcinomas were formerly believed to develop from basal cells and squamous-cell carcinomas from prickle cells, but it is now believed that there is no essential histogenetic difference between them and that cutaneous epithelial cells are pluripotential throughout life.

Both basal- and squamous-cell carcinomas are derived from the same pluripotential epidermal or adnexal epithelial cells, but the basal-cell lesions develop toward higher organ differentiation and the squamous-cell toward lower. Basal-cell carcinomas make an abortive effort to form adnexal structures, whereas the course of squamous-cell lesions is toward dedifferentiation and anaplasia. The former tend to be sustained locally, and the latter may be beyond local regulatory forces so they may metastasize.

Another feature pointing up the adnexal relationship of basal-cell carcinomas is that they have both stromal and epithelial elements. Thus, squamous-cell carcinomas may be regarded as solely epithelial, while adnexal neoplasms are fibroepithelial.

Although most tumors are entirely of one type or the other, some lesions may demonstrate histologic features of both types and are sometimes referred to as basosquamous.

GRADING

The degree of malignancy of cancer cells can be graded, to some extent, on the basis of their morphologic characteristics. Many factors must be considered in assessing cellular activity or unrest. These include mitosis and amitosis; variation in cell size and particularly the presence of large, spheroidal nuclei with or without prominent nucleoli; decrease in cell cytoplasm in relation to the nucleus; hyperchromatosis with the nuclei having particular avidity for the basic dyes; lack of polarity of the cells; invasive properties of the cells; and the paucity of cellular products laid down by the particular cells from which the tumor arises, such as various kinds of fibers (collagen, reticulin, elastin, myoglia), keratin, melanin, and similar substances. In a tumor with a glandular structure, dedifferentiation is indicated by the degree of variance between the tumor cell and the parent cell.

CLINICAL APPEARANCE AND COURSE

Skin carcinomas occur in persons between 50 and 55 years of age, on the average, and the incidence is somewhat higher in men. They usually arise in sunlight-damaged skin but also occur in otherwise normal skin with no specific cause. The tumors tend to occur at sites where the epithelium undergoes a transition, e.g., the lid margin where the epidermis undergoes transition to conjunctiva. When such tumors seem to be due to chronic irritation, they may be multiple and diffuse over the facial skin. The irritation may result from repeated exposure to the elements, particularly sun, over long periods. In rare instances it may possibly result from inadequate cleansing of skin that is habitually covered with mineral dust, ashes, grease, or oil.

The dermatitis associated with chronic blepharitis, conjunctivitis, or constant tearing could also be predisposing to carcinomas. The senile keratoses that may develop into carcinomas are multiple, localized, slightly elevated, dry, scaly areas. Carcinomas have also developed as late sequelae of radiation in seemingly trivial doses for disfiguring skin eruptions.

Basal- and squamous-cell carcinomas in pure form have essentially the same clinical appearance except that whitish elements in the squamous-cell type, due to keratin production, appear as various degrees of a striking pearly-white translucency (Fig. 1–1A, see p. 3). An indurated, elevated, sharply demarcated nodule with an irregular or undulating surface is seen in both types of tumor, either at the lid margin or adjacent to it (Fig. 1–1B, see p. 3). The lesion infiltrates the skin but is freely movable unless it is located on the lid margin. As the nodule enlarges, the overlying skin seems to thin out, become glossier, and develop telangiectases. Ulceration occurs with enlargement of the lesion or may be present from the onset. Sometimes a papilloma develops into a carcinoma. The basal-cell type, particularly in dark-skinned individuals, may show varying degrees of pigment. If the pigmentation is quite marked, a nevus or a malignant melanoma may be suspected (Fig. 1–1C, see p. 3).

A hereditary type of multiple basal-cell carcinoma associated with systemic abnormalities such as bone cysts, ectopic calcification, and skeletal abnormalities has been reported.[47]

Inflammation may be a prominent feature of carcinoma of the meibomian glands, confusing the clinical picture. Presumably, occlusion of the ducts of the gland is a causative factor. In the advanced stage, the tumor sometimes grows outward as a bulky, fungating lesion, or it may invade and even erode the lid without producing any appreciable mass, or even penetrate the deeper orbital structures including the bone. Some carcinomas show an early and marked propensity for invading orbital structures without manifesting an ulcerative tendency.

In a series of 364 basal-cell epitheliomas diagnosed microscopically, almost half (misdiagnosed clinically as benign) contained large cysts and one-third contained small cysts. In contrast, only one-tenth of solid tumors in this group were misdiagnosed clinically.[51]

The lesion often involves the inner canthus either primarily or by invasion (Fig. 1–2, see p. 3). If either the punctum or canaliculus becomes involved, epiphora results.

HAIR FOLLICLE TUMORS

The usual tumors arising from hair follicles—folliculoma and trichoepithelioma (Fig. 1–3) —appear as single or multiple, small, firm, yellowish lesions in the skin of the lids as well as the forehead, side of the nose and cheeks, and less frequently the neck, scalp, and shoulders. In many cases they are noted early in life, grow very slowly to the size of a pinhead or pea, and usually remain stationary. Some of them sprout abnormal hairs. A case was reported in which the patient noticed the tumor because of a tuft of abnormally light hairs or cilia which increased in number and length.[32]

The lesions are a type of benign basal-cell adenoma; their cells usually vary markedly in degree of differentiation toward hair follicle

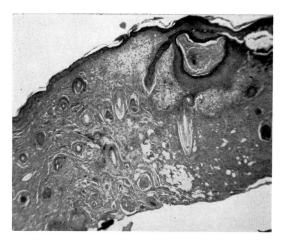

FIG. 1–3. Hair follicle epithelioma (trichoepithelioma) of the lid. An elevated smooth, yellowish lesion 4 mm in diameter, resembling a xanthelasma, was noted on the skin of the lower lid in a 58-year-old woman. Some of the epithelial downgrowths, when examined microscopically, contained small hair shafts.

structure. In some instances many immature follicles with rudimentary hair shafts are present; in others there may be some keratinization and cysts with keratin.

Brooke's tumor, a hereditary type of trichoepithelioma, is cystic and multiple; it has a predilection for the nasolabial folds but is also found on the eyelids and brow.[3,78]

PILOMATRIXOMA (BENIGN CALCIFYING EPITHELIOMA OF MALHERBE)

This well-localized hard nodule of the lid, particularly the upper, and the brow is 1 to 3 cm in diameter and freely movable but adherent to the overlying skin (Fig. 1–4). A number of representative cases have been reported.[2,38,61]

I described such a lesion in 1925 as "recurrent tumor of brow with unusual histologic findings." The tumor that recurred five years after excision was larger than the original one. Benign calcifying epithelioma had not been recognized as an entity at that time. With the help of Verhoeff and Fuchs, this case was interpreted as a reaction to an incompletely excised dermoid cyst. The tumor is generally confused with a sebaceous cyst or an adnexal epithelioma.

Histologically, eosin-staining necrotic masses of squamous-cell epithelium are held together by fibrous stroma that invades the necrotic and often calcified epithelium. The lesion is sharply encapsulated, entirely benign, and can usually be surgically excised in its entirety without difficulty.

Pilomatrixoma is believed to be a type of embryonic structure composed of primary germ cells with a tendency to differentiate into immature hair cells. Helwig[27] coined the term *pilomatrixoma* for this benign tumor of hair follicles, and it is now in wide use.

SWEAT GLAND TUMORS

Benign tumors arising from the sweat glands—syringoma, syringocystadenoma, and cylindroma—are single or multiple, pinhead-to pea-sized, yellowish or waxy-looking lesions usually found in young people. Histologically, their glandular acini resemble those of sweat glands (Fig. 1–5) and tend to form cysts filled with clear fluid.

The sweat glands of the lids, called glands of Moll, are classified as apocrine rather than exocrine, because of their mode of secretion. Apocrine glands are located primarily in the axilla, around the nipples, and in the perigenital and perianal regions. The apocrine sweat gland carcinomas are slow-growing and anaplastic.

FIG. 1–4. Benign calcifying epithelioma. A mass on the left midbrow in a 32-year-old woman enlarged over a 2-year period and was excised. It gradually recurred, reaching 1 cm in diameter. The section shows strands of necrotic epidermal epithelium surrounded by connective tissue infiltrated with a few chronic inflammatory cells and foreign-body giant cells.

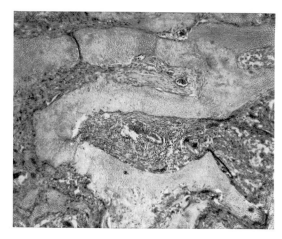

Wherever apocrine sweat glands are found, a special type of carcinoma often called "extramammary Paget's disease" may develop. This is difficult to diagnose because of the tumor's small size in relation to the widespread intraepithelial involvement of the surface epithelium. Since the glands of Moll are modified apocrine glands, it is not surprising that a carcinoma arising from them may resemble extramammary Paget's disease.[64]

SEBACEOUS (MEIBOMIAN AND ZEIS) GLAND TUMORS

Tumors arising from sebaceous (meibomian and Zeis) glands of the lid, eyebrow, and caruncle may be adenomas (Fig. 1–6), epitheliomas, or carcinomas (Fig. 1–7, see p. 4). Initially the lesion may be confused with a chalazion or a hordeolum because of its inflammatory nature. Some product of the tumor growth seems to lead to inflammation which can mask its neoplastic nature. In certain cases I believe the primary lesion is actually a chalazion with or without suppuration. Incision with curettage produces the usual friable granulation tissue with or without pus. The area remains inflamed and in time a frank epithelioma or carcinoma develops. Since the inflammation is possibly a factor in precipitating the tumor, I believe that any lump in the lid behaving differently from the usual chalazion should be considered suspect and a biopsy taken.

A study of 16 patients with meibomian gland carcinoma revealed only 4 who had effective therapy initially; the other 12 underwent a total of 22 surgical procedures before the true nature of the lesion was appreciated.[64]

Meibomian gland carcinomas in 8 patients were first diagnosed and treated as chalazions.[66] They had been present from five months to five years (an average of two years) before appropriate treatment was started. Metastasis to regional lymph nodes occurred in two cases.

In a series of 88 cases,[5,6] the caruncle was the primary site of origin in 8, the eyebrow in 2, and the eyelid in 78. The majority arose in the upper lid from the meibomian glands. Twelve of the 88 patients had been treated for chronic blepharoconjunctivitis before the correct diagnosis was made; in 7 the sebaceous glands of both upper and lower lids were involved as well as pagetoid or carcinoma-*in-situ* changes in the conjunctiva, cornea, and

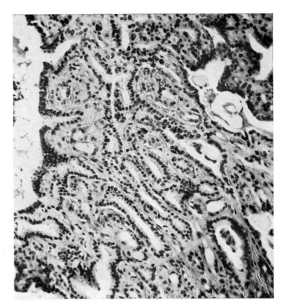

FIG. 1–5. Sweat gland epithelioma of the lid. A slow-growing mass 5 × 8 mm in a 53-year-old man extended around the margin of the lid and involved its entire thickness. The epithelial structure resembled that of a sweat gland.

FIG. 1–6. Sebaceous gland adenoma. Section from an excised nontender mass which had been noted in the brow of a 70-year-old woman for 6 months.

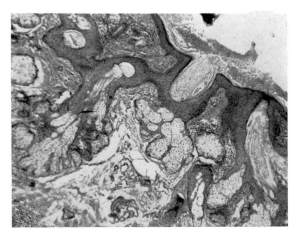

adnexal tissues of the lid. Orbital invasion occurred in 17% of the cases; the tumor-related mortality in the series was 13.5%. The multicentric origin of this tumor in a single lid has been described.[10]

Five reported cases of multiple sebaceous neoplasms of the skin were associated with multiple visceral cancers, particularly adenocarcinoma of the colon. The visceral lesions were present for years before the skin lesions appeared.[57] In one case the multiple sebaceous neoplasms were associated with metastatic endometrial carcinoma[4] and in another with carcinoma of the colon in a father and son.[30]

In one reported case an apparently simple cutaneous horn of the lid margin masked an underlying occult sebaceous carcinoma of the eyelid.[8]

DIFFERENTIAL DIAGNOSIS

Simulating lesions must be considered in the differential diagnosis of lid tumors. In a review of 115 eyelid lesions originally diagnosed histologically as squamous-cell carcinomas, only 12 were considered to have been correctly identified.[34] "Overdiagnosis" of such lesions has been emphasized.[83]

The conditions most frequently confused with squamous-cell carcinoma are senile and seborrheic keratoses, inverted follicular and other benign keratoses, keratoacanthoma, pseudoepitheliomatous hyperplasia induced by an inflammatory process, intraepithelial epithelioma or carcinoma *in situ* (Bowen's disease), basal-cell carcinoma, adnexal-cell carcinoma, pilomatrixoma (benign calcifying epithelioma of Malherbe), and adenoacanthoma.

Keratoacanthoma

Keratoacanthoma[55] is important because it is frequently mistaken, both clinically and histologically, for basal-cell or squamous-cell carcinoma. The usual clinical picture is that of a rapidly enlarging, nodular, umbilicated lesion occurring more often in the lower lid (Fig. 1–8). The central crater is filled with keratin. The lesion reaches its maximal diameter of 1–2 cm in four to eight weeks and involutes spontaneously, leaving only a faint scar.

A less common, generalized form may progress throughout the patient's life.[18]

A keratoacanthoma sometimes merges into a carcinoma and is misdiagnosed histologically; therefore cases originally diagnosed as keratoacanthoma should be closely followed.[44]

Well-documented cases of keratoacanthoma of the bulbar conjunctiva have been reported.[73] I examined a 48-year-old patient who suddenly developed a lesion of the bulbar conjunctiva which extended around the limbus from 2 o'clock to 5:30. The clinical appearance was consistent with that of a squamous-cell carcinoma. The lesion was diagnosed histologically as a keratoacanthoma and disappeared without treatment within three and a half months; no trace could be found on close examination.

Since chemical carcinogens can produce similar lesions in various animals, it has been suggested that they might also produce at least some keratoacanthomas in man.[21] The lesion's rapid growth and tendency to spontaneous regression suggest a viral origin, and, in fact, viruslike particles have been demonstrated by electron microscopy.[9,19,80]

If the lesion fails to regress after a period of observation, treatment should be instituted, preferably conservative surgical excision. Temporization may be in order for large lesions at a site that would involve extensive and disfiguring surgery, since spontaneous regression usually occurs. However, an adequate biopsy should be taken to rule out the possibility of squamous-cell carcinoma. In some reported cases fatalities occurred because a squamous-cell carcinoma was not recognized in the curable stage. Small suspected keratoacanthomas should be excised before they attain a size making surgical removal difficult.

Successful treatment by radiation has been reported.[20]

Seborrheic Keratosis

Seborrheic keratosis, another common lesion in the acanthoma group, is characterized by intraepidermal basal-cell proliferation with pigmentation and keratin cysts. It usually appears as a raised, broad plateau or mound in the lid, frequently along the cilia line. A greasy surface encrusted with dirt, as well as melanin in the cells, gives the lesion a brown or dark color, sometimes leading to confusion with melanoma. It is not considered precancerous.

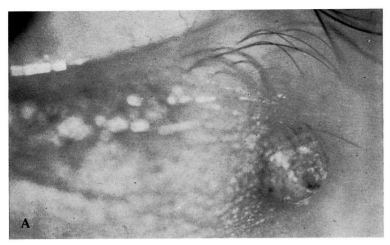

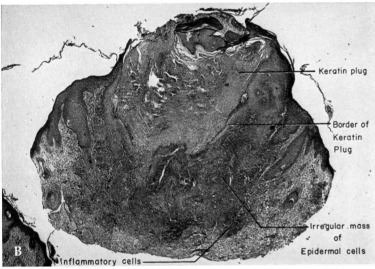

FIG. 1–8. Keratocanthoma of the lower lid. **A.**
The umbilicated center is apparent clinically in
a tumor that developed in a 33-year-old man
over a period of four weeks. **B.** Microscopic
section through the center of the tumor.
(Courtesy of L. Christensen and T. B.
Fitzpatrick.[11])

Inverted follicular keratosis. This form of
seborrheic keratosis or pseudoepitheliomatous
hyperplasia has a predilection for the face[27]
and frequently involves the lids, particularly
their margins (Fig. 1–9). The papillary or
nodular projection may be confused both
clinically and histologically with a carcinoma
and therefore lead to unnecessary surgery. It
is considered to be a keratinizing process that
has become inverted and to have no malignant
potential.

The clinical term *cutaneous horn* has been
suggested for an elongated, sometimes
pedunculated mass of keratin and keratinous
debris (Fig. 1–10). It may develop from senile
keratosis or may overlie a keratoacanthoma,
inverted follicular keratosis, squamous-cell
carcinoma, or other skin lesions.[5]

Chalazion or Hordeolum with Pseudoepitheliomatous Hyperplasia

If tissue is taken from a suspected chalazion
or hordeolum for biopsy, interpretation may
be difficult because of dyskeratosis, hyperkeratosis, and epithelial proliferation (pseudo-
epitheliomatous hyperplasia), particularly at
the junction of conjunctiva and skin.

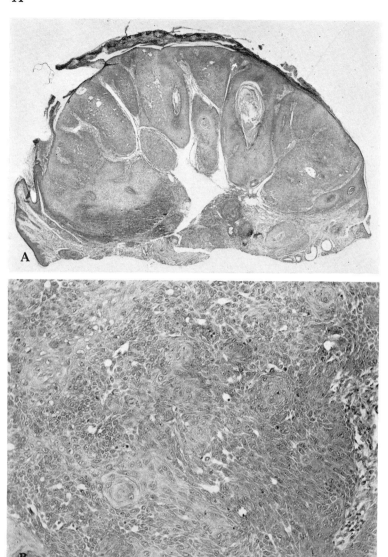

FIG. 1–9. Inverted follicular keratosis of the lid margin. **A.** Low-power view of a section from a lesion present in a 63-year-old man for over a year which was clinically diagnosed as a basal-cell carcinoma. **B.** Under higher magnification typical "squamous eddies" are visible. (Zimmerman LE: In Ackerman LV (ed): Surgical Pathology. St Louis, CV Mosby, 1959)

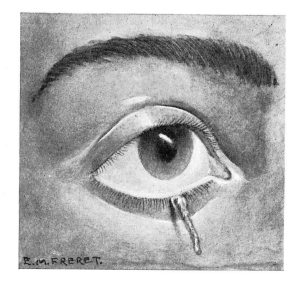

FIG. 1–10. Keratin horn on the lower lid.

Nevi

Confusion sometimes arises between nevi and skin cancers because some nevi have papillomatous patterns and because the epithelium may show extensive cystic pseudo-epitheliomatous downgrowths. Furthermore, a papilloma or a basal-cell carcinoma may be pigmented in dark-skinned individuals and thus resemble a nevus or a melanoma (See ch. 7, Pigmented Tumors).

Miscellaneous Conditions

Granuloma, molluscum contagiosum, rhinosporidium granuloma,[62] sebaceous cyst, sudoriferous cyst, and traumatic or congenital inclusion cyst[56] on rare occasions simulate an epithelioma.

TREATMENT

Treatment would be simple if the goals were only curing the disease and saving the patient's life. But the additional considerations of the patient's eye function and cosmetic result make the choice of treatment very important.

Lid carcinomas can undoubtedly be cured by radiation in adequate dosage. The problem is to administer a sufficient amount to arrest the growth with minimal deleterious effects.

When lid carcinomas are treated by radiation, localized loss of cilia and a break in continuity of the lid margin may occur. The break is due for the most part to a localized absorption of the elastic tissue in the lid margin. This may cause only a slight marginal depression or an actual notch in the lid margin. Also, there may be atrophy of the adjacent skin with some bleaching of the pigment and telangiectasis. One of the most distressing complications is keratinization of the conjunctiva and cornea resulting in constant desquamation of keratin in the eye; this usually produces irritation and tearing. Such epithelial changes on the cornea result in punctate opacities that stain with fluorescein. No matter how carefully the radiation therapy is given there is some risk of cataract, not necessarily complete opacity of the lens leading to loss of vision, but the far more common localized stationary posterior cortical opacity that reduces the vision to about 20/30 or 20/40. This may develop insidiously over a long period of time, with little or no complaint from the patient who does not associate it with the radiation treatment.

Far-advanced carcinoma of the lid may require combined radiation and surgery for the best possible functional and cosmetic results. The patient shown in Figure 1–11 had a bulky, fungating basal-cell carcinoma that involved practically the entire lower eyelid and inner canthus. The growth was arrested by fractionated x-ray treatment with protective shielding of the eye, and the cosmetic problem was handled by surgery. Although there was considerable destruction of the lid substance, it would have been much greater after a wide surgical excision. The defect was repaired by the greater resection technique to be discussed later.

Irradiation is the sole recourse in certain far-advanced inoperable carcinomas of the eyelid. The tumor may extend deeply into the orbit, invading bone or the nasal cavity and penetrating into the subcutaneous tissue of the cheek and forehead. The lesions may have recurred or persisted after repeated attempts at surgical removal or after inadequate radiation therapy. If the patient has already received a large total dose, radiation treatment in these advanced cases may be merely palliative. In most instances, however, the disease can be permanently eradicated by aggressive x-ray therapy, although the high dosage required may result in loss of the eye and formation of an avascular surface over the denuded bone which never completely heals. This unfortunate result is still preferable to a steadily eroding cancer.

A bulky tumor mass on the lid is best treated by excising the projecting portion down to the skin level, then instituting x-ray therapy. The initial excision permits more accurate direction of the beam to the base of the lesion and makes the line of junction between normal and neoplastic tissue more readily discernible. This combined surgical and x-ray therapy is, of course, restricted to extremely large fungating lesions in which mechanical difficulties due to the very bulk of the tumor hinder other effective treatment.

Surgical Treatment

Basal-cell carcinomas that are diagnosed early and surgically excised seldom result in fatality. Plastic repair following excision is indicated for the majority. Surgery is usually imperative when such lesions recur after irradi-

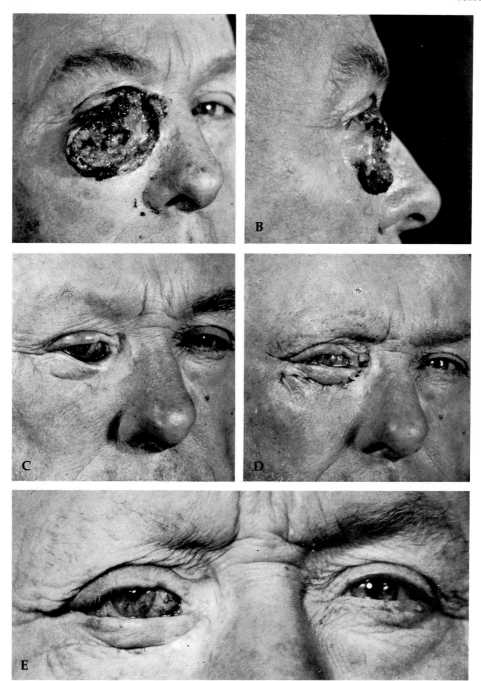

FIG. 1–11. Large, fungating basal-cell epithelioma of the upper and lower lid treated by x ray and surgery. Appearance before treatment **(A, B)**, after x-ray therapy **(C)**, and five days after the greater resection with sutures still in place **(D)**. The result two years after completion of treatment is shown in **E**.

ation. Even when neglected or inadequately treated in the early stages, most carcinomatous lesions of the lids can be controlled, although radical and therefore disfiguring surgery may be required.

Less than 6% mortality was reported for patients with lid carcinomas treated at the Memorial Center for Cancer and Allied Diseases.[39] The fatalities were due largely to metastasis of squamous-cell carcinomas, less often to complications of basal-cell carcinomas.

Among 1197 excised basal cell carcinomas, marginal extension of the tumor was noted in 66 cases, 4 of which were on the eyelid. All 23 recurrences in the 66 cases were successfully managed by reexcision or radiation therapy. A conservative policy of close observation was therefore suggested for patients showing marginal extension of excised lesions, with secondary treatment reserved for cases of recurrence.[22]

In another long-term follow-up[50] on 209 of 273 patients with histologically confirmed basal-cell eyelid carcinomas treated surgically, the recurrence rate was 12% and the death rate 2%.

Before excising a basal-cell carcinoma, it is very important to try to determine its extent. This is best done by grasping the lesion with the index finger in the conjunctival cul-de-sac and the thumb on the outer surface. After determining where the normal lid tissue begins, the excision should extend some distance beyond this site. After excision and plastic repair there should be no break in continuity of the lid margin or the cilia line at the site of the lid closure.

The lower lid is more often involved, and this is fortunate for it is easier to repair. The techniques described here apply to the lower lid, with mention of any modifications needed to apply them to the upper lid.

There are many techniques for excision of lid tumors. When the skin of the lid is primarily involved, a simple excision with or without a skin graft suffices. However, the majority of lid tumors arise in or around the lid margin, necessitating plastic repair. Two techniques will be described: the lesser and the greater resections.

When an epithelioma is incompletely removed by excisional biopsy, the tumor site may be hard to recognize if further resection proves necessary. This impasse can be prevented by cutting the cilia over the area to be resected when the excisional biopsy is done.

Whether a lid tumor has been totally excised may be determined at the time of surgery by preparing frozen sections.[57]

If the tumor is at the inner canthus, efforts should be made to preserve the upper or lower canaliculus if possible. When one or the other must be sacrificed, epiphora becomes annoying only when irritants such as wind, dust, or cold provoke excessive tearing. Sacrifice of the upper canaliculus is better tolerated.

The lesser procedure is adequate for lesions requiring resection of up to one-third of the lid. In fact, it is adequate for the large majority of lesions, particularly in older patients with lax lids.

Technique for the lesser resection (Fig. 1–12). General anesthesia is preferable although both local infiltrative and block anesthesia are satisfactory. With a Graefe knife the lid is halved on each side of the lesion for 2–3 mm. The halving should start several millimeters beyond the point to which the lesion is believed to extend.* The outer half of the lid should include skin, cilia, and orbicularis muscle, with conjunctiva and tarsus on the inner half.

A traction suture passed through the lesion facilitates manipulation. The lesion is excised by removing the desired amount of lid in square or rectangular shape. This consists of a block resection of the entire thickness of the lid including the conjunctiva. A square or rectangle is better than a V excision because less lid margin is sacrificed; also the cut edges of the tarsus are virtually parallel and can be approximated accurately. The anterior half of the lid margin at one edge is excised, and the posterior half at the other edge. An external canthotomy is then done, with the skin incision directed slightly upward to follow the contour of the lower lid. Scissors are inserted into the canthotomy opening, and all fibers of the ligament that fix the lid are severed. It is important to release all of them, so that the lid can fill the defect. This is best accomplished by putting the lid on the stretch and palpating to detect any remaining unsevered fibers.

A double-arm silk suture is placed through the posterior lip of the halved portion (the tarsus) and carried through the anterior lip

* Drawings for both operative procedures show the excision close to the lesion, a nevus. How far from the lesion the excision should be made depends, of course, on the individual case.

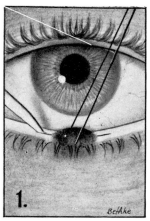
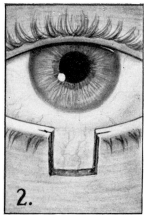
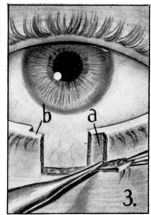
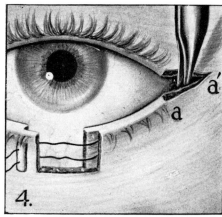
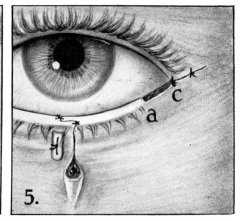
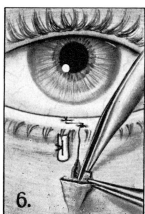
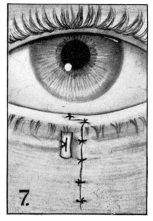

FIG. 1–12. Steps in the technique for lesser resection of the lid. **1.** A traction suture is placed through the lid margin at the site of the lesion, and the lid is halved on each side of it. **2.** Resection of the affected part of the lid. **3.** The outer half of the lid margin (*a*) and the inner half (*b*) are removed preparatory to approximation of the lid edges by the halving procedures. **4.** A double-arm suture is placed through the tarsus and skin, and an external canthotomy is carried out from *a* to *a'*. **5.** The lid margins are approximated by the double-arm suture tied over a rubber peg; the new lid margin extends from *a* to *c*. **6.** A triangular piece of redundant skin is excised to prevent puckering. **7.** The lid margins and skin edges are approximated by fine interrupted silk sutures.

(the skin). It should be placed so that there is overcorrection when the halved edges come together. Release of the lateral portion of the lid at the external canthus should be sufficient for the halved edges to approximate easily without tension on the suture. The double-arm suture is then tied over a rubber peg, leaving puckered skin below the lid approximation. A triangular piece of this skin is excised, and the edges are sutured. The main suture merely approximates the halved margins; fine sutures are needed for accurate closure, particularly along the lid margin. An interrupted silk suture is placed to mark the new external canthus; several similar sutures approximate the skin edges over the site of the external canthotomy. The space from *a* to *c* (Fig. 1–12) in this same step is the newly formed lid margin; no further suturing is needed along the edge. This technique is applicable to the upper lid as well.

For small lesions, requiring a 4–6 mm resection of the lid margin, the defect can usually be repaired without resorting to external canthotomy and release of the canthal ligament (Fig. 1–13).

Technique for the greater resection (Fig. 1–14). A more extensive operation is indicated for excising a lesion requiring resection of more than one-third the length of the lid. Halving is carried out as described for the lesser procedure.

A traction suture passed through the lesion facilitates manipulation of the lid. The conjunctiva is dissected from the posterior surface of the lid to the cul-de-sac. As much of the conjunctiva as possible is salvaged; all can usually be saved except the portion firmly adherent to the tarsus. The dissected free conjunctiva is now pushed down into the cul-de-sac and left there until the operation is completed. The amount of the lid to be included in the resection and sliding graft is outlined on the skin with a scalpel. Incisions in this area should diverge temporally to broaden the base of the graft for nutritional purposes.

The vertical incision through the lid nasally is now completed, along with the horizontal incisions; the portion to be resected and also the portion to be included in the sliding graft are dissected free into the temporal region. The extent of this dissection depends on the size of the defect to be filled by the sliding graft.

Up to this point, unless the lesion is ulcer-

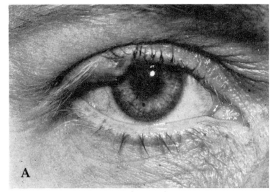

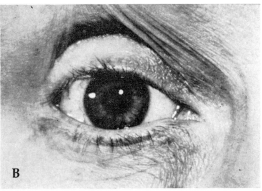

FIG. 1–13. Basal-cell epithelioma of the upper lid treated by the lesser resection. **A.** Preoperative appearance. **B.** Postoperative appearance (the skin of the upper lid is retracted to expose the approximated margins).

ated or infected, the portion of the lid to be resected has been left intact, to facilitate manipulation of the lid during the dissection. That portion is now excised and the remaining lid margins are prepared for the halving procedure as described for the lesser resection. The anterior half (cilia, skin, and orbicularis muscle) or the temporal edge is excised over the region which was halved, and the posterior half (tarsus and conjunctiva) of the nasal edge is also excised over the region which was halved. The skin and cilia are left on the nasal side so that they can benefit from the established blood supply of this part of the lid.

The portion of the sliding graft that will participate in the new part of the lower lid should be thin but become progressively thicker toward its base in the interest of blood supply. With the skin sufficiently undermined and fascial attachments of the temporal flap freed, the graft should slide

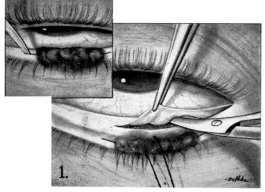

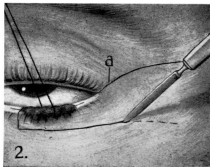

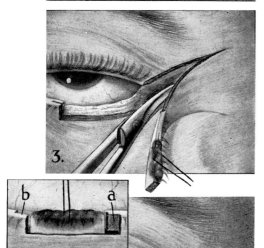

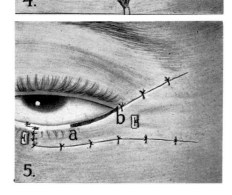

FIG. 1–14. Steps in the technique for greater resection of the lid. **1.** A traction suture is placed through the lesion, and the palpebral conjunctiva is dissected back. Inset shows halving of the lid margin, which is done on both sides of the lesion. **2.** The skin incisions; *a* shows the extent of the upper incision. **3.** The lid is severed, and the dissection is carried into the temporal region. The palpebral conjunctiva to be salvaged has been tucked into the cul-de-sac. **4.** The affected part of the lid is now excised. Inset shows the excised portion and halving of the lid margins at *a* and *b*. A double-arm suture *c* is placed through the lid and the periosteum at the orbital margin to facilitate sliding the skin flap nasally. **5.** To complete the operation, the skin is closed with fine silk sutures. The new lid margin extends from *a* to *b*. No sutures are required to join the palpebral conjunctival edge to the lid margin.

FIG. 1–15. Result following greater resection of the right lower lid for a basal-cell epithelioma which had recurred after x-ray therapy.

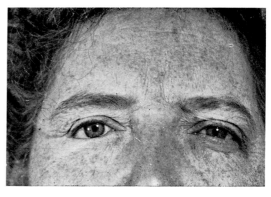

comfortably to fill the defect. As shown in Figure 1–14, a double-arm 4-0 silk suture is passed through the periosteum at the orbital margin (step 4a) and then through the temporal flap in such a way that when the suture is tied, the temporal flap can slide far enough nasally to fill the defect. This suture is tied over a rubber peg (step 5). A double-arm 5-0 silk suture is then placed through the complementing halves of the lid margin (step 5b) so there will be some overcorrection of the junction, as described for the lesser resection. The suture is also tied over a rubber peg. No tension should be put on the suture and it should be tied loosely, minimizing the risk of interfering with nutrition of the tip of the graft and possibly producing a slough. Interrupted silk sutures unite the skin margins.

It is essential to place an interrupted silk suture accurately, to determine the new external canthus properly (step 5b). The new lid margin now lies between the points designated *a* and *b* in step 5 (Fig. 1–14). The free edge of the conjunctiva, which was reflected into the cul-de-sac away from the operative site, is now placed opposite the new lid margin. I have found it better not to suture the conjunctiva to the skin margin.

When the graft is pulled toward the defect to be filled, some excess skin may result in puckering. It is not necessary to excise this skin fold unless it is bulky; almost any amount of puckering flattens out and leaves no blemish.

When the lid defect to be filled is rather large, the upper horizontal incision is inadequate as the lid margin tends to evert. This tendency is overcome by making the lower horizontal incision as well. A result obtained using this technique is shown in Figure 1–15.

The same procedure is applicable to the upper lid. Regardless of the extent of the lid resection, the resected portion should always be wide enough for the upper horizontal incision to extend along the normal horizontal fold of the upper lid. While the technique described here is suitable for any size defect in the lower lid, even one involving the entire lower lid, it cannot be used to repair a defect involving more than half of the upper lid.

In performing any halving procedure on the lid, the joining of tarsus and tarsus is more satisfactory than tarsus and skin. However, when the lesion to be excised is so close to the external or internal canthus that no tarsus is available on one side, it is necessary to attach tarsus to skin. Also, when one edge is beyond the termination of the tarsus so that it does not include tarsal tissue, approximation of the two lid edges is less accurate because the double-arm suture yields more on the side without tarsal tissue. In such cases the sliding graft should be more extensively freed to permit a generous release of the lid.

When the lesion on the upper or lower lid is adjacent to the inner or outer canthus, there is no lid on one side to be attached to the other lid margin. A satisfactory result can

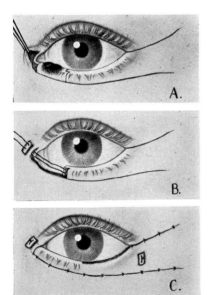

FIG. 1–16. Resection for removal of a lesion involving the inner canthus. **A.** The skin, deeply undermined to receive the halved lid margin, is raised with forceps. **B.** After the lesion is excised, a double-arm silk suture is passed through the halved lid margin and anchored deep under the skin flap. **C.** One double-arm suture is tied over a peg (left), and another similarly tied (right) anchors the skin flap to the periosteum at the external orbital margin.

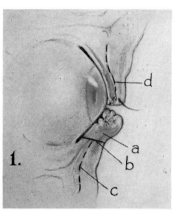

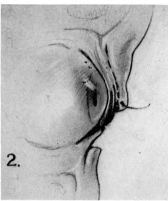

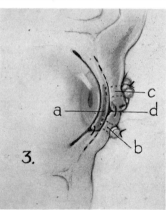

FIG. 1–17. The Hughes operation as applied to the lower lid.[28] **1.** The tumor *a* is excised along line *b;* the lower lid is halved along line *c,* and the upper lid along line *d.* **2.** The tumor has been excised. **3.** The posterior leaves of both lids are sutured to the tarsus *h* by double-arm sutures tied over pegs as shown at *e* and *f.* In this way half of the tarsus of the upper lid remains *in situ* and half is in the lower lid. The margins of the two lids are approximated by a suture at *g* which marks the new palpebral aperture.

be obtained in such cases by anchoring the lid margin under the skin to the canthal ligament or periosteum in an overcorrected position (Fig. 1–16). This technique can be used with both the lesser and greater resections.

Hughes operation (Fig. 1–17). This procedure[28] is useful for lesions requiring resection of the entire lower lid and, less satisfactorily, of the entire upper lid, or for lesser degrees of resection of either lid. The basic principle is division of the unaffected lid into an anterior half consisting of skin, cilia, and orbicularis muscle and a posterior half consisting of conjunctiva and tarsus. These two halves are sutured to the remaining corresponding halves of the lid from which the tumor was removed. The operation is also suitable for partial lid resection; a result is shown in Figure 1–7B (see p. 4).

Hughes has emphasized[28a] that the attachment of Mueller's muscle to the tarsus must be severed, the sliding flap freed so that it lies loosely in position to form the new lower lid; and, after the fissure is opened, the tarsal layers must be placed so that they protrude 1 mm beyond the skin edges.

Other Techniques. When the tumor is too far advanced to preserve function of the eye, *e.g.,* when it involves most of the lid and has extended into the orbit (Fig. 1–18, see p. 4), exenteration of the orbit is indicated.

When a very extensive cancer of the lids invades the nose and sinuses, it ceases to be solely an ophthalmologic problem. Tumors that straddle the external or the internal canthus, involving both the upper and lower lids in varying degrees, usually require extensive plastic surgery depending on their location and size.

A suggested technique for chemosurgical excision of eyelid and canthal tumors[42] includes a system of marking specimens in a coded pattern with various stains (Mercurochrome, Prussian blue, and India ink). The tumor site is fixed *in vivo* with zinc chloride; the area is pared from the unfixed underlying tissue and examined microscopically. The pathologist can then accurately localize areas positive for tumor, as a guide to the surgeon's staged excisions. An offshoot of this method[12] for tumors of the lid margin is essentially staged excisions without prior fixation. In both techniques the site is allowed to heal by granulation. This type of marking and coding is proving useful in special cases.

Radiation

Treatment of basal-cell carcinoma by radiation is described in the section Radiotherapy of Ocular and Orbital Tumors by Dr. Patricia Tretter, in Chapter 12.

PROGNOSIS

A patient with an untreated basal-cell carcinoma of the eyelid may live 10 or 20 years or even more before fatal complications set in, such as deep invasion of the orbit, erosion of bone, and intracranial extension. Metastases are unlikely. The course of squamous-cell carcinoma of the eyelid is usually shorter; the disease, if untreated, may result in death from metastases. Lid carcinomas may extend to the regional lymph nodes, most frequently those in the preauricular region, with the upper and lower deep cervical nodes next most frequently affected.

CARCINOMAS OF THE CONJUNCTIVA

Epidermization or dyskeratosis of the conjunctiva, corneal epithelium, or any mucous membrane represents a change to keratinized epithelium, either occurring spontaneously or caused by inflammation, irradiation, exposure to chemicals such as arsenic, or prolonged exposure to air. This change may presage leukoplakia, intraepithelial epithelioma (Bowen's disease), or papilloma. Frank carcinomas may develop from any of the three. Epidermization usually extends well beyond the carcinoma, and if not excised with the main lesion it is a potential focus for recurrence.

Three cases of epibulbar squamous-cell tumors characterized by diffuse growth with-

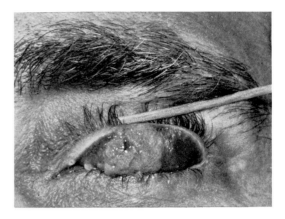

FIG. 1–20. Diffuse squamous-cell epithelioma of the palpebral conjunctiva of the upper lid.

out tumefaction and by marked inflammation that clinically obscured their dyskeratotic nature have been reported.[29]

In the conjunctiva, squamous-cell carcinomas occur about ten times more frequently than the basal-cell type. They usually arise at the limbus (Fig. 1–19, see p. 4) and spread to the cornea and adjacent bulbar conjunctiva (Fig. 1–20). A limbal carcinoma sometimes invades the sclera and, very infrequently, the cornea (Fig. 1–21) inasmuch as Bowman's membrane usually acts as a barrier to corneal invasion. In extremely rare cases the tumor extends through the sclera to the intraocular structures.

CLINICAL APPEARANCE AND COURSE

A papilloma is at times confused with a squamous-cell carcinoma; in the transitional stage it may be difficult to determine, even on histologic examination, whether it is a papilloma or an early squamous-cell carcinoma.

The lesion is localized and elevated; its rather characteristic white color, due to the keratin content, may give the tumor a striking pearly appearance. Large nutrient conjunctival vessels course toward it.

Leukoplakia, very common on the oral mucous membrane, is found less frequently on the conjunctiva. A focal area of epithelial hyperplasia and keratinization, it is usually seen at the limbus temporally but may also appear on the bulbar conjunctiva (Fig. 1–22). The slightly elevated white plaque is easily overlooked and is sometimes mistaken for a pinguecula. However, a leukoplakial lesion is

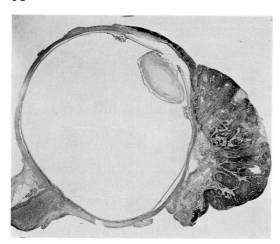

FIG. 1–21. Squamous-cell epithelioma of the limbus with secondary extension to the cornea. A gradually enlarging mass, noted on the right eye of a 67-year-old woman for two years, had extended over the entire corneal surface, replacing the lamellae.

FIG. 1–22. Leukoplakia of the bulbar conjunctiva at the limbus.

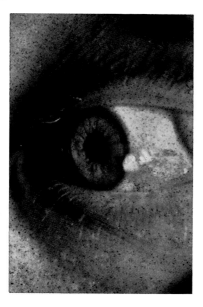

white and superficial, whereas a pinguecula is yellow and subepithelial. Leukoplakia is viewed as precancerous and may be the forerunner of squamous-cell epithelioma. *Leukokeratosis* and *acanthosis* are terms sometimes used for the precancerous lesion at a more advanced stage in which there is considerable keratinization and a mild chronic inflammatory reaction. Increased vascularization and inflammation in a precancerous lesion have been considered signs of active growth.[65]

As carcinomas tend to arise at sites of epithelial transition, their predilection for the limbus is consistent. Also, chronic irritation is a precipitating factor. It is interesting to note that squamous-cell carcinomas of the conjunctiva, as well as benign leukoplakia, tend to develop in the palpebral aperture, usually on the temporal side where there is exposure. The incidence is significantly high in elderly men. Since these carcinomas are solar-related, they occur more frequently in tropical than in temperate zones.

The possible relationship between pterygia and conjunctival carcinoma has been pointed out.[60] Most of the carcinomas studied arose within the palpebral aperture at the medial limbus and showed evidence of submucosal collagen degeneration. Contralateral pterygia were noted in about one-third of the cases. Precancerous changes have been found in sections of pterygia.

Diffuse epithelial tumors of the conjunctiva frequently masquerade as chronic infectious conjunctivitis or keratoconjunctivitis.[68] A unilateral chronic conjunctivitis resistant to treatment, punctate keratitis, and a diffuse thickening and inflammation of the tarsal plate form a suspicious triad[67] in which a biopsy is mandatory. Cytologic smears of epithelial scrapings stained and fixed by the Papanicolaou method have been recommended.[17]

Basal-cell carcinomas of the conjunctiva have no particular distinguishing characteristics except that they tend to be flat. They may arise from either the bulbar or palpebral conjunctiva, and have no predilection for the limbus.

In a report based on 93 cases of limbal tumors[1] there were 48 carcinomas, 28 papillomas, and 17 dyskeratotic cancerous lesions. Most of the epithelial tumors of the limbus were in the palpebral fissure—78 of them in male patients. Four papillomas and four carcinomas appeared at the site of, and immediately following, an injury. Epidermization of adjacent epithelium with or without dyskeratosis in 12 of the 28 papillomas and 35 of the 48 frank carcinomas among the limbal tumors suggested that it is an important precursor of either benign or malignant tumors. Thirty-nine of the 48 carcinomas were of the squamous-cell type, 8 of the papillary squamous-cell type, and 1 was a basal-cell epithelioma.

Pingueculas and pterygia, viewed by some as potentially precancerous, appear to progress from the usual elevated lesion located nasally or rarely temporally at the limbus to an invading carcinoma.[1,69] In one series of 100 pterygia[60] there were 12 cases of carcinoma and 17 cases of carcinoma *in situ*.

The term *precancerous epithelioma* has been proposed for the hyperactive epithelium over the pterygium.[76] The epithelial changes of a pterygium are always accompanied by typical degenerative changes of the stroma consisting of coiling and fragmentation of the collagen fibers which form amorphous hyaloid masses.

A hereditary dyskeratosis of the perilimbal conjunctiva, invariably associated with comparable lesions of the oral mucosa, has been described in patients from Halifax County, North Carolina.[71,72,77] Similar lesions involving the bulbar conjunctiva in a mother and daughter were reported.[79] Although the daughter was born in Philadelphia, the mother came from Halifax County.

TREATMENT

The treatment of squamous- and basal-cell epitheliomas of the conjunctiva depends largely on their location and size. Excision is indicated when the lesion is well localized. If it involves the limbus, heat cautery or cryotherapy may be applied at the sulcus between the cornea and sclera after the excision, which may not have included all tumor tissue at that point. As stated earlier, Bowman's membrane offers considerable resistance to growth, and therefore the tumor may advance over the cornea and involve the pupillary area without invading the stroma. Complete excision is thus possible in some cases where the growth seems to be quite far advanced.

If the tumor seems to show invasive tendencies in the sclera at the time of surgery, enucleation may be necessary, or an excision supplemented with radiation. Some ophthal-

mologists have advocated superficial lamellar keratectomy or sclerectomy.

If a primary or recurrent tumor has been excised over most of the limbal circumference, the patient may develop secondary glaucoma presumably due to disturbance of the aqueous outflow from cicatricial contracture.

In a series previously cited[1] simple excision sufficed in 23 of the 48 cases of carcimoma of the limbus; additional excision was necessary in 2 cases. Enucleation was carried out in the other 23 patients. Only one death was attributed to the tumor, and the evidence was presumptive in this case. The authors concluded that local excision is adequate unless recurrences persist, when enucleation or exenteration may be necessary. They advised against preoperative or postoperative irradiation.

Leukoplakic lesions and large exophytic epithelial tumors of the conjunctiva and cornea may increase in size without deep invasion of the underlying tissue or metastasis to the regional nodes, thus often making total excision possible without sacrificing the eye.[83] In this group only carcinomas of the palpebral conjunctiva metastasize.[29,83]

PAPILLOMAS

Papillomas favor sites where the epithelium undergoes a transition; hence in ophthalmology they are rarely seen except at the lid margin and at the limbus (Figs. 1–23, 1–24, see p. 5).

They are recognized clinically by their mulberrylike or cauliflowerlike surface and their tendency to be pedunculated. In people with dark skin the presence of melanin in the basal layer of the epithelium may make them pigmented. A papilloma may be so markedly pigmented in blacks as to be mistaken for a melanoma (Fig. 1–24, see p. 5).

Papillomas are classified according to whether or not they are caused by a viral infection. The infectious type is usually called a verruca and tends to be multiple. When the conjunctiva is involved, particularly in young people, the lesion may be diffuse, multiple, or both. If located on the lid margin, it sometimes gives rise to a contact lesion on the bulbar conjunctiva or the opposite lid margin.

A type of recurrent juvenile squamous-cell papilloma of the conjunctiva has its counterpart in the trachea and larynx. The lesions are usually multiple and may recur after excision. The prognosis is good even after one or more excisions. The lesions are neither invasive nor metastatic and are considered to be of an infectious nature. They are frequently encountered in the lower cul-de-sac, particularly near the inner canthus, the canaliculus, and the lacrimal sac.[15] A juvenile papilloma of the eyelid that seemed to extend from the nose has been reported.[35]

A 5-year-old black girl with multiple verrucae involving the palpebral and bulbar conjunctiva failed to respond to three months of local and systemic treatment,[46] which was continued, however, and the lesions disappeared completely within the next three months. According to another report,[25] recurrent conjunctival papillomas were successfully treated by cryotherapy in a 7-year-old white girl.

Histologically, the viral and nonviral papillomas are similar (Fig. 1–23B, see p. 5). In a series cited before,[1] 25 of the 28 papillomas of the limbus consisted of an epidermal type of epithelium and the other 3 of a conjunctival type. A nonviral papilloma tends to develop into a squamous-cell carcinoma, and in some instances it is difficult to put the lesion into either classification. In fact, 8 of the 48 cases of carcinoma of the limbus in this series were classified as the papillary squamous-cell type.

TREATMENT

Excision flush with the surface is adequate treatment for a papilloma. Eighteen of the 28 cases of limbal papilloma[1] were treated by local excision; there was only one recurrence. Eight eyes were enucleated because of extensive corneal involvement. It is quite possible, however, that they might have been saved; since the papilloma grows entirely above the surface, excision to Bowman's membrane may be sufficient. Although the tumors can be eradicated by radiation (Fig. 1–24, see p. 5), the possible secondary effects make this treatment less desirable than excision.

Conjunctival papillomas, with features presumably of the infectious type, have been reported in 3- and 5-year-old sisters.[75]

INTRAEPITHELIAL EPITHELIOMAS (BOWEN'S DISEASE)

Intraepithelial epitheliomas occur on the cornea, conjunctiva, and skin of the lids. They are often called Bowen's disease, but some authorities believe this term should be reserved for lesions of the skin, including the eyelid, and not used for lesions of the mucous membrane such as occur on the conjunctiva or cornea.[84] Ophthalmologists most often encounter intraepithelial epitheliomas on the cornea and conjunctiva as diffuse, slightly elevated, vascularized, granulomatous- or gelatinous-looking lesions (Fig. 1–25, see p. 6). They arise from the epithelium and may be confined within it for years without breaking through the basement layer or showing infiltrative tendencies. They are capable of metastasizing, however. An accompanying inflammatory reaction may mask their neoplastic character. One case in a published series started in a trachomatous pannus (Fig. 1–26, see p. 6), another in an eye injured 14 years earlier (Fig. 1–27), and still another in an eye burned 13 years earlier which became ulcerated within 3 years.[40] There was no previous injury, inflammation, irradiation, or exposure in two cases. In another report, one-third of such lesions arose from a site of preexisting disease.[37]

The patients' average age in reported cases was 60 years, and more males were affected. The disease usually started at the limbus and was characteristically unilateral, although bilateral cases have been encountered.

The hyperplasia in Bowen's disease is intraepithelial. The basal cells proliferate, lose their neat palisaded arrangement, and may form elongated pegs; these basal cells remain intact as a layer, however, and no actual invasive tendencies are noted. An abrupt transition between the normal and the hyperplastic tissue is typical (Fig. 1–25B, see p. 6, and Fig. 1–27B). The cellular variations that characterize this disease are marked variations in size, shape, staining properties, and loss of cell polarity. The so-called monster cells are of two types: a) those with a very large single nucleus and b) those with multiple nuclei clumped together, indicating amitosis—sometimes called "clumped cells of Bowen." Mitotic figures are common. Darier's *corps ronds* are large cells with deeply eosinophilic cytoplasm; a very large vacuole completely surrounding the nucleus gives the cells a double-ringed appearance (Fig. 1–27C). They are regarded as having undergone partial, premature keratinization before reaching the surface layer. Other cells may undergo complete, premature keratinization. Actual keratin pearls are sometimes seen. Concentric

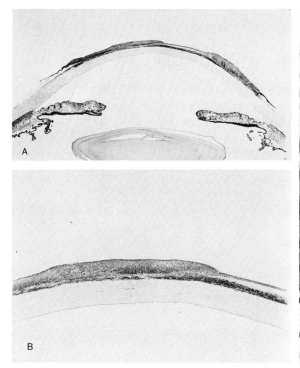

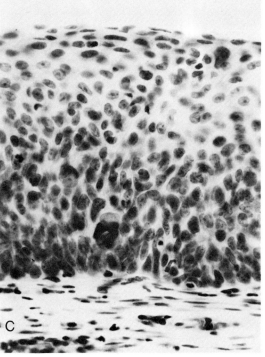

FIG. 1–27. Intraepithelial epithelioma of the cornea. A 67-year-old woman had a red painful eye following an injury 14 years earlier. The cornea showed a dense superficial opacity with many blood vessels growing in from the limbus. The corneal epithelium was elevated, particularly from 5 to 9 o'clock, and the possibility of Bowen's disease was considered. **A.** Low-power view shows diffuse thickening of the corneal epithelium. **B.** Higher magnification reveals an abrupt transition from normal to epitheliomatous corneal epithelium, and dense infiltration of lymphocytes in superficial corneal lamellae. **C.** Still higher magnification shows the structure of the epitheliomatous lesion. (Courtesy of J. S. McGavic.[40])

laminae of squamous cells show gradually increasing cornification toward the center. Some lesions exhibit hyperkeratosis and granule formation (parakeratosis) along the surface. Intercellular bridges are at times noted. Lymphocytes, plasma cells, and histiocytes are present beneath the epithelium (Fig. 1–25B, see p. 6).

Bowen's disease is variously classified as intraepithelial epithelioma or carcinoma *in situ* and as a precancerous lesion which becomes malignant in 40% of the mucous membrane lesions and in 3% of the skin lesions.[63]

In about half the cases the disease begins insidiously at the site of a chronic inflammatory process or some previous pathologic change and may go unrecognized. The fact that the lesion is frequently flat and diffuse also adds to difficulty in diagnosing its neoplastic nature.

A surprisingly high percentage of primary cancers elsewhere in the skin or in the internal organs are associated with Bowen's disease.[23,37] The finding that 80% of patients with Bowen's disease have one or more primary internal cancers or a primary skin cancer with metastasis has led some investigators to consider it a manifestation of a systemic carcinogenic disease process.[24]

The cancerous change of the lesion in Bowen's disease is always slow and is manifested in one of two clinical forms: an atypical squamous-cell carcinoma arising from a portion of the lesion and forming an ulcerating or fungating mass, or metastasis without clinical evidence of local invasion.

Carcinoma *in situ* recurs after excision in about 20% of the cases affecting the conjunctiva and cornea. The tumor is diffuse, making it difficult to determine, at the time of excision, the exact limits of its extension. Also, some etiologic factors may continue to affect the remaining conjunctiva after surgery. Eight patients with such recurrences were treated by an extensive *en bloc* excision of the conjunctiva as well as lamellar scleral and corneal resection at the limbus.[59] There were no recurrences after 15 to 51 months follow-up.

DIFFERENTIAL DIAGNOSIS

Among conditions clinically resembling Bowen's disease are a) corneal pannus from any cause, b) filtering cicatrix of the cornea, c) Mooren's ulcer, d) fatty degeneration of the cornea, e) epithelial dystrophy of the cornea, and f) pterygium. Although suspected clinically, the diagnosis can be established definitely only by microscopic examination of the tissue.

Lesions with histologic characteristics somewhat similar to Bowen's disease are a) basal- and squamous-cell carcinomas, especially in the early stages before there is a break in the basement layer; b) xeroderma pigmentosum; c) arsenical keratosis; arsenic is believed to play a role in the pathogenesis of some cases of Bowen's disease; d) precancerous melanosis and cancerous melanosis of the conjunctiva and skin; e) senile keratosis; f) radiation dermatitis and carcinoma; g) leukoplakia; and h) cancers of workers in contact with paraffin and allied substances.

TREATMENT

The treatment of choice is complete surgical excision; removal of a portion of the tumor for biopsy purposes is not contraindicated. The tumors are not very sensitive to radiation therapy and are so diffuse that the target area would have to be extensive. Treatment with chemicals or actual cautery is considered inadequate and perhaps dangerous, as it may provide a stimulus to malignant change.

Since the tumors do not tend to infiltrate deeply, small lesions are not difficult to excise. A lesion confined to the cornea can be stripped away from Bowman's membrane leaving clear cornea. Complete excision of a lesion extending diffusely over the conjunctiva may require enucleation and, if the palpebral conjunctiva is involved, possible loss of the eyelid. Excision of conjunctiva alone may suffice, but symblepharon is likely to follow unless adequate grafts are made.

Even though the lesion in Bowen's disease may remain a long time *in situ* without showing invasion or metastasis, its malignant potential should be considered in outlining the treatment. Temporizing is more in order here than with a true basal- or squamous-cell carcinoma, but if the lesion is not completely controlled it may prove to have more than local significance.

When the tumor involves the skin of the lids, it is usually localized and may be confused with a flat papilloma or a nevus. Microscopically, an intraepithelial epithelioma of the skin of the lid resembles thickened epithelium with hyperplastic deranged pegs formed by the rete cells.

XERODERMA PIGMENTOSUM

Xeroderma pigmentosum (Fig. 1–28, see pp. 6, 7), although primarily a disease of the skin and mucous membranes, frequently causes ocular complications. The skin shows an abnormal reaction to light, producing potentially cancerous lesions. Many of the affected patients are offspring of consanguineous marriages. The skin seems normal at birth, but after exposure to sunlight the child develops an acute erythema differing from ordinary sunburn only in that it is induced by less sunlight and disappears more slowly. This is followed by a diffuse pigmentation resembling freckles, irregular in outline and in varying degrees of intensity. The skin becomes dry, scaly, and atrophic, and small stellate telangiectases appear. Multiple verrucae sometimes develop later on the pigmented maculae; they may fuse but rarely become very large. They ulcerate, fungate, and take on active malignant characteristics. The disease peaks between the sixth and seventh years, and death usually occurs before the twenty-first year. The growths are carcinomas of various types; in one series 21 of 55 cases were malignant.[43]

TUMORS OF THE LACRIMAL SAC

Over 100 cases of neoplasms arising in the lacrimal sac fossa, largely squamous-cell carcinomas or malignant lymphomas, were reviewed.[31] One of the author's six cases was an intraepithelial epithelioma (Bowen's disease), and one was a Kaposi's sarcoma. Hypertrophic changes follow most inflammations of the lacrimal sac. These may take the form of granulomas or of polyps.[7] All reported cases of lacrimal sac tumors up to

1964, a total of 184, were analyzed and two others added.[54]

The clinical course of tumors of the lacrimal sac is marked by epiphora, swelling, and extension of the process outside of the immediate area of the sac. The swelling at times may be accompanied by some dacryocystitis. Even with considerable swelling the lacrimal canaliculus may be patent. Although diagnostic x rays with the aid of contrast media are of value, the final diagnosis depends upon microscopic examination of biopsy tissue.

About 50% of tumors of the lacrimal sac are said to be in the papilloma-carcinoma group; the histologic picture is identical with that of solid cylindrical-cell carcinomas arising from the respiratory epithelium in the nasal and paranasal cavities.[2] The authors of this report[2] suggested use of the term *malignant cylindrical-cell carcinoma* instead of *papilloma* for these growths, since the so-called papillomas arising from the lacrimal sac epithelium have a different formation and structure from true papillomas and are probably malignant from the outset.

Melanomas of the lacrimal sac are rare. Papillomas and carcinomas were the two main classifications in a clinicopathologic study of primary epithelial neoplasms of the lacrimal sac.[58] Eight of the 13 lesions in another series[26] were of epithelial origin; 2 of the remaining 5 were malignant melanomas, 2 reticuloses, and 1 an angiosarcoma.

It has been recommended that both lacrimal canaliculi be excised even if not involved in the tumor.[49]

Dacryocystography is indicated for patients with suspected carcinoma of the tear sac, especially in the presence of unexplained epiphora, bleeding disproportionate to the ease of probing, or unsuccessful irrigation despite passing of the probe.[41]

TUMORS OF THE CARUNCLE AND SEMILUNAR FOLD

It must be remembered that the caruncle may be the seat of any tumor or cyst occurring in the conjunctiva or in the skin because the surface epithelium of the caruncle and the semilunar fold is mucous membrane, and the caruncle itself harbors all skin elements including hair follicles, sebaceous glands, and sweat glands.

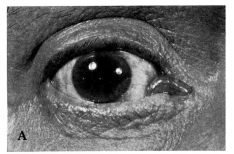

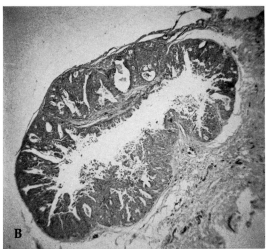

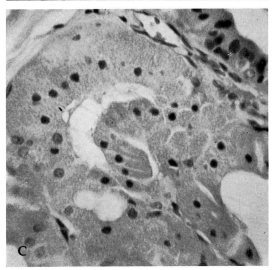

FIG. 1–29. Oncocytoma of the caruncle. **A.** Clinical appearance. **B.** Low-power view of section from tumor. **C.** Higher magnification shows the cell structure. (Courtesy of T. T. Noguchi.)

ONCOCYTOMA (OXYPHILIC ADENOMA)

Oncocytoma, a rare benign tumor, seems to have a predilection for the caruncle[45,48,53] (Fig. 1–29). The tumor usually appears as a small hyperplastic nodule, seldom as a true neoplasm. The possibility of an oncocytic variant of acinous-cell carcinoma has been suggested, and an oncocytic papillary cystadenoma of both lacrimal caruncles described.[74] An oncocytoma which developed in the caruncle of an 80-year-old woman was histologically identical with a parotid gland tumor removed from her nine years earlier.[16] Two cases of adenolymphomalike tumors of the lacrimal caruncle and the larynx have been described.[36]

The tumor is composed of granular aci-dophilic cells called oncocytes which seem to arise from the ductile epithelium. They are found principally in the salivary and lacrimal glands but also at times in the trachea, pharynx, esophagus, buccal mucosa, pancreas, hypophysis, breast, thyroid, parathyroid, testes, fallopian tubes, liver, and stomach. Since oncocytes have been found in normal lacrimal glands, it is surprising that oncocytomas seldom develop there or in the lacrimal sac.

Oncocytoma occurring in salivary glands is referred to as Warthin's tumor or papillary cystadenoma lymphomatosum.

The treatment of choice for these usually symptomless nodules is excision, and the prognosis is good.

REFERENCES

1. ASH JE, WILDER HC: Epithelial tumors of the limbus. Am J Ophthalmol 25:926–932, 1942
2. ASHTON N, CHOYCE DP, FISON LG: Carcinoma of the lacrimal sac. Br J Ophthalmol 35:366–376, 1951
3. BISHOP DW: Trichoepithelioma. Arch Ophthalmol 74:4–8, 1965
4. BITRAN J, PELLETTIERE EV: Multiple sebaceous gland tumors and internal carcinoma: Torre's syndrome. Cancer 33:835–836, 1974
5. BONIUK M, ZIMMERMAN LE: Eyelid tumors with reference to lesions confused with squamous cell carcinoma. II. Inverted follicular keratosis. Arch Ophthalmol 69:698–707, 1963
6. BONIUK M, ZIMMERMAN LE: Sebaceous carcinoma of the eyelid, eyebrow, caruncle and orbit. Trans Am Acad Ophthalmol Otolaryngol 72:619–642, 1968
7. BOUZAS A: Polyps of the lacrimal sac. Arch Ophthalmol 66:236–240, 1961
8. BRAUNINGER GE, HOOD I, WORTHEN DM: Sebaceous carcinoma of lid margin masquerading as cutaneous horn. Arch Ophthalmol 90:380–381, 1973
9. BURKET JM, CAPLAN RM: Multiple self-healing epithelioma. Arch Dermatol 90:7–11, 1964
10. CAVANAGH HD, GREEN WR, GOLDBERG HK: Multicentric sebaceous adenocarcinoma of the Meibomian gland. Am J Ophthalmol 77:326–332, 1974
11. CHRISTENSEN L, FITZPATRICK TB: Keratoacanthoma of the ocular adnexa. Arch Ophthalmol 53:857–859, 1955
12. CIES WA, BAYLIS HI: Complications of Mohs' chemosurgical excision of eyelid and canthal tumors. Am J Ophthalmol 80:116–122, 1975
13. COLE JG: Histologically controlled excision of eyelid tumors. Am J Ophthalmol 70:240–244, 1970
14. COOPER WC: Personal communication
15. CRAWFORD JS: Papilloma of lacrimal sac. Am J Ophthalmol 51:1303–1304, 1961
16. DEUTSCH AR, DUCKWORTH JK: Onkocytoma (oxyphilic adenoma) of the caruncle. Am J Ophthalmol 64:458–461, 1967
17. DYKSTRA PC, DYKSTRA BA: The cytologic diagnosis of carcinoma and related lesions of the ocular conjunctiva and cornea. Trans Am Acad Ophthalmol Otolaryngol 73:979–995, 1969
18. EPSTEIN W, KLIGMAN AM: The pathogenesis of milia and benign tumors of the skin. J Invest Dermatol 26:1–11, 1956
19. EREAUX LP, SCHOPFLOCHER P, FOURNIER CJ: Keratoacanthoma. Arch Dermatol 71:73–83, 1955
20. FINNEY R: Treatment of molluscum sebaceum. Lancet 2:1358, 1953
21. GHADIALLY FN, BARTON BW, KERRIDGE DF: The etiology of keratoacanthoma. Cancer 16:603–611, 1963
22. GOODING CA, WHITE G, YATSUHASHI M: Significance of marginal extension in excised basal-cell carcinoma. New Eng J Med 273:923–924, 1965
23. GRAHAM JH, HELWIG EB: Bowen's disease and its relationship to systemic cancer. Arch Dermatol Syphilol 80:133–159, 1959
24. GRAHAM JH, HELWIG EB: Bowen's disease and its relationship to systemic cancer. Arch Dermatol Syphilol 83:738–758, 1961
25. HARKEY ME, METZ HS: Cryotherapy of conjunctival papillomata. Am J Ophthalmol 66:872–874, 1968
26. HARRY J, ASHTON N: The pathology of tumours of the lacrimal sac. Trans Ophthalmol Soc UK 88:19–35, 1968
27. HELWIG EB: Seminar on the Skin: Neoplasms and Dermatoses. Proc 20th Seminar Am Soc Clin Pathol, Washington DC, 1954
28. HUGHES WE: Reconstructive Surgery of the Eyelids. St. Louis, CV Mosby, 1954
28a. HUGHES WE: Personal communication

29. IRVINE RA JR: Diffuse epibulbar squamous-cell epithelioma. Am J Ophthalmol 64:550–554, 1967
30. JAKOBIEC ·FA: Sebaceous adenoma of the eyelid and visceral malignancy. Am J Ophthalmol 952–960, 1974
31. JONES IS: Tumors of the lacrimal sac. Am J Ophthalmol 42:261–266, 1956
32. KEYES JEL, QUEEN FB: Trichoepithelioma of eyelid. Am J Ophthalmol 28:189–191, 1945
33. KLIGMAN AM, PINKUS H: The histogenesis of nevoid tumors of the skin. Arch Dermatol Syphilol 81:922–930, 1960
34. KWITKO ML, BONIUK M, ZIMMERMAN LE: Eyelid tumors with reference to lesions confused with squamous-cell carcinoma. I. Incidence and errors in diagnosis. Arch Ophthalmol 69:693–697, 1963
35. KYRIAKOU K: Juvenile papillomata of the eyelids. Bull Soc Hellen Ophthalmol 23:68–69, 1955
36. LENNOX B, TIMPERLEY WR, MURRAY D, KELLETT HS: Adenolymphomalike tumours of the lacrimal caruncle and the larynx. J Pathol Bacteriol 96:321–326, 1968
37. LOCKE JC: Bowen's disease (intraepithelial epithelioma) of the cornea and conjunctiva; a clinicopathologic study. Am J Ophthalmol 41:801–809, 1956
38. LOHSE K, TOST M: Epithelioma calcificans "Malherbe." Acta Ophthalmol (Kbh) 45:876–882, 1967
39. MARTIN HE: Cancer of the eyelids. Arch Ophthalmol 22:1–20, 1939
40. McGAVIC JS: Intraepithelial epithelioma of the cornea and conjunctiva (Bowen's disease). Am J Ophthalmol 25:167–176, 1942
41. MILDER B, SMITH ME: Carcinoma of lacrimal sac. Am J Ophthalmol 65:782–784, 1968
42. MOHS FE: Chemosurgery for microscopically controlled excision of skin cancer. J Surg Oncol 3:257, 1971
43. MORTADA A: Incidence of lid, conjunctival, and orbital malignant tumours in xeroderma pigmentosa in Egypt. Bull Ophthalmol Soc Egypt 61:231–236, 1968
44. NEUMAN Z, GILADI A: Plea for a radical approach in so-called keratoacanthoma of the eyelid. Plast Reconstr Surg 47:231–233, 1971
45. NOGUCHI TT, LONSER ER: Oncocytoma (oxyphil-cell adenoma) of the caruncle of the eyelid. Arch Pathol 69:516–519, 1960
46. NOOJIN RO: Multiple ophthalmic verrucae. Arch Dermatol 97:176–177, 1968
47. NOVER A, KORTING GW: About the familial basal-cell nevus. Klin Monatsbl Augenheilkd 156:621–628, 1970
48. PARKHILL E: Oncocytoma of caruncle. Case presentation before Ophthalmic Pathology Club, Armed Forces Institute of Pathology, Washington DC, 1956
49. PAXTON BR, DAVIDORF FH, MAKLEY TA JR: Carcinoma of lacrimal canaliculi and lacrimal sac. Arch Ophthalmol 84: 749–753, 1970
50. PAYNE JW, DUKE JR, BUTNER R, EIFRIG DE: Basal cell carcinoma of the eyelids; a long-term follow-up study. Arch Ophthalmol 81:553–558, 1969
51. PETERSON RA, AABERG TM, SMITH TR: Solid vs cystic basal cell epitheliomas of the eyelids; correlation of clinical and pathological diagnoses. Arch Ophthalmol 79:31–32, 1968
52. PINKUS H: Premalignant fibroepithelial tumors of the skin. Arch Dermatol Syphilol 67:598–615, 1953
53. RADNÓT M: Seltene Geschwülste der Caruncula lacrimalis. Ophthalmologica 113:270–275, 1947
54. RADNÓT M, GALL J: Tumors of the lacrimal sac (Tumoren des Tränensackes). Ophthalmologica 151:1–22, 1966
55. ROOK AJ, WHIMSTER IW: Le keratoacanthome. Arch Belg Dermatol Syphiligr 6:137–146, 1950
56. RUEDEMANN AD JR: A corneoscleral epithelial inclusion cyst. Am J Ophthalmol 41:316–317, 1956
57. RULON DB, HELWIG EB: Multiple sebaceous neoplasms of the skin; an association with multiple visceral carcinomas, especially of the colon. Am J Clin Pathol 60:745–752, 1973
58. RYAN SJ, FONT RL: Primary epithelial neoplasms of the lacrimal sac. Am J Ophthalmol 76:73–88, 1973
59. SANDERS N, BEDOTTO C: Recurrent carcinoma in situ of the conjunctiva and cornea (Bowen's disease). Am J Ophthalmol 74:688–693, 1972
60. SEVEL D, SEALY R: Pterygia and carcinoma of the conjunctiva. Trans Ophthalmol Soc UK 88:567–578, 1968
61. SOBIESKA-CLAROWA H, DUDEK W: A case of Malherbe's mummifying epithelioma. Klin Oczna 40:241–244, 1970 (Polish)
62. SOOD NN, RAO SN: Rhinosporidium granuloma of the conjunctiva. J Pediat Ophthalmol 6:142–144, 1969
63. STOUT AP: Malignant manifestations of Bowen's disease. New York J Med 39:801–809, 1939
64. STRAATSMA BR: Meibomian gland tumors. Arch Ophthalmol 56:71–93, 1956
65. SWAN KC, EMMENS TH, CHRISTENSEN L: Experiences with tumors of the limbus. Trans Am Acad Ophthalmol 52:458–469, 1947–1948
66. SWEEBE EC, COGAN DG: Adenocarcinoma of the meibomian gland. Arch Ophthalmol 61:130–138, 1959
67. THEODORE FH: Conjunctival carcinoma masquerading as chronic conjunctivitis. Eye Ear Nose Throat Monthly 46:1419–1420, 1967
68. THYGESON P: Observations on conjunctival neoplasms masquerading as chronic conjunctivitis or keratitis. Trans Am Acad Ophthalmol Otolaryngol 73:969–978, 1969
69. TICHO U, BEN-SIRA I: Clinical and pathologic correlation of non-pigmentary tumors of the conjunctiva and pingueculas among Africans. Am J Ophthalmol 70:757–763, 1970
70. TS'O MOM, ALBERT DM: Pathological conditions of the retinal pigment epithelium; neoplasms and nodular neoplastic lesions. Arch Ophthalmol 88:27–38, 1972
71. VON SALLMANN L, PATON D: Hereditary dyskeratosis of the perilimbal conjunctiva. Trans Am Ophthalmol Soc 57:53–62, 1959
72. VON SALLMANN L, PATON D: Hereditary benign intraepithelial dyskeratosis. I. Ocular manifestations. Arch Ophthalmol 63:421–429, 1960
73. WHORTON CM, PATTERSON JB: Carcinoma of Moll's glands with extramammary Paget's disease of the eyelid. Cancer 8:1009–1015, 1955

74. WILKERSON JA, WINQUIST PG: Bilateral papillary cystadenomas of the lacrimal caruncle. Arch Pathol 88:549–552, 1969

75. WILSON FM II, OSTLER HB: Conjunctival papillomas in siblings. Am J Ophthalmol 77:103–107, 1974

76. WINTER FC, KLEH TR: Precancerous epithelioma of the limbus. Arch Ophthalmol 64:208–215, 1960

77. WITKOP CJ JR, SHANKLE CH, GRAHAM JB, MURRAY MR, RUCKNAGEL OL, BYERLY BH: Hereditary benign intraepithelial dyskeratosis. II. Oral manifestations and hereditary transmission. Arch Pathol 70:696–711, 1960

78. WOLKEN SH, SPIVEY BE, BLODI FC: Hereditary adenoid cystic epithelioma (Brooke's tumor). Am J Ophthalmol 68:26–34, 1969

79. YANOFF M: Hereditary benign intraepithelial dyskeratosis. Arch Ophthalmol 79:291–293, 1968

80. ZELICKSON AS, LYNCH FW: Electron microscopy of virus-like particles in a keratoacanthoma. J Invest Dermatol 37:79–83, 1961

81. ZIMMERMAN LE: Surgical pathology of eyes and ocular adnexa. In Ackerman LV (ed): Surgical Pathology. St. Louis, CV Mosby, 1959

82. ZIMMERMAN LE: Squamous cell carcinoma and related lesions of the bulbar conjunctiva. In Boniuk M (ed): Ocular and Adnexal Tumors. St. Louis, CV Mosby, 1964

83. ZIMMERMAN LE: Changing concepts concerning the malignancy of ocular tumors. Arch Ophthalmol 78:166–173, 1967

84. ZIMMERMAN LE: Personal communication

2

EPITHELIAL TUMORS
OF THE UVEA

Tumors arising from the ocular tissues that stem embryologically from the optic vesicle are all neurogenous, although all do not have counterparts elsewhere in the nervous system. Figure 2–1 shows the optic vesicle divided into three sections representing anlagen of the epithelial elements of the choroid, ciliary body, and iris. We shall discuss here the tumors whose parent tissues have their anlage in A) the pigment epithelium of the retina, B) the pigment epithelium of the ciliary body, and iris. We shall discuss here the and E) the nonpigment layers of the ciliary body. Tumors arising from the anlage of the dilator and sphincter muscles of the iris C) are discussed in Chapter 9, Leiomyoma, and those arising from the anlage of the retina proper F) are discussed in Chapter 3, Retinoblastoma and Other Neuroectodermal Tumors of the Retina.

The pigment epithelium of the retina, ciliary body, and iris proliferates on slight provocation.[42] If sufficiently provoked by pathologic processes, the hyperplasia may take the form of large plaques of tissue with characteristics of either the mother epithelial cell or metaplastic fibrous tissue. For example, a woman who had recurrent attacks of iridocyclitis from childhood complained, after age 50, of steadily decreasing vision until she became blind within a few years. The left eye was enucleated because of severe pain (Fig. 2–2). This tendency for hyperplasia to take the form of large tumorlike plaques of tissue is apparent in microscopic sections of eyes with all kinds of pathologic conditions. It is largely responsible for repair by adhesions between the retina and the choroid after surgery for a detached retina. The hyperplastic pigment cells seem to account for all acquired pigment seen in the fundus.

In contrast, melanocytes of the choroid do not reproduce their kind if they are destroyed. Therefore, it can be said that all acquired nonneoplastic pigmentation (excluding hemosiderin) of the fundus comes from the pigment epithelial cells; it may be associated with choroidal tumors but more often follows inflammations and degenerative processes. Because this profuse proliferation occurs so readily, lesions caused by inflammation and degenerative processes frequently have a dark color which may make them difficult to distinguish clinically from melanomas. Inflammation may not only lead to proliferation of the pigment epithelium into plaques of tissue, but also make it take on active neoplastic charactistics leading to carcinoma.

The proliferative proclivity of the pigment epithelium is also observed in tissue cultures. When some pigment epithelium is inadvertently included in cultures of the normal choroid, growth is manifest in 48 hours and outstrips the growth of other tissues.[43]

A reactive epithelial hyperplasia and an epithelial neoplasia may be difficult to differentiate; even expert pathologists at times disagree on the diagnosis. Tumors may start as hyperplasias provoked by noxious stimuli, and then almost imperceptibly change until they eventually assume neoplastic or even malignant characteristics. A neoplasm may be considered an abnormal mass of tissue whose growth exceeds and is uncoordinated with that of normal tissue and persists after the cessation of the stimulus that evoked it. The hallmark of a neoplasm is persistent growth after withdrawal of this stimulus.

Epithelial tumors that arise in chronically inflamed eyes and in otherwise normal eyes seem to have the same cytologic picture: large epithelial cells with oval nuclei arranged in tubes and cords interspersed with eosin-staining homogeneous material—a cuticular product of the epithelium. They show local invasiveness but are not known to have metastasized or to have extended out of the scleral coat.

TUMORS OF THE RETINAL PIGMENT EPITHELIUM

The histologic distinction between epithelial neoplasms and inflammatory epithelial hyperplasia is often difficult; it has been suggested that such lesions be arranged on a graduated scale with obvious hyperplasias of inflammatory origin in which active inflammatory processes are dominant, at one extreme, and obvious epithelial neoplasms at the other extreme.[22] In between there would be many tissue formations showing a more even balance between histologically inflammatory and neoplastic elements.

In a review of 19 cases of tumors of the retinal pigment epithelium, 10 were benign and 9 malignant.[18] Malignant lesions were found more often in patients over 40. The malignancy in such cases was usually low grade and the prognosis favorable in the apparent absence of invasion beyond the choroid or lamina cribrosa at the time of enucleation.

A histopathologic study of 11 primary neoplasms of the retinal pigment epithelium was reported.[59] Heavily pigmented, large polyhedral cells containing intracellular vacuoles were demonstrated in an adenoma by electron microscopy.[17]

TUMORS OF THE NEUROEPITHELIUM OF THE CILIARY BODY

The ciliary body and its processes are covered by two layers of epithelium, the inner one usually nonpigmented and the outer one pigmented. There is justification for treating the two layers as one, however. In pathologic processes, as well as in normal eyes, the inner layer is sometimes pigmented and both layers participate in the same tumor. In a classical contribution to our understanding of neuroepithelial tumors of the ciliary body over 100 cases were reviewed.[64] The tumors were classified as follows:

Congenital
  Glioneuroma

  Medulloepithelioma (diktyoma) $\begin{cases} \text{benign} \\ \text{malignant} \end{cases}$

  Teratoid medulloepithelioma

  (diktyoma) $\begin{cases} \text{benign} \\ \text{malignant} \end{cases}$
Acquired
  Pseudoadenomatous hyperplasia
  Adenoma (benign epithelioma)
  Adenocarcinoma

Glioneuromas are congenital choristomatous malformations in which essentially mature glial and neuronal elements have re-

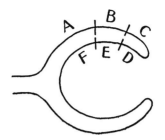

FIG. 2–1. The secondary optic vesicle showing anlagen of various structures. **A.** Pigment epithelium of the retina. **B.** Pigment epithelium of the ciliary body. **C.** Dilator and sphincter muscles of the iris. **D.** Pigment epithelium of the iris. **E.** Nonpigmented epithelium of the ciliary body. **F.** Retina.

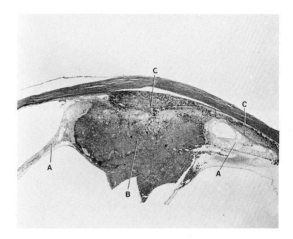

FIG. 2–2. Hyperplasia of the retinal pigment epithelium from an inflammatory process of childhood resulting in a large tumorlike mass. In a section from the left eye of a 56-year-old woman, the hyperplasia at points *C* still resembles the mother cells but at *B* becomes a large plaque of metaplastic fibrous tissue interspersed with pigment. Complete gliosis of the adherent retina is seen at points *A*. Some bone formation was noted in old scar tissue elsewhere in the eye. The cornea shows old degenerating scar tissue with calcium deposits. Peripheral anterior synechiae, occlusion of the pupil, and complete glaucomatous cupping of the disc were among other findings. Verhoeff and others who studied this section concurred in the diagnosis of a pure hyperplasia of the pigment epithelium into a tumorlike mass. (Courtesy of J. G. Johnstone and the Armed Forces Institute of Pathology.)

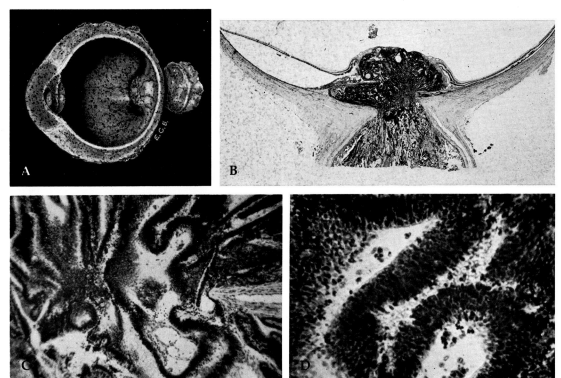

FIG. 2–3. Medulloepithelioma (diktyoma) of the optic nerve. **A.** Interior of the enucleated globe, after removal of a calotte, shows enlarged optic nerve. **B.** Cross section of the involved optic nerve. **C.** Characteristic structure resembling embryonic retina with a general pattern of the primary and secondary optic vesicles. **D.** Portion from the center of **B** under higher magnification.

placed portions of the iris and ciliary body that failed to develop normally. Instead, we find well-differentiated masses of tissue resembling brain. These tumors may accompany congenital colobomas of the iris and the ciliary body[29] as well as colobomas of the optic nerve. The malignant counterpart of this tumor is the spongioneuroblastoma.

MEDULLOEPITHELIOMAS (DIKTYOMAS)

Medulloepitheliomas (diktyomas) are embryonic tumors which usually originate in the ciliary epithelium (pars ciliaris retinae) and in rare instances in the optic nerve. A typical medulloepithelioma of the optic nerve in a 4½-year-old boy is shown in Figure 2–3. Findings were a drooping left upper lid,

marked swelling of the left disc, no light perception, and no proptosis. Four months later the swelling had progressed markedly, and there was a 1–2 mm exophthalmos. Death ensued from intracranial extension of the lesion.[41] A malignant teratoid medulloepithelioma of the optic nerve was described in a 6-year-old girl who showed no evidence of metastasis 18 months after exenteration and removal of the intracanalicular and intracranial portions of the nerve.[21]

In one reported case a tumor with numerous membranes and tubules of pigment epithelium was believed to represent abnormal differentiation of a medulloepithelioma into pigment epithelium of the inner layer of the secondary optic vesicle.[26] This seems quite possible since the pigment epithelium of the iris stems from the same layer. In another case[35] a medulloepithelioma in the posterior part of the eye of an 18-month-old girl showed malignant changes with infiltration of the retinal pigment epithelium, choroid, and sclera. The maldeveloped anterior ocular segment contained no tumor. Benign hamartomatous elements were intimately associated

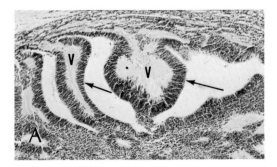
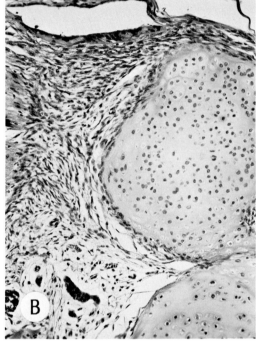
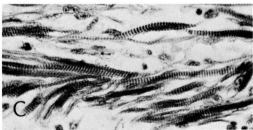

FIG. 2–4. Benign teratoid medulloepithelioma. **A.** Anlage of the retina containing primitive vitreous. **B.** Hyaline cartilage. **C.** Cytoplasmic cross-striations of skeletal muscle. (Courtesy of L. E. Zimmerman.[64])

with persistent hyperplastic primary vitreous.

Although this tumor characteristically simulates embryonic retina, it may grow as a solid mass of cells which include rosettes and thus resemble a retinoblastoma.

The teratoid type of medulloepithelioma has heteroplastic elements not usually observed in the eye, such as cartilage, bone, brain tissue, and skeletal muscle in addition to the medulloepitheliomatous components.[65]

Elements of a benign teratoid medulloepithelioma are shown in Figure 2–4.

The heteroplastic mesodermal elements of cartilage and skeletal muscle are possibly derived from the mesoderm which enters through a colobomatous defect in the medullary epithelium. Also, the heteroplastic teratoid tissue may possibly arise from the neuroectoderm itself, from which some embryologists suggest that heteroplastic mesodermal elements such as cartilage and skeletal muscle may stem.[55] They view the mesenchyme in a functional sense rather than as a genetic entity. This mesenchyme derived from various epithelia is referred to as mesectoderm.

The previous edition of this text reflected the prevailing view that medulloepitheliomas of the ciliary body were of two types: embryonal (diktyoma) and adult. This distinction was based on the incorrect premise that the medullary epithelium of the optic vesicle persists in an undifferentiated form as nonpigmented epithelium of the ciliary body and that an adult medulloepithelioma arises from this layer. What was formerly called an adult medulloepithelioma arising from this embryonal medullary epithelium is now viewed as an acquired adenoma or carcinoma[64] or as a benign or malignant epithelioma[5] arising from fully differentiated ciliary epithelium which has undergone neoplastic changes, often preceded by reactive hyperplasia.[64]

Medulloepithelioma may show elements resembling medullary epithelium, embryonic retina, primary vitreous, and neuroglia from the inner layer of the secondary optic vesicle, as well as various components of the outer layer of this vesicle, such as ciliary epithelium and retinal pigment epithelium. The tumor therefore presents a pattern of organoid epithelial structures in a mesenchymal stroma. The vitreous element can be demonstrated by the Alcian blue stain for acid mucopolysaccharide.[64]

FIG. 2–5. Diktyoma (congenital medulloepithelioma) of the ciliary body and iris. A mass in the right eye of a 2½-year-old boy had enlarged progressively since birth. **A.** The clinical appearance. **B.** Low-power view. (Courtesy of A. G. DeVoe.)

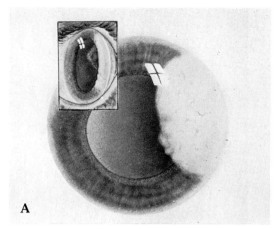

A

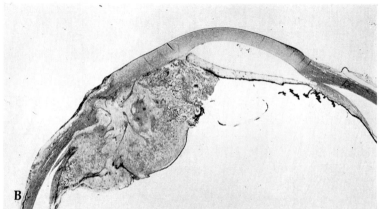

B

Clinical Course

A medulloepithelioma may grow as a localized tumor mass (Fig. 2–5), but more often it tends to form a simple covering of the visible affected structures or, when extending into cavities, to develop in a cystic or netlike arrangement. Relatively early in its growth this tumor, which usually lies on surfaces, may interfere with filtration, leading to glaucoma and subsequent buphthalmos. Eventually, however, tumor tissue penetrates the involved structures and follows its destructive course.

Age at Onset

A medulloepithelioma is usually detected in infancy or early childhood, but may be present at birth. Among our cases, ocular symptoms or signs were first noted at an average age of 3 years and 8 months. One patient was a newborn whose eye was carefully examined because of microphthalmos, and the oldest was age 9.

There is no fitting description of the clinical appearance. A medulloepithelioma may arise from the ciliary body or the iris or both, grow anteriorly, cover the lens surface and the posterior surface of the iris, and fill the anterior chamber, or it may grow posteriorly and form a large mass detaching the retina. Sometimes years elapse before it is diagnosed and the eye is removed. Enucleation is sometimes performed only after the patient develops extraocular extension or glaucoma.

In contrast to retinoblastoma, medulloepithelioma is never bilateral or multicentric, and there is no evidence of a hereditary factor.[11]

The tumor may occur in a microphthalmic eye, or the globe may become atrophic or phthisical and be removed with a diagnosis of uveitis. In one case a small undetected medulloepithelioma of the ciliary body ruptured the lens capsule, resulting in inflammation and second glaucoma which then dominated the clinical picture.[38]

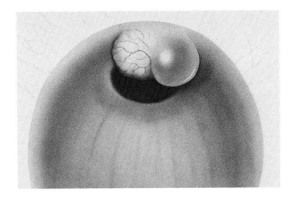

FIG. 2–6. Teratoid medulloepithelioma (diktyoma). This partly solid, partly cystic lesion extends through the pupil.

FIG. 2–7. Shrunken, calcified, dislocated lens back of the iris simulating a medulloepithelioma (diktyoma) of the ciliary body.

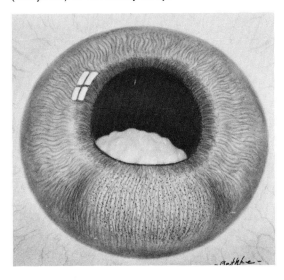

Differential Diagnosis

Since the tumor may occur in a somewhat microphthalmic eye and be present at birth, it is sometimes confused with congenital anomalies, particularly those related to remains of the hyaloid system. A medulloepithelioma in an 18-month-old girl, believed to have originated in a persistent rest of the primitive epithelium of Bergmeister's papilla, has been described.[35]

A medulloepithelioma must be suspected in any case of unilateral buphthalmos, especially if there appears to be a diffuse tumor or cystic tissue in the anterior chamber. Another cause for suspicion is any cystic formation in and around the anterior chamber (Fig. 2–6). A cyst that had become detached from the main tumor was seen floating in the anterior chamber in one instance.[53] A dislocated cataractous lens, especially when calcified, may be difficult to differentiate from medulloepithelioma (Fig. 2–7).

Prognosis

Although this tumor is malignant, its growth is usually slow. It may invade the surrounding structures including the sclera. In one case the patient's white pupil was noted at age 3, the tumor was diagnosed at age 10, but the eye was removed only when an extrabulbar mass appeared at age 19;[46] in another the tumor was suspected at birth and progressed in size but was not removed until the patient was 16 years old;[4] and in still another buphthalmos was apparent at birth but the eye was not removed until the child was 11 years old.[40]

Pathology

The tumor may grow as membranes comprising a single row of nuclei. A limiting membrane on the proximal border of the cells has been considered analogous to the external limiting membrane of the retina.[60] The single-cell membranes correspond to the nonpigmented layer of the ciliary epithelium. They sometimes grow forward as folds which on cross section appear as double rows of nuclei (Fig. 2–8). The various types of membranes and cell layers are folded, show invagination of varying degree, and become fused. Sectioned at various angles, they present quite a bizarre picture. However, they have one constant feature: the proximal surface of the tumor membrane is free while the distal surface borders on the connective tissue stroma. When the cell bands circumscribe a cavity or lumen, the proximal surface tends to face the lumen, which is either empty or filled with a coagulum and thus corresponds to the cavity of the primary optic vesicle. When occasionally the membranes fold in the opposite manner, the distal surface encloses the lumen. The lumen in these instances is filled either by fine fibrous tissue, by tissue resembling

FIG. 2–8. Medulloepithelioma (diktyoma) arising from the epithelium of the ciliary body. **A.** Low magnification. **B.** High magnification. (Courtesy of J. Meller.)

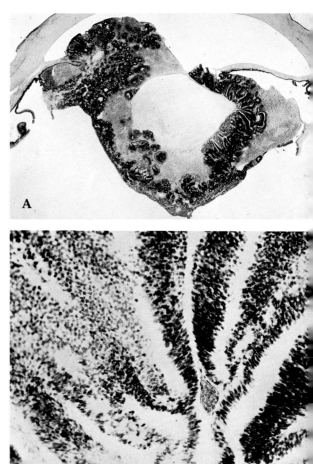

FIG. 2–9. Hyperplasia of the pigment epithelium into metaplastic fibrous tissue at the ora serrata. This patient had an old detachment of the retina.

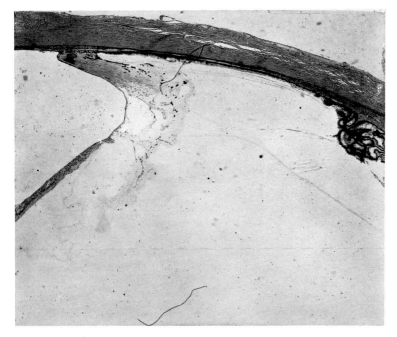

vitreous, or by blood vessels; it then corresponds to the cavity of the secondary optic cup filled with the anlage of vitreous.

Mitotic figures can be seen at the margin of the cell layers, which correspond to the outer surface of the inner layer of the optic vesicle. This margin often shows a fine membranous structure over which extend short blunt protoplasmic processes resembling rods and cones. These cell layers of cancerous tissue thus resemble the cross section of an embryonic retina before the nuclei in the individual layers have undergone differentiation. In the human embryo this differentiation occurs before the sixth week, shortly after invagination of the primary into the secondary optic vesicle.

Medulloepitheliomas have no stroma. In some places the remains of invaded tissue may act as the stroma, but no stromal element is discernible where the tumor grows along a surface. Its malignant nature is evident from the histologic features and its infiltrating and destructive characteristics.

Treatment

Treatment can range from enucleation of the eye to exenteration of the orbit and even more extensive surgery when contiguous structures are involved.

PSEUDOADENOMATOUS HYPERPLASIAS

Pseudoadenomatous hyperplasias usually develop after a long-standing inflammatory process, perhaps abetted by glaucoma or trauma, although some appear to be primary. Also, in eyes with an old detachment of the retina, a plaque of pigmented fibrous tissue (*Ringschweile*) may be seen at the ora serrata (Fig. 2–9). This represents a proliferation of the ciliary epithelium into metaplastic fibrous tissue, supposedly caused by the constant tug of the detached retina at the site where it adheres to the ciliary body.

True neoplasms occasionally develop from these epithelial hyperplasias. They may be benign (adenomas) or malignant (adenocarci-

FIG. 2–10. Medulloepithelioma (adult type) arising from the epithelium of the corona ciliaris. Section of the enucleated eye shows invasion and substantial replacement of the ciliary muscle and processes by the tumor. Its extension into the anterior chamber from the scleral spur *a* to *b* pushed forward the root of the iris, filling the filtration angle and forming two large thin-walled cysts *c* and *c'*. Small calcified areas are seen in the delicate stroma. The nonpigmented epithelium participated to some extent in the tumor growth, which was secondary to an inflammatory process from an old injury. (Courtesy of J. N. Dow and the Armed Forces Institute of Pathology.)

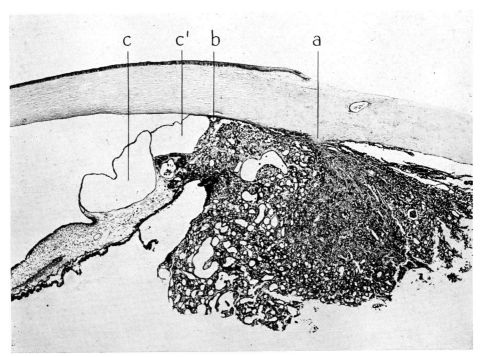

nomas). Either type usually develops in an eye that has suffered a severe exogenous or endogenous inflammation, as shown by such residual effects as organized inflammatory membranes. True neoplasms are often encountered in adults who have had a blind and atrophic eye since childhood. The fact that cells of the tumor may invade already-formed, organized fibrous tissue or bone is further evidence that the process was initiated by inflammation.

A medulloepithelioma of the adult type developed in a woman who had a penetrating injury of the right eye at age 16. Visual loss gradually became more marked until the eye became blind when she was 41. Four years later the severely painful eye was enucleated (Fig. 2–10).

Many instances of true tumors developing in the wake of old intraocular pathologic processes have been reported.

Some cases described as primary hyperplasias around the disc may actually be neoplasms.[28]

Malignant tumors of the retinal pigment epithelium have been produced experimentally.[1]

ADENOMAS (BENIGN EPITHELIOMAS)

These tumors usually produce no symptoms but are detected in the microscopic examination of eyes removed for other reasons (Fig.

2–11). Although they have been considered congenital, some authors view them as acquired.[62,64] They are usually round to oval with a maximal diameter of about 1 mm. They may be embedded in a ciliary process, sometimes near its apex, causing thickening so that it protrudes farther into the posterior chamber than is true with the other processes.

In structure, the lesion is characterized by invagination of both the nonpigmented and pigmented layers into the substance of the ciliary process. This results in an ampulla-shaped cavity with its hilus or orifice facing the surface of the ciliary process (Fig. 2–12). All membranous outgrowths of the nonpigmented epithelial layer, which fill the invaginated cavity, form an epithelial network. The network's interstices are filled not with the usual connective tissue characteristic of adenomas, but with a homogeneous eosin-staining material which is no doubt produced by the epithelium, although its exact nature is unknown. It does not give the characteristic staining reaction for mucus with the use of thionine and mucicarmine. The homogeneous substance in the retiform spaces of the epithelium can constitute an appreciable portion of the tumor, resembling extensive cystic degeneration. The pigmented epithelial layer surrounds the tumor but does not participate in its formation.

In one study 16 unsuspected ciliary body adenomas were found in 14 eye-bank eyes from 12 patients.[25]

A benign ciliary epithelioma cannot be considered an adenoma in the usual sense because the connective tissue stroma is not a

FIG. 2–11. Adenoma of the ciliary processes in an eye removed because of choroidal malignant melanoma. The hilus is seen at *a*.

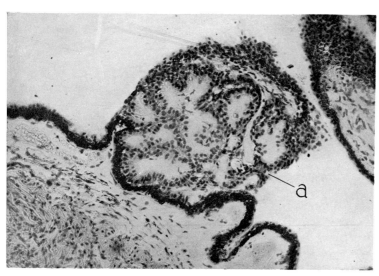

part of its structure. In both tumors, the epithelium itself grows into the surrounding tissue. In a true adenoma, however, the epithelial cells surround a lumen, whereas in this tumor the epithelium projects from the surface like papillomas except that no connective tissue is formed. Actually, the term *benign epithelioma of the ciliary body* is preferable to *adenoma*, which is commonly employed.

A benign epithelioma near the optic disc, comparable with those usually seen in the ciliary body, has been described.[63]

MALIGNANT EPITHELIOMAS

Adenocarcinomas are usually detected when they expand sufficiently to press on the equator of the lens and produce a cataract. Such a tumor was found near the ciliary body in a 20-year-old man who complained of blurred vision (Fig. 2–13.) In other instances adenocarcinomas infiltrate the root of the iris and are detected because of secondary iris changes.

A 63-year-old man had noted failing vision in the left eye for three years. Examination revealed a dense cataract and a dark mass near the ciliary body which pushed the iris forward (Fig. 2–14, see p. 7). These neoplasms may also manifest themselves by pushing the root of the iris forward against the cornea, sometimes producing secondary glaucoma. They may be mistaken for primary malignant melanomas of the iris. Their malig-

FIG. 2–12. Adenoma of the ciliary body. The otherwise normal eye was removed because a basal-cell epithelioma of the lid had extended into the orbit. **A.** The hilus is seen at *a*. **B.** Area indicated as *a* under higher magnification.

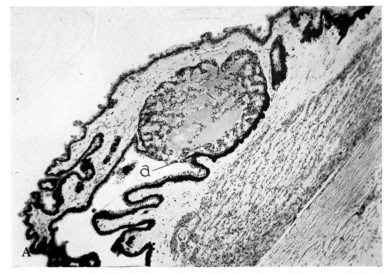

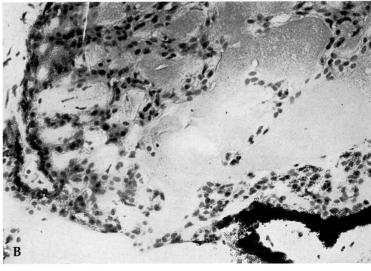

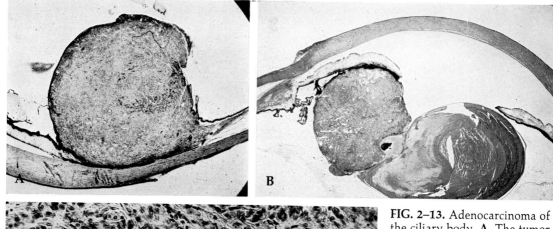

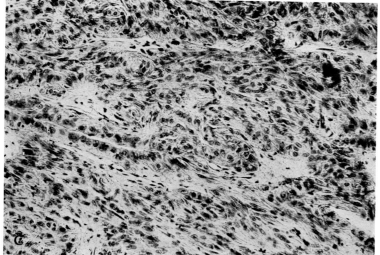

FIG. 2–13. Adenocarcinoma of the ciliary body. **A.** The tumor has two ciliary processes on the right. **B.** Pressure on the lens is evident when the tumor is cut. **C.** Structure of the tumor under higher magnification. (Courtesy of J. A. C. Wadsworth.[62])

nant tendency seems to be confined to the eyes; they expand and infiltrate adjacent tissues but do not spread distally.

These tumors certainly develop either from an adenoma or as the sequela of an old or recent inflammation.[24,56,62] Histologically, they appear as localized masses with the general structure of adenomas except for their tissue dedifferentiation and invasive properties (Fig. 2–13).

TUMORS OF THE PIGMENT EPITHELIUM OF THE IRIS

The nonpigmented epithelium of the ciliary body is continued onto the iris as the pigment epithelium. Medulloepitheliomas as well as benign and malignant tumors composed of pigment epithelium may arise from this layer alone in the iris (Figs. 2–15, 2–16). The pigment epithelium of the ciliary body is continued onto the iris as smooth muscle, which may give rise to conditions ranging from leiomyomas to frank pigment epithelium. Often the same tumor shows all these cytologic variations. Some authors have even questioned whether a true leiomyoma could arise from this neurogenous smooth muscle, as they believe most if not all such tumors are neurinomas.[8]

A number of cases of benign epithelioma of the iris have been reported (Fig. 2–17). This is the counterpart of benign epithelioma (adenoma) of the ciliary body.

Although these tumors lack stroma, they are permeated by blood vessels that stem from the adjacent iris stroma (Fig. 2–18). They are particularly likely to occur in the sphincter region of the iris where the so-called pigment spurs are found. These spurs have a predilection for the periphery of the

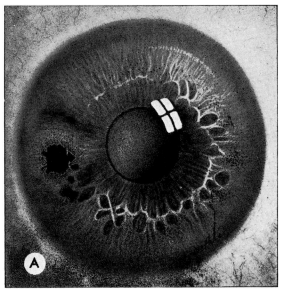

FIG. 2–15. Benign melanoma of the iris arising from the pigment epithelium. A pigmented lesion was noted in the left eye of a 55-year-old woman during a routine examination. **A.** The velvety black pigment on the anterior surface was only the "tip of the iceberg," the major part of the lesion being submerged in the stroma. Pigment dust, representing migrant pigment epithelial or clump cells, dots the surface near the collarette as well as at the tumor site. **B.** Low-power view of a section through the tumor. **C.** Blanched section. **D.** High-power view of the portion outlined in **C.**

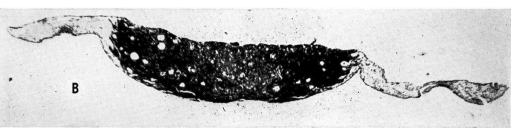

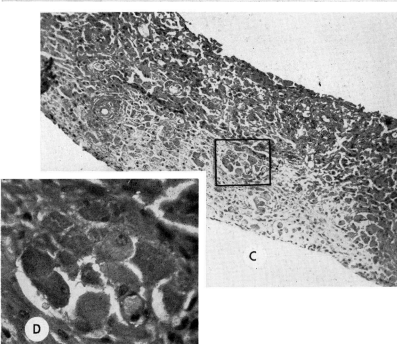

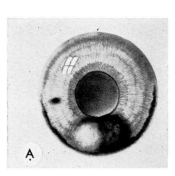
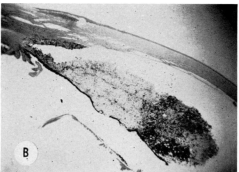

FIG. 2–16. Carcinoma of the pigment epithelium of the iris. A 65-year-old man consulted an ophthalmologist one week after noting a spot in the right eye. **A.** The black elevated mass with a grayish center, diagnosed as malignant melanoma of the iris, was excised. The patient died eight months later of generalized carcinomatosis. Study of lung, liver, and spleen sections obtained at autopsy revealed carcinoma probably primary in the lung and unrelated to the eye lesion. The type of growth and some of the iris tissue cultures indicated origin in the pigment epithelium. **B.** Low-power view of section through the tumor.

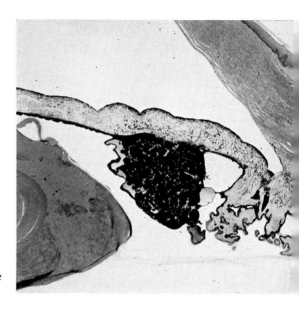

FIG. 2–17. Adenoma of the pigment epithelium of the iris. A small black tumor arising from the posterior surface of the iris was noted in a 60-year-old woman. The lens was opaque over the tumor site. Microscopy revealed no blood vessels in the tumor and very little connective tissue stroma. Cells in depigmented sections resembled those of the pigment epithelium of the iris. (Courtesy of V. Morax.[33])

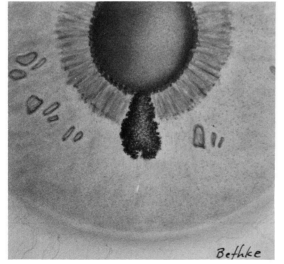

FIG. 2–18. Adenoma of the pigment epithelium of the iris. The tumor has a papillomatous or mulberry appearance. It is continuous with the normal pigment epithelium on the posterior surface (partially desquamated during preparation of the sections). Blood vessels course through the tumor but no actual stroma is apparent. Some hyaloid material (cuticular product) is consistent with most lesions of the pigment epithelium. Bleached sections showed the tumor cells to be epithelium in an adenomatous arrangement.

sphincter muscle. At times they represent actual invagination of the pigment epithelium into the stroma. Some authorities consider pigment disturbances such as spurs and invagination to be the source of benign epitheliomas. The pupillary margin is another preferred site for benign epitheliomas of the iris pigment epithelium. They are localized, heavily pigmented, and have convoluted surfaces (Fig. 2–19, see p. 7). Such localized black nodules are normally seen at the upper and lower borders of the oval pupils of *Ungulata*, particularly the horse, where they are referred to as *corpora nigra*. In the human eye they may be atavistic or develop where pigment has proliferated owing to imperfect closure of the fetal cleft.

Because these tumors are certainly benign they are examined microscopically only occasionally, when removed during an iridectomy for cataract extraction. The fact that pigment epithelium secretes a cuticular product accounted for hyaloid deposits in one case.[3] In another case[51] the specimen was included in an iridectomy; there were blood vessels and some hyaloid material but no stroma.

I know of no unequivocal case of malignant epithelioma of the iris comparable with the lesion seen in the ciliary body. However, typical tumors belonging to this group arise in the region between the ciliary body and the iris, involving both structures about equally. These tumors probably arose from a benign epithelioma of the ciliary body and extended secondarily to the iris.

In two reported cases primary neoplasms of the pigment epithelium of the iris were mistaken for malignant melanomas of the ciliary body.[34] One of the lesions was associated with hyperplasia of the pigment epithelium of the pupillary margin of both eyes. The criteria for a medulloepithelioma arising from the iris pigment epithelium, a counterpart of medulloepithelium of the ciliary body, have long been known. Another tumor that may belong to this group[52] showed areas of cells resembling a retinoblastoma. A glioneuroma was found arising from the margin of a congenital coloboma of the iris and ciliary body in a newborn infant.[47]

Since the pigment epithelium of the ciliary body is continued onto the iris as the dilator and sphincter muscle layer, tumors arising in this layer will be discussed in Chapter 9, Leimoyoma. However, certain rare iris tumors contain elements resembling smooth muscle, neuroepithelium, and pigment epithelium. Iris tumors arising from the pigment epithelial layer may therefore contain areas resembling a leiomyoma or a neuroepithelioma (retinoblastoma, medulloepithelioma), alone or in combination.

The author of a treatise on iris tumors[48] believed that 3 of his 11 cases had originated in elements of the pigment epithelial layer but had differentiated sufficiently to show their neurogenous nature and belonged either to the retinoblastoma or to the leiomyoma group.

In some of our cultures of iris melanomas[43] cells were noted with characteristics between those of pigment epithelium and smooth muscle.

One type of benign melanoma of the iris pigment epithelium has unusual clinical features. Most of the tumor cells are embedded in the stroma of the iris, with only a small part of the black tumor visible on the anterior surface (Fig. 2–15). To my knowledge, this iceberg type of iris melanoma is entirely benign. In fact, it may be another instance of a lesion of the pigment epithelium that lies in the border between hyperplasia and neoplasia. No history or sign of inflammation, glaucoma, or trauma has been found associated with these tumors. The involved iris may show an unusual number of clump cells appearing as pigment dust, especially in the region of the collarette (Fig. 2–15), or freckles composed of pigment epithelium may be present.

Adenocarcinomas may also arise in the pigment epithelium of the iris (Fig. 2–16).

HYPERPLASIAS OF THE RETINAL PIGMENT EPITHELIUM

Congenital hyperplasias (benign melanomas) of the retinal pigment epithelium are unilateral, isolated, flat, dark gray to black, and sharply demarcated. The lesions are irregularly round or oval, and of 1 to 3 disc diameters. Such a lesion, discovered incidentally during the fundal examination in a 61-year-old woman,[43] is shown in Figure 2–20. The normal retinal vessels usually course over the lesion undisturbed but are at times sheathed or actually surrounded by some pigment which extends along and around the perivascular spaces. Small nonpigmented foci with rather sharp borders are occasionally seen. The lesion has no growth potential, and no field defects can be elicited. The involved eye

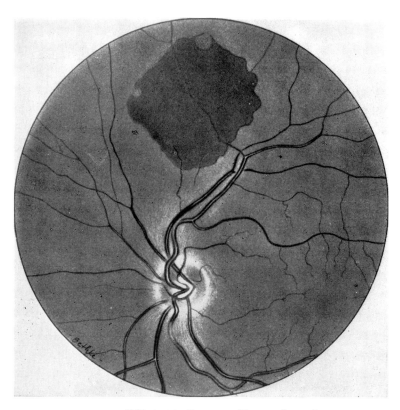

FIG. 2–20. Congenital hyperplasia (benign melanoma) of the retinal pigment epithelium. The flat, irregularly square lesion of 3 dd is dark gray. Two pigmented lacunae are seen around the sharp border. Retinal vessels cross undisturbed. (A. B. Reese and I. S. Jones.[44])

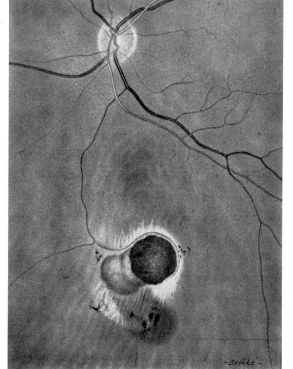

FIG. 2–21. Postinflammatory hyperplasia of the pigment epithelium. A markedly elevated black stalk of tissue below the disc protrudes so far forward into the vitreous that it casts a shadow from the ophthalmoscope light. An old area of inactive choroiditis lies around this focus of proliferated epithelium. This case is interpreted as hyperplasia of the pigment epithelium secondary to a choroiditis. (Courtesy of Max Fratkin.)

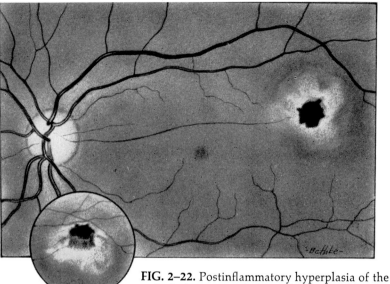

FIG. 2–22. Postinflammatory hyperplasia of the retinal pigment epithelium. A 30-year-old woman, treated six years earlier for an inflammation in the fundus of the left eye, showed a jet-black mass between 2 and 3 o'clock at the equator of the fundus. The stalk of tissue protrudes far forward into the vitreous, the flat base has an atrophic area, and some pigment proliferation has resulted from an old inactive choroiditis. Inset indicates height of lesion. This case is interpreted as a massive hyperplasia of the pigment epithelium. (Courtesy of William Roth.)

seems otherwise comparable with the normal fellow eye. There are no foci elsewhere in the fundus suggesting choroiditis or any other pathologic process.

The most common site for primary hyperplasia of the retinal pigment epithelium is around the disc, usually in young people. Since clinical progress may be manifest without active tumor growth, it is at times considered a progressive tumor and incorrectly diagnosed as melanoma, melanocytoma, glioma, angiomatosis, or choroidal hemangioma, leading to enucleation of the eye. Histologically, the lesion appears as a reticular proliferation of the pigment epithelium at the margin of the disc. Sometimes the pigment content is minimal or clinically unrecognized; in such instances the eye has been enucleated because of a suspected retinoblastoma or a glioma of the optic nerve.[7,54]

Among other conditions that must be considered in the differential diagnosis are melanocytoma of the disc, peripapillary choroidal hemangioma, and inflammation. Excrescences or masses laid down by pigment epithelium seem to account for some of the bizarre filigree patterns leading to an incorrect diagnosis. These confusing clinical vagaries seem to be related to the hyalin cuticular product of the pigment epithelium.

Histologic examination establishes the diagnosis as hyperplasia of the pigment epi-

thelium. In the choroid, under the hyperplastic epithelium, the melanocytes appear more pigmented than elsewhere but seem to be neither abnormal nor especially abundant.

Primary hyperplasias of the pigment epithelium may occur with no apparent provocation for the proliferation. The postinflammatory proliferation may produce an elevated dark mass which is rarely uniform but tends to be either accentuated at the periphery or mottled. Other postinflammatory sequelae are frequently noted elsewhere in the same fundus or that of the fellow eye.

Any noxious stimulus in the choroid may provoke a proliferative reaction in the overlying pigment epithelium. This may be due to inflammation such as choroiditis or uveitis, or induced by trauma such as surgery or diathermy for detached retina. When such hyperplasias assume tumor proportions, the question of a malignant melanoma arises (Figs. 2–21, 2–22). The pigmented mass is characteristically jet black; it extends into the vitreous abruptly with very little base, around which some atrophic and pigment changes are usually noted, particularly after a choroiditis.

A choroidal melanoma, especially if necrotic, may incite sufficient pigment proliferation to disguise the lesion. Also, macular degeneration of the disciform type may have a large element of pigment proliferation, lending a dark color and the clinical appearance of a melanoma.

An analysis of 16 cases arising from the retinal pigment epithelium, from our files and the literature, revealed 7 that occurred around the disc, seeming to indicate a predilection for the juxtapapillary area. In cases I have encountered the lesion appeared as an elevated localized mass on or around the disc (Fig. 2–23). Only in recent years has this juxtapapillary lesion been appreciated. Four reported cases of proliferation of the juxtapapillary retinal pigment epithelium simulating malignant melanoma of the nerve head[61] were all characterized by disturbance in and near the disc, slight elevation of the affected tissues but no definite tumefaction, fine retinal folds radiating from the lesion to the macula, a stationary or slowly progressive course, and enlargement of the blind spot with deterioration of vision.

A case of primary hyperplasia of the retinal pigment epithelium was characterized by juxtapapillary growth and clinical progression without true malignancy or metastasis, a type believed to occur principally in young people.[31] A peripapillary tumor arising from the retinal pigment epithelium had histologic features resembling those found in both adenocarcinomas and reactive hyperplasias arising there.[20] Other juxtapapillary cases have been reported.[6,11,44,45,58] In one instance the lesion was located away from the disc.[14]

HYPERPLASIAS OF THE EPITHELIUM OF THE CILIARY BODY

Acquired hyperplasias of the epithelium of the ciliary body occur in response to an inflammatory process or trauma (Fig. 2–24), and as in the retina, the resulting plaques may attain a considerable size. I have never encountered any large enough to be confused with a neoplasm.

Congenital hyperplasias of the epithelium of the ciliary body no doubt occur, but I have not recognized the condition clinically and do not know if it has ever been detected microscopically.

HYPERPLASIAS OF THE PIGMENT EPITHELIUM OF THE IRIS

The rather large excrescences occasionally seen in the pigment epithelium around the pupillary margin may become detached and lie on the iris surface in the lower part of the filtration angle. Such an implant may increase in size and simulate a melanoma. Also, in a congenital coloboma of the iris, the pigment epithelium may form large excrescences at the margin of the lesion and even partially or entirely fill the colobomatous area.

A 58-year-old man had an elevated black nodule on the iris of the left eye. Examination revealed apparently noncystic pigment excrescences in both eyes, which were otherwise normal (Fig. 2–25). The patient had no history of trauma or use of local eye medications.

Acquired hyperplasias commonly develop following inflammation of the iris, with the pigment epithelium in some cases extending onto the anterior lens capsule. The pigment epithelium may also proliferate across the entire pupillary area after an uneventful cataract extraction—intracapsular[39] or extracapsular,[10] even one with the usual postoperative reaction. Vision may be sufficiently reduced to warrant a discission operation. The

FIG. 2–23. Primary hyperplasia of the retinal pigment epithelium. Adjacent to the disc in an otherwise normal eye, the lesion showed extensive drusenlike material produced by the epithelium, simulating a malignant melanoma. (Courtesy of James W. May.)

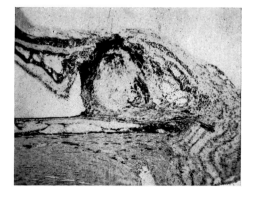

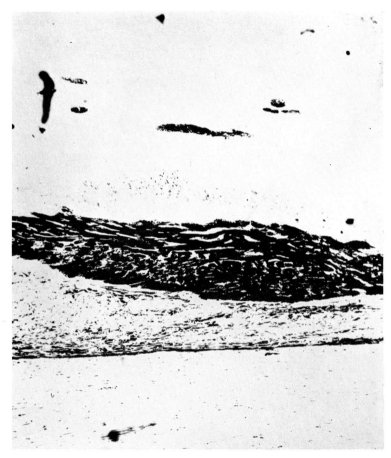

FIG. 2–24. Hyperplasia of the epithelium of the ciliary body. The eye was removed because of secondary glaucoma following an old perforating injury.

FIG. 2–25. Pigment excrescences around the pupillary margins of the iris in both eyes. In a 58-year-old man one of these excrescences (interpreted as atavistic remains) had become dislodged and implanted at the periphery of the iris of the left eye where it proliferated, leading to an ophthalmologic examination.

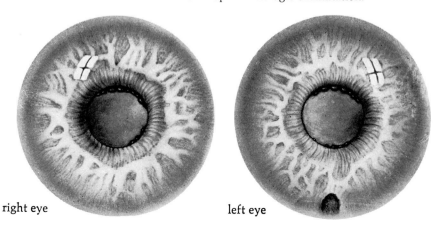

right eye   left eye

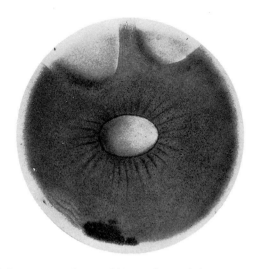

FIG. 2–26. Seeding and hyperplasia of the pigment epithelium following surgery. A patient who had two operations for primary glaucoma showed some seeding of the pigment epithelium on the anterior surface of the iris. The epithelium had proliferated, forming a black plaque from 6 to 7 o'clock.

FIG. 2–27. Hyperplasia of the pigment epithelium of the iris. Proliferation of the pigment epithelium at the pupillary margin, following prolonged use of diisopropyl fluorophosphate (DFP), was mistaken for malignant melanoma and the eye was enucleated. (Courtesy of L. Christensen.[12])

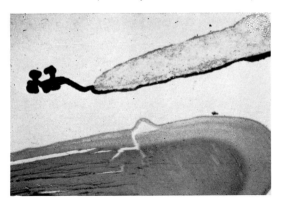

pupillary area in a reported case[10] was so black that a melanoma was suspected. Flecks of pigment epithelium abraded during cataract extraction may lodge on the posterior surface of the cornea and proliferate to the extent that vision is seriously impaired. Moreover, such flecks may lodge on the anterior surface of the iris after surgery and proliferate, simulating a melanoma (Fig. 2–26).

In some instances excrescences of the pigment epithelium are quite marked around the pupillary margin after the use of strong miotics, particularly anticholinesterases. Secondary cystic changes may accompany the proliferation. In a reported case[12] marked proliferation and cystic changes in a child treated with diisopropylfluorophosphate (DFP) led to a diagnosis of iris melanoma and enucleation of the eye (Fig. 2–27). In other cases[57] a nodule was seeded on the iris surface, and a free nodule was deposited in the lower portion of the angle where it enlarged.

In addition to the hyperplasias which either accompany or are secondary to various conditions, there may be primary hyperplasias. Pigmented epithelial cells may migrate into the iris stroma as clump cells in the region of the sphincter muscle. There are instances where, in an otherwise normal eye, pigment epithelial cells migrate to the anterior surface of the iris and proliferate sufficiently to produce a melanotic spot resembling a true melanoma. These lesions have the velvety black appearance of the pigment epithelium normally seen around the pupillary margin, whereas most melanomas and the usual freckles, which are due to thickening of the anterior limiting layer of the iris, are light brown.

In one of several cases I have encountered, an area was large enough to be noted by the patient. This 35-year-old woman had been aware of a black spot on the iris of the right eye for some time. She insisted that the spot be removed because her father had had a malignant melanoma of the iris and ciliary body, requiring enucleation. An iridectomy ruled out a true growing melanoma of the iris. Microscopic sections revealed pigment epithelium traceable by a tract of epithelial cells to the posterior pigmented epithelial layer. The clinical diagnosis of benign hyperplasia of the pigment epithelium was confirmed histologically (Fig. 2–28). Similar cases were mentioned by others.[30,57]

CYSTS OF THE EPITHELIUM OF THE RETINA, CILIARY BODY, AND IRIS

RETINA

To my knowledge no cases have been reported of cysts of the retinal pigment epithelium, unless the blood cysts or hematomas occurring in the macular region may be classified as such. These hematomas constitute an important group because they at first closely resemble melanomas, and the patient usually consults an ophthalmologist because of sudden visual loss. The lesion develops at the posterior pole but not necessarily in the macula proper. It may be in the extramacular region or even nasal to the disc. The only feature not consistent with a melanoma is some degree of hemorrhage at the periphery. Histologically, this hemorrhage, which is under the pigment epithelium, seems to come from a thin vascular layer which, for some unknown reason, is interposed between the pigment epithelium and the lamina vitrea. Many eyes with such hematomas have been removed because of a mistaken diagnosis of malignant melanoma. Within weeks the hemorrhage dominates the clinical picture, and the true nature of the condition can be more readily perceived.

CILIARY BODY

Single or multiple intraepithelial cysts are frequently noted in the ciliary body. Such multiple cysts are commonly found in cases of multiple myeloma.[49] When small they are usually undetected or merely noted in a routine microscopic examination of the globe and are clinically unimportant. When large they may resemble melanomas of the ciliary body and iris. The inferior temporal quadrant is the preferred site.[13,19]

In a routine microscopic examination of eyes removed for various reasons, single or multiple globular cysts may be found in the valleys between the ciliary processes (Fig. 2–29). They arise mainly from the anterior portion of the corona ciliaris at the base of the iris; the wall is composed partly of nonpigmented and partly of pigmented layers of the ciliary epithelium. The cysts therefore represent a localized separation of the two epithelial layers and are actually pseudocysts.

The cysts are filled with a clear fluid, most of which is evacuated when the microscopic section is prepared. They are not necessarily

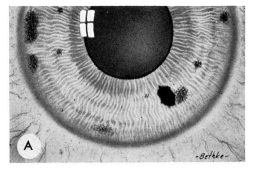

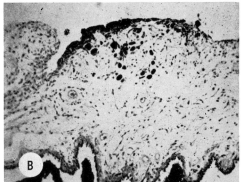

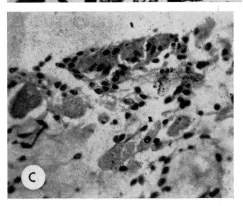

FIG. 2–28. Hyperplasia of the pigment epithelium of the iris. **A.** A flat plaque of proliferated pigment epithelium on the anterior surface of the iris in an otherwise normal eye simulated a true melanoma. **B.** Low-power view showing the accumulation and proliferation of pigment epithelial cells on the anterior surface and an aggregate in the adjacent stroma. **C.** Depigmented section showing the cells to be pigment epithelium.

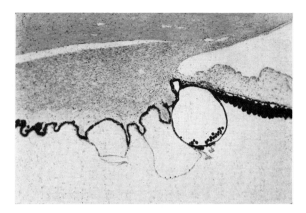

FIG. 2–29. Multiple intraepithelial cysts of the ciliary body and iris. The cyst at the base of the iris contained free pigment epithelial cells. This type probably sometimes becomes detached and lies free in the anterior chamber or vitreous.

confined to the corona ciliaris but may involve the same epithelial layers over the periphery of the iris and over the pars plana of the ciliary body. When in the former location, the entire epithelial wall is pigmented; when in the latter location, the cysts are flat instead of globular and the inner layer is nonpigmented. The incidence of these cysts cannot be estimated, but modified forms are frequently encountered in histologic sections.

The internal and external layers of the secondary optic vesicle are not united but lie in apposition. In the postnatal eye the structures derived from the internal layer also lie in apposition to those derived from the external layer. In the posterior portion of the eye, an actual separation of the two layers represents a detachment of the retina. In the region of the iris and ciliary body the two layers are not united, and their separation is referred to as an intraepithelial cyst.

Small ciliary body cysts have no clinical significance, but large lesions may manifest themselves in several ways. The periphery of the iris is at times pushed forward, which causes bulging of the iris stroma and a distinct localized narrowing or obliteration of the angle. This process may even obstruct the filtration angle enough to produce glaucoma. The cyst may push the anterior surface of the iris against the posterior surface of the cornea. In this case the resulting friction at times incites proliferation and pigment changes that make the lesion resemble a melanoma. This explanation would seem to

apply to a reported case of melanoma of the ciliary body and iris[32] in which there was a difference of opinion about the diagnosis. After studying the sections I believe it was primarily a cyst of the ciliary body with secondary iris changes. In rare instances, the cyst wall extends through the periphery of the iris and can be seen in the anterior chamber.

When the cyst arises from its usual site in the corona ciliaris, it has a smooth surface and a dark color due chiefly to its inaccessibility; it transilluminates and may be tremulous. If it indents the lens, secondary localized cataractous changes may be observed. A bright focal light thrown on the cyst may penetrate it sufficiently to elicit a reddish reflex from the underlying uvea. Also, magnified ciliary processes may be identified posterior to the cyst. Because of the clear fluid content and lack of pigment in the epithelium composing the inner wall, transillumination may have a refractive quality which accentuates the cyst—a sharp contrast to the transillumination picture of a melanoma. The advantage of studying these cysts with the gonioscope has been stressed.[50] I have followed an intraepithelial cyst of the ciliary body which finally ruptured spontaneously.

In most of our cases there was no appreciable enlargement of the cysts over a period of years. They are usually considered significant only because of possible confusion with neoplasms or because very rarely they produce glaucoma.

Authors who reviewed intraepithelial cysts of the pars plana of the ciliary body found at autopsy in 53 patients[2] considered them helpful in interpreting abnormalities at the periphery of the fundus, but found no evidence that they cause complications. A free-floating cyst in the vitreous, presumably intraepithelial and originating in the pars plana of the ciliary body, has been reported.[23]

IRIS

The iris cysts that mainly concern us are the intraepithelial type which may be mistaken for melanomas. These cysts represent an incomplete obliteration or reestablishment of the space between the two layers of the secondary optic vesicle. The same layers separate to produce intraepithelial cysts in the ciliary body. In the iris the outer layer of the cyst is composed of pigment epithelium, while in the ciliary body it is composed of

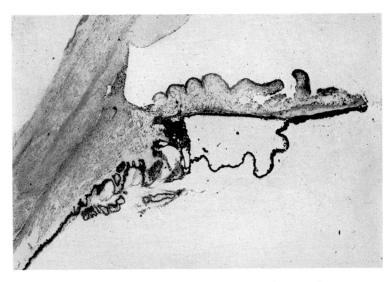

FIG. 2–31. Intraepithelial cyst of the iris. This cyst simulated a melanoma, leading to enucleation. (Courtesy of J. Mandelbaum.)

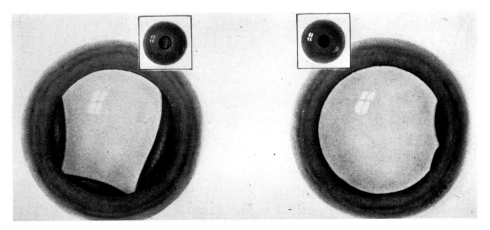

FIG. 2–32. Bilateral multiple intraepithelial cysts of the iris. Right eye: In the normally contracted iris (inset) a cyst is barely seen nasally, but three cysts are manifested with the pupil dilated. Left eye: In the normally contracted iris (inset) no cysts are seen, but two cysts are manifested temporally with the pupil dilated. (Courtesy of A. Callahan.)

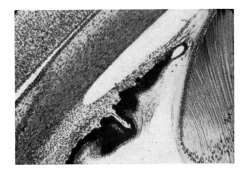

FIG. 2–33. Ring sinus cyst of the iris in a 70 mm human fetus (Courtesy of G. K. Smelser.)

nonpigmented epithelium. Therefore, such cysts in the iris have a black surface and do not transilluminate.

A cyst in the peripheral portion of the iris usually pushes the anterior surface of the iris forward, producing a localized globular protrusion occasionally with pigment changes in the overlying stroma due to migration of pigmented epithelial cells (Fig. 2–30, see p. 8). In other cases the cyst extends through the iris periphery into the anterior chamber.[15,19] When the cyst is more centrally located, the iris may not bulge forward; the cyst then appears as a black globular mass behind the iris (Fig. 2–31). The cyst is more or less concealed by a pupil in its natural or contracted state, but in a dilated pupil it everts and appears much more prominent in the pupillary area (Fig. 2–32).

Such an iris cyst may not be detected in the normal or contracted state of the pupil, or it may be seen only at one site on the pupillary margin. But in the dilated pupil this site becomes more visible, and several other small cysts are at times noted in the same eye or in both eyes (Fig. 2–32). These iris cysts are often confused with iris melanomas because they are black and do not transilluminate. Important features in the differential diagnosis are that the cysts evert when the pupil is dilated; they are usually multiple, not only in the same eye but also in the fellow eye; they do not splint the iris in dilatation; and they do not push the overlying iris stroma forward or produce secondary changes in it.

Intraepithelial cysts may become detached and settle at the pupillary margin. They are probably vestiges of the marginal ring sinus of Szily (Figs. 2–33, 2–34, 2–35). Such a cyst may arise in the anterior chamber, leading to suspicion of a tumor (Fig. 2–36), or it may originate in elongated strands of iris pigment epithelium at the root of the iris posteriorly or from a medulloepithelioma of the ciliary body. In some instances it reaches the vitreous through the base of the iris where there is no hyaloid membrane. It can be seen by ophthalmoscopy, and here too a tumor may be suspected (Fig. 2–29). When an intraepithelial cyst enlarges sufficiently to threaten the patient's vision, it should be removed.[9] In a reported case the cyst arose from the iris pigment epithelium.[16]

Another type of iris cyst which is less frequently mistaken for a tumor is the congenital nonpigmented stromal cyst.[36] It is lined with neuroepithelium which comes from mis-

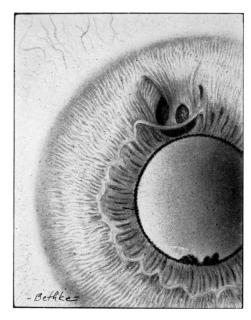

FIG. 2–34. Ring sinus cysts of the iris. Cyst at 12 o'clock transmitted light; there were two similar cysts at 6 o'clock.

FIG. 2–35. Ring sinus cyst of the iris. A 21-year-old man had noted a dark-brown spot on the left iris for some time which proved to be a globular cyst moored to the iris nasally at the pupillary margin. Inset: Slit-lamp beam passes through the cyst.

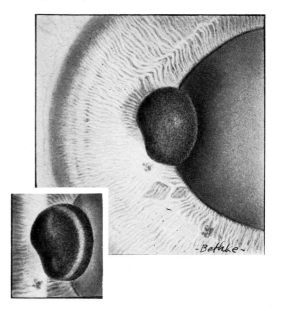

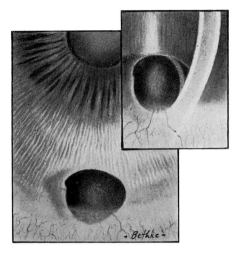

FIG. 2–36. Cyst of the pigment epithelium free in the anterior chamber. The cyst, which was in the lower portion of the chamber, moved with head movements. Inset: Slit-lamp beam passes through the cyst.

placed islands of surface ectoderm. This tissue is thought to be unused neuroectoderm—left over from the differentiation of iris muscles.[27] These stromal cysts in infants may regress spontaneously or be excised. However, in some instances glaucoma, spontaneous rupture, or an incorrect diagnosis of tumor leads to enucleation of the eye.[37]

REFERENCES

1. ALBERT DM, Ts'o MOM, RABSON AS: Experimental malignant tumors from retinal pigment epithelium. Arch Ophthalmol 88:70–74, 1972
2. ALLEN RA, STRAATSMA BR: Cysts of the posterior ciliary body (pars plana). Arch Ophthalmol 66: 302–313, 1961
3. ANARGYROS E: Melanom der Iris. Arch Augenheilkd 46:62–66, 1903
4. ANDERSEN SR: Medulloepitheliomas, diktyoma, and malignant epithelioma of the ciliary body. Acta Ophthalmol 26:313–330, 1948
5. ANDERSEN SR: Differentiation features in some retinal tumors and in dysplastic retinal conditions. Am J Ophthalmol 71:231–241, 1971
6. BEC P: Tumeurs papillaires développées aux dépens de l'epithélium pigmentaire de la rétine. Bull Soc Ophtalmol Fr 67:423–434, 1967
7. BLODI FC, REULING FH, SORNSON ET: Pseudomelanocytoma at the optic nervehead; an adenoma of the retinal pigment epithelium. Arch Ophthalmol 73:353–355, 1965
8. BÖKE W: Zur kenntnis der gutartigen Iristumoren. Graefes Arch Klin Ophthalmol 157:368–379, 1956
9. BROWNING CW, SWAN KC: Experiences with some tumors of the iris. Trans Pac Coast Otoophthalmol Soc 29:107–132, 1948
10. BRUECKNER A: Pigment-Nachstar. Klin Monatsbl Augenheilkd 27:461–463, 1919
11. CARDELL BS, STARBUCK MJ: Diktyoma. Br J Ophthalmol 43:217–224, 1959
12. CHRISTENSEN L: The histopathology of iris changes induced by miotics. Arch Ophthalmol 55:666–671, 1956
13. DAVIDSON SI: Spontaneous cysts of ciliary body. Br J Ophthalmol 44:461–466, 1960
14. DUKE JR, MAUMENEE AE: An unusual tumor of the retinal pigment epithelium. Am J Ophthalmol 47:311–317, 1959
15. ELSCHNIG H: Ziliarkörperzyste. Klin Monatsbl Augenheilkd 74:476–483, 1925
16. FINE BS: Free-floating pigmented cyst in the anterior chamber; a clinicohistopathologic report. Am J Ophthalmol 67:493–500, 1969
17. FONT RL, ZIMMERMAN LE, FINE BS: Adenoma of the retinal pigment epithelium; histochemical and electron microscopic observations. Am J Ophthalmol 73:544–554, 1972
18. GARNER A: Tumors of the retinal pigment epithelium. Br J Ophthalmol 54:715–723, 1970
19. GARRON LK: Cysts of the iris. ciliary body, and retina that simulate malignant melanoma with retinal detachment. Trans Pac Coast Otoophthalmol Soc 34:125–136, 1953
20. GRAHAM GC: Juxtapapillary retinal pigment tumor. Arch Ophthalmol 85:299–301, 1971
21. GREEN WR, ILIFF WJ, TROTTER RR: Malignant teratoid medulloepithelioma of the optic nerve. Arch Ophthalmol 91:451–454, 1974
22. GREER CH: Epithelial tumours of the retinal pigment epithelium. Trans Ophthalmol Soc UK 72: 265–277, 1952
23. HAGLER WS: Free floating cysts. Feature photo. Arch Ophthalmol 78:400–401, 1967
24. HARRIS JL, GUMICIO CC, OHANION MB: Adenocarcinoma of the ciliary epithelium. Arch Ophthalmol 80:217–219, 1968
25. ILIFF WJ, GREEN WR: The incidence and histology of Fuch's adenoma. Arch Ophthalmol 88: 249–254, 1972
26. KLIEN B: Diktyoma retinae. Arch Ophthalmol 22:432–438, 1939
27. KLIEN BA, TANNER GS: Congenital epithelial cyst of the iris stroma. Am J Ophthalmol 55:291–295, 1963
28. KREIBIG: Personal communication
29. KUHLENBECK H, HAYMAKER W: Neuro-ectodermal tumors containing neoplastic neuronal elements: ganglioneuroma, spongioneuroblastoma and glioneuroma, with a clinicopathologic report of 11 cases, and a discussion of their origin and classification. Milit Surg 99:273, 1946
30. LAVAL J: Benign pigment-epithelium tumor of the iris. Arch Ophthalmol 48:66–74, 1952

31. MACHEMER R: Primary hyperplasia of the retinal pigment epithelium. Graefes Arch Klin Ophthalmol 167:284–295, 1964

32. MEEK RE: Sarcoma of the iris (complicated by a cyst). Arch Ophthalmol 8:864–870, 1932

33. MORAX V: Epithelioma pigmente et sarcome de l'iris. Bull Soc Ophtalmol Fr, pp 102–106, 1925

34. MORRIS DA, HENKIND P: Neoplasms of the iris pigment epithelium. Am J Ophthalmol 66:31–41, 1968

35. MULLANEY J: Primary malignant medulloepithelioma of the retinal stalk. Am J Ophthalmol 77:499–504, 1974

36. MULLANEY J, FITZPATRICK C: Idiopathic cyst of the iris stroma. Am J Ophthalmol 76:64–68, 1973

37. NAUMANN G, GREEN GR: Spontaneous nonpigmented iris cysts. Arch Ophthalmol 78:496–500, 1967

38. NEWELL FW: Diktyoma of the ciliary body. Trans Am Acad Ophthalmol Otolaryngol 60:406–412, 1956

39. RADNÓT M: Contribution to data on sight disturbances caused by proliferation of pigment epithelium. Br J Ophthalmol 32:423–426, 1948

40. REDSLOB E: Neuroépitheliome gliomateux de la retine; contribution a l'étude de l'histogénèse des tumeurs rétinennes. Bull Cancer (Paris) 12:573–584, 1923

41. REESE AB: Medulloepithelioma (dictyoma) of the optic nerve. Am J Ophthalmol 44:4–6, 1957

42. REESE AB: The role of the pigment epithelium in ocular pathology. Am J Ophthalmol 50:1066–1084, 1960

43. REESE AB, EHRLICH G: The culture of uveal melanomas. Am J Ophthalmol 46:163–174, 1958

44. REESE AB, JONES IS: Benign melanomas of the retinal pigment epithelium. Am J Ophthalmol 42:207–212, 1956

45. REIN G: On melanoblastoma of the papilla and tumors of retinal epithelium. Graefes Arch Klin Ophthalmol 161:519–531, 1960

46. RUBINO A: I tumori della pars ciliaris retinae (dictiomi di Fuchs). Ann Ottalmol Clin Ocul 69:385–437, 1941

47. RYCHENER R: Cited by Kuhlenbeck H, Haymaker W, in reference 29

48. SALIM I: De neurogene facetten van iris tumors. Amsterdam, NV Drukkerij Dico, 1956

49. SANDERS TE, PODOS SM, ROSENBAUM LJ: Intraocular manifestations of multiple myeloma. Arch Ophthalmol 77:789–794, 1967

50. SCHEIE HG: Gonioscopy in the diagnosis of tumors of the iris and ciliary body, with emphasis on intra-epithelial cysts. Trans Am Ophthalmol Soc 51:313–331, 1953

51. SCHMIDT R: Ein epithelialer Tumor der Iris. Arch Augenheilkd 108:457–463, 1934

52. SEEFELDER R: Ein Beitrag zu den Geschwulstbildungen des retinalen Epithels. Graefes Arch Klin Ophthalmol 105:271–278, 1921

53. SPICER WTH, GREEVES RA: Multiple cysts in the anterior chamber derived from a congenital cystic growth of the ciliary epithelium. Proc R Soc Med (Ophthalmol Sect) 8:9–26, 1914–1915

54. SPIERS F, JENSEN OA: Pseudo-epitheliomatous hyperplasia of the retinal pigment epithelium. Acta Ophthalmol (Kbh) 41:722–727, 1963

55. STARCK D: Embryologie, ein Lehrbuch auf allgemein biologischer Grundlage. Stuttgart, Springer-Verlag, 1965, pp 193, 387, 395, 577

56. STREETEN BW, McGRAW JL: Tumor of the ciliary pigment epithelium. Am J Ophthalmol 74:420–429, 1972

57. SWAN KC: Iris pigment nodules complicating miotic therapy. Am J Ophthalmol 37:886–889, 1954

58. THEOBALD GD, FLOYD G, KIRK HQ: Hyperplasia of the retinal pigment epithelium. Am J Ophthalmol 45:235–240, 1958

59. TS'O MOM, ALBERT DM: Pathological condition of the retinal pigment epithelium; neoplasms and nodular non-neoplastic lesions. Arch Ophthalmol 88:27–38, 1972

60. VERHOEFF FH: A rare tumor arising from the pars ciliaris retinae (terato-neuroma) of a nature hitherto unrecognized, and its relation to the so-called glioma retinae. Trans Am Ophthalmol Soc 10:351–377, 1904

61. VOGEL MH, ZIMMERMAN LE, GASS JDM: Proliferation of the juxtapapillary retinal pigment epithelium simulating malignant melanoma. Doc Ophthalmol 26:461–481, 1969

62. WADSWORTH JAC: Epithelial tumors of the ciliary body. Am J Ophthalmol 32:1487–1501, 1949

63. WOLTER JR: Fuchs' epithelioma of the posterior retina. Am J Ophthalmol 57:835–838, 1964

64. ZIMMERMAN LE: Verhoeff's "terato-neuroma"; a critical reappraisal in light of new observations and current concepts of embryonic tumors. Am J Ophthalmol 72:1039–1057, 1971

65. ZIMMERMAN LE, FONT RL, ANDERSEN SR: Rhabdomyosarcomatous differentiation in malignant intraocular medulloepitheliomas. Cancer 30:817–835, 1972

3

RETINOBLASTOMA AND OTHER NEUROECTODERMAL TUMORS OF THE RETINA

Retinoblastoma's interesting and stormy history warrants a brief review. From the earliest reports suggestive of the disease, there has been strong controversy as to its origin, symptoms, genetic influence, treatment, and prognosis.[17] Hayes, a London surgeon, appears to have described the first case of retinoblastoma in 1765, including the peculiar fundal reflex noted early in the disease and optic nerve involvement. Such terms as amaurotic cat's eye, scrofula, fungus hematodes, soft cancer, and neuroepithelioma were in vogue from time to time.

Wardrop of Edinburgh in 1809 established retinoblastoma as an entity, gave a good clinical description of 35 cases, and was the first to advocate early enucleation as a life-saving measure. "It is an experiment, at all events, which still merits trial," he wrote, "and were I in any case to be assured of the existence of the disease in the early stage, I would have no hesitation in urging the performance of the operation." He felt that if the optic nerve was in a healthy state "success could be hoped for."

This view was hotly disputed for almost 50 years. Scarpa, the great Italian surgeon, in 1816 stated that the complete extirpation of the eye, "although performed on the first appearance of the disease under the form of a yellowish spot, is useless and rather accelerates the death of the patient."

Guthrie, three times president of the Royal College of Surgeons, in 1823 spoke of fungus hematodes as "a fatal disease, inasmuch as the removal of the eye has not, I believe, hitherto succeeded in arresting its progress when it has been so fully formed at the bottom of the eye to show distinctly its nature."

Advances rapidly followed the advent of the microscope and ophthalmoscope and the introduction of chloroform anesthesia. Virchow in 1864 correctly identified retinoblastoma as a neoplasm which he called glioma of the retina, but unfortunately he equated it with gliomas of the brain, for which radiation is known to be unavailing. Indeed, the hazards and technical difficulties in the early days of radiation, as well as the large doses given, resulted in numerous complications.

Verhoeff's term *retinoblastoma*, adopted after much discussion by the American Ophthalmological Society in 1926, is commonly used in the United States and Great Britain. Many ophthalmologists on the Continent still prefer the term *glioma of the retina*, although it seems less descriptive because of its implied identification with glioma of the brain.

When the tumor was established as a retinoblastoma and not a glioma, its radiosensitivity was soon appreciated, ushering in an era of effective treatment. Despite strongly divergent opinions regarding each step in various therapeutic measures, progress has been steady, culminating in a sharp rise in cure rate within the past few decades.

This malignant tumor arising from the nuclear layers of the retina develops characteristically from multiple foci in one or both eyes. It is congenital but usually not recognized at birth. The fact that it may be manifest in one eye many months before the other suggests a varying growth rate from one focus to another and sometimes delay of active growth until after birth. Such tumors have been reported in animals.[51]

Neuroblastoma (sympathicoblastoma) of the peripheral nervous system as well as medulloblastoma of the central nervous system have much in common with retinoblastoma. All three are highly malignant neuroblastic neoplasms of infants and young children and display similar histologic characteristics of partial or complete rosette formation. Two of our patients with retinoblastoma have developed neuroblastomas. Retinoblastoma and neuroblastoma both undergo marked necrosis and calcification, tend to regress spontaneously, are radiosensitive, and affect the same age groups; medulloblastoma also occurs in these age groups, is radiosensitive and frequently undergoes necrosis.

While there is probably some fundamental reason why similar neoplasms are found in the retina, brain, and peripheral nervous system of infants and children, justifying the use of a common term, it seems wise on the basis of present knowledge to consider them separate neoplasms and to call the retinal tumor retinoblastoma.

Incidence

Various incidence figures have been reported for different countries: 1 case of retinoblastoma per 14,000 births in Holland, 1 per 17,000 in Norway, 1 per 19,000 in both Finland and Denmark, and 1 per 20,500 in the Republic of Ireland.[5] One case was found in every 23,000 births in Michigan[21] and 1 for every 2154 infants admitted to a pediatric hospital in Mexico.[38]

Age

The average age at the time of diagnosis in our series was 18 months, and treatment was begun at the average age of 16 months. In two cases the disease was present at birth; the oldest patient was 34 years of age. Well-documented cases have been reported in patients from 29 to 62 years of age.[2,8,30]

Association with IQ

Statistical surveys have suggested that patients blinded by the tumor have above-average intelligence.[18,69] However, mental retardation has also been reported in this group.[61]

Bilaterality

In bilateral cases the retinoblastoma originates from separate sites in the two eyes; it is extremely rare for the disease to extend from one eye to the other via the optic chiasm. The large proportion of bilateral cases at our clinic (80%, compared with about 30% in most series) reflects the high percentage of referrals and our particular interest in retinoblastoma. In one-third of the cases the lesion was originally diagnosed in only one eye. This finding highlights the importance of a thorough examination of both eyes under general anesthesia, preferably by indirect ophthalmoscopy and indentation of the sclera for a view of the peripheral fundus. Small intraretinal tumors are more difficult to detect in heavily pigmented fundi. Occasionally both eyes are about equally affected, but usually the disease is much more advanced in one eye.

CLASSIFICATION

The retina stems from the optic vesicle, an outpocketing of the neural tube from which the central nervous system is derived. Since the retina and central nervous system are formed from the same type of cells, they could be expected to harbor the same tumors. In fact, the primitive medullary epithelium of the neural tube lines both the primitive cerebral vesicle and the optic nerve.

All tumors of the central nervous system, except blood-vessel tumors, develop basically from one embryologic layer, the neuroectoderm. Its most primitive cells, which make up the medullary epithelium lining the neural tube and optic vesicle, can develop into either nerve tissue or supporting tissue. The less primitive, more differentiated cells have already declared themselves as progenitors of the retina. Thus, tumors arising from the central nervous system or retina may be composed of very malignant undifferentiated cells (medulloblastoma, retinoblastoma), of benign differentiated cells (glioma, neurocytoma), or of cells at any intermediate stage of differentiation (neuroepithelioma, medulloepithelioma). Virtually all such neuroectodermal tumors are composed of primitive cells, usually with a highly mixed cell content.

A histiogenic classification of brain tumors[4] is based on the fact that the medullary epithelium lining the neural tube in the embryo differentiates into three types of cells: neuroblasts, which develop into nerve tissue; spongioblasts, which develop into supporting tissue, the majority becoming astrocytes and a lesser proportion becoming ependymal cells; and medulloblasts, which are primitive undifferentiated cells whose fate is unknown but may lie in the direction of glial or nerve tissue. With the use of gold and silver staining methods to differentiate these various cells, the tumor types were classified according to the predominating cells.

Attempts have been made to show that comparable tumors arise in the retina.[39,60] Such a parallel is certainly reasonable in principle, and the efforts of these investigators have resulted in basic, if not complete, agreement.

THEORY OF THE ORIGIN OF TUMORS

The formerly widely held concept that tumors arise from misplaced embryonic cell rests has been supplanted by the concept that truly primitive or embryonic cells do not persist in fully developed adult tissue or organs, and that cancer develops from normal cells that have dedifferentiated into immature anaplastic cells. The specialized function of these anaplastic cells diminishes or disappears, and their reproductive capacity usually increases. Instead of an embryonic cell there is an entirely new type, a cancer cell, which may be even less differentiated than the normal embryonic cell.

Some authors contributed to the concept that retinal tumors originate from the glial or supporting cells, either astrocytes or Mueller's fibers or both.[39] The nuclei of Mueller's fibers are in the inner nuclear layer of the retina; astrocytes are found not only in this layer but also in the ganglion-cell and nerve-fiber layers. Retinal tumors therefore arise most often in the inner nuclear layer, less often in the ganglion-cell and nerve-fiber layers, and rarely in the outer nuclear layer where few glial cells have been demonstrated.

In accord with the view that neoplasms arise from cells capable of reproduction and not from mature specialized cells, it is logical to expect retinal tumors to arise from cells still able to reproduce or regenerate. It is generally agreed that in the retina, as in the central nervous system, the highly specialized nerve or ganglion cells are completely formed at birth and never reproduce, whereas the less-specialized glial or supporting cells retain their power of reproduction, and therefore neoplasms are perhaps of glial origin.

HISTOPATHOLOGY

A retinoblastoma is composed of undifferentiated anaplastic cells that are uniformly small, round or polygonal, and have a scanty or almost invisible cytoplasm that stains poorly. Their relatively large nuclei, rich in chromatin, stain deeply with hematoxylin; sometimes a sparse amount of cytoplasm is located on one side of the cell, giving it a carrot shape suggesting an embryonic retinal cell. The stroma in these tumors is sparse, and the tumor cells show little cohesion.

When silver-impregnated preparations were used to identify several stages in the histogenesis of the retinoblastoma cell, spon-gioblasts as well as adult astroblasts and astrocytes were found.[37] However, in other hands[39] special stains revealed no cell processes or fibrils indicating either glial or nerve tissue; indeed, the primitive cells failed to show any specialized functional differentiation. According to one investigator,[22] neuroblasts have never been demonstrated.

For practical purposes there are only two types of retinoblastoma: by far the most common is composed of highly undifferentiated retinoblasts; the other, composed partially of somewhat more differentiated cells characterized by rosette formation, is often called a neuroepithelioma. Since the latter never appears in a pure form but merely as a modification of the first type, their pathologic characteristics can be considered together.

A retinoblastoma may arise in the internal nuclear layer, the nerve-fiber and ganglion-cell layers, or the external nuclear layer. When arising from the external layer it tends to grow in the subretinal space, pushes the retina inward, and in the early stages may gain access to the vitreous cavity. It is frequently referred to clinically as the exophytum type (Fig. 3–1). If arising from inner layers, the tumor mass extends early into the vitreous cavity and is frequently referred to clinically as the endophytum type.

In most instances it is impossible to determine from which retinal layer the tumor originated, inasmuch as it extends from one to another by direct invasion. One section

FIG. 3–1. Two foci of exophytum retinoblastoma. The tumor masses protrude from the posterior surface of the retina, not toward the vitreous; the smaller mass might be barely visible by ophthalmoscope.

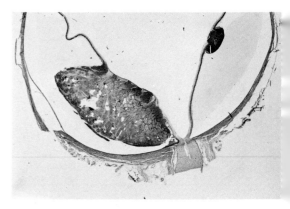

through an invaded area may suggest its origin in that layer, while an adjacent section may show extension from another layer. The picture is sometimes further confused by tumor seeds and perhaps by neoplastic emboli.

Multiple Foci

A common and important feature of the tumor is its multiple origins. Eighty-four percent of retinoblastoma patients have multiple tumors, sometimes five or more, in the affected retina (Fig. 3–2). These multiple foci are independent, not disseminated from a primary focus or from the other eye. They should not be confused with tumor implants or intraretinal metastases.

In rare instances the entire retina seems to be replaced by cancer cells (Fig. 3–3).

The supposedly new foci that may be noted after the original tumor has been treated by contact radiation seem to represent previously undetected independent areas of tumor. In a series of 43 cases, such areas were found in 26 eyes after the original focus had been treated.[57] Multiple foci have been attributed to a possible induction factor produced by the original focus.[62]

Necrosis and Perivascular Growth

In retinoblastoma the cancer cells are frequently arranged around the many newly formed vascular channels (Fig. 3–4). A perivascular cuff of 8 to 15 viable tumor cells around a capillary is sometimes confused with a true rosette. Elsewhere the tumor shows either necrosis or a lesser degree of cell degeneration. The necrotic areas, which appear amorphous and granular and stain with eosin, are in marked contrast to the perivascular viable areas. The necrotic foci may contain large phagocytic cells rich in lipid. The nuclei in tumor cells that have not yet necrosed may become pyknotic and show karyorrhexis and karyolysis. Necrotic retinoblastoma tissue may produce a uveitis or endophthalmitis which so confuses the clinical picture that retinoblastoma is not suspected.

The perivascular arrangement of the tumor cells was at first believed to result from the rapid growth of cancer cells that outdistanced their blood supply, but the same arrangement is sometimes found in early tumors. Such a cell distribution tends to predominate when the tumor is confined to the vitreous cavity. Pressure on the tumor within the confines of the globe is probably not an important factor in the degeneration of cells, because choroidal extension of the tumor shows little perivascular degeneration.[39]

Rosettes, Fleurettes and Pseudorosettes

The neuroepitheliomatous type of retinoblastoma that shows photoreceptor differentiation into rosettes (Fig. 3–5) and fleurettes seems more resistent to radiation than anaplastic retinoblastoma, a finding that supports the general principle that the radiosensitivity of cells varies inversely with their degree of differentiation.[63,64,65] Fleurettes can be seen by light and electron microscopy (Fig. 3–6).

Pseudorosettes may also show such arrangements as perivascular growth (Fig. 3–4), particularly around a small vascular channel, or a small group of tumor cells that degenerate and leave a clear space containing cellular debris surrounded by a ring of viable cells.

Implantation Growths

Since retinoblastomas have little stroma, the cells tend to disseminate throughout the eye. Globules of tumor tissue at times permeate the vitreous cavity, where they receive sufficient nutrition to remain viable and even to grow. Implantation growths may be found at any site where nutrition is adequate. The most common site is the choroidal surface (Fig. 3–7); others are the surface of the retina (Fig. 3–8) and the posterior surface of the cornea in the region of the angle.

The entire surface of the iris is sometimes covered by a layer of retinoblastoma cells (Fig. 3–9). Those along the choroidal surface may break through the lamina vitrea and gain access to the choroid (Fig. 3–7); in this event the choroid's rich blood supply offers an excellent medium for rapid growth and extension of the tumor (Fig. 3–10). A characteristic finding is necrosis of the central portion of the implantation focus which is surrounded by viable cancer cells (Fig. 3–11).

As mentioned earlier, tumor seeds may collect under the retina at the ora serrata and grow as separate foci. Clinically, when seen late in the course of treatment they may be considered new tumor foci. When these are located in the periphery, they may not be reached by radiation, in which case their ac-

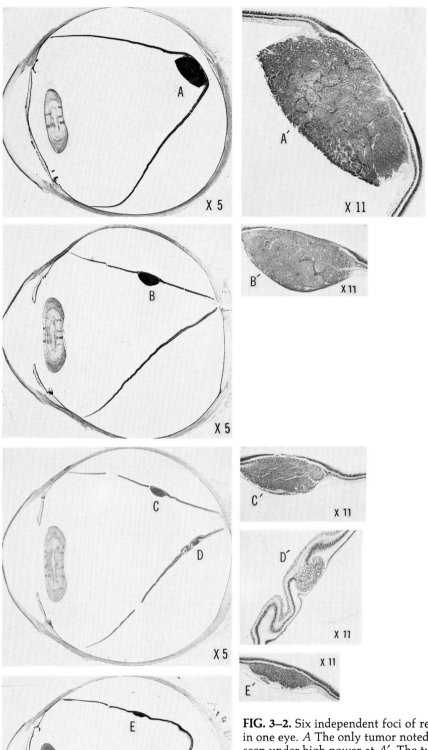

FIG. 3–2. Six independent foci of retinoblastoma in one eye. *A* The only tumor noted clinically, seen under high power at *A'*. The tumors at *B,B'* and *C,C'* were detected after the globe was opened and inspected with the dissecting microscope. The tumors at *D,D'* and *E,E'* were discovered in sections prepared for light microscopy. A tiny tumor in the macular area is not pictured. Two tumors were located at the ora; three showed marked rosette formation. (Courtesy of L. E. Zimmerman.)

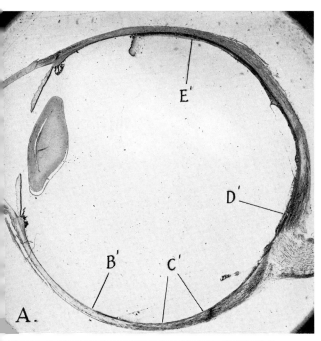

FIG. 3–3. Flat diffuse retinoblastoma. **A.** Survey of involved retina. Photomicrographs: **B.** Sector B'. **C.** Two sites at C' showing rosettes. **D.** The macula at D' seen with the fovea. **E.** Sector E'.

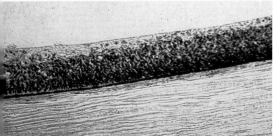

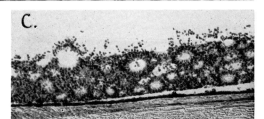

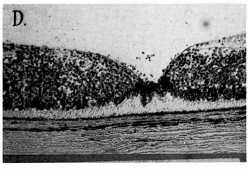

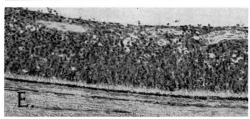

FIG. 3–4. Section of retinoblastoma showing perivascular growth. The light areas between the tumor foci represent necrosis, and the dark amorphous areas are calcium. Inset shows cancer cells surrounding a small vascular channel. This type of pseudorosette may closely resemble a true rosette.

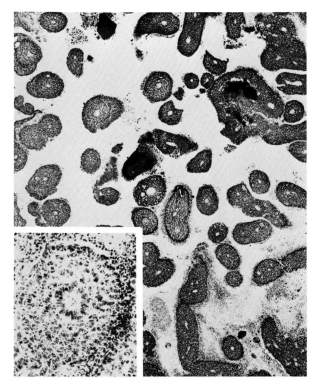

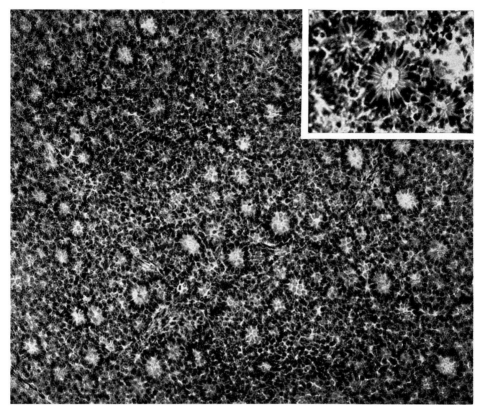

FIG. 3–5. Section of neuroepitheliomatous type
of retinoblastoma with many rosettes. Inset
shows a highly magnified rosette.

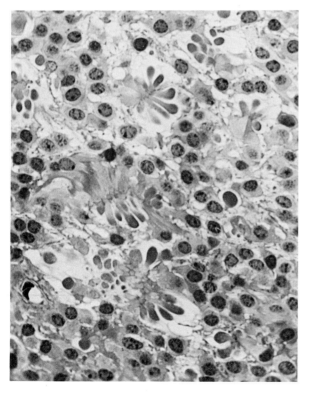

FIG. 3–6. Photoreceptor cell elements called
fleurettes. These fleurettes have been studied by
light and electron microscopy. (Courtesy of
M. O. M. Ts'o, L. E. Zimmerman and B. Fine.[63])

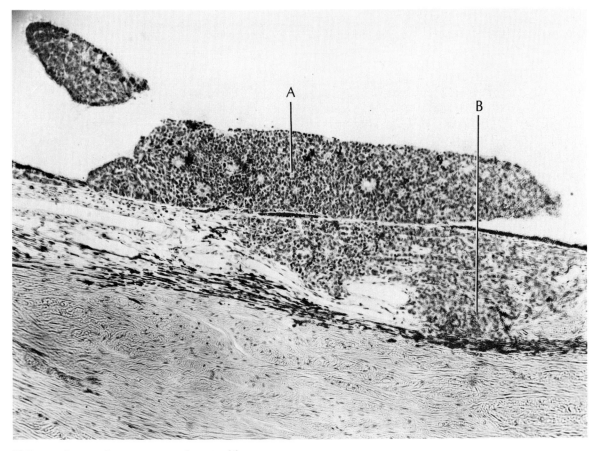

FIG. 3–7. Section from an eye with retinoblastoma showing implantation growth and choroidal extension. Implantation growth (*a*) with rosettes follows the choroidal surface. Most of the pigment epithelium is missing below (*b*), and the tumor has extended through the lamina vitrea into the choroid.

FIG. 3–8. Section from an eye with retinoblastoma showing an implantation growth. The implantation growth (*a*) extends along the inner retinal surface in the foveal region; the tumor proper is seen at *b*.

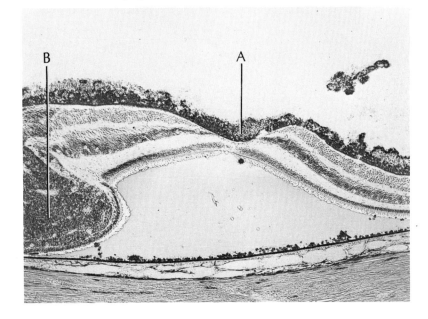

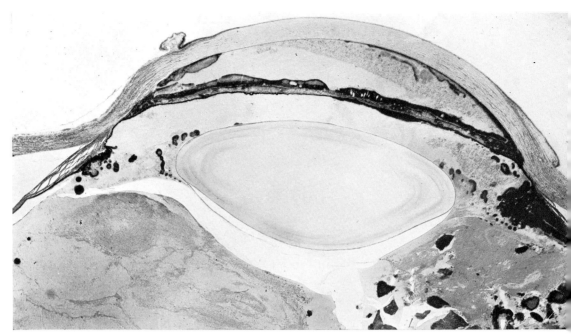

FIG. 3–9. Anterior sector of an eye with retinoblastoma showing implantation growths. Tumor tissue is seen along the surface of the iris, the ciliary body, the cornea, and the zonules. The bulk of the tumor and also the central portion of the implantation growth are necrotic.

FIG. 3–10. Section of an eye in which a retinoblastoma gained access to the vascular choroid, where it grew rapidly. The portion under the retina regressed after x-ray therapy.

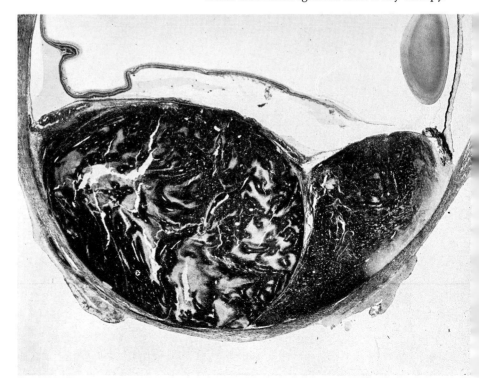

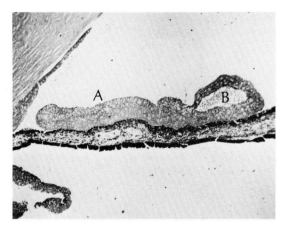

FIG. 3–11. Implantation growth of retinoblastoma along the anterior surface of the iris. The huge growth extends from *a* to *b*; at *b* there is an area of necrosis. This tumor seed led to the correct diagnosis.

FIG. 3–12. Invasion of the optic nerve by retinoblastoma. **A.** Tumor invasion beyond the lamina cribrosa. **B.** Shows the average depth of tumor extension when such invasion occurs. **C.** Retinoblastoma has completely replaced the normal optic-nerve bundles. (**A.** Courtesy of Armed Forces Institute of Pathology.)

tivity continues after successful arrest of the tumor at the primary site or sites.

An implantation growth of retinoblastoma transferred from a donor eye to the eye of an adult host during a successful corneal transplant operation has been described.[24] A 54-year-old woman had undergone keratoplasty on the right eye. The graft was taken from the cornea of an eye containing retinoblastoma. The graft remained viable and clear, and the visual result was good. One and a half years later the host eye developed what seemed to be a hypopyon iritis with secondary glaucoma. Enucleation was performed, and microscopic examination revealed retinoblastoma tissue growing in the anterior segment.

Extension into the Optic Nerve

The tumor's predilection for invading the optic nerve and the clinical significance of such invasion are well known. It occurs especially when glaucoma is present.[55] Results of a microscopic study of optic nerve invasion in enucleated eyes containing retinoblastoma were compiled for three different periods: 1878–1929, 1934–1947, and 1963–1973. These studies[44,45,46] revealed that an increased effort to remove an adequate portion of the optic nerve during enucleation resulted in a steady rise in the percentage of cases showing no residual tumor in the portion of the nerve left in the orbit.

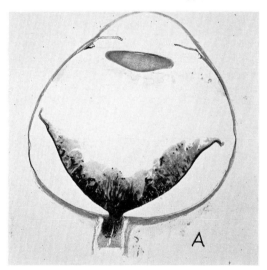

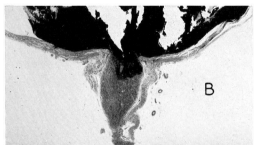

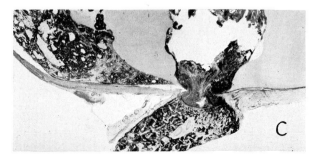

In series 1 (1878–1929, which included 119 enucleated eyes) retinoblastoma cells had extended into the optic nerve in 53%, compared with 27% for series 2 (1934–1947—116 eyes), and 25% for series 3 (1963–1973—319 eyes). In series 1, only 47% of the total cases showed a tumor-free portion of optic nerve remaining in the orbit after enucleation. In series 2 this figure had risen to 73% and in series 3 to 75%.

The prognostic value of careful attention to optic nerve invasion is strikingly demonstrated in a histopathologic study of 300 cases at the Armed Forces Institute of Pathology.[70] The author reported a 91.6% survival when the tumor had not invaded the optic nerve, a 55.6% survival when invasion stopped short of the plane of surgical transection, but only 36% when the tumor had reached this plane.

The tumor rarely extends more than a few millimeters beyond the lamina cribrosa. If the extension is as much as 10 mm, it gains access to the subarachnoid space at the site where the central vessels leave the nerve and spreads rapidly to the chiasm and brain.

Tumor invasion of the nerve begins in the base of the physiologic or glaucomatous cup around the central vessels (Fig. 3–12); in three specimens tumor cells were found in the lumen of one of these vessels. The size of the tumor does not seem related to its potential for extending into the nerve, since small as well as large tumors may do so.

At times the optic nerve bundles and their septa retain their size and shape even though the nerve fibers have been replaced by tumor tissue. On the other hand, the tumor does not tend to invade fibrous tissue. When the optic nerve is atrophic, the hypertrophied septal tissue appears to offer a barrier to invasion, and extension through the sclera to the extraocular structures occurs late if at all, and only if the growth is massive.

Extension into the Choroid

In about 25% of cases the tumor invades the choroid, usually when far advanced. It reaches the choroid by means of implantation growths along the choroidal surface or around the margin of the optic nerve where the lamina vitrea terminates. In the highly vascular choroid the cancer cells flourish; the tumor may extend throughout the entire uveal tract, resulting in a large mass overshadowing the affected retinal area. Indeed,

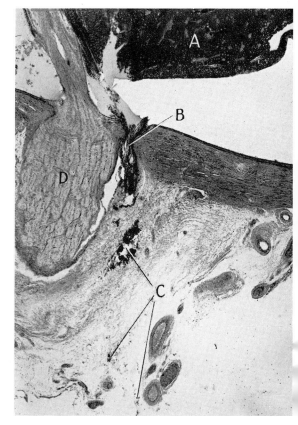

FIG. 3–13. Extension of retinoblastoma from the choroid out of the globe. The choroid is heavily invaded (A) by the tumor, which extends through the sclera along the optic nerve (B) and into the orbit (C). The optic nerve is shown at D.

FIG. 3–14. An advanced untreated case of retinoblastoma. (Courtesy of F. Palomino-Dena.)

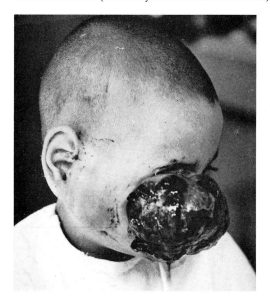

in some cases the retinal element shows marked necrosis and regression while the choroidal element becomes established as the dominant lesion.

Extension into the Orbit

Orbital extensions are responsible for orbital recurrences and should be suspected in advanced cases, especially when secondary glaucoma is present. A choroidal tumor may gain access to the orbit through the emissaria, manifesting itself not necessarily as a conglomerate mass but perhaps as discrete cells. In such instances there may be a question whether the cells are an artifact arising from cutting and preparation of the specimen. When studying sections to determine whether the tumor has spread beyond the globe, several avenues other than the optic nerve are possible. It is well to consider that once the tumor reaches the choroid it may extend through the emissaria as well as directly into the vaginal space through the thin border tissue separating the choroid from the nerve (Fig. 3–13). Untreated tumors may grow to a large size (Fig. 3–14).

DIAGNOSIS

Retinoblastoma is rarely diagnosed in these very young patients in an early stage unless a family history of the disease leads to examination of the eyes under general anesthesia.

Presenting signs or symptoms that lead to the detection of retinoblastoma in 65% of the cases are as follows, in order of frequency:

1. Leukocoria (white pupillary or cat's-eye reflex)
2. Esotropia or exotropia
3. Red, painful eye with or without glaucoma
4. Poor vision

Leukocoria

The most common early overt manifestation is a white pupillary reflex or a mass back of the lens (Fig. 3–15). This cat's-eye reflex is only one of many conditions in the so-called leukocoria group; others will be discussed under differential diagnosis. It cannot be overemphasized that a white pupil may mean serious trouble and must be immediately investigated.

A 3–4 dd tumor in the macular region may produce a light reflex and be apparent when the patient looks straight toward the observer. Tumors located at the periphery of the fundus are seen only if larger and when the patient looks in a certain direction. This explains why the parents may be aware of the light reflex in the eye at home while it is missed by the pediatrician or ophthalmologist. The cat's-eye reflex has been noted in 50% of our total cases (more than 1250) and much more frequently in recent years probably because of publicized warnings of its importance.[19]

Esotropia or Exotropia

Esotropia and, more rarely, exotropia may be due to poor vision from involvement of the macular area by the tumor. If the child is too young to cooperate during an adequate examination of the fundus before squint surgery, the nonfixing eye should be thoroughly examined with the ophthalmoscope while the child is under general anesthesia for the muscle operation.

Red, Painful Eye with or without Glaucoma

This complication is usually due to intraocular inflammation or angle obstruction from tumor necrosis. The glaucoma tends to appear suddenly and, with conservative treatment, proves transitory.

Poor Vision

Visual loss is usually due to macular involvement, cloudy vitreous, inflammation, or cataract.

FIG. 3–15. Typical appearance of leukocoria in retinoblastoma.

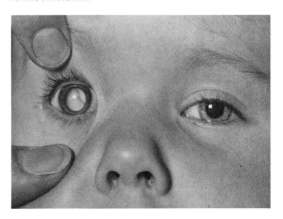

In addition, the following findings in a child may arouse suspicion of retinoblastoma: secondary glaucoma, unequal size of the pupils, a family history of the disease, characteristic color of the tumor, seeds in the vitreous, implantation growths, orbital cellulitis, anisocoria, heterochromia iridis, hyphema, hypopyon iritis, uveitis, and endophthalmitis.

The eye itself is usually normal in size with an anterior chamber of normal depth. To date I have had no irrefutable evidence that microphthalmos was already present when the retinoblastoma developed.

Secondary Glaucoma

Glaucoma at times ensues, causing corneal changes that prevent an accurate view of the interior of the eye. The glaucoma eventually leads to buphthalmos. In some cases, development of a cataract in the late stages further confuses the diagnosis.

Family History of the Disease

Because of the strong hereditary factor in retinoblastoma, all siblings of patients and all children of survivors must have a thorough examination of the fundi under general anesthesia, to be repeated at regular intervals. The same holds for children with a suspect family history, e.g., an unexplained enuclea-

tion or eye disease. (A separate section on Genetics of Retinoblastoma by F. David Kitchin appears at the end of this chapter.)

Color

Of diagnostic importance is the characteristic pale pink of the tumor in which newly formed blood vessels extend over the surface or into its substance (Fig. 3–16, see p. 8). In some cases, however, the lesion appears white and avascular. An early intraretinal or exophytum retinoblastoma may appear as a poorly demarcated, light-colored zone (Fig. 3–17, see p. 9).

Seeds in the Vitreous

Multiple globules of dull, white to light gray, disseminated tumor seeds may be present in the vitreous (Fig. 3–18) or over the surface of the retina, emanating from the site where the tumor first breaks through its confines. A vitreous densely packed with seeds varying in size from dustlike particles to large masses may obscure the view of the tumor, making the diagnosis more difficult.

Implantation Growths

The more advanced tumors may be accompanied by implantation growths recognizable as white foci over the iris, in the angle of the

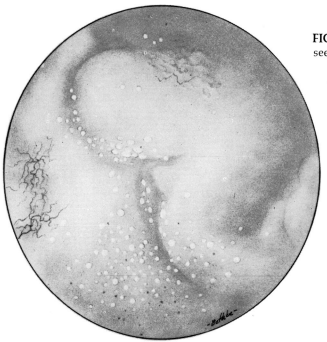

FIG. 3–18. Advanced retinoblastoma with tumor seeds in the vitreous.

anterior chamber (Fig. 3–19), along the dependent portion of the posterior surface of the cornea appearing as a hypopyon, on the surface of the retina, and in the vitreous.

Extension of Retinoblastoma to the Choroid, Optic Nerve, and Orbit

A tumor that reaches the choroid usually grows rapidly by virtue of the rich vascular supply. It become a protruding globular mass, outstripping or concealing the retinal tumor.

Extrascleral extension via the emissaria or through scleral necrosis, with orbital involvement and even exophthalmos, may be a late manifestation.

When the tumor invades the optic nerve, x rays only rarely show enlargement of the optic foramen. Thus, negative films do not exclude optic nerve invasion.

Examination of Subretinal and Anterior Chamber Fluids

Subretinal fluid has been withdrawn for diagnostic purposes in difficult cases, but I consider the practice questionable because of the risk of tumor seeding. When subretinal fluid is obtained with the use of a rather large-bore beveled needle, the fluid may escape through the bevel portion after the point of the needle pierces the sclera. To minimize the possibility of seeding tumor cells into the surrounding tissue, a needle with a bore large enough to take a plunger may be inserted, with plunger in place, through an incision one-fourth to four-fifths of the scleral thickness. A double-arm purse-string suture previously placed around the insertion site is tightened when the needle is withdrawn after the fluid has been obtained.

It has been suggested that detection of catecholamines in the urine of retinoblastoma patients may be of diagnostic value,[10] but this has not yet been well established.

It has been shown the LDH (lactic dehydrogenase) can be measured simply and that its ratio in aqueous humor provides an index to intraocular necrosis and perhaps tumor metabolism. Elevated ratios have been reported in retinoblastoma.[41]

Aspiration of the anterior chamber to obtain material for stained smears is another diagnostic aid that has been recommended. Four reported cases of very diffuse retino-

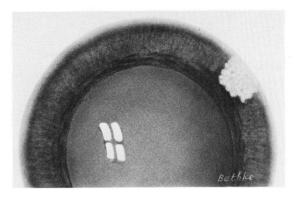

FIG. 3–19. Retinoblastoma seeded on the iris. Implantation growth on the left iris in an 11-month-old infant.

blastoma with hypopyon were diagnosed by identifying the tumor cells in material from the anterior chamber.[52] These four patients and two others with a similar history[31,67] were older than most retinoblastoma patients, and the clinical appearance suggested iritis or choroiditis.

Miscellaneous Comments

Heterochromia of the iris, particularly hemosiderosis, contraindicates the presence of retinoblastoma.

The ^{32}P test is of limited value in diagnosing retinoblastoma.

In an infant or child, any blind eye that shows advanced pathologic changes whose nature cannot be defined because of vitreous opacities, cataractous changes, or a cloudy cornea may harbor a retinoblastoma and should be enucleated.

When it is difficult to visualize the fundus, B-scan ultrasonography may confirm the presence or absence of a mass in the posterior segment and thus help to differentiate retinoblastoma from simulating lesions. (See the section on Ultrasonic Evaluation of Ocular and Orbital Tumors by D. Jackson Coleman in Chapter 12.)

In the advanced stages, retinoblastoma and some other leukocorias cannot be distinguished unequivocally. If a satisfactory examination of the interior of the eye is possible, the diagnosis should invariably be established.

In older children the diagnosis of retinoblastoma may be delayed because of unusual eye manifestations such as a) a globular avascular tumor at the periphery of the retina near the ora serrata which grows slowly over a six- to eight-year period; the presenting signs are vitreous floaters or decreased vision;[19] b) white clumps of cells seen in the anterior chamber requiring paracentesis to establish the diagnosis;[6] or c) growth of the diffuse type.

Among 618 reviewed cases of retinoblastoma 6.6% were diagnosed initially as primary ocular manifestations with no suspicion of a neoplasm, and 8.3% were considered to be other lesions—a total of 14.9% of erroneous diagnoses.[56]

Among 19 cases of retinal detachment in children under age 15 who had enucleations, more than half were misdiagnosed as retinoblastoma.[29]

Examination of the Fellow Eye

When retinoblastoma has been diagnosed in one eye, the other eye should be thoroughly examined, ideally under general anesthesia with dilatation of the pupil. The disease occurs bilaterally in 25%–30% of cases. A small tumor, which may be merely a grayish, poorly demarcated zone of about 1 dd, may easily be overlooked in the fellow eye. The bilateral feature is often not appreciated at the initial examination. Some of our earlier statistics showed that the tumor was undetected in the eye with less-advanced disease in over 40% of the cases. Early detection is ob-

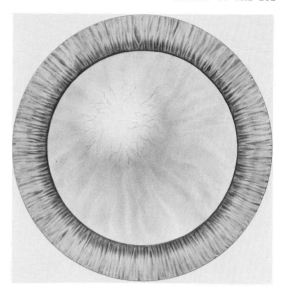

FIG. 3–20. *Toxocara canis* endophthalmitis. Examination of a child revealed complete detachment of the retina, hazy vitreous, and an indistinct mass in the upper temporal quadrant with exudate and retinal folds radiating to it. The diagnosis was suspected clinically, and the larva was identified microscopically as *Toxocara canis*.

FIG. 3–21. *Toxocara canis* granuloma of the macula. A 16-year-old girl had an elevated white lesion in the right macula surrounded by white retinal deposits (residual edema). The white area was more elevated at the central, cream-colored core, which on retroillumination was believed to be an encysted larva. The girl and her mother had both been treated in previous years for intestinal worms.

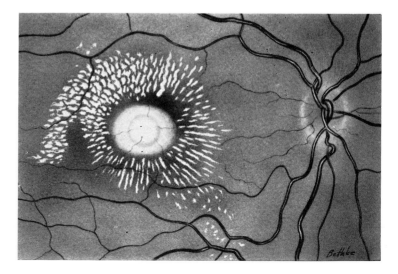

viously of the utmost importance, since the smaller the lesion the better the chance of effective treatment. We believe that patients who have had one eye removed should have the other eye examined under general anesthesia at least three times at three-month intervals, then at six-month intervals for the next year or so.

The binocular indirect ophthalmoscope is preferred to the direct ophthalmoscope because of the lower magnification and better contrast. Also, the periphery of the retina as far as the ora serrata in all quadrants can be examined by scleral indentation. Since we have been using these techniques we have found an increasing number of tumors at the periphery of the retina, seemingly explaining why so-called new tumor sites and recurrences are frequently noted there. Some tumor sites at the periphery result from migration of tumor cells in the subretinal space to the ora serrata where they start to grow.

DIFFERENTIAL DIAGNOSIS

The following conditions should be considered in the differential diagnosis of retinoblastoma:

1. Larval granulomatosis
2. Retrolental fibroplasia
3. Persistent hyperplastic primary vitreous
4. Retinal dysplasia
5. Metastatic retinitis
6. Coats's disease
7. Massive retinal fibrosis
8. Medullated nerve fibers
9. Congenital chorioretinal coloboma
10. Retinal astrocytoma
11. Congenital retinal detachment with or without retinoschisis

Vitreous or anterior chamber hermorrhage from hemorrhagic disease of the newborn or from persistent hyaloid artery may mask retinoblastoma.

Vascular changes simulating an angiomatous tumor may be induced by retinoblastoma anywhere in the fundus. When the tumor is at the periphery, von Hippel–Lindau disease may be suspected.

Retinoblastoma may manifest a flat type of growth which Ashton called diffuse infiltrating retinoblastoma. Among reported cases is the one that appears in Figure 3–3. Such lesions characteristically occur in an older than usual age group and clinically resemble iritis or choroiditis. They are said to be invariably

unilateral and to carry a generally good prognosis.[34] Hypopyon is frequently present, suggesting an anterior chamber aspiration biopsy as a possible diagnostic aid.

Larval Granuloma Due to Toxocara canis

Twenty-four of 46 eyes enucleated for suspected retinoblastoma had an endophthalmitis characterized by a massive focal inflammatory process localized at one site in the vitreous and retina. Exudative vitreous strands radiated to the lesion's focal area (Fig. 3–20), but vitreous opacities at times obscured the details. In each case a nematode was found which was believed to be a third-stage larva of the hookworm.[68] If the vitreous clears, it is possible to see details of the localized retina puckered by contracture. One patient had previously been treated for intestinal worms (Fig. 3–21).

Ashton's recognition that a localized, white, globular mass in the macular area resembling a retinoblastoma was due to *Toxocara canis* changed the clinical scope of intraocular nematode infestation.[3] He later identified the same parasite in three similar lesions.

The clinical picture ranges from the type described by Ashton to advanced cases with complete detachment of the retina from cicatricial contracture in an old blind eye. The degree of inflammation and extent of pathologic change seem to depend on whether the larva is still alive. The living organism induces a minimal response and the dead organism a maximal response.

The host for these *Toxocara* infections may be the dog or the cat, but to my knowledge no cases in ophthalmology have been reported implicating the cat. Young children who play with or around dogs may inadvertently ingest the embryonated eggs of *Toxocara canis* deposited in the animals' stools. The adult nematode is estimated to be present in the small intestine of up to 90% of puppies. The eggs contain infective larvae which hatch in the child's intestine and may in time reach the eye.

Organized *Toxocara* granuloma is the lesion that most often simulates retinoblastoma. Both conditions affect young people, producing a mass in the fundus. The diagnostic features of *Toxocara* granuloma are

1. History of the child's close relationship to a dog

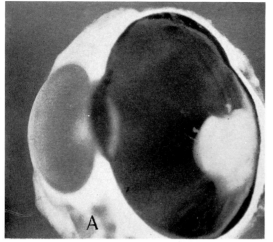

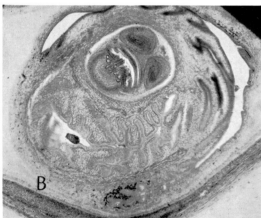

2. History of dirt-eating
3. Overt evidence of worms in either the child or the animal
4. Active inflammation or its sequelae (uveitis or endophthalmitis) associated with the fundal lesion in which a central core often contains the larva

The larvae usually enter the eye through the short ciliary arteries, and the lesion is noted clinically in the macular and peripapillary areas. When the larvae enter the central retinal artery, they may lodge in a temporal arteriole and give rise to a characteristic granuloma at the retinal periphery.[26]

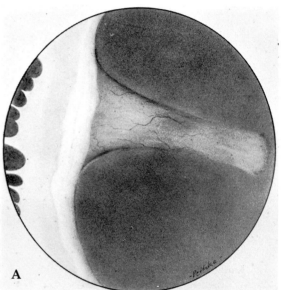

FIG. 3–22. Large mushroom-shaped granuloma in the macular area due to the larva of *Taenia solium*. **A.** The globe of a 5-year-old girl, with a calotte removed, shows an elevated white mass simulating a retinoblastoma. **B.** Section through the mass shows a larva between the retina and the choroid. (Courtesy of I. S. Jones.)

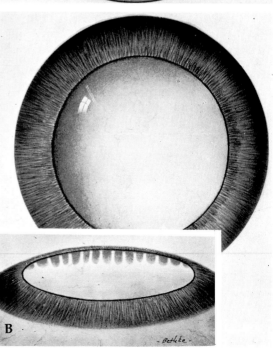

FIG. 3–23. Retrolental fibroplasia. **A.** In a case of grade III cicatricial retrolental fibroplasia a retinal fold extends from the disc to a mass of fibrous tissue temporally. At the temporal periphery are ciliary processes. **B.** In a grade V case the pupillary area is covered by vascularized white tissue. The inset shows the ciliary processes at the periphery of the retrolental tissue.

In a summary of 245 cases of ocular *Toxocara canis*, the author[11] differentiated its characteristics and stated that there are no serologic tests for the infection, although anti-A and anti-B levels seem to offer a promising approach. In fact, the diagnosis is difficult to confirm even in enucleated eyes; the larvae in a granuloma with abundant eosinophils may dissolve in time, and the remaining larval fragments defy detection at a later stage even with serial sectioning of the eye. As the eye is usually irreparably damaged before the diagnosis is made, treatment tends to be unavailing. However, thiabendazole and steroids have been effective in some early cases.[11]

Children with proved *Toxocara* granulomas in the retina or choroid seldom have other clinical manifestations of visceral larva migrans.[19]

I have seen two cases of unilateral exophthalmos in children which seemed to be due to *Toxocara* granulomatosis from larvae implanted in the orbit.

A case I first reported in 1936 was described in the last edition of this text as a massive retinal fibrosis in a 5-year-old boy blind in the left eye since birth. Ashton requested the block from this old case, remounted it in fresh celloidin, examined 110 sections, and found a larval fragment in the central part of the overlying retina. Thus, I unwittingly reported the first case of retinal granuloma due to *Toxocara* which Ashton diagnosed more than 30 years later.

Larval Granulomatosis due to Cysticercus

In ocular granuloma due to cysticercus the intestinal tapeworm can be demonstrated simultaneously in only 19%–25% of the cases. The eosinophil count may be elevated or normal. A cestode, cysticercus cellulosae, was found in one of our cases.[66] The clinical picture simulates retinoblastoma in the same way as does *Toxocara* granuloma (Fig. 3–22). The complement fixation test and the Casoni skin test represent rather nonspecific "group" reactions, but they are significant because they are positive in the great majority of ocular cases.

Retrolental Fibroplasia

For more than two decades retrolental fibroplasia was the condition most often confused with retinoblastoma, but this is no longer true. Since the characteristics of retrolental fibroplasia have become well known, the incidence has been drastically reduced by monitoring the oxygen saturation of the blood of newborns. Nevertheless, cases are seen occasionally in full-term as well as premature infants, with no apparent oxygen factor. The differential diagnosis should be clear.

Retrolental fibroplasia first becomes evident in its cicatricial stage between the third and fifth months of life, typically in premature infants given oxygen. It is bilateral, occurring in eyes with some degree of microphthalmos and shallow anterior chambers. It usually appears as a grayish, opaque, vascularized mass of tissue which occupies the anterior part of the vitreous just posterior to the lens, thus preventing visualization of the interior of the eye. In a less severe form, opaque tissue appears at the periphery of some quadrant of the fundus (temporally in 90% of cases). This tissue incorporates a fold of the retina and extends back to the disc (Fig. 3–23). Long ciliary processes almost always occur at the periphery of the white tissue, an important diagnostic feature never seen in retinoblastoma. These ciliary processes are visible because the ciliary body is pulled centrally by the contracting fibrous tissue; in persistent hyperplastic vitreous the ciliary processes are visible because they are abnormally long.

Iris changes such as atrophy, posterior synechiae, and pupillary membrane are frequently noted in eyes with retrolental fibroplasia. No calcium is detected clinically or by x ray. The iris-lens diaphragm sometimes advances sufficiently to touch the cornea and produce opacification, often associated with secondary glaucoma and resultant buphthalmos. In this event the interior of the eye cannot be visualized, but the disease can usually be diagnosed on the basis of the lesion in the fellow eye or by other identifying features.

Long ciliary processes are invariably seen at the periphery of a lens that is usually smaller than normal; their presence is helpful in differentiating this condition from retinoblastoma. There is a degree of microphthalmos, although sometimes so slight as to be detected only by carefully comparing the two eyes. The lens capsule may have a dehiscence at the posterior pole, resulting in cataractous changes which eventually involve the entire lens. The swollen lens advances forward against the cornea, glaucoma ensues, and the eye is lost. This sequence of events can usu-

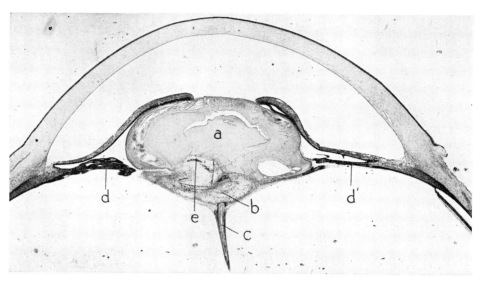

FIG. 3–25. Persistent hyperplastic primary vitreous. Anterior sector of the globe shows the hyaloid artery (*c*) posterior to the retrolental tissue (*b*), rupture of the capsule of the lens (*a*) at the posterior pole (*e*), and long ciliary processes (*d-d'*) extending up to the fibrous tissue.

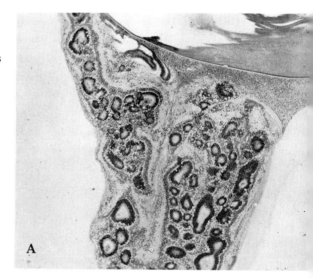

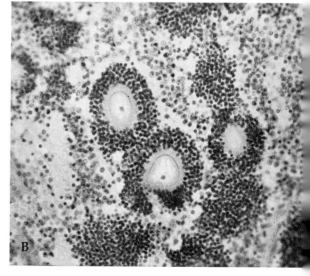

FIG. 3–26. Retinal dysplasia. **A.** Dysplastic retina and persistent retrolental fibrovascular tissue in a 2-month-old male infant. Examination revealed opaque vascular tissue back of the lens and an irregularly dilated pupil due to remnants of the pupillary membrane. He had multiple anomalies, was mentally retarded, and died at 6 months of age. **B.** Rosettes showed a central lumen, an abortive rod and cone layer, a fine limiting membrane, and a layer of dark nuclei. (A. B. Reese and B. R. Straatsma.[50])

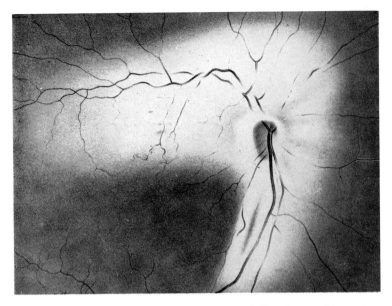

FIG. 3–28. Extensive medullated nerve fibers. A white reflex in the pupil led to the suspicion of retinoblastoma.

ally be prevented if the lens is removed in time by a needling operation.

Persistent Hyperplastic Primary Vitreous

This condition is unilateral and usually detected in full-term infants immediately after birth on the basis of leukocoria[47,48] (Fig. 3–24, see p. 9). It more closely resembles retinoblastoma than does any other form of leukocoria. Situated on the posterior surface of the lens, it sometimes shows an anterior concavity, is densest in the center and thinnest at the periphery.

A characteristic feature is the presence of obvious blood vessels in the iris stroma. The hyaloid artery, always evident in the microscopic sections (Fig. 3–25), can sometimes be seen clinically. Persistence of the hyaloid artery or of any part of the hyaloid system may lead to spontaneous hemorrhage into the vitreous when the infant is about 6 months old. When a definitive diagnosis cannot be made, enucleation of a useless and disfiguring eye is indicated.

Retinal Dysplasia

Retinal dysplasia, a developmental aberration present at birth in full-term infants, seems to belong in the 13–15 trisomy syndrome, char-acterized by an extra chromosome in the D group of paired chromosomes. The syndrome is manifested by multiple congenital abnormalities such as cleft palate, umbilical hernia, polydactylism, and defects of the cardiovascular and central nervous systems. Other ocular malformations besides retinal dysplasia include extreme microphthalmos, iris coloboma, partial aniridia, and cataracts.[49,50]

Fifteen cases with eye defects were reviewed, and the authors added three others.[13] All six eyes in their three patients showed intraocular cartilage which they considered a significant and characteristic feature.

Retinal dysplasia is differentiated from retinoblastoma by several features: the presence of opaque tissue adherent to the posterior surface of the lens; grayish-white tissue in the vitreous representing the elevated malformed retina (Fig. 3–26); a shallow anterior chamber and some degree of microphthalmos, often very slight; frequent association with systemic anomalies or with mental retardation.

Metastatic Retinitis

Any of the childhood infectious diseases may give rise to a metastatic embolus to the retina. The resulting subclinical, symptomless, localized inflammatory reaction subsides

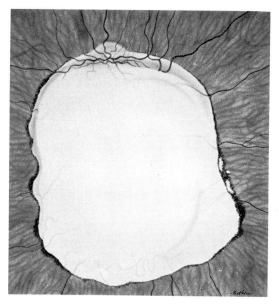

FIG. 3–29. Congenital coloboma of the choroid and retina. Retinoblastoma was suspected in this 7-year-old boy because of leukocoria.

undetected. Organization and contracture later lead to detachment of the retina and to a leukocoria (Fig. 3–27, see p. 9). The correct diagnosis is facilitated by noting sequelae of the inflammatory reaction in the retina, vitreous, or anterior sector of the eye. The vitreous is usually cloudy so that the lesion appears as an indistinct white haze.

Coats's Disease

Coats's disease is discussed in Chapter 8, Angiomatous Tumors.

Massive Retinal Fibrosis

In this type of leukocoria the organization of an undetected massive retinal hemorrhage occurring at birth results in a grayish-white mass protruding from the retina.

A 10% incidence of retinal hemorrhage has been reported in all newborns.[16] Another study revealed bloody spinal fluid in 46 of 500 infants born consecutively,[54] suggesting about a 10% incidence of intracranial hemorrhage, usually without any signs that would arouse suspicion. The predisposing factors seem to be prolonged labor (especially with late instead of early use of forceps in delivery), premature or breech delivery, spontaneous or precipitate birth, too strenuous efforts at resuscitation, asphyxia, and interference with fetal or placental circulation, as by pressure on the umbilical cord or premature separation of the placenta.

An important factor leading to retinal hemorrhage in newborns seems to be increased thoracic pressure during delivery. This pressure is transmitted to the terminal vessels of the head by the valveless veins of the thorax.

In rare instances a massive intracranial hemorrhage in a newborn has led to death or to permanent serious malfunction of the central nervous system, particularly cerebral spastic paralysis associated with mental retardation. As the retinal circulation is a continuation of the intracranial system, it is not surprising that a similar massive hemorrhage may occur occasionally in the retina of newborns; organization of the hemorrhage leads to the clinical picture of massive retinal fibrosis. This condition was probably included in Coats's description of the heterogeneous group of lesions known as Coats's disease.

Medullated Nerve Fibers

I have seen a number of infants with such extensive medullated nerve fibers of the retina that a leukocoria led the parents to seek medical advice. The lesion appeared as a large, flat, white area in the nerve-fiber layer at the posterior pole of the fundus (Fig. 3–28) and in some instances has been confused with a retinoblastoma.

Congenital Chorioretinal Coloboma

A large congenital coloboma of the retina and choroid baring the white sclera (Fig. 3–29) gives a leukocoria and may be confused with a retinoblastoma. The chance of a misdiagnosis is minimized by examining the eye with the indirect ophthalmoscope.[15]

Retinal Astrocytoma

An astrocytoma of the fiber layer of the retina may be confused with a retinoblastoma. (See Ch. 4, Glioma of the Optic Nerve, Retina, and Orbit.)

Congenital Detachment of the Retina with or without Retinoschisis

When first seen by an ophthalmologist, retinoblastoma often fills a large portion of at

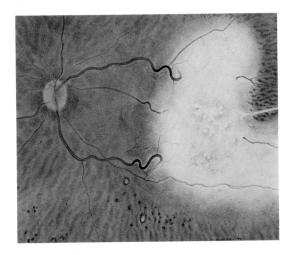

FIG. 3–30. Clinical appearance of calcium formation in retinoblastoma.

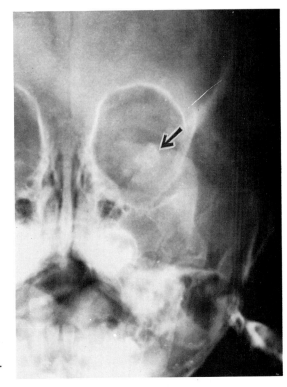

FIG. 3–31. X-ray demonstration of calcium in a retinoblastoma. Arrow points to calcium deposit. (Courtesy of S. L. Trokel.)

FIG. 3–32. Phases of regression in a retinoblastoma treated by x ray and chemotherapy. **A.** Before treatment, the eye showed one small focus of calcium. **B.** Three weeks after treatment was begun, the tumor had shrunk and showed several calcium foci as well as pigment changes. **C.** After four weeks the tumor was reduced essentially to calcium. **D.** Ten months later there had been considerable absorption of calcium.

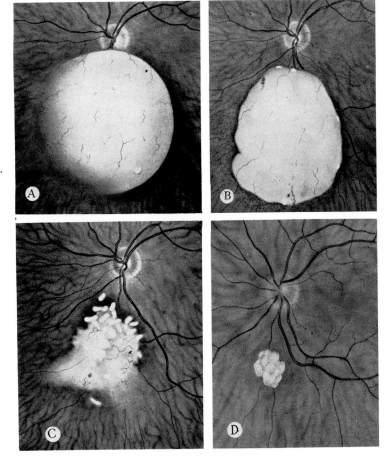

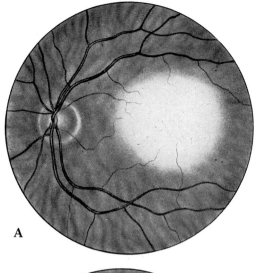

A

FIG. 3–33. Virtually complete absorption of cottage-cheeselike calcium residue of a retinoblastoma treated by x ray and chemotherapy. **A.** Tumor in the macular area before treatment. **B.** Calcium residue three weeks after treatment was initiated. **C.** Three months later the only visible remains of calcium were three pinpoint flecks.

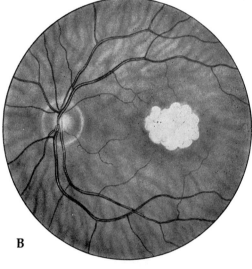

B

FIG. 3–34. Avascular type of residue of a retinoblastoma successfully treated by x ray and chemotherapy. **A.** Three areas of tumor before treatment. **B.** Three years later the lesions were somewhat smaller, were completely avascular, and had little or no visible calcium.

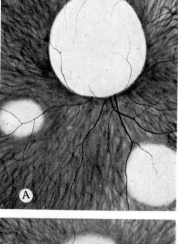

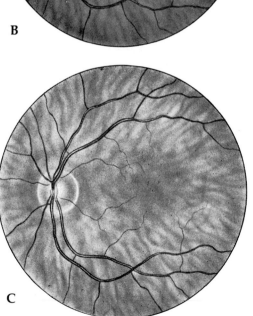

C

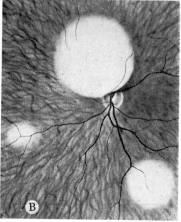

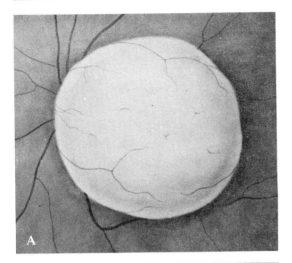

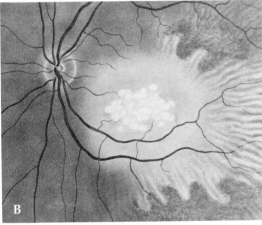

FIG. 3–35. Mixed type of residue of a retinoblastoma treated by x ray and chemotherapy. **A.** Before treatment the tumor obscured the optic disc. **B.** Three years later the central part of the tumor had regressed to a mass of calcium surrounded by a grayish zone, then by an atrophic area with the choroidal vessels and a black collar of proliferated pigment epithelium visible above and below.

least one eye. The more common endophytum type, which arises primarily from the inner layers of the retina, grows out into the vitreous cavity. Diagnosis is facilitated by the presence of actual tumor tissue for direct inspection. In contrast, the exophytum type arises from the outer layers of the retina and may not lend itself to direct inspection. When small, it appears as an indistinct, poorly demarcated, slightly grayish zone (Fig. 3–17, see p. 9). When large, the tumor grows for

the most part under the retina, ultimately causing a funnel-shaped detachment.

One portion of the detached retina may be translucent, in contrast to the relatively opaque and often calcareous remaining portion. Since no other pathologic basis for the retinal separation can be demonstrated in the vitreous or elsewhere, it is logical to conclude in such a case that some solid tissue is pushing the retina away from the underlying choroid.

In doubtful cases it may be possible to demonstrate such a relatively solid portion of a totally detached retina by ultrasonogram. Transillumination is not a helpful diagnostic aid.

DNA-CALCIUM COMPLEX

In retinoblastoma with areas of necrosis in which nuclear DNA is released, free globules of the DNA may be found in the extracellular spaces, in blood vessel walls, and in areas of calcification.[35,36] When calcium is bound to DNA, radiopaque masses may form.

The DNA-calcium complex can be recognized clinically to some degree in almost all cases of retinoblastoma and is, in fact, the most important diagnostic aid. It also serves as an index of tumor regression. The clinical appearance depends on the depth of the calcium (Fig. 3–30). When viewed directly it is pearly white and sharply demarcated; when a little below the surface it appears chalky white and the borders are poorly demarcated; when somewhat deeper it is a fuzzy white zone.

The fact that the white cottage-cheese effect appears in about the fifth week of tumor regression following treatment, and that in many cases ophthalmoscopy reveals its complete disappearance, provides evidence that DNA is largely responsible. Neither finding would be expected if calcium per se were the principal factor.

Since DNA-calcium deposition is pathognomonic of retinoblastoma, the importance of recognizing it clinically cannot be overemphasized. When diagnosis is difficult, as with the exophytum type with a funnel-shaped retinal detachment, recognition of even a small focus of calcium can be decisive. X rays can also be helpful in detecting the calcium (Fig. 3–31). In about 75% of cases it appears as a mottled, granular shadow. Fortunately, the shadows of calcium deposits due to other eye diseases either look different or are seen in a different age group.

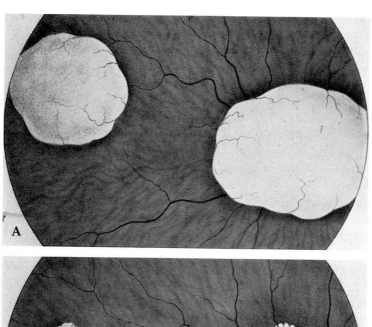

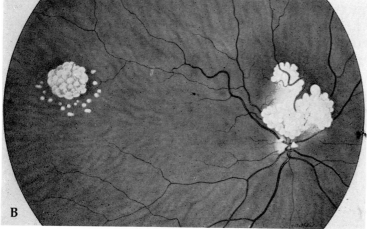

FIG. 3–36. Regression of a retinoblastoma treated by x ray and chemotherapy. **A.** Before treatment, the larger of the two foci of retinoblastoma covered the site of the disc. **B.** Six months after treatment was initiated, both tumors were reduced to a cottage-cheeselike calcium residue, and calcium seeds were seen in the surrounding vitreous.

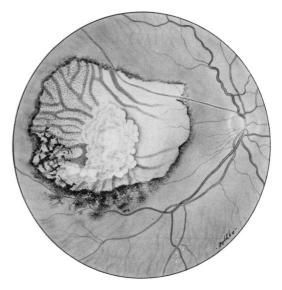

FIG. 3–37. Spontaneous regression of retinoblastoma. Typical mound of cottage-cheeselike calcium in the macular area in a 45-year-old untreated man. The surrounding atrophic zone shows the pattern of choroidal vessels. Proliferated pigment epithelium forms a collar around the lesion. (Courtesy of J. H. Dunnington.)

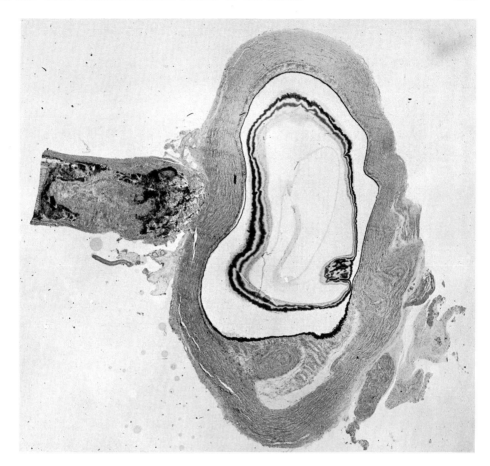

FIG. 3–38. Spontaneous regression of a retinoblastoma. Section of an eye that became phthisical because of spontaneous regression of the tumor. Among the findings was complete sterilization of the intraocular portion, whereas the portion that had invaded the optic nerve remained viable, leading to recurrence in the orbit after enucleation.

Calcium's potential for growth inhibition is suggested by its presence in necrotic areas of spontaneously regressed retinoblastomas. Absorption of the DNA-calcium takes place over a period of about one year (Figs. 3–32, 3–33).

Much rarer types of regression are a grayish-white, avascular mass smaller than the original tumor (Fig. 3–34) or a mass with a calcified center surrounded by grayish, homogeneous, avascular tissue and, beyond that, by a zone of atrophy and pigment disturbance (Fig. 3–35).

After treatment, the tumor breakdown into DNA-calcium may result in dispersion of white granules of this complex into the vitreous (Fig. 3–36) and over the periphery of the retina, especially below.

SECONDARY CHANGES

When the growth is extensive, secondary glaucoma and buphthalmos may ensue, with the lens becoming cataractous. In some instances tumor necrosis produces uveitis and endophthalmitis.

Although extensive necrosis of retinoblastoma is very common, it is less likely to give rise to an inflammatory reaction than even a small focus of necrosis of a uveal melanoma.

SPONTANEOUS REGRESSION

Many well-authenticated cases of spontaneous cure of retinoblastoma have been reported, with follow-up periods ranging from 5 to 13 years. The diagnosis was established microscopically in almost all instances.

On ophthalmoscopic examination, the spontaneously arrested lesions appear to be identical with the arrested processes we have observed in patients treated with irradiation and chemotherapy. The "crumbly, chalklike white masses"[32] or cottage-cheese appearance undoubtedly refers to the unabsorbed residual DNA-calcium content (Fig. 3–37).

Three regression patterns have been recognized[19] in treated and spontaneously regressed cases of retinoblastoma: a) Cottage-cheese appearance due to the DNA-calcium complex; tumors of about 4 dd may disappear entirely. b) Shrinkage of the tumor to a gray, homogeneous, avascular mass with atrophic pigmented annula around the base. c) Appearance combining a and b.

In a reported case[28] one eye was enucleated and the diagnosis of retinoblastoma established. The other eye became completely filled with retinoblastoma in a short time, and the globe was buphthalmic. The parents refused enucleation of the second eye. Eleven years later, during a follow-up study, the patient was found to be well and living in an institution for the blind. The eye had become phthisical, and permission was given for an enucleation. Microscopic examination revealed advanced degenerative changes, including a good deal of calcium and bone, but no evidence of viable retinoblastoma cells.

The histopathologic findings in 700 eyes with retinoblastoma from the Armed Forces Institute of Pathology files showed that 8 had healed spontaneously as the result of complete necrosis; the small shrunken globe could not be distinguished clinically from phthisis bulbi developing after either trauma or infection.[40]

In a young child the possibility of spontaneous regression of a retinoblastoma must be kept in mind as the underlying cause of an atrophic or phthisical eye that cannot be attributed to some known pathologic process, such as an injury or inflammation. Sometimes the tumor in the shrunken globe is incompletely arrested and later resumes growth, or the tumor is completely arrested but an extraocular extension remains viable and manifests itself later. In one tragic case brought to my attention the phthisical eye was removed for cosmetic reasons, there being no suspicion of retinoblastoma (Fig. 3–38). Several months later the surgeon excised what he thought to be a postoperative granuloma in the orbit but failed to examine the tissue microscopically. The lesion recurred and was excised. On microscopic examination it proved to be a retinoblastoma.

The spontaneous regression and cure of a retinoblastoma have been attributed to the tumor's outgrowing its blood supply and becoming necrotic, with toxic products in turn causing further destruction—a cycle that eventually arrests and eliminates the lesion. Although certainly not the sole cause of regression, this cycle can be a contributing factor by stimulating host-resistant antigens. A "quiet, uniform, and simultaneous regression" of three untreated tumor sites was described in one patient.[32]

TREATMENT

The treatment should be predicated on the retinoblastoma's multiple origins. When the tumor appears to diffuse throughout the retina, leaving scarcely any normal sector (Fig. 3–3), we must consider the entire retina to be potentially involved. In this event any attack on a single visible tumor focus—*e.g.*, with radiation, radon seeds or plaques, light coagulation, or diathermy—is usually destined to failure.

The problem of achieving anesthesia suitable for a 5- to 10-minute ophthalmoscopic examination of these ambulatory children has been solved by the use of Fluothane (1,1,1-trifluoro-2-bromo-2-chloroethane). Most patients can leave for home in 15 minutes; only 1% must remain longer because of vomiting. All treated patients are examined in this way at two- to four-month intervals for about three years, at five- or six-month intervals for the next two years, then annually. If they had to be hospitalized for the usual general anesthesia with its long and sometimes unpleasant recovery, this program would not be practical.

CHARTING OF LESIONS

As the principal objective at follow-up examinations is to determine whether there is evidence of regression or active growth, accurate charting of the lesions at each visit—as to size, location, DNA-calcium content, vascularity, and seeding—is important. New sites of active growth may appear on or around the previous lesion. Areas that were more or less avascular may show vascularization. An active focus is pinkish in contrast to the dull grayish white of an arrested tumor.

Treatment of retinoblastoma is discussed in two sections in Chapter 12: Diathermy,

Light Coagulation, and Cryotherapy in the Management of Intraocular Tumors, by Robert M. Ellsworth, and Radiotherapy of Ocular and Orbital Tumors, by Patricia Tretter.

Treatment is directed toward five types of cases: unilateral, bilateral, residual tumor tissue in the orbit at the time of enucleation, recurrent tumor in the orbit, and tumor extension to the cranial cavity of distal metastases.

UNILATERAL TUMOR

Unilateral cases are usually far advanced when detected except in certain circumstances, *e.g.*, when the tumor arises in or around the macula causing an esotropia which prompts the parents to seek medical advice, when a sibling of a retinoblastoma patient has an early precautionary fundal examination, or when a child of a retinoblastoma survivor has an early fundal examination.

Enucleation

Enucleation is indicated in the usual advanced unilateral case. It is important to obtain a long enough portion of optic nerve to place the operative section beyond any possible tumor extension into it. If only a 2 or 3 mm section is removed from a nerve invaded by tumor, there will probably be some cells in the remaining portion. Experience has shown that the nerve stump should be approximately 10 mm long. The following procedure should ensure an adequate length of nerve.

A heavy traction suture is passed through the insertion stumps of the internal and external rectus muscles so as to engage some of the adjacent sclera. The globe is pulled forcibly outward with the traction sutures. With the optic nerve placed under tension, the scissors blades are pressed backward along the nasal wall of the orbit. It must be remembered that the optic foramen which the optic nerve traverses in straight back along the nasal wall. The points of the scissors are therefore guided backward toward the optic foramen. When severing the nerve, care should be taken not to cut into the muscle funnel near its apex, causing excessive bleeding and allowing orbital fat to enter the funnel and thus preventing a good cosmetic result.

After the globe is enucleated, a plastic implant is placed in the muscle funnel. Al-though an implant tends to mask an early orbital recurrence of the tumor, the large majority of patients do not suffer this fate. An implant not only improves the cosmetic result but also seems to promote more normal development of the bony orbit. If the postoperative microscopic examination reveals that there is probably residual tumor tissue in the portion of the optic nerve remaining in the orbit, or microscopic examination of the eye shows choroidal extension with tumor left in the orbit, an implant of a material other than plastic is removed if radiation treatment is instituted.

Immediately after enucleation the optic nerve is severed from the globe flush with the sclera, and biopy material is prepared. Sections are cut from the proximal, distal, and central portions to determine whether there has been tumor extension and, if so, whether the nerve was severed beyond it.

If the tumor in the enucleated eye appears on gross examination to be far advanced and choroidal extension is suspected, especially if the picture is complicated by secondary glaucoma and buphthalmos, immediately prepared paraffin sections in the region of the posterior emissaria are in order, in an attempt to rule out orbital extension.

Orbital recurrence is most unlikely when microscopic sections of the optic nerve immediately after enucleation show no tumor invasion and there is no gross or microscopic evidence of extraocular tumor extension. In such cases prophylactic radiation therapy of the orbit is inadvisable. On the other hand, indications of residual tumor call for further treatment.

A combined intracranial and orbital operation for retinoblastoma was at one time advocated, in which the first step was to excise the intracranial portion of the optic nerve between the chiasm and the optic foramen.[42] In my opinion the rationale for this procedure is unsound, as it is no longer generally believed that retinoblastoma deaths are due largely if not solely to intracranial extension from the optic nerve.

Advocates of the combined intracranial and orbital operation evidently conceived of the tumor's invading the optic nerve and extending back, within its confines, to the intracranial cavity. Actually, the tumor usually extends into the nerve proper only a few millimeters posterior to the lamina cribrosa. In order to reach the cranium, it would have to extend 10 mm into the nerve and gain access

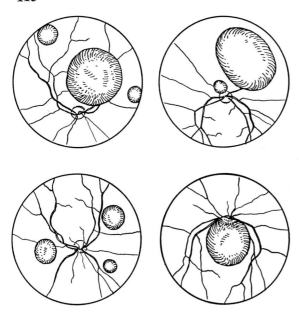

FIG. 3–39. Scale drawings of eyes, three with multiple sites of retinoblastoma, considered favorable for treatment. Radiation and chemotherapy resulted in cure with no recurrence after over ten years.

degree of differentiation of the tumor cells. The longer the tumor exists, the more undifferentiated the cytology becomes, *i.e.*, the fewer rosettes form.[12] The more differentiated tumors are less radiosensitive.[19,65] In a study of serial sections of enucleated eyes of retinoblastoma patients followed at least five years,[43] choroidal invasion was found to be both more common and less dangerous than previously believed.

The following is a classification of retinoblastomas into groups I to V with the prognosis for each:

Group I—Very favorable (Fig. 3-39)
  a. Solitary tumor, less than 4 disc diameters in size, at or behind the equator
  b. Multiple tumors, none over 4 disc diameters in size, all at or behind the equator
Group II—Favorable
  a. Solitary tumor, 4 to 10 disc diameters in size, at or behind the equator
  b. Multiple tumors, 4 to 10 disc diameters in size, behind the equator
Group III—Doubtful
  a. Any lesion anterior to the equator
  b. Solitary tumors larger than 10 disc diameters behind the equator
Group IV—Unfavorable (Fig. 3-40)
  a. Multiple tumors, some larger than 10 disc diameters
  b. Any lesion extending anteriorly to the ora serrata
Group V—Very unfavorable
  a. Massive tumors involving over half the retina
  b. Vitreous seeding

The results in 192 cases treated between 1960 and 1965 (Table 3–1) were based on Ellsworth's comprehensive study at our tumor clinic.[19]

Although the prognosis in unilateral cases should be better than in bilateral cases where there may be greater risk of metastasis and extraocular extension, in our series the overall mortality is roughly 18%–20% in both groups.

to the subarachnoid space at the site where the central vessels exit from the nerve. A tumor reaching the subarachnoid space by this route, or by direct extension from the optic nerve, spreads not only in the involved optic nerve but also to the chiasm and to various cranial sites. By this time excision of the intracranial portion of the nerve would not include the entire intracranial extension.

If biopsy material from the removed portion of the nerve is immediately prepared and examined microscopically, it will be known within hours whether or not the operative incision was made beyond any tumor extension into the nerve.

Prognosis

The prognosis for patients having had enucleation for unilateral disease is difficult to assess for several reasons. First, at the time of surgery the tumors may be either very small or large enough to fill most of the globe. Some are not detected early; the correct diagnosis may be delayed while the child is treated for other conditions, and some parents procrastinate about seeking or acting on medical advice. Still more important is the question of whether the tumor has invaded the optic nerve or reached the choroid, increasing the likelihood of orbital invasion and metastasis.

Another factor bearing on prognosis is the

BILATERAL TUMOR

Enucleation

Enucleation of both eyes is necessary when the disease is so extensive that no vision can be saved in either by any means. In fact, delay in complete eradication of the growth unquestionably increases the risk of dissemination. If the disease is allowed to take its course, the tumor's progressive growth usually leads to a painful, marked enlargement of the globes which protrude between the lids. Corneal ulceration, perforation of the globe, and sepsis often ensue, with so much local pain that both eyes must be removed to give the patient relief. Leaving in the eyes until removal is obligatory serves no useful purpose and permits the certain wide dissemination of the growth, whereas immediate bilateral enucleation may be lifesaving.

When the child's useful vision is irrevocably lost in both eyes, the parents have the choice of bilateral enucleation or allowing the disease to take its inevitably fatal course. Life expectancy is shorter when the tumor invades the cranial cavity directly or via the sinuses than when distal metastases develop.

Advocates of bilateral enucleation consider it more humane to try to cure the disease, even though the child will be blind, than to let him face a few weeks of rapidly diminishing vision before blindness ensues and then undergo severe pain before death. They feel that it is presumptuous for the parents, the physician, or a lay committee to choose death for a child rather than life without sight. Few adults even if blind since childhood would agree that death is preferable. Still some parents feel that a loved child should not have to fight for a place in this strongly competitive world without sight. The fact that they have, or can have, other children may influence their decision.

In most bilateral cases the disease is more advanced in one eye, which is enucleated, but the tumor may be arrested and useful vision salvaged in the fellow eye. This challenge has been met with varying degrees of success by treatment with different types of radiation, diathermy, light coagulation, cryotherapy, radon seeds and radioactive cobalt applicators. (See sections in Chapter 12: Radiotherapy of Ocular and Orbital Tumors, by Patricia Tretter, and Diathermy, Light Coagulation, and Cryotherapy in the Management of Intraocular Tumors, by Robert M. Ellsworth.)

Radon Seeds

Stallard[27,58] pioneered in the development of techniques for treatment of retinoblastoma by high-energy radiation from radon seeds implanted in the tumor area. It is clear from reports[25,59] that radon seeds can cure small retinoblastomas, but cobalt applicators are easier to handle and deliver a more predictable type of radiation.[20]

Orthovoltage

Although retinoblastoma is radiosensitive, the retinal tissue from which it arises is fortunately relatively radioresistant. Blood vessels supplying the retina may be affected, sometimes causing complications with large doses, but retinoblastoma is often completely devitalized by a radiation dose well tolerated by the blood vessels, skin, subcutaneous fat, and bone. It would indeed be a simple matter to arrest such a tumor if it were readily accessible to radiation and did not lie close to the radiosensitive ciliary body, lens, and cornea. A radiation dose lethal to the tumor de-

FIG. 3–40. Scale drawings of eyes with retinoblastomas considered unfavorable for treatment. **A.** This eye has six tumors of 1 to 5 dd. **B.** This eye has one tumor of at least 5 dd and a large detachment of the retina which undoubtedly concealed other sites. **C.** Three large tumors are present as well as tumor seeds in the vitreous. **D.** This eye has one small and three large tumors as well as tumor seeds in the vitreous.

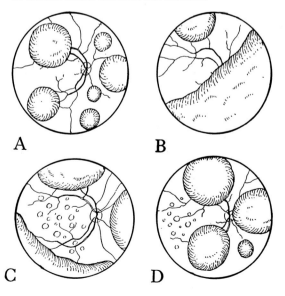

stroys the vision if it passes through the anterior chamber of the eye. Indeed, so sensitive is this sector that even a small fraction of the prescribed dose from an improperly directed beam could result in loss of the globe. The object is to direct a lethal radiation dose to the site of the lesion in the posterior sector without damaging the vulnerable anterior sector.

Chemotherapy

In the past decade there has been a revolution in cancer chemotherapy. Synergistic combinations have been developed, techniques of administration worked out, and the killing effect on tumor cells determined. Chemotherapy was formerly considered a last-resort attack on metastatic disease but is now used in early cancer.

The drugs that have proved effective are nitrogen m u s t a r d , triethylenemelamine (TEM), 5-fluorouracil, cyclophosphamide (Cytoxan), vincristine, and adriamycin. Uracil mustard, melphalan, and hydroxyurea were found to be ineffective. No systematic trials have yet been conducted.

Treatment of Primary Intraocular Disease. In the past, anticancer drugs have been given by intraarterial infusion into the carotid or ophthalmic arteries. The procedures are difficult and risky and should be used only when other methods have failed.

There is no sure way of detecting the patients at greatest risk from metastatic disease; but large tumors anteriorly or over the optic nerve, massive posterior choroidal extension, extension through the scleral emissaria, and cells on the scleral surface appear to be a threat to life. Adjuvant chemotherapy should be started soon after surgery and continued for at least 15 months in these high-risk patients even though metastasis is not clinically apparent. The treatment consists of vincristine 50μg/kg IV and cyclophosphamide (Cytoxan 30 mg/kg IV, both on day 1. This cycle is repeated at 21-day intervals for 15 months.

Treatment of Extraocular Extension and Widespread Metastatic Disease. Children with orbital disease or metastatic disease outside of the CNS are treated by excisional biopsy followed by orbital irradiation (5000 rads to the entire orbit). They are given vincristine 50μg/

kg IV, Cytoxan 20 mg/kg IV, and adriamycin 2 mg/kg IV on day 1 and day 21. These three agents are repeated at 21-day intervals from day 1 for 15 months, except that adriamycin is discontinued after the cumulative dose reaches 16 mg/kg.

A third group includes patients with gross or microscopic disease at the cut end of the optic nerve or other CNS involvement. If the disease is limited to microscopic evidence of involvement of the cut end of the optic nerve, 5000 rads is delivered to the orbit. However, if there is gross involvement of the cut end of the optic nerve or more extensive disease of the CNS 3000 rads is delivered to the entire brain besides 5000 rads to the orbit. Both of these patient groups are given six doses of methotrexate 0.5 mg/kg intrathecally at weekly intervals beginning on day 1.

Patients with widespread metastatic disease may have long remissions on anticancer drugs. It is hoped that the above-described drug regimens will reduce the present high mortality rate.

Follow-up Period

Five years has been generally considered the minimal period for a cancer "cure." We feel that the chance of resumed growth is extremely remote after three years in retinoblastoma patients. Since the tumor is in transparent media and usually is entirely visible with the ophthalmoscope using magnification, in most instances six months is adequate to tell whether it has been arrested. We have seen rare cases showing active growth after one to two years. In two of three "freak" cases there was recurrent growth in the bones and soft tissues around the orbit 6 and 18 years after x-ray treatment; the third patient developed intractable glaucoma 9 years later, leading to enucleation, and had a recurrent tumor in the nose and sinuses after another 5-year period.

It is difficult to explain this late tumor activation, but some retinoblastoma cells must remain in a state of suspended viability for many years, as reported in other types of cancer. For example, patients with malignant melanoma of the uvea have developed the disease in the liver or other structures 20 to 25 years after enucleation. In one of our cases, retinoblastoma was arrested for 8 years after completion of treatment. The patient had 20/20 vision and attended school during

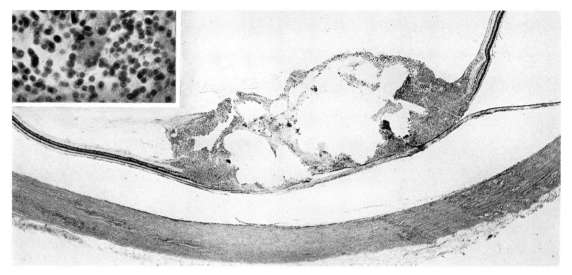

FIG. 3–41. Section of an eye with retinoblastoma treated by radiation. The tumor was arrested for eight years; the patient had normal vision and attended school. He then developed a fatal rhabdomyosarcoma in the temporal muscle over the site of the temporal portal. On examination of the eye, obtained at autopsy, the majority of the tumor mass had been reduced to calcium which dropped out during preparation of the section, accounting for the clear central areas. Inset shows tumor cells at the periphery of the calcium, which do not appear necrotic although they had lost their growth potential.

this time. He then developed a postradiation rhabdomyosarcoma in the temporalis muscle over the site of the temporal radiation portal, which proved fatal. Microscopic examination of the eye revealed that the radiated retinoblastoma was composed of calcium and tumor cells that appeared viable but for 8 years had evidently lost their power to proliferate (Fig. 3–41).

Reduced vision after irradiation for retinoblastoma may be mistakenly interpreted as regrowth of the tumor, whereas it actually stems from hemorrhage secondary to postradiation vascular changes.[7]

Management of Patients Responding Poorly to Initial Treatment

Anoxic cells, both normal and neoplastic, have long been known to be less radiosensitive than well-oxygenated cells. Also, retinoblastomas are thought to have a relatively poor blood supply, as evidenced by necrosis and calcification.

Six children in our clinic who had not responded to two courses of radiation were treated with hyperbaric oxygen radiation. Despite some dramatic results we are not now using this method, which is extremely complicated, time-consuming, and has a considerable element of risk.

In some retinoblastoma cases resistant to treatment, the cells are possibly differentiated into complete or partial rosettes, placing them in the category of neuroepitheliomas, which are less amenable than undifferentiated tumors.

Some retinoblastomas resume growth after one type of treatment but respond well to another. In very far advanced and seemingly hopeless cases, perseverance with treatment is justified on the premise that the body may develop some host resistance to the tumor. If it can be controlled to some degree until this immunizing process shares the battle, an unexpected cure sometimes results. That such an antigenic process has come to the rescue is attested by well-documented spontaneous remissions in cases not only of retinoblastoma but also of neuroblastoma.

Choroidal Extension After Irradiation

A tumor that reaches the highly vascular choroid grows rapidly and responds poorly to irradiation. This complication in the choroid may be first noted clinically six to nine months after treatment is initiated. A diffuse, yellowish-white, elevated area sometimes appears along the border of or encircling the previously observed retinal lesion, or adjacent to the disc. It continues to broaden and heighten until the large globular mass protrudes into the vitreous. The retinal tumor may be identified on its surface.

The following case shows the typical course of choroidal involvement: A large area of retinoblastoma occupied the lower temporal portion of the right fundus, and a number of tumor fragments floated in the vitreous. Regression was satisfactory after two months of radiotherapy. Then around the main lesion, composed largely of dense, pearly-white areas of calcium, appeared a condition first interpreted as a retinal detachment. The fundal picture no longer resembled retinoblastoma. After another month what seemed to be a large bullous retinal detachment had developed over the temporal half of the fundus where, far toward the periphery, the site of the retinal growth was visible as a localized area of calcium extending over the protruding retinal surface. Still another month later, the supposed bullous detachment was larger and more elevated, and a wide disinsertion was noted. At this point, arrested retinoblastoma with wide secondary retinal detachment was diagnosed.

Three weeks later the patient had his last radiation treatment. Within 12 hours he developed glaucoma with sudden severe pain in the eye. At his monthly checkup, a week after this complication, the interior of the eye could not be visualized. Many blood vessels were noted in the iris; the anterior chamber was shallow and the iris seemed pushed forward against the cornea at 12 o'clock. An enucleation without implant was performed five months after treatment was started. The pathology report showed retinoblastoma with extension into the choroid and secondary glaucoma (Fig. 3–10).

RESIDUAL TUMOR

A distinction should be made between residual and recurrent retinoblastoma in the orbit. If proper measures are taken in cases of residual cancer, the prognosis is good. However, if the cancer recurs the prognosis is extremely poor. A subtotal exenteration is often curative in patients with residual orbital cancer, but even a total exenteration is usually ineffective in those with recurrent orbital cancer.

RECURRENT TUMOR IN THE ORBIT

A recurrence of the tumor in the orbit results from a residual tumor focus that was undetected until it grew sufficiently to be visible or palpable. This occurs from tumor left in the optic nerve or from extraocular extension a few months after enucleation, even though random sections of the globe revealed neither extension of the tumor through the emissaria nor involvement of the optic nerve. A few tumor cells had obviously extended beyond the globe and would have been noticed in serial sections, which should always be prepared when the choroid is invaded.

An appreciable number of patients with orbital recurrence probably have developed distal metastatic foci that were undetected; therefore local treatment would be unavailing. But since heroic treatment occasionally succeeds, it should be undertaken. In one authenticated cure, a lesion confirmed by biopsy had been treated over a 3½-year period by exenteration, x ray, and intramuscular TEM. Our series includes two cures 7 and 20 years, respectively, after exenteration and irradiation, but unfortunately no biopsy was taken from the orbital mass in either instance. These three cases are the only ones with a favorable outcome among 32 patients treated for recurrent retinoblastoma of the orbit.

METASTASES

Metastases are treated palliatively by pursuing the sites as they are detected. If untreated the areas may enlarge sufficiently to ulcerate, with a foul-smelling discharge. Although the treatment is admittedly hopeless, it seems advisable for the patient's comfort during his remaining months of life. Three children, two from our series and one from Memorial Hospital For Cancer and Allied Diseases, New York, have survived six months, one year, and nearly two years, respectively, with metastases.

Metastatic foci may appear simultaneously with orbital recurrence. Occasionally, if the size and location of the lesion permit, radiation can be given through the same portals as when the frontal, temporal, and maxillary bones are invaded. In other instances separate portals are required, with the risk of overlapping of the treatment areas.

Most of the areas requiring treatment are in the face, skull, or long bones. When the jaw is being treated, strict oral hygiene measures must be observed because of the considerable reaction in the mucous membranes. Such patients, who are usually hospitalized, need frequent mouthwashing and cleansing of ulcerated areas.

Depilation occurs when the skull is treated. After a few treatments, the underlying lesion may no longer be palpable.

Visceral metastases rarely achieve a size to be appreciated clinically, and do not seem to interfere with function. Because new metastatic foci continue to appear, the dosage to any one site should be kept as low as possible. The larger the area, the lower the total dose. Reduction in the size of tumor foci in the mandible frequently relieves trismus, enabling the patient to eat solid food.

ASSOCIATED INTRACRANIAL MALIGNANCY

In addition to a tendency to develop soft-tissue malignant tumors, children with hereditary retinoblastoma may carry the risk of developing independent malignant tumors of the central nervous system.[26a]

CAUSES OF DEATH

Retinoblastoma is by no means purely local or confined to the eye and cranium; this highly malignant disease tends to be disseminated widely by way of the bloodstream.

In an analysis of 17 autopsies performed at the Institute of Ophthalmology and the Memorial Center for Cancer and Allied Diseases,[33] it was found that while 91% of the patients had some form of intracranial involvement, only 47% died with the disease confined to the head or spinal cord. In the remaining 53%, the lymph nodes were involved in 47%, the skull bones in 53%, distal bones in 53%, and the viscera in 47%.

Figures from another center agree closely.[12] Metastasis to the distal bones was common. In one described case[14] the tumor spread from one eye by direct continuity to the meningeal sheaths and optic nerve of the opposite eye.

Retinoblastoma patients who survive their original tumor have a high incidence of second nonocular malignancies, appearing between 1 and 40 years after successful treatment of the original lesion. A review of 2309 cases in our clinic and in the files of the Armed Forces Institute of Pathology revealed that the second tumors occurred almost exclusively in patients who had had bilateral disease and were 85% fatal. These tumors were osteogenic sarcomas (usually of the femur), fibrosarcomas, and less commonly malignant melanomas, basal-cell carcinomas, and rhabdomyosarcomas. It is estimated that children who have survived after treatment of retinoblastoma are about 300 times more likely than the rest of the population to develop osteogenic sarcoma of the femur and 1000 times more likely to have osteogenic sarcoma of the skull.

From this study it can be anticipated that 15%–20% of children who survive after treatment for bilateral retinoblastoma will develop a second fatal neoplasm years afterward.[1]

OTHER NEUROECTODERMAL TUMORS OF THE RETINA

Some authors[39] have used the widely accepted term *glioma* to include all brain tumors of neuroectodermal origin, from the well-differentiated astrocytomas to the highly undifferentiated spongioblastomas and medulloblastomas. They offered the following classification of gliomas of the retina: a) the retinoblastoma type—the highly undifferentiated tumors resembling neuroblastomas or medulloblastomas; b) the neuroepithelioma type—tumors showing slight or partial differentiation, as indicated by the rosette or fibril formation that characterizes the primitive spongioblastic cell; and c) the astrocytoma type—well-differentiated tumors, very rare in the retina, and composed primarily of cells nearly as well differentiated as the normal astrocyte.

Following the same general pattern, another author[9] graded these tumors from IV to I: grade IV, the usual retinoblastomas with no cell differentiation; grade III, tumors indicating differentiation by either complete or partial rosette or fibril formation; grade II, an indeterminate group showing more differentiation; and grade I, true gliomas composed of more or less mature astrocytes.

NEUROEPITHELIOMA

Neuroepitheliomas, or rather the neuroepitheliomatous type of retinoblastoma, tend to arise in the external nuclear layers of the retina. They do not occur in pure form; their cellular characteristics and rosette formation are noted only in certain areas of the tumor, which are always composed principally of retinoblasts. Some degree of rosette formation is seen in about half of all retinoblastomas, although it rarely predominates and is never present throughout the tumor. This type of retinoblastoma is comparable with the very rare neuroepithelioma of the brain, in which the same kind of rosette formation is found.

MEDULLOEPITHELIOMA

The highly undifferentiated medulloepitheliomas of the central nervous system are far more malignant than the relatively differentiated medulloepitheliomas of the eye. (See Chapter 2, Epithelial Tumors of the Uvea.)

RETINAL ANLAGE TUMOR

The retinal anlage tumor—also called pigmented retinoblastoma, retinoblastic teratoma, melanotic progonoma, and pigmented ameloblastoma—seems to be composed of tissue elements of the embryonic retina: pigmented cells and neurocytes. The pigment-bearing cells resemble primitive retinal pigment epithelium. The arrangement of the neurocytes suggests crude optic vesicles, and neurofibrils can be demonstrated by Cajal's stain.

These tumors are generally believed to arise from misplaced retinal anlagen. In reported cases they were noted in the first year of life, and the course was benign. Almost all arose in the maxilla, but a few involved the mandible and other sites such as the anterior fontanelle, the epididymis, the fourth ventricle, the uterus and ovaries, and the soft parts of the shoulder.

Before they were characterized as retinal anlage tumors,[23] they were considered a peculiar type of melanoma whose exact nature was unknown or odontogenic lesions called melanoameloblastoma.[53] They have occurred in the orbit and been mistaken for melanomas. In any event, it is well to be alert to their possible presence in or around the eye.

GENETICS OF RETINOBLASTOMA

F. David Kitchin

In a biologic situation as complicated as retinoblastoma, it is hardly surprising that the genetic features were slow to be appreciated. Retinoblastoma is a malignant neoplasm expressed in early life and, when untreated, kills before sexual maturity. Thus, even in this century when mendelian genetics were being avidly applied to man, most examples of retinoblastoma were found to be sporadic, and only a few familial. Those rare families that did show vertical transmission down through the generations did so because survivors into adult life had been generated by therapeutic enucleation, a failure of the gene to manifest itself fully (low penetrance), or the rare occurrence of self-curative spontaneous regression.

Over the years the slow accumulation of hereditary data, combined with better diagnosis and increased survival, have permitted more precise analysis. Information is now available concerning the incidence of the disease within populations, the manner of transmission, and the penetrance of the gene, as well as its locus and associated effects. Furthermore, it has become apparent that the disease behaves differently in those affected unilaterally and those affected bilaterally, not only in the proportion of each kind in the population, but also in the numbers of sporadic and familial examples within each group. Particularly, it has been realized that sporadic unilateral retinoblastoma is not a homogeneous category, but probably represents a mixture of germinal and somatic mutations.

FREQUENCY OF RETINOBLASTOMA

In various population surveys, including Germany, Ireland, Japan, the Netherlands, Switzerland, the United Kingdom, and the United States from 1950 to 1960, estimates of frequency have been made that ranged from 1 in 30,000 to 1 in 15,000 live births.

Since the frequency of a dominant trait in a population is a measure of an equilibrium between the rate at which abnormal genes are being produced (mutation) and the rate at which they are eliminated by lowered reproductive rate (biologic fitness), it would seem likely that the equilibrium has altered in recent years. Many more children who are the recipients of germinal mutations now survive to reproductive years and can contribute abnormal genes to future generations. The increase in the frequency that necessarily ensues has been shown in the data from a survey in the Netherlands that is noteworthy for its completeness. In 1927–1929 the frequency was 1 in 34,000 live births, and in the years 1950–1959 it was 1 in 15,230. Since the mutation rate probably remains static, the most likely explanation is increased biologic fitness. Theoretically, if the fitness increases from zero, i.e., 100% early mortality, to about 50% normal, then a new equilibrium will be reached where the frequency of the gene in the population is about four times the mutation rate. In retinoblastoma, the lowest estimate of mutation rate $m = 6$–7×10^{-6} per locus per generation, or 1 in 71,000 children born has the mutation, which will increase at $4m$ to about 1 in 17,000 children. These figures, of course, apply only to the genetic form of retinoblastoma, since it is assumed that somatic mutation occurs in a population at a relatively fixed rate and makes no contribution to the frequency in subsequent generations.

Therefore, we can be reasonably certain that improved treatment and survival will not increase the frequency of the disease alarmingly, provided we assure a biologic fitness held at about 50%–70% of normal. This it would seem possible to achieve by careful genetic counseling.

FAMILIAL RETINOBLASTOMA

In families with a clear concentration of examples of retinoblastoma, pedigree analysis reveals whether the gene is expressed in the heterozygous state, so-called dominant inheritance, or only in the homozygous state, recessive inheritance.

Since the foundation of the Eye Tumor Clinic at the Edward S. Harkness Eye Institute, New York, some 108 sibships have been documented, representing 10% of all cases

TABLE 3–1. Results of 192 Cases of Retinoblastoma (1960–1965)

	Number of cases	Cure rate (%)
Group I	20	95
Group II	32	87
Group III	24	67
Group IV	32	69
Group V	74	34
Orbit	10	30

TABLE 3–2. Retinoblastoma Pedigrees

	Sibships		
	New York*	Nether-landst	Total
1. Affected parent			
Bilateral	28	7	35
Unilateral	35	11	46
2. Normal parent			
Distant relatives affected	30		30
Two or more affected sibs	15		15
	108	18	126

* Edward S. Harkness Eye Institute, Columbia-Presbyterian Medical Center.
† Schappert-Kimmijser, J., Hemmes, G.D., and Nijland, R. (1966).[76]

TABLE 3–3. Bilaterality in Hereditary Retinoblastoma

Pedigree type	Bilaterality in affected children (%)
1. Affected parent	
Bilateral	95
Unilateral	92
2. Normal parents	
Distant relatives affected	83
Two or more affected sibs	60

TABLE 3–4. Manifestation (2p) of Retinoblastoma

Sibship type	No.	2p	SE
Selected*			
Parent affected			
Bilaterally	28	86.1% (113.4)	26.5
Unilaterally	25	46.7% (60.4)	20.2
Carrier	45	40.9%	11.7
Unselected†	11	98.4%	23.1

* With a propositus or a parent or grandparent of a propositus.
† With an affected parent but not containing a propositus, parent or grandparent of a propositus.
Figures in parentheses refer to the pedigrees published from the Netherlands (Table 3–2).

seen. They have been divided into several categories: those with a parent affected bilaterally or unilaterally and those with normal parents, further subdivided into those with or without distant relatives affected, i.e., carrier and putative carrier parents (Table 3–2).

In sibships with an affected parent, the children are almost always affected bilaterally, but in sibships with phenotypically normal parents the proportion drops substantially—a finding suggesting that modifying factors may be operating within this class (Table 3–3).

The general vertical pattern of the kindreds and the finding of five examples of three-generation pedigrees is consistent with a hypothesis of dominant transmission in the majority of families, with the exception of the sibships with two or more affected children and normal parents. Here the pattern is horizontal and suggests the possibility of recessive inheritance.

These hypotheses can be tested by segregation analysis, which in essence calculates the ratio (p) of affected to unaffected within each sibship, after due allowance has been made statistically for the biases of selection, the number of ascertainments, and sibship size.[72] The segregation ratio (p) of each class of sibships can be calculated and compared with the expected value for autosomal dominant inheritance, $p = 0.5$, and recessive inheritance, $p = 0.25$, with manifestation or penetrance $2p$.

The results of such analysis confirm the hypothesis of dominant inheritance in families where the parent is affected bilaterally ($p = 0.43$, manifestation 86%) and for unselected families ($p = 0.49$, manifestation 98%). The unilaterally affected parents, however, have fewer affected children, $p = 0.23–0.32$, manifestation 46%–60%, even though the children usually have bilateral disease. In the sibships with carrier parents, if we assume dominant inheritance, a similarly low manifestation, $2p = 0.40$, is found.

In the sibships with clear vertical transmission, we have to fall back on an explanation of modifying genes at other loci, or environmental factors as yet undetermined, to account for this low manifestation. In the sibships with a horizontal pattern, recessive inheritance cannot be entirely excluded, but if entertained certain consequences ensue and will be discussed later. The results appear in Table 3–4.

SPORADIC RETINOBLASTOMA

Rare dominant traits, when lethal at an early age, do not allow familial aggregations to occur, so that the majority of examples in a population would be expected to be sporadic. Thus, if children with sporadic retinoblastoma are the expression of the first germinal mutation in the family, the hypothesis would be tested by examining the proportion of affected to unaffected children they produce if they survive to adulthood and procreate. Several such studies have been done; the most complete and unbiased are summarized in Table 3–5 where the survivors have been divided into bilateral and unilateral examples of the disease.

These data clearly show that adult bilateral survivors behave as recipients of a germinal mutation, since affected and unaffected children are produced in equal proportions. Unilateral survivors do not behave this way, although they do show a concentration of affected children in a certain number of families. Using the data of Schappert-Kimmijser et al.[76] (Table 3–5), we can calculate, from the manifestation previously derived from our unilateral familial cases (46%), that a further 5 families would by chance have had no affected children, in spite of carrying the mutation. Thus, in this group of sporadic unilateral retinoblastoma survivors, 15 (10 + 5) families (23%) were probably germinal mutations, and 53 families (77%) with no affected children were possibly somatic mutations.

These calculations do not totally exclude the possibility of an extremely poorly penetrant dominant mutation, but to account for such a finding we should have to postulate a manifestation as low as 18%, and this is inconsistent with the data collected from our

TABLE 3–6. Retinoblastoma Type and Laterality (%)

	Bilateral	Unilateral	Total
Hereditary	25–30	15–20	40–50
Nonhereditary	0	50–60	50–60
Total	25–30	70–75	100

families. One further explanation that concerns the nature of the mutational event will be discussed later.

The proportion of examples of retinoblastoma that are clearly due to a germinal mutation expressed in the heterozygous state to those in which there is no evidence of a germinal mutation is shown in Table 3–6.

CHROMOSOMAL DEFECTS AND RETINOBLASTOMA

The numerous chromosomal studies of unselected cases of retinoblastoma have shown no consistent abnormalities. However, in the genetic literature there have been several examples of a syndrome of multiple congenital defects with deletion of a small portion of the long arm of one of the D group (Nos. 13–15) chromosome. This syndrome, designated Dq-, has been associated with retinoblastoma in slightly over half the reported cases and recently was reported in one example of a related D chromosome abnormality, Dr (ring chromosome of the D group).

These children have many congenital defects that first prompted the chromosome analysis. The defects involve many systems and include psychomotor retardation, skeletal abnormalities (e.g., small or absent thumbs), eye defects (e.g., microphthalmia, coloboma,

TABLE 3–5. Retinoblastoma in Children of Survivors of Sporadic Retinoblastoma

Author	No. of parents	Having healthy children	Having affected children	No. of children	Healthy	Affected
Bilateral						
Vogel (1957)[78]	2	2	0	3	3	0
Schappert-Kimmijser et al. (1966)[76]	7	2	5	22	10	12
Ellsworth (1969)[71]	5	3	2	5	3	2
Sorsby (1972)[77]	10	3	7	14	6	8
	24	10	14	44	22	22
Unilateral						
Schappert-Kimmijser et al. (1966)[76]	68	58	10	177	161	16

ptosis, epicanthus), congenital heart disease, and renal and alimentary abnormalities.

In one example[79] the affected chromosome has been identified by using Giemsa banding methods, and it appears that a small subterminal portion of the long arm of chromosome 13 is missing. This evidence seems to suggest that the locus for retinoblastoma is on the long arm of chromosome 13 and that in some children the mutational event is a microscopically visible deletion of this locus. Theoretically, deletions in chromosomes can be as small as single base deletion of the DNA strand giving rise to a frame-shift abnormality, or large enough to be visible under the light microscope. In the latter case one would anticipate associated defects (such as psychomotor retardation), since a large portion of the genome is affected.

To this end it has long been recognized that retinoblastoma families have a five- to ten-fold higher incidence of mental retardation than normal families. This increase may be accounted for by assuming that in some children rather more than a point mutation of the DNA has occurred and that the mental retardation is the consequence of either the addition or subtraction of a sizable portion of the total genome.

It is also possible that the deleted portion of the chromosome is not lost completely but translocated to another chromosome. The possibility of balanced translocation gives rise to the interesting likelihood of irregular transmission, below theoretical proportions, due to gamete selection. In this event a sperm or ovum carrying the abnormal genetic complement is at a disadvantage during fertilization. If the normal or the balanced complement results, the children will be phenotypically normal, but if the unbalanced form segregates, the resulting children will either have a deletion of, or be trisomic for, a small portion of the long arm of chromosome 13.

Such occurrences could account for the not inconsiderable number of families with sporadic retinoblastoma that have on exhaustive inquiry been shown to be linked by common distant ancestors to other families with sporadic cases. Several pedigrees of this kind have been published,[75] and the manifestation is calculated to be as low as 20% in those families with collateral cases of retinoblastoma and common ancestors. A balanced translocation in a parent could also explain the occasional occurrence of children with the features of trisomy 13 who apparently have normal chromosomes, since the translocated portion of the long arm may not be large enough to be easily recognized microscopically unless banding stains are used. Such situations are illustrated in Figure 3–42.

MUTATION AND RETINOBLASTOMA

As discussed earlier the majority of examples of familial retinoblastoma seem to result from the inheritance of a single major gene expressed in the heterozygous state. But if we conclude from the chromosome evidence that the mutation in retinoblastoma is a deletion of one gene at a locus, we are faced with a puzzling genetic situation, for the locus consists of two homologous genes on paired chromosomes. Two hypotheses might satisfy these conditions.

1. The deletion of a dominant allele releases the restraint on a remaining recessive abnormal allele, and allows unhindered gene expression in the hemizygous state. From this it follows that in subsequent generations the children of such parents will be phenotypically normal and carriers of one recessive allele. Expression of the recessive allele in future generations requires either a further mutation that deletes the dominant allele or development of the homozygous state. The latter can be achieved only by the mating of two heterozygotes. Generally speaking, in rare recessive diseases, an undue proportion of consanguineous marriages is usually found. This has not been demonstrated in any published pedigrees of retinoblastoma and makes recessive inheritance an unlikely explanation.

2. The second explanation requires a second mutation at the retinoblastoma locus postzygotically (somatic mutation), which effectively interferes with the function of the remaining normal gene; a two-mutation or "two-hit" hypothesis. In the familial form of retinoblastoma the first hit would be a germinal mutation which renders all cells in the zygote defective, and the second hit would occur in some of these genetically preconditioned retinal cells. In the nonhereditary form of the disease both mutations are assumed to be somatic and to occur in a single retinal cell at some period before these cells become permanently postmitotic, i.e., in early infancy.

Evidence has been offered to support the hypothesis of a "two-hit" generation of neoplasia by an ingenious statistical analysis.[74]

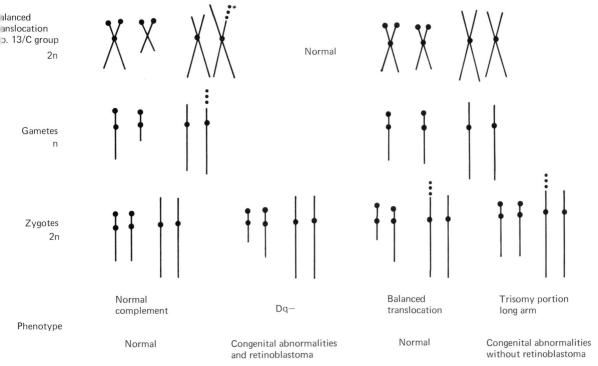

Balanced
translocation
o. 13/C group
2n

Normal

Gametes
n

Zygotes
2n

| Normal complement | Dq− | Balanced translocation | Trisomy portion long arm |

Phenotype

| Normal | Congenital abnormalities and retinoblastoma | Normal | Congenital abnormalities without retinoblastoma |

FIG. 3–42. Chromosome translocation and retinoblastoma. Asterisk indicates that the deleted long arm of No. 13 (dotted) is translocated from the second pair to the short arm of a C group chromosome.

This author calculated that the mutation rate for both hits is approximately the same. In the hereditary form of the disease, with an initial germinal mutation, all retinal cells are at risk and so it is usual for the neoplasms to be multicentric and expressed bilaterally in early life. In our series the mean number of tumors distributed between the two eyes in bilateral cases is five. In the nonhereditary dual somatic mutation form, it is likely that the neoplasm represents a clone derived from one retinal cell and thus is unicentric and expressed at a somewhat later time in development. At present there is no direct evidence for a monoclonal origin of nonhereditary retinoblastoma, but technical methods are available for testing the hypothesis. There is, in addition, no evidence concerning the cause of the mutation and whether it is due to one or more of the main classes of mutagens, viruses, chemicals, or ionizing radiation.

ASSOCIATED EFFECTS OF THE RETINOBLASTOMA GENE

It is a genetic commonplace to recognize that the effects of a single abnormal gene may be extremely varied. Unrelated effects are re-ferred to as pleiotropic and are seen at a clinical level in many dominantly inherited conditions. The syndrome Dq- previously described is not quite in this class, since many genes are probably eliminated by the deletion, but it is now becoming apparent that survivors of retinoblastoma, after a long latent period, seem to be at risk for further neoplasms.

A careful follow-up of children treated at the Edward S. Harkness Eye Institute has revealed a disturbingly large number of such cases. In the majority, the second neoplasm occurred in the field of radiation, and since early radiation doses were high, a certain number of radiation-induced neoplasms were expected. But in a number of cases a second neoplasm was observed outside the radiation field, even in children who had received no radiotherapy. In particular, the incidence of osteogenic sarcoma of the long bones (9 cases) was striking and statistically highly significant. These findings are shown in Table 3–7.

TABLE 3–7. Second Tumors in Bilateral Retinoblastoma Survivors (n ~ 800)

Type	Within radiation field	Outside field	Total
Sarcoma			
Soft tissue	17	1	18
Bone	18	9	27
Thyroid		2*	2
Wilms's tumor		1	1
Ewing's tumor		2	2
Epidermoid tumor	2		2
Astrocytoma, benign		1	1
Malignant melanoma		1	1
Unclassifiable	2		2
	39	17	56

* Includes one unilateral case.
Kitchin and Ellsworth, 1975.[73]

The most outstanding feature of the analysis was that all but one of the children who developed a second primary neoplasm had the hereditary form of the disease. Consequently, it is difficult to avoid the conclusion that the retinoblastoma gene has pleiotropic effects, one of which is to increase the liability to neoplastic change at sites other than the eye, of which the most frequent is osteogenic sarcoma of long bones.

GENETIC COUNSELING

It is quite clear that the risks vary with the different genetic situations in each family.

Familial Retinoblastoma

If the retinoblastoma patient is a familial case, i.e., a parent or one or more siblings affected, each of his children will have a 50% or 1 in 2 chance of receiving the mutant gene. The manifestation of the disease is sufficiently high to make any modification of these odds of no practical importance. Although we found lower manifestation in the children of a unilaterally affected or carrier parent, cautious genetic counseling is indicated for their children because no data are yet available, and the risk should be considered 1 in 2.

An unaffected subject in a hereditary situation has a chance of carrying the gene for retinoblastoma but not manifesting its effects. The chances of being a carrier, if calculated from the lowest level of manifestation, are

found to be 1 in 8 with a 5% or 1 in 20 chance of the children of the carrier developing retinoblastoma.

We do not advise parents whether or not to have children, but give the odds and qualify them. A 1 in 2 risk we consider high and 1 in 20 or less we consider low, inasmuch as there is a 1 in 50 general overall risk of any pregnancy resulting in a serious congenital or developmental abnormality. We point out the usual time when the disease becomes clinically apparent and advise that any newborn child at risk should have an ophthalmologic examination, with dilatation of the pupils, within the first two days. If the findings are normal, a more extensive examination with scleral indentation under general anesthesia is usually done a month to six weeks later. The frequency of subsequent examinations will depend on the findings at that time.[7]

Sporadic Retinoblastoma

Unilateral. About 20% of sporadic cases of unilateral retinoblastoma (Table 3–6) are due to germinal mutations that by chance affect only one eye. The remaining 80% are not hereditary (somatic mutations) and cannot transmit the disease. We cannot separate these classes, except when multiple discrete tumors are seen in one eye, in which case it is highly unlikely that more than one clone of cells could arise by somatic mutation alone. Thus, multiple unilateral disease represents a germinal mutation and the parents are counseled accordingly. For the remainder the combined chance of having an affected child is about 1 in 12 or 8% an intermediate risk category. As in the hereditary group, careful regular ophthalmologic examination is advised. Production of an affected child reveals the hereditary basis, and all subsequent children will fall into the high-risk group, 1 in 2.

Bilateral. A bilaterally affected patient (Table 3–4) has received a germinal mutation, and his children will be in the high-risk group, 1 in 2.

In two situations the risk figures are empirical: a) In a family with one affected child and no other members with retinoblastoma, there is a chance of subsequent children being affected since one parent may be a carrier. There is no way to identify such a person, but this seems to be a rare possibility. Extensive data from the Netherlands show that only 1.1% of subsequent children were affected. However, results of one study indicate a slightly higher risk in bilateral rather than in unilateral sporadic cases. Before counseling, it is imperative to examine both parents for evidence of spontaneous regression. b) There is also the rare possibility that an unaffected sibling of a child with sporadic retinoblastoma, like one of his parents, may be a carrier. Although few data are available, the risk appears to be extremely low, 1 in 100 or less.

REFERENCES

1. ABRAMSON DH, ELLSWORTH RM, ZIMMERMAN LE: Nonocular cancer in retinoblastoma survivors. Trans Am Acad Ophthalmol Otolaryngol (in press)
2. ARSENI C, OPRESCO I: Unusual anatomo-clinical aspects in a case of retinoblastoma. Ann Anat Pathol 4:129–135, 1959
3. ASHTON N: Larval granulomatosis of the retina due to Toxocara. Br J Ophthalmol 44:129–148, 1960
4. BAILEY P, CUSHING H: A Classification of the Tumors of the Glioma Group on a Histologic Basis with a Correlated Study of Prognosis. Philadelphia, Lippincott, 1926
5. BARRY G, MULLANEY J: Retinoblastoma in the Republic of Ireland (1955–1970). Trans Ophthalmol Soc UK 91:839–855, 1971
6. BINDER PS: Unusual manifestations of retinoblastoma. Am J Ophthalmol 77:674–679, 1974
7. BLODI FC, WATZKE RC: A clinicopathologic report on treated retinoblastoma. Am J Ophthalmol 71:193–197, 1971
8. BONIUK M, GIRARD LJ: Spontaneous regression of bilateral retinoblastoma. Trans Am Acad Ophthalmol Otolaryngol 73:194–198, 1969
9. BRODERS AC: Practical points on the microscopic grading of carcinoma. New York J Med 32:667–671, 1932
10. BROWN, DH: The urinary excretion of vanilmandelic acid (VMA) and homovanillic acid (HVA) in children with retinoblastoma. Am J Ophthalmol 62:239–243, 1966
11. BROWN DH: Ocular Toxocara canis. Part II. Clinical review. J Pediatr Ophthalmol 7:182–191, 1970
12. CARBAJAL UM: Metastasis in retinoblastoma. Am J Ophthalmol 48:47–69, 1959
13. COGAN DG, KUWABARA T: Ocular pathology of the 13–15 trisomy syndrome. Arch Ophthalmol 72:246–253, 1964
14. DEBUEN S: Retinoblastoma with spread by direct continuity to the contralateral optic nerve. Am J Ophthalmol 49: 815–819, 1960
15. DEBUEN S, FENTON RH: Coloboma of the optic disk mistaken clinically for retinoblastoma. Survey Ophthalmol 10:7–14, 1965
16. DEVRIES WM: Het oog van den zuigeling. Ned Tijdschr Geneeskd 1:325, 1901
17. DUNPHY EB: The story of retinoblastoma. Trans Am Acad Ophthalmol Otolaryngol 68:249–264, 1964
18. ELDRIDGE R, O'MEARA K, KITCHIN D: Superior intelligence in sighted retinoblastoma patients and their families. J Med Genet 9:331–335, 1972
19. ELLSWORTH RM: The practical management of retinoblastoma. Trans Am Ophthalmol Soc 67: 462–534, 1969
20. ELLSWORTH RM: Personal communication
21. FALLS HF, NEEL JV: Genetics of retinoblastoma. Arch Ophthalmol 46:367–389, 1951
22. GRINKER RR: Gliomas of the retina, including the results of studies with silver impregnations. Arch Ophthalmol 5:920–935, 1931
23. HALPERT B, PATZER R: Maxillary tumor of retinal anlage. Surgery 22:837–841, 1947
24. HATA B: Glioma development in aging eye into which the cornea of a glioma patient has been transplanted. Acta Soc Ophthalmol Jap 43:1763, 1929.
25. HENDERSON JW, VAN HERIK M: Multicentric unilateral retinoblastoma treatment by radon with seven-year cure. Am J Ophthalmol 61:1140–1145, 1966
26. IRVINE WC, IRVINE AR: Nematode endophthalmitis with Toxocara canis. Am J Ophthalmol 47:185–191, 1959
26a. JAKOBIEC FA, TS'O MOM, DANIS P, ZIMMERMAN LE: Retinoblastoma and intracranial malignancy. Unpublished observations
27. JONES AE, STALLARD HB: The eye and orbit. In Treatment of Cancer in Clinical Practice. Edinburgh and London, E&S Livingston Ltd, 1959
28. KNIEPER C: Ein Fall von doppelseitigem glioma retinae mit Enucleation des einen und nummehr fast 11-jähriger Atrophie des andern Auges. Graefes Arch Klin Ophthalmol 78:310–330, 1911
29. KOGAN LL, BONIUK M: Causes for enucleation in childhood with special reference to pseudogliomas and unsuspected retinoblastomas. Int Ophthalmol Clin 2:507–524, 1962
30. MAKLEY TA JR: Retinoblastoma in a 52-year-old man. Arch Ophthalmol 69:325–327, 1963
31. MANSCHOT WA: Difficulties in the clinical diagnosis of retinoblastoma. Ophthalmologica 132: 162–164, 1956
32. MELLER J: On the retrogression of retinal glioma. Am J Ophthalmol 32:193–199, 1915
33. MERRIAM GR JR: Retinoblastoma; analysis of 17 autopsies. Arch Ophthalmol 44:71–108, 1950
34. MORGAN G: Diffuse infiltrating retinoblastoma. Br J Ophthalmol 55:600–606, 1971
35. MULLANEY J: DNA in retinoblastoma. Lancet 2:918, 1968
36. MULLANEY J: Retinoblastoma with DNA precipitation. Arch Ophthalmol 82:454–456, 1969
37. MUNOZ-URRA F: Ueber die feine Gewebsstruktur des Glioms der Netzhaut. Graefes Arch Klin Ophthalmol 112:133–151, 1923
38. PALOMINO-DENA F, VILLEGAS-LEON L, MURILLO-FAJARDO R, SILVA-ZERON S, SALAS M, VERGAS L: Estado actual del problema del retinoblastoma. Ann Oftalmol 27:117–161, 228–242, 1954
39. PARKHILL EM, BENEDICT WL: Gliomas of the

retina; a histopathologic study. Am J Ophthalmol 24:1354–1373, 1941

40. PARKS MM, ZIMMERMAN LE: Retinoblastoma. Clin Proc Child Hosp DC 16:77–84, 1960

41. PORTER R, SKILLEN AW: Lactic dehydrogenase activity in the aqueous humour of eyes containing malignant melanoma. Br J Ophthalmol 56:709–710, 1972

42. RAY BS, MCLEAN JM: Combined intracranial and orbital operation for retinoblastomas. Arch Ophthalmol 30:437–445, 1943

43. REDLER LD, ELLSWORTH RM: Prognostic importance of choroidal invasion in retinoblastoma. Arch Ophthalmol 90:294–296, 1973

44. REESE AB: Extension of glioma (retinoblastoma) into the optic nerve. Arch Ophthalmol 5:269–272, 1931

45. REESE AB: Invasion of the optic nerve by retinoblastoma. Arch Ophthalmol 40:533–557, 1948

46. REESE AB: Unpublished data

47. REESE AB: Persistence and hyperplasia of primary vitreous; retrolental fibroplasia—two entities. Arch Ophthalmol 41:527–552, 1949

48. REESE AB: Persistent hyperplastic primary vitreous. Am J Ophthalmol 40:317–331, 1955

49. REESE AB, BLODI FC: Retinal dysplasia. Am J Ophthalmol 33:23–32, 1950

50. REESE AB, STRAATSMA BR: Retinal dysplasia. Am J Ophthalmol 45:199–211, 1958

51. SAUNDERS LZ, BARRON CN: Primary pigmented intraocular tumors in animals. Cancer Res 18:234–245, 1958

52. SCHOFIELD PB: Diffuse infiltrating retinoblastoma. Br J Ophthalmol 44:35–41, 1960

53. SHAFER WG, FRISSELL CT: The melanoameloblastoma and retinal anlage tumors. Cancer 6:360–364, 1953

54. SHARPE W, MACLAIRE AS: Further observations of intracranial hemorrhage in the newborn. Surg Gynecol Obstet 41:583–588, 1925

55. SPENCER WH: Primary neoplasms of the optic nerve and its sheaths: clinical features and current concepts of pathogenetic mechanisms. Trans Am Ophthalmol Soc 70:490–528, 1972

56. STAFFORD WR, YANOFF M, PARNELL BL: Retinoblastomas initially misdiagnosed as primary ocular inflammations. Arch Ophthalmol 82:771–773, 1969

57. STALLARD HB: Multiple islands of retinoblastoma. Br J Ophthalmol 39:241–243, 1955

58. STALLARD HB: Glioma retinae treated by radon seeds. Br Med J 2:962–964, 1936

59. SUCKLING RD: The treatment of retinoblastomata with radon rings. Trans Ophthalmol Soc New Zeal 17:43–48, 1965

60. SUSSMAN W: Intraocular tumors. Br J Ophthalmol 22:722–737, 1938

61. TARKKANEN A: Occurrence of mental retardation in patients with retinoblastoma. Acta Ophthalmol 51:67–71, 1973

62. TENG CC, KATZIN HM: The evidence for a retinoblastoma induction factor. Am J Ophthalmol 39:20–29, 1955

63. TS'O MOM, ZIMMERMAN LE, FINE BS: The nature of retinoblastoma. I. Photoreceptor differentiation: a clinical and histopathologic study. Am J Ophthalmol 69:339–349, 1970

64. TS'O MOM, FINE BS, ZIMMERMAN LE: II. Photoreceptor differentiation: an electron microscopic study. Am J Ophthalmol 69:350–359, 1970

65. TSUKAHARA I: A histopathological study on the prognosis and radiosensitivity of retinoblastoma. Arch Ophthalmol 63:1005–1008, 1960

66. WADSWORTH JAC: Personal communication

67. WEIZENBLATT S: Differential diagnostic difficulties in atypical retinoblastoma. Arch Ophthalmol 58:699–709, 1957

68. WILDER HC: Nematode endophthalmitis. Trans Am Acad Ophthalmol 55:99–109, 1950

69. WILLIAMS M: Superior intelligence of children blinded from retinoblastoma. Arch Dis Child 43:204–210, 1968

70. ZIMMERMAN LE: Retinoblastoma including a report of illustrative cases. Med Ann DC 38:366–374, 1969

GENETICS OF RETINOBLASTOMA

71. ELLSWORTH RM: The practical management of retinoblastoma. Trans Am Ophthalmol Soc 67:462–534, 1969

72. FISHER RA: The effects of methods of ascertainment upon the estimation of frequencies. Ann Eugen (Lond) 6:13, 1934

73. KITCHIN FD, ELLSWORTH RM: The pleiotropic effects of the gene for retinoblastoma. J Med Genet 11:244–246, 1974

74. KNUDSON AG: Mutation and cancer: statistical study of retinoblastoma. Proc Natl Acad Sci USA 68:820–823, 1971

75. MACKLIN MT: A study of retinoblastoma in Ohio. Am J Hum Genet 12:1–43, 1960

76. SCHAPPERT-KIMMIJSER J, HEMMES GD, NIJLAND R: The heredity of retinoblastoma. Ophthalmologica 151:197–213, 1966

77. SORSBY A: Bilateral retinoblastoma: a dominantly inherited affection. Br Med J 2:580–583, 1972

78. VOGEL F: Neue Untersuchungen zur Genetik des Retinoblastoms. Z Menschl Vereb Konstit Lehre 34:205–236, 1957

79. WILSON MG, TOWNER JW, FUKIMOTO A: Retinoblastoma and D-chromosome deletions. Am J Hum Genet 25:57–61, 1973

4

GLIOMA OF THE OPTIC NERVE, RETINA, AND ORBIT

OPTIC NERVE

The optic nerve, unlike a peripheral nerve, is a tract comparable with the intracerebral pathways of the brain except that it is subdivided into bundles of nerve fibers by vascular fibrous septa that enter from the pia. The nerve fibers are further separated by a glial network with cells similar to those in the central nervous system. These cells are of three types: astrocytes, oligodendrocytes, and microglia. Cajal's staining method with gold chloride, del Río-Hortega's with silver carbonate, or Weil-Davenport's with ammoniacal silver is necessary to bring out the cytologic details.

The astrocytes have a large cell body with cytoplasmic extensions (Fig. 4–1).

The oligodendrocytes can be demonstrated with the hematoxylin-eosin stain. In longitudinal sections they appear as rows of cells with small round nuclei arranged in parallel columns. Short, wavy protoplasmic processes are sometimes revealed with use of special stains. These processes are believed to form an intimate contact with the individual myelinated nerve fibers[11,27] and to be implicated in the elaboration or maintenance of myelin and thus analogous to the Schwann cells of the peripheral nerves (see Ch. 6, Tumors of the Peripheral Nerves). In support of this view, oligodendrocytes were not demonstrable in the unmyelinated portion of the optic nerve internal to the lamina cribrosa,[8] although they were reported to constitute 75% of the glial elements of the optic nerve.[13]

The interstitial cells of the microglia were extensively studied by del Río-Hortega and are sometimes called Hortega cells. He felt that they have some motility which is especially marked in the presence of inflammation. Considered to be of mesodermal origin, they are more sparse than the astrocytes and oligodendrocytes. The nuclei are small and oval or elongated with short delicate branches. These cells are also the phagocytes of the central nervous system.

TYPES OF GLIOMA

There are three types of glioma of the central nervous system: astrocytoma, by far the most common; oligodendroglioma; and ependymoma. Gliomas are not always pure in type but frequently have varying elements of astrocytes, oligodendrocytes, and microglia. The oligodendroglioma in an essentially pure form occurs in the optic nerve but very rarely. I have encountered only one tumor that appeared to be composed entirely of oligodendrocytes, an oligodendroglioma of the optic nerve that I reported at the 1961 meeting of the Verhoeff Society (Fig. 4–2). This 19-year-old girl had progressive blurring of vision and exophthalmos of the right eye, which after two years had 20/200 vision. No mass was palpable. She denied diplopia and had no skin pigmentation or nodules suggesting neurofibromatosis. The lateral wall of the orbit was resected and a 27 × 15 × 15 mm tumor, which had replaced the optic nerve, was removed. The clinical diagnosis of astrocytoma of the optic nerve was confirmed histologically by several neuropathologists.

A tumor composed predominantly of oligodendrocytes and Schwann cells, both producing myelin, has been reported,[23] as well as nine tumors in which the oligodendroglial and schwannian elements were equally represented.[24,25] Since oligodendroglia is concerned with the elaboration of myelin, not normally found in the retina, it is surprising that a number of cases of oligodendroglioma of the retina have been published.[3,21,38] All were clinically diagnosed as retinoblastomas.

Ependymomas of the eye as such have not been described in the literature, although histologic structures in the medulloepitheliomas arising from the uveal epithelium seem to resemble those seen in ependymomas. This is to be expected, as medulloepitheliomas of the eye and ependymomas of the central nervous system have a common stem cell.

There have been no reports of tumors arising from the microglia. Because gliomas arise from preexisting adult cells by a process of

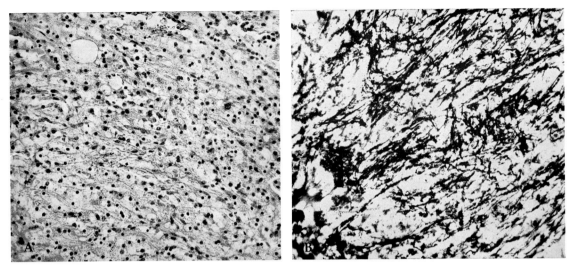

FIG. 4–1. Glioma of the optic nerve. **A.** Hematoxylin and eosin stain. **B.** Cajal stain.

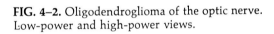

FIG. 4–2. Oligodendroglioma of the optic nerve. Low-power and high-power views.

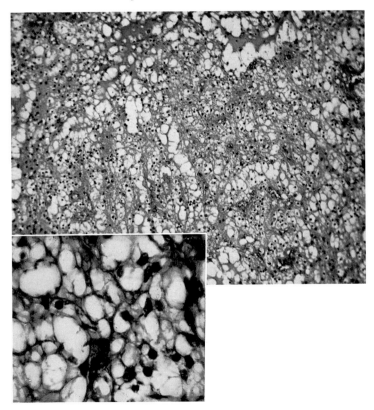

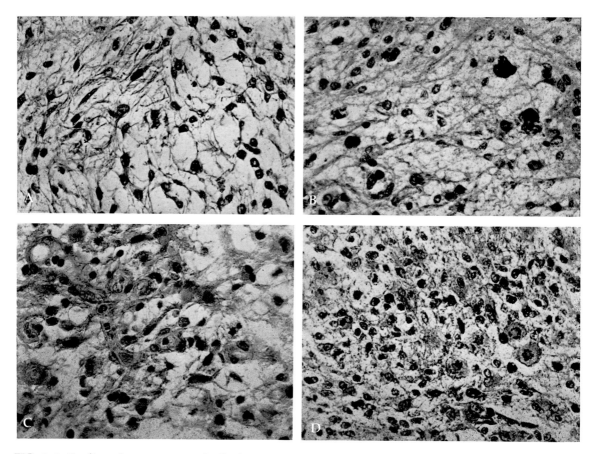

FIG. 4–3. Grading of astrocytomas. **A.** Grade 1—relatively acellular tumor with no giant cells, giant nuclei, or mitotic figures; cells and nuclei show no pleomorphism; glial fibrils are sparse. **B.** Grade 2—tumor with many glial fibrils, several giant nuclei, some pleomorphism, but no mitotic figures. **C.** Grade 3—tumor with glial fibrils, pleomorphism, giant cells, and mitotic figures as well as tissue edema. **D.** Grade 4—highly malignant tumor with hyperchromatic nuclei, many bizarre mitotic figures, and proliferation of the vascular endothelium; no giant cells or marked pleomorphism. (Courtesy of H. J. Svien et al.[30])

dedifferentiation or anaplasia, and the degree of malignancy is commensurate with the degree of dedifferentiation, it has been proposed that they be graded 1 to 4 on the basis of cellular dedifferentiation.[30] Grade 1, the least malignant, is the most common brain tumor occurring in children; grades 3 and 4, the most malignant, constitute more than 90% of all brain tumors in elderly patients (Fig. 4–3).

Piloid gliomas are composed of long, straight, hairlike cells instead of the usual stellate cells. Most gliomas of the optic nerve and chiasm belong in this group.

PATHOLOGY

Glioma of the optic nerve has been viewed as a degenerative gliomatosis. The markedly reduced vision and early optic atrophy associated with glioma of the optic nerve suggest that the primary lesion is a degenerative process in the nerve itself, while glial proliferation and tumor formation are secondary manifestations. These tumors have also been considered neuroectodermal, belonging in the hamartomatous group, or transitional to teratoid medulloepitheliomas.

Five different stages in the evolution of gliomas of the optic nerve have been described:[10] a) generalized hyperplasia of the astrocytes and oligodendrocytes; b) extension of the growth through the pial sheath with hyperplasia of the arachnoid cells forming a tumorlike growth (this is a separate proliferative process subsequent to, and apparently dependent upon, the first stage); c) extension of the tumor cells farther into the sheath of the optic nerve with penetration and infiltration of the mass formed by the arachnoid cells, the two tissue elements becoming so intermingled that it is difficult to distinguish them; d) destruction of most of the landmarks by a haphazard intermixture of glial and arachnoid cells; and e) loss of landmarks within the nerve stem and sheath, and perhaps malignancy.

Meningeal fibromatosis in the subarachnoid space secondary to an adjacent glioma is an important feature of the disease. Clinically, this collateral change makes it difficult to determine the extent of the basic neoplastic process.

The tumors may have accumulations of so-called cytoid bodies. It is generally agreed that these bodies, resembling ganglion cells in size and appearance, result from some change in the neuroglial cells.

Other features that may occur in glioma are calcium deposits and cystic spaces filled with a mucinous substance.

Squeezing of the optic nerve during surgery at times leads to extrusion of myelin into the nerve head, and the resulting artifact may be confused with a true tumor of the nerve head.[6]

FREQUENCY

Approximately two-thirds of the reported cases of primary tumors of the optic nerve are gliomas and one-third are meningiomas.

DIAGNOSIS

Glioma of the optic nerve is usually manifested as a unilateral exophthalmos in young people (Fig. 4–4). Progress of the lesion is extremely slow, and there are no ocular symptoms; the only change is poor vision caused by optic atrophy. In some instances, instead of a fundal picture of simple optic atrophy, the disc becomes elevated. When the elevation is slight it may have the appearance of a papilledema, although it usually represents actual tumor extension which may be quite marked.

In the early stage the disease may be insidious. For example, blurring of one disc was noted in the routine examination of a young child with normal vision and no exophthalmos. The eye was 2.5 diopters hyperopic, and

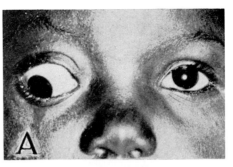

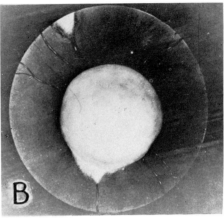

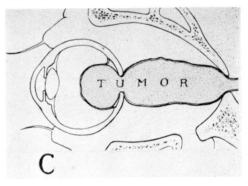

FIG. 4–4. Glioma of the right optic nerve. **A.** Exophthalmos in an infant girl. **B.** Fundus shows a tumor mass on the optic disc. **C.** Schema indicates its position and extent. (Courtesy of J. M. Wilson and W. D. Farmer.[37])

the fellow eye was emmetropic. In four months optimal vision was 20/40. There was a slight exophthalmos, some retinal striae were observed at the posterior pole, and blurring of the disc was more marked. An astrocytoma of the optic nerve was removed surgically. Another patient with a large astrocytoma of the optic nerve had no pallor or other clinical evidence of nerve changes. In early cases the proptosis is axial, but in advanced cases the eye may deviate downward and inward. The tumor may be palpable through the upper lid nasally.

The disease is characteristically unilateral, although bilateral cases have been reported, one in a patient 79 years of age.[7] When both optic nerves are involved, the tumor may have spread from one to the other by way of the chiasm or may have had multiple origins.

X rays frequently show an enlarged optic foramen (see Ch. 17, Fig. 17–10H) or a neck-like shadow resembling a gourd in the region of the sella turcica, extending from the body of the sella under the anterior clinoid process. This change has been attributed chiefly to erosion of the optic canal.

The tumor process in the optic nerve may extend back to and involve the optic chiasm, thereby frequently causing changes in the visual field of the fellow eye. This finding is, of course, valuable in planning treatment.

Among conditions to be considered in the differential diagnosis are meningioma, pituitary tumor, and cysts of the intracranial portion of the optic nerve.

A review of 25 cases of primary intraorbital meningioma at the Armed Forces Institute of Pathology[22] revealed the average age of the patients to be 31.7 years; 10 were under age 20, and 6 under age 10. Since glioma affects the optic nerve itself, vision is affected early and severely. In meningioma, however, the optic nerve is affected through compression; if there is visual disturbance it occurs later and is less severe than in glioma. A glioma of the optic nerve involving the chiasm may be confused with a tumor of the pituitary, but central vision in the fellow eye is normal or only slightly altered. Conversely, patients with glioma of the chiasm usually have markedly reduced vision in the fellow eye.

Two described cases of astrocytoma of the retina were diagnosed clinically as retinoblastoma.[5] Other cases were considered cysts of the intracranial portion of the optic nerve, from observations made at the time of intracranial surgery.[14]

TREATMENT

There are two conflicting opinions regarding the nature, natural history, and treatment of glioma of the optic nerve and optic tracts. The older concept gained wide acceptance and still has many adherents who recommend that a tumor limited to a single optic nerve be resected from the globe to the chiasm to prevent chiasmal extension (Fig. 4–5). In a comprehensive report on 97 cases of glioma of the optic nerve, optic disc, or both,[18] the chiasm was involved in 60%, the intracranial portion of the optic nerve in 25%, and the tumor was confined to the orbit in 15%. The cases were not divided into adult and juvenile types.

The disease has a variable natural history, and radiotherapy effectively controls progressive symptoms in some cases, according to the study.[18] Of the 97 patients, 90 were given radiation, 62 postoperatively and 28 as the sole therapy; the other 7 were treated by primary transcranial and orbital resection of the optic nerve without radiation. Radiotherapy was not instituted when there was a clean resection margin without histologic evidence of residual tumor at the proximal end of the resected nerve. All 7 patients with total resection were tumor-free and well from 1 to 5 years later.

The overall survival rate for postoperative patients receiving radiotherapy was 75%—5 years; 63%—10 years; 50%—20 years; 43% —25 years. Among the 28 patients treated by irradiation alone who survived more than 5 years, 68% showed visual improvement.

Of the 97 cases in this series, 18 developed obstructive hydrocephalus. Since they had ventriculopleural or ventriculoatrial shunting procedures, the prognosis for life and vision was, of course, poor, although 4 of the 18 patients survived 1½ to 10 years. Only 5 of them had presented with proptosis. The vast majority had piloid astrocytomas, and one infant harbored a highly anaplastic malignant astrocytoma, grade 4.

In the opinion of others, however, optic gliomas should be excised only to control proptosis in a blind eye; the patient's visual impairment at the time of diagnosis changes little thereafter; life cannot be prolonged by surgery; and irradiation has no influence on the natural history.[19] These authors consider the tumor to be congenital, nonneoplastic, and self-limiting with a good chance of the patient's long survival even in the event of chiasmal and hypothalamic involvement. Their conclusions were based on a long-term follow-up (3 to 41 years) of 36 children. In 19 of them ophthalmic symptoms had led to the diagnosis of a tumor in the anterior optic pathways. The diagnosis was confirmed in 15 of the 19 cases before 5 years of age, but ocular symptoms in the other 4 were unex-

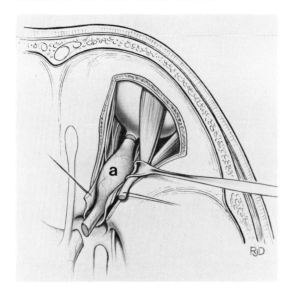

FIG. 4–5. Technique for removing a glioma of the optic nerve by the transcranial route through the orbital roof. The superior rectus and levator muscles are severed at their insertion and retracted. The optic nerve bearing the glioma (*a*) is resected from the globe to the chiasm. (Courtesy of E. M. Housepian.[17])

plained until they were between 10 and 40 years of age. The 12 patients with hypothalamic signs all had a tumor of the chiasm and anterior third ventricle. When the condition was diagnosed, 45% of the patients already had severe visual loss, whereas 40% had good or excellent vision. Since this ratio remained constant during 10–20 years of follow-up, the authors concluded that optic gliomas tend to enlarge and cause symptoms early in life but remain static thereafter. These tumors appear to belong to the congenital glial group seen in the cerebellum, medulla, corpus callosum, and spinal cord.[4,11] What is interpreted as tumor growth may be attributed to the collateral hyperplasia of adjacent glial and connective tissue[36] and to the production of intracellular and extracellular mucosubstance.[1]

Many investigators have called attention to the limited growth of optic nerve gliomas. Even incomplete excisions through an orbitotomy resulted in cures. In the future this factor of self-limiting growth must be evaluated in the treatment. The fact that spontaneous improvement can occur makes evaluation difficult, however.[32]

Gliomas of the optic nerve may behave like other tumors of infants and children by progressing perhaps at a rapid rate and then spontaneously regressing, at times to the point of complete inactivity. Such tumors are infantile hemangioma, lymphangioma, xanthogranuloma, Coats's disease, juvenile lipomatoses and fibromatoses, nodular fasciitis, and neuroblastoma. In this event, treatment of optic nerve glioma before the chiasm becomes involved may effectively slow the process until the regressive phase begins.

The accepted view regarding cancer cells is that mature cells dedifferentiate to immature anaplastic or cancer cells. The tumors of early childhood just cited might be regarded as instances where the process is reversed, the tumor cells differentiating into mature benign cells. This seems to be true even in cases of neuroblastoma with highly malignant cytologic characteristics and extensive metastases, which may regress to a completely benign ganglioneuroma.

Glioma of the optic nerve is in the province of the neurosurgeon. I subscribe to a transfrontal craniotomy after resection of the orbital roof and confirmation of the diagnosis by inspection of the chiasmal and prechiasmal areas.[16] If excision seems indicated the procedure is as follows: The insertion of the levator muscle is severed at the annulus and reflected. The third, fifth, sixth, and sometimes fourth cranial nerves can be identified and avoided. The optic nerve is then excised from the chiasm to the globe.

When chiasmal involvement is noted or suspected at the time of surgery, irradiation is indicated.

Gliomas of the optic nerve and tract may involve four sites, either primarily or secondarily: the orbital portion of the nerve, the intracanalicular portion, the prechiasmal intracranial portion, and the chiasm and the neighboring structures of the hypothalamus and third ventricle.

Treatment would be arbitrary if the involved area could be readily delineated clinically. A tumor confined to the orbit can be approached through the lateral orbital wall. A transcranial approach should be employed for a tumor limited to the intracanalicular or cranial portion of the optic nerve. Irradiation, with or without surgery, is the treatment of choice for a tumor of the chiasm and adnexa.

Unfortunately, it is difficult to select the most appropriate treatment because the extent of the tumor cannot be accurately determined. Also, more of the lesion's bulk may be due to fibromatosis than to the actual neoplastic element. For instance, the tumor proper may be confined to the orbit, whereas the collateral fibromatosis may result in enlargement of the optic foramen, as seen in x rays. This may explain a cure in a patient with an enlarged optic foramen by an excision through the lateral wall of the orbit.

When the patient's age permits, a visual field of the fellow eye should be taken, in an attempt to rule out chiasmal involvement. If there is still doubt, a transcranial exploration may be advisable. In cases where excision is not indicated or advisable, decompression of the bony roof of the optic foramen may alleviate constriction of the optic nerve and thus slow optic atrophy and prolong the period of useful vision.

After excision of an optic nerve harboring a glioma, sequelae in the fundus in addition to optic atrophy seem to depend on the site of the excision. When it is flush with the sclera and the posterior ciliary arteries and nerves are severed or injured, fundal changes are marked. When it is at a level posterior to the site in the optic nerve where the central vessels enter, which occurs usually in the transcranial operation, the resulting fundal changes in addition to optic atrophy may be negligible. Minimal changes have been attributed in some instances to probable anastomosis of the retinal and ciliary vessels. This conclusion was based on observation of a patient three and a half years postoperatively whose retinal arteries seemed filled with blood. The fundus was normal in color and there were no marked pigment changes. Another patient who had a similar operation showed extensive pigment changes in the fundus six months postoperatively, with large masses of pigment cells accumulated over the retina and the disc. The vessels were extremely narrow and apparently contained no blood. The fundal changes were virtually the same two and a half years postoperatively.

Extensive pigment changes are usually observed in the fundus after excision of the optic nerve, with large masses of pigmented epithelial cells over the retina and the disc, perhaps with retinitis proliferans, iridocyclitis, and secondary glaucoma leading ultimately to enucleation. Verhoeff's histologic examination of an eye from which a large tumor of the optic nerve had been excised some years earlier revealed atrophy of both the choroid and the retina; the retina was pigmented as a result of cells migrating from the proliferated pigment epithelium. Since obstruction of the central vessels alone does not cause such changes, they were assumed to result from severing of the posterior ciliary arteries.[35]

Although good results were reported in a series of patients with glioma of the optic nerve and chiasm treated with radiation, a longer follow-up led to correction of the earlier impression.[31] Eight of the nine patients with proptosis subsequently required surgery; among those who showed visual improvement after radiation, vision later declined even to the stage of blindness. Some of the patients whose disease appeared to have been arrested died. The authors therefore concluded that patients with indications of chiasmal involvement should be treated by radiation, which seemed to improve their vision for several years.

PROGNOSIS

In five reported cases of astrocytoma of the optic nerve there was no recurrence 15 to 24 years after excision of the tumor through the lateral orbital wall.[20] In several others there was no recurrence 3½ to 18 years after excision of the tumor.[10] In two patients who had a lateral orbitotomy, postoperative x rays showed a decreased diameter of the previously enlarged optic canal.[2] A recurrence that had become massive 22 years after enucleation of the eyeball in a proved case of glioma of the optic nerve was described in a patient who had meanwhile led a comparatively normal life.[12]

RELATION TO VON RECKLINGHAUSEN'S DISEASE

The relationship between optic nerve tumors and von Recklinghausen's disease has been widely recognized. In the latter disease there may be diffuse hyperplasia or benign neoplasia of the connective tissue, meningeal and glial elements in the central or peripheral nervous system.[29] These diffuse hyperplasias of the optic nerve may lead to enlargement of the optic foramen without visual loss. Malignant changes developed in 13% of such patients in one series.[15]

As the stem cell of von Recklinghausen's disease is the Schwann cell, not present in the optic nerve, which is a cranial nerve, it seems inconsistent for the nerve to participate in this systemic disease.

Some authors have considered oligodendroglia of the central nervous system (which includes the optic nerve) comparable with Schwann cells of the peripheral nerves, since both types of cells function by elaborating and maintaining the myelin sheaths of the nerves. Both were believed to participate in von Recklinghausen's disease—in which case a tumor in the optic nerve would be essentially an oligodendrocytoma.[11]

Multiple cranial nerve tumors may accompany von Recklinghausen's disease, the optic nerve being the least frequently and the acoustic nerve the most frequently affected. In one review of 37 authentic cases of optic nerve tumors associated with this disease, 15 of the patients had bilateral involvement of the nerve, and 16 had some form of intracranial involvement.[10] This author believed that optic nerve tumors were more often associated with minor peripheral manifestations of von Recklinghausen's disease, or with the most abortive types, than with the typical variety. The manifestations may be limited to café-au-lait spots or easily overlooked tumors of the skin. In instances where there is evidence of the disease in the patient's family history, the optic nerve tumor could be a *forme fruste*. The age range was 2 to 52 years.

An early estimate that about 10% of optic nerve tumors are associated with von Recklinghausen's disease is considered too low, because the tumors usually accompany the easily overlooked manifestations of the disease. Also, 60%–75% of all optic nerve tumors occur during the first decade of life, generally before the disease becomes systemically apparent. Early manifestations of von Recklinghausen's disease in young patients are often subtle. I have seen 11 histologically confirmed cases of either glioma of the optic nerve or neurofibroma of the orbit that were suspected preoperatively because of inconspicuous skin lesions, such as café-au-lait spots, elephantiasis neuromatosa, or multiple skin neurofibromas consistent with this disease.

As mentioned earlier, proliferation in the arachnoid accompanying gliomatous tumors of the nerve appears to be a secondary process. However, a primary meningioma of the optic nerve sheath may be associated with von Recklinghausen's disease. It may also occur with a neurofibroma of the orbit (see Ch. 5, Fig. 5–4).

A probable case of neurofibromatosis has been reported in which numerous tumors involved the brain, spinal cord, and cranial and peripheral nerves.[28] Three types of central nervous system tumors were found at autopsy: a meningioma of the left optic nerve, a neurofibroma of the roots of the spinal and cranial nerves, and a glioma of the spinal cord and right frontal lobe.

THE RETINA

Since the inner layers of the retina contain astrocytes, it may harbor a true glioma comparable with the common gliomas of the brain (Fig. 4–6), though the retinal lesion is extremely rare.[3] The few cases in the literature suggest that retinal astrocytomas tend to develop in the second and third decades of life, are not particularly invasive locally, and do not tend to metastasize.

Glioma of the retina must be considered in the differential diagnosis of retinoblastoma. Both may occur as solitary or multiple lesions and be unilateral or bilateral. The presence of a systemic disease such as tuberous sclerosis or neurofibromatosis or a history of precocious puberty is helpful in the diagnosis.[5]

Also, a larval granuloma may simulate a glioma of the retina.

RELATION OF TUMORS OF THE OPTIC NERVE AND RETINA TO TUBEROUS SCLEROSIS

Tuberous sclerosis is discussed here because it is composed essentially of glial tissue; it has some neoplastic characteristics; clinically and microscopically it shows the ocular characteristics of a tumorlike lesion of the retina and optic disc; and the retinal lesion may be a true glioma. Tuberous sclerosis (Bourneville's disease), multiple neurofibromatosis (von Recklinghausen's disease), angiomatosis (von Hippel–Lindau disease), and the Sturge-Weber syndrome all have some characteristics in common, depending on the tissue or structure involved. Tuberous sclerosis involves the cerebrum; multiple neurofibromatosis involves the cranial, peripheral, and sympathetic nerves; angiomatosis involves

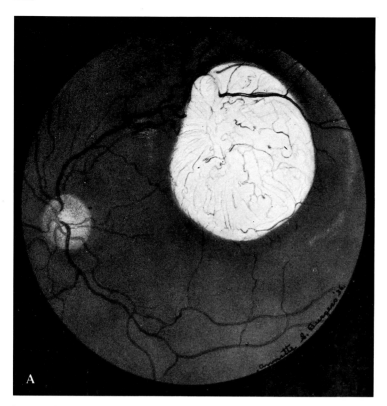

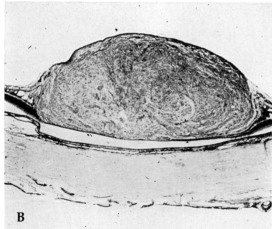

FIG. 4–6. Glioma of the retina. **A.** Clinical appearance. **B.** Lesion under low magnification. **C.** High-power magnification reveals the characteristic astrocytes. (Courtesy of J. M. McLean.[26])

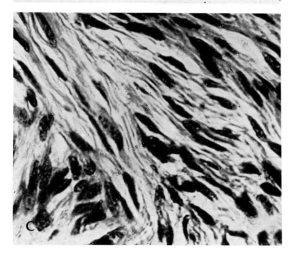

the cerebellum, medulla, and spinal cord; and the Sturge-Weber syndrome may manifest an intracranial, a facial, or an ipsilateral choroidal hemangioma. All are considered congenital heredofamilial anomalies, the principal signs being cutaneous lesions, tumefactions, and cysts combined with other congenital malformations elsewhere, especially in the central nervous system. The patient may have spina bifida, ectopia testis, or syndactylia and often skin manifestations. The term *phakomatoses* (*phakos* = mother spot) was suggested for the entire group.[33]

Glioma of the retina in a case thought to be tuberous sclerosis is shown in Figure 4–7. A 6-month-old infant was having convulsions several times daily. The physical examination was negative except for a retinal tumor in the right eye.

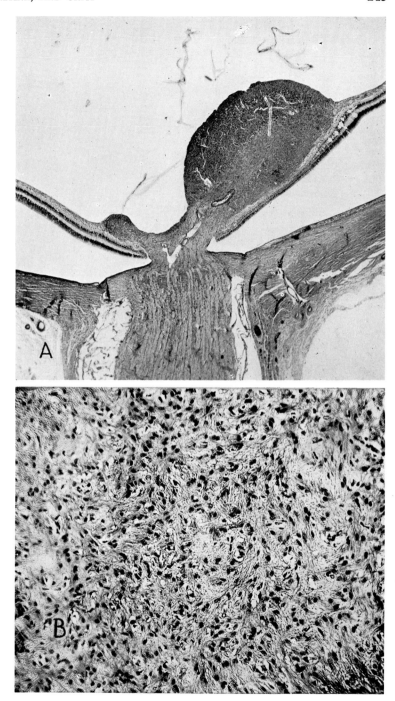

FIG. 4–7. Glioma of the retina in a case thought to be tuberous sclerosis. A round, elevated, grayish-white mass on the temporal side of the optic disc in a 6-month-old infant was somewhat larger than the disc and covered with capillary-sized vessels. **A.** At low magnification, the tumor is seen extending over the surface of the disc. **B.** High magnification reveals its cytologic characteristics. (Courtesy of J. S. McLean.)

PATHOLOGY

Macroscopically, the cerebrum contains numerous whitish, slightly prominent nodules; they sometimes degenerate in the center, forming small cysts, but more often form calcareous foci. Microscopically, these sclerotic nodules show considerable overgrowth of glial cells as well as immature embryonic cells resembling neuronal or glial cells. An outstanding feature is the marked tendency of these lesions to form calcium and hyalin.

CLINICAL COURSE

Tuberous sclerosis may begin as developmental delay, particularly in walking and talking. The mental defect may be obvious by the third year, and the cutaneous manifestations sometimes appear in the first decade.

CLINICAL VARIANTS

The disease has many clinical variants and *formes frustes*. A study of the patient's siblings and progenitors usually reveals a much higher incidence of abortive forms than of the pure form.

When some members of a family have tuberous sclerosis with systemic manifestations, another member may have a typical retinal tumor only. One such tumor was described in the eye of a 21-year-old woman who had no other signs or symptoms of tuberous sclerosis, although five of her siblings were later found to have an advanced form of the disease.[34] Six years later her retinal tumor was somewhat larger, and a few similar ones had appeared. She had meanwhile married and was the mother of six children, of whom three had retinal tumors and one was subject to frequent epileptic seizures. It has been suggested that finding only one typical tumor justifies a positive diagnosis of tuberous sclerosis.

CUTANEOUS COMPLICATIONS

Adenoma sebaceum appears as a papular rash on the face in conjunction with the disease. Reddish to brownish spots are seen in a butterfly-shaped arrangement noted first in the nasolabial folds, then over the entire nose, and finally over the cheeks in the infraorbital region.

ASSOCIATED SYSTEMIC DISEASE

Mixed tumors of the kidney, usually multiple and bilateral, are at times associated with tuberous sclerosis. According to some authors,[9] the tumors occurred in 80% of all cases but were rarely diagnosed clinically.

INVOLVEMENT OF THE OPTIC NERVE AND RETINA

The association of tumors of the retina and optic nerve with tuberous sclerosis has long been known. Either single or multiple and whitish to yellowish in color, they vary greatly in size, sometimes being elevated 4 or more diopters (Fig. 4–8, see p. 10). The surface is usually mulberrylike or nodular. Mulberrylike tumors also occur in the disc and retina.

Multiple foci of increased density, sometimes noted in skull x rays, represent the often calcified cerebral lesions characteristic of tuberous sclerosis.

RELATION OF TUMORS OF THE OPTIC NERVE AND THE RETINA TO NEUROFIBROMATOSIS

See Chapter 6, Tumors of the Peripheral Nerves.

REFERENCES

1. ANDERSON DR, SPENCER WH: Ultrastructural and histochemical observations of optic nerve gliomas. Arch Ophthalmol 83:324–325, 1970
2. BERKE RN: A modified Krönlein operation. Arch Ophthalmol 51:609–632, 1954
3. BONIUK M, BISHOP DW: Oligodendroglioma of the retina. Survey Ophthalmol 13:284–289, 1969
4. BUCY PC, THIEMAN PW: Astrocytomas of the cerebellum; a study of a series of patients operated upon over 28 years ago. Arch Neurol 18:14–19, 1968
5. CLEASBY GW, FUNG WE, SHEKTER WB: Astrocytoma of the retina; report of two cases. Am J Ophthalmol (Suppl) 64:633–637, 1967
6. COGAN DG, KUWABARA T: Myelin artifacts. Am J Ophthalmol (Suppl) 64: 622–626, 1967

7. CONDON JR, ROSE FC: Optic nerve glioma. Br J Ophthalmol 51:703–706, 1967

8. CONE W, MACMILLAN JA: The optic nerve and papilla. In Penfield WC (ed): Cytology and Cellular Pathology of the Central Nervous System, Vol 2. New York, Hoeber-Harper, 1932, pp 837–901

9. CRITCHLEY M, EARL CJC: Tuberose sclerosis and allied conditions. Brain 55:311–346, 1932

10. DAVIS FA: Primary tumors of the optic nerve (a phenomenon of Recklinghausen's disease). Arch Ophthalmol 23:735–831, 957–1022, 1949

11. Del Río-Hortega P: Anatomia Microscópia de los Tumores del Sistema Nervioso Central y Periferico. Madrid, S.A. Blass, 1934

12. DONAHUE HC: An exceptional lesion of the orbit. Arch Ophthalmol 54:259–261, 1955

13. ENRIQUEZ L: Oligodendroglia de las vias opticas. Boll Soc Espan Hist Nat 26:301, 1926

14. HOLT H: Cysts of the intracranial portion of the optic nerve. Am J Ophthalmol 61:1166–1170, 1966

15. HOSOI K: Multiple neurofibromatosis (von Recklinghausen's disease) with special reference to malignant transformation. Arch Surg 22:58, 1931

16. HOUSEPIAN EM: Surgical treatment of unilateral optic nerve gliomas. J Neurosurg 31:604–607, 1969

17. HOUSEPIAN EM: Tumors of the orbit. In Mark VH (ed): Practice of Surgery: Neurosurgery. Hagerstown, Md, Harper & Row, 1972, Ch 12, pp 1–24

18. HOUSEPIAN EM, WOOD EH, CHANG CH: Obstructive hydrocephalus and optic glioma in childhood. Presented at the European Society for Pediatric Neurosurgery, Versailles, France, 1970.

19. HOYT WF, BAGHDASSARIAN SA: Optic glioma of childhood; natural history and rationale for conservative management. Br J Ophthalmol 53:793–798, 1969

20. HUDSON AC: Primary tumors of the optic nerve. R Lond Ophthalmol Hosp Rep 18:317–439, 1910–1912

21. HUGGERT A, HULTQUIST GT: True glioma of the retina (a case of probable oligodendroglioma). Ophthalmologica 133:193–202, 1947

22. KARP LA, ZIMMERMAN LE, BORIT A: Primary intraorbital meningiomas. Arch Ophthalmol 91:24–28, 1974

23. LISS L, WOLTER JR: The histology of the glioma of the optic nerve. Arch Ophthalmol 58:689–694, 1957

24. LUNDBERG Å: Ueber die primaren Tumoren des Sehnerven und der Sehnervenkreuzung. Orebro, Lindska boktryckeriet, 1935

25. LUNDBERG Å: Ueber Oligodendrozytome des Sehnervs. Acta Ophthalmol (Kbh) 14:271–277, 1936

26. MCLEAN JM: Astrocytoma (true glioma) of the retina. Arch Ophthalmol 18:255–262, 1937

27. PENFIELD W: Cytology and Cellular Pathology of the Nervous System. New York, Hoeber-Harper, 1932

28. SHAPLAND CD, GREENFIELD JG: A case of neurofibromatosis with meningeal tumor involving the left optic nerve. Trans Ophthalmol Soc UK 55:257–279, 1935

29. SPENCER WH, BORIT A: Diffuse hyperplasia of the optic nerve in von Recklinghausen's disease. Am J Ophthalmol 64:638–642, 1967

30. SVIEN HJ, MABON RF, KERNOHAN JW, ADSON AW: A simplified classification of gliomas, based on the concept of anaplasia. Surg Clin North Am 29:1169–1187, 1949

31. TAVERAS JM, MOUNT LA, WOOD EH: The value of radiation therapy in the management of glioma of the optic nerves and chiasm. Radiology 66:518–528, 1956

32. TYM R: Piloid gliomas of the anterior optic pathways. Br J Surg 49:322–331, 1961

33. VAN DER HOEVE J: Augengeschwülste bei der tuberosen Hirnskleröse (Bourneville) und verwandten Krankheiten. Graefes Arch Klin Ophthalmol 111:1–16, 1923

34. VAN DER HOEVE J: Les phakomatoses de Bourneville, de Recklinghausen et de von Hippel-Lindau. J Belge Neurol Psychiat 33:752–762, 1933

35. VERHOEFF FH: Primary intraneural tumors (gliomas) of the optic nerve; a histologic study of eleven cases, including a case showing cystic involvement of the optic disk, with demonstration of the origin of cytoid bodies of the retina and cavernous atrophy of the optic nerve. Arch Ophthalmol 51:120–140, 239–254, 1922

36. VERHOEFF FH: Tumors of the optic nerve. In Penfield WC (ed): Cytology and Cellular Pathology of the Nervous System, Vol 3. New York, Hoeber-Harper, 1932, pp 1029–1039

37. WILSON JM, Farmer WD: Glioma of the optic nerve. A critical review; report of two cases with autopsy observations in one. Arch Ophthalmol 23:605–618, 1940

38. WINTER F: Case presented at the Verhoeff Society meeting, 1968

5

MENINGIOMA

Meningiomas are thought to arise from the "cap cells" or meningocytes found in clusters at the tip of the arachnoid villi.[14] The meningocytes are essentially neuroectodermal in origin. Although they predominate in these tumors, a stromal feature of mesenchymal origin is generally acknowledged, This feature, derived from the pia, the arachnoid, or the dura, contains several elements including collagen, blood vessels, and fibroglia.

The tumor tends to assume one of two forms: globular (compressing nerve tissue) or *en plaque* (spreading across nerve tissue).

INCIDENCE

Meningiomas constitute about 17% of all tumors of the central nervous system. Although they appear predominantly in women about 45 years of age, they are not uncommon in children under age 15. A report on 25 patients with primary intraorbital meningiomas showed that in children they occur more commonly and are more aggressive than meningiomas elsewhere.[12]

In our analysis of 504 consecutive cases of expanding lesions of the orbit (Ch. 17, Table 1), meningioma was twelfth on the list of causes with 17 cases, accounting for 3% of the total.

CLASSIFICATION

Meningiomas have been classified into nine types:[2] mesenchymal, angioblastic, meningotheliomatous, psammomatous, osteoblastic, fibroblastic, melanoblastic, sarcomatous, and lipomatous. However, some authors[14] believe that all meningiomas fall into three major categories—meningotheliomatous, psammomatous, and stromal or fibroblastic—or even two, since the psammomatous meningiomas are variants of the meningotheliomatous type. They favor reserving the term *meningioma* for a tumor containing meningotheliomatous cells (Fig. 5–1), and question the inclusion of angioblastic, melanoblastic, osteoblas-

tic, and lipomatous tumors since they are not specific for the meninges.

According to another report,[18] meningeal hemangiopericytoma should not be considered an entity distinct from meningioma.

It will be recalled that the anlage of the head is represented by a layer of mesenchyme stretching between the primitive nervous system and the skin. The greater part of this mesenchyme remains as an undifferentiated layer of tissue occupying the space between the primitive brain tissue and the developing bony tissue of the skull. Thus, it represents the primordium of all the meningeal coverings as well as that of the periosteum. A portion of this so-called skeletoneural intertissue of Hallerstein later differentiates into the anlage of the skull periosteum, the dura, and the leptomeninges, which subsequently become the arachnoid and the pia. At one stage in development of the meninges, therefore, the anlage of the bone-producing periosteum, the collagen-producing dura, the endothelium-producing arachnoid, and the blood-vessel-producing pia is a single mesenchymal layer.

One concept of meningiomas is based on a phylogenetic theory:[9] the tumors stem from primitive meningeal rests incorporating the primordia of different layers of the mature meninges as well as that of the periosteum. They may therefore exhibit the characteristics of one or more of the meningeal component layers or embody in varying degrees all of them, including even bony structure from the periosteal anlage. The early stages of meningeal differentiation coincide with cell migration from the neural crest, so that neuroblasts, spongioblasts, and even melanoblasts may become enmeshed in the mesodermal primordium of the meninges. This concept would explain the fact that meningiomal components occasionally resemble neuroblastoma, spongioblastoma, or melanoma.

As the meninges covering the orbital portion of the optic nerve amount to only a small fraction of the meninges covering the brain

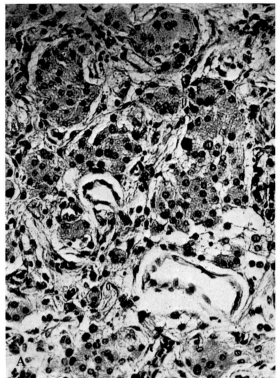
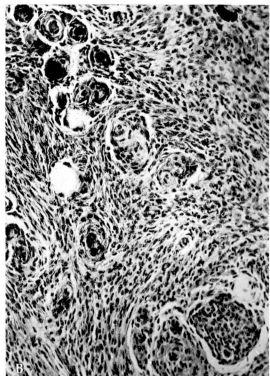

FIG. 5–1. Meningotheliomatous meningioma. **A.** Whorls and psammoma bodies are seen in various stages of formation and (at bottom) some elements of fibrous meningioma. **B.** Higher magnification of section from another case shows small islands of indistinctly outlined tumor cells with nuclei varying in size and chromatin content. This meningioma, of low-grade malignancy, has loose stroma, well-formed blood vessels, and no mitotic figures. (Courtesy of J. W. Kernohan and G. P. Sayre.[14])

and spinal cord, primary tumors arising from the orbital meninges are relatively rare. In fact, most meningiomas encountered in the orbit originate in the cranium. In many instances, however, it is impossible to determine whether the tumor is primary in the orbit or in the cranium. In a series of 52 orbital meningiomas, 17 were considered primary in the orbit and 35 were thought to have invaded the orbit from the cranium.[3] Even in the face of strong clinical evidence that a lesion is primary in the orbit, a cranial origin cannot be definitely ruled out.

Over one-third of intracranial meningiomas arise at the sphenoidal ridge, as an *en plaque* growth. They often invade the orbit early at its apex, either by direct growth through the bone or, less frequently, by extension along the nerve sheath, and become manifest because of orbital symptoms.

The large majority of orbital meningiomas are either of this intracranial type or primary tumors arising from the arachnoid around the optic canal or the posterior pole of the eyeball. Less frequently they arise from ectopic arachnoid in the dura, the periosteum, or the orbit (Fig. 5–2). The tumor is frequently lo-cated between the orbit and the cranium, in which case the primary site is of academic interest only.

A meningioma may have multiple origins. In a reported case the tumor arose from the optic nerve sheaths and from several cranial sites.[13]

ECTOPIC OR EXTRACRANIAL MENINGIOMA

Ectopic or extracranial meningiomas may develop in the region of the glabella or bridge of the nose.[15] They arise from small fragments of arachnoid cells that protruded through the glabella before the bones fused. These tumors may also appear in the orbit at the site of an encephalocele or a meningocele.

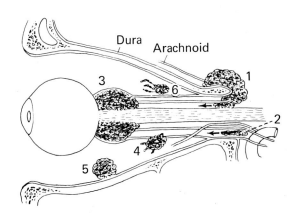

From arachnoid
   1 — Intracranial
   2 — Around canal
   3 — Around posterior
      pole of the eye

From ectopic arachnoid
   4 — In dura
   5 — In periosteum
   6 — In orbit

FIG. 5–2. Origins of orbital meningiomas. (Adapted from F. B. Walsh, by permission.)

RELATION TO VON RECKLINGHAUSEN'S DISEASE

A meningioma may be a feature of neurofibromatosis (von Recklinghausen's disease). A 17-year-old boy with no vision in the left eye for one year showed slight exophthalmos, no light perception, elevation and pallor of the left optic nerve, but no palpable mass in the orbit. A nodule from an arm and one from the chest were diagnosed as neurofibroma. A large tumor of the optic nerve, which had replaced three-fourths of its orbital portion, was removed. At the apex of the orbit the nerve assumed its normal size and consistency. The pathologic diagnosis was meningioma of the optic nerve sheath as a feature of neurofibromatosis (Fig. 5–3).

At a school eye testing, a 6-year-old girl was found to have no vision in the left eye. An ophthalmologic examination showed 15/70 vision in the fellow eye and lesions in both, diagnosed as meningiomas of the optic nerve in the left and possibly astrocytoma in the right (Fig. 5–4). A Krönlein operation included enucleation of the left eye and excision of the entire optic nerve, which was enlarged.

CLINICAL TYPES OF MENINGIOMA

Three clinical types are of interest to the ophthalmologist: suprasellar meningiomas, presellar meningiomas, and sphenoid-ridge meningiomas. The last-named group may be subdivided into lesions of the inner third, the middle third, and the outer third of the sphenoid ridge. The outer-third tumors are further subdivided according to whether the growth pattern is globular or *en plaque*. Finally, there may be overlapping symptoms; because of the small area involved, the symptoms of one type may simulate those of an adjacent growth. The chronologic appearance of the signs and symptoms may thus be important.

Suprasellar Meningioma

These usually globular tumors arise at the tuberculum in front of the sella and extend above it.[6] A field defect, usually bitemporal hemianopsia produced early in the course of

FIG. 5–3. Meningioma of the optic nerve sheath confined to the orbit, associated with von Recklinghausen's disease. **A.** Location of the tumor and its size in relation to the globe. **B.** High-power cytologic view.

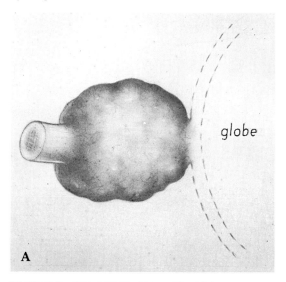

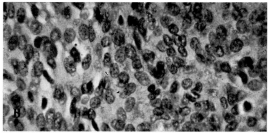

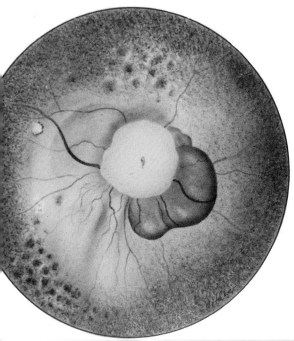

FIG. 5–4. Meningioma of the optic nerve associated with von Recklinghausen's disease of the orbit. **A.** In the left eye, the fundus shows a highly elevated, dumbbell-shaped mass obscuring the nerve head. Most of the base was under the retina and appeared cystic on transillumination; the remaining part projected into the vitreous as a chalky-white knob. X rays revealed many calcium deposits anterior to and above the sella turcica. This eye was smaller that the fellow eye, had a 4 mm proptosis and increased soft-tissue density of the orbit. The markedly enlarged left optic canal measured 8 mm. **B.** In the right eye the fundus showed a solitary, grayish-white, avascular, slightly elevated intraretinal mass of about 3 dd nasal to the nerve head. **C.** Cross section shows the optic nerve compressed by the meningioma and by areas of neurofibromatosis of the orbit. **D.** Psammoma bodies are visible under high-power magnification.

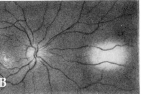

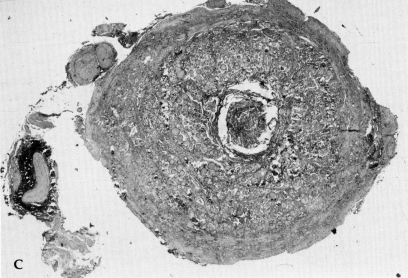

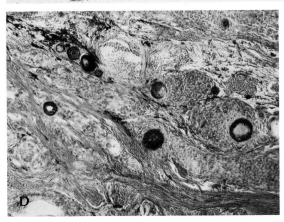

the tumor, calls attention to it while it is still small. One nerve may be more involved than the other, and the symptoms tend to become protean if the tumor is allowed to grow. Early surgical excision is often curative.

Presellar Meningioma

Presellar meningiomas arise from the olfactory groove and usually lead sequentially to unilateral optic atrophy, anosmia, papilledema on the side opposite to the atrophy (Gower-Kennedy syndrome), and perhaps chiasmal symptoms later.

Sphenoid-Ridge Meningioma

The distinct clinical picture of the meningiomas arising at different sites of the sphenoid ridge has been described.[6] Those arising from the inner third are related to the lesser sphenoidal wing and the anterior clinoid process. The usual symptoms, developing sequentially, are unilateral visual loss with optic atrophy, a nasal hemianopsic field defect on the affected side, unilateral exophthalmos, contralateral papilledema, abducens paralysis, other ocular muscle paralyses, and olfactory hallucinations. The symptoms of optic nerve meningiomas, whether arising there primarily or secondarily, are similar to those noted in tumors of the inner third of the sphenoid ridge.

Meningiomas of the middle third of the sphenoid ridge are asymptomatic when small. If they extend into the brain, a psychosis may be the first sign, and in some cases visual and olfactory hallucinations. Contralateral homonymous hemianopsia, unilateral optic atrophy, the Gower-Kennedy syndrome, and various ocular muscle paralyses appear in sequence, with unilateral proptosis a late symptom.

Outer-third tumors of the globular type usually cause headaches, convulsions, and psychoses but no eye symptoms, while those of the *en plaque* type produce unilateral exophthalmos, swelling of the temple and, late in the course, a decline in vision.

About 80% of sphenoid-ridge meningiomas are associated with bone destruction or hyperostosis, or both.

DIAGNOSIS

The patient may consult an ophthalmologist because of poor vision, unilateral exophthal-

mos, or both. In two reported series,[10,11] 66% of the patients had lost vision completely in one eye before the tumor was detected.

The importance of careful evaluation of the visual fields in making an early diagnosis has been stressed.[4] A homonymous hemianopsia, rather than a bitemporal chiasmal defect, was found in 75% of cases. These tumors are thought to cause no characteristic field defect.[7]

Optic atrophy may be one of the earliest ophthalmic signs,[8] and a frequent finding is a unilateral, long-standing visual disturbance in patients whose tumor is in the region of the anterior clinoid process.[19]

Meningiomas primary within the orbit seem to occur more frequently in children than in adults. A delay in the proper diagnosis is quite common. When there is any evidence of neurofibromatosis, glioma of the optic nerve is the first possibility to be considered, but the tumor may be a meningioma. Indeed, glioma, meningioma, and neurofibroma of the orbit may occur in the same patient (Fig. 5–4). Normal vision does not necessarily rule out glioma of the optic nerve.

The vagaries of meningiomas arising around the intracranial portion of the optic nerve have been noted.[17] The symptoms follow an episodic course and include a bilateral central scotoma simulating toxic amblyopia. The tumor may be first noticed during pregnancy, presumably because growth is accelerated.[21]

The tumor is locally invasive but does not metastasize. When originating in the cranium it may spread to the orbit, or the reverse may be true. The optic nerve as well as the disc, sclera, choroid, and retina may be involved.

Since the tumor tends to invade contiguous bone, hyperostosis is common and, with acquired tumor tissue, is a factor in the development of exophthalmos. Hyperostosis of the lateral orbital wall is occasionally recognized by bulging of the temporal fossa. Hyperostosis has been said to result from growth of the tumor into and through the haversian canal system of the bone.[6] The bone becomes irritated, resulting in osteoplastic proliferation. Lesions arising from the sphenoid ridge frequently show an *en plaque* type of growth with hyperostosis a prominent feature.

The importance of detecting hyperostosis by x rays at any point along the sphenoid ridge or around the optic canal has been stressed.[16] At first this may appear as a slight thickening of the bone with smooth cortical surfaces and no visible spicule formation. When the lesion is on the inner half of the ridge, the thickening may at first be confined to the lesser wing of the sphenoid. Hyperostosis in the early stages is often of a porous nature, increasing in density with later bony overgrowth until it simulates an osteoma. Other manifestations are bone destruction or pressure atrophy or both.

However, absence of hyperostosis does not rule out a diagnosis of meningioma. Also, overgrowth of bone may result from tumors of other types.

In a described case, a very small meningioma of the optic nerve was diagnosed through positive contrast orbitography which showed enlargement of the nerve.[5] Neither x ray nor carotid angiography was helpful in making the diagnosis in this patient, who presented with visual loss and papilledema but no other significant signs suggesting orbital tumor.

TREATMENT (See also Chapter 17)

In general, orbital meningiomas in children and adults are treated similarly except that temporization or orbital decompression by removal of the roof to relieve the exophthalmos, or removal of some of the bony optic foramen and canal to relieve pressure on the optic nerve, may be permissible in adults, some of whom have the tumor 20 to 30 years before function of the eye is jeopardized. However, it is usually unwise to withhold surgery when meningioma occurs in children as a feature of neurofibromatosis because of the expected accelerated growth in this age group.

The transcranial approach is indicated for tumors that extend to the apex of the orbit and may in places infiltrate the periosteum. This procedure includes removal of the orbital roof. The defect in the roof should be covered with a piece of mesh or a plate; otherwise, the frontal lobe may prolapse if an exenteration is carried out later.[20] If the findings suggest the need for orbital exenteration, it can be performed ten days to two weeks later.

Primary meningiomas of the orbit, which are rare, almost always originate from within the dural sleeve, but have been reported as arising on the outside.[1] They are more common in young people than in adults and more likely to be an early manifestation of neurofibromatosis, in which event they are especially progressive and usually require surgery. The Krönlein approach may be used except when the optic canal is involved, in which case the transcranial approach is indicated.

Early meningiomas of the lateral portion of the sphenoid ridge respond better to surgical treatment than those in the middle portion. With improved facilities for filling large bone defects, tumors located medially around the base of the brain and chiasm may be successfully excised.

If the cornea is threatened by exposure due to exophthalmos, lid adhesions may be necessary. In patients with marked exophthalmos and visual loss because of optic atrophy, enucleation may be desirable for cosmetic reasons. Some of the orbital tissue can be excised from time to time if the socket becomes too shallow to hold the prosthesis.

Irradiation is of no value in the treatment of meningiomas.

PROGNOSIS

When surgical excision is required in cases of meningioma primary in the orbit in young people, total visual loss in the affected eye can seldom be avoided. The same is true of primary meningiomas in the region of the optic canal. Orbital meningioma or optic nerve glioma with even minimal evidence of neurofibromatosis carries a poorer prognosis than without this complication, regarding both retention of vision and length of survival.

REFERENCES

1. AGERS T: Cited by Walsh FB in reference 20
2. BAILEY P, BUCY PC: The origin and nature of meningeal tumors. Am J Cancer 15:15–54, 1931
3. BENEDICT WL: Surgical treatment of tumors and cysts of the orbit. Am J Ophthalmol 32:763–773, 1949
4. BIRGE HL: Meningiomas: an ophthalmic problem. Am J Ophthalmol 32:763–773, 1949
5. BRANDT DE, BEISNER DH: Meningioma of the optic nerve; diagnosis by orbitography. Arch Ophthalmol 84:477–480, 1970
6. CUSHING H, EISENHARDT L: Meningiomas: Their Classification, Regional Behavior, Life History, and Surgical End-Results. Springfield, Ill, Charles C Thomas, 1938
7. DUNN SN, WALSH FB: Meningioma (dural endo-

thelioma) of the optic nerve. Arch Ophthalmol 56:702–707, 1956

8. GIBSON GG: Discussion in Grant FC, reference 10
9. GLOBUS JH: Meningiomas: the origin, divergence in structure, and relationship to contiguous tissues in light of phylogenesis and ontogenesis of meninges; with suggestion of a simplified classification of meningeal neoplasms. Arch Neurol Psychiat 36:667–712, 1937
10. GRANT FC: Meningioma of the tuberculum sellae. Arch Ophthalmol 49:365–367, 1953
11. GRANT FC, HEDGES TR: Ocular findings in meningiomas of the tuberculum sellae. Arch Ophthalmol 56:163–170, 1956
12. KARP LA, ZIMMERMAN LE, BORIT A, SPENCER W: Primary intraorbital meningiomas. Arch Ophthalmol 91:24–28, 1974
13. KERNOHAN JW, PARKER HL: Case of Recklinghausen's disease with observations on associated formation of tumors. J Nerv Ment Dis 76:313–330, 1932
14. KERNOHAN JW, SAYRE GP: Tumors of the Central Nervous System. In Atlas of Tumor Pathology, Section 10, Fascicles 35 and 37, Armed Forces Institute of Pathology, published by the National Research Council, Washington DC, 1952
15. NEW GB, DEVINE KD: Neurogenic tumors of the nose and throat. Trans Am Laryngol Assoc 67:137–149, 1946; also Arch Otolaryngol 46:163–179, 1947
16. PFEIFFER RL: Roentgenography of exophthalmos with notes on the roentgen ray in ophthalmology. Am J Ophthalmol 26:724–741, 816–833, 928–942, 1943
17. RUCKER CS, KEARNS TP: Mistaken diagnoses in some cases of meningioma. Am J Ophthalmol 51:15–19, 1961
18. RUSSELL DS, RUBENSTEIN LJ: Pathology of Tumours of the Nervous System. Baltimore, Williams & Wilkins, 1965
19. UIHLEIN A, WEYAND RD: Meningiomas of anterior clinoid process as a cause of unilateral loss of vision; surgical considerations. Arch Ophthalmol 49:261–270, 1953
20. WALSH FB: Meningiomas, primary within the orbit and optic canal. In Smith, JL (ed): Neuro-Ophthalmology, Symposium of the University of Miami and the Bascom Palmer Eye Institute, Hallandale, Fla, Huffman Pub Co, Vol 5, pp 240–266, 1969
21. WEYAND RD, MACCARTY CS, WILSON RB: Effect of pregnancy on intracranial meningiomas occuring about the optic chiasm. Surg Clin North Am 31:1225–1233, 1951

6

TUMORS OF THE
PERIPHERAL NERVES

All peripheral nerves are sheathed with a fibrous syncytium of Schwann cells after they leave the central nervous system. Most tumors of the peripheral nerves stem from these Schwann cells: neurofibroma, neurilemoma, malignant schwannoma, neurogliogenic tumor, and amputation neuroma. The group also includes some rarer choroidal tumors: solitary neurofibroma, Schwann-cell melanoma, and neurofibromatosis.

NEUROFIBROMATOSIS

Neurofibromatosis or multiple fibromas (von Recklinghausen's disease) is a systemic contion characterized by diffuse proliferation of the Schwann cells of the peripheral nerves. This complex multiple-tumor syndrome should be viewed as a congenital aberration. The lesions develop over an extensive area of the nervous system, in some instances apparently involving the entire system.

Normally, Schwann cells do not produce pigment. But in pathologic states the cells may produce melanin as well as a metaplastic striated muscle, bone, or cartilage and fat. A Schwann-cell tumor situated along the trunk of a nerve is usually nonpigmented, encapsulated, and benign. In ophthalmology, such a lesion is found most often in the orbit but sometimes in the uvea and is called a neurilemoma. On the other hand, a diffuse tumor arising from both the nerve trunk and the sensory terminals is associated with pigment production and is usually called a neurofibroma.

HEREDITY

The disease is inherited as a simple dominant trait[29] or an autosomal dominant trait with a very high rate of genetic mutation.[16] The history of two patients with ocular involvement in von Recklinghausen's disease showed a dominant mode of inheritance over two generations.[49] The disease has been reported in identical twins and in six successive generations.

Among the various primary manifestations in this disease are the following:

1. A localized acapsular nodule on the surface of the skin or mucous membrane due to proliferation at a nerve terminal.
2. A diffuse thickening and hypertrophy of the skin and sometimes the mucosa, making the integument hang in baggy folds. This so-called elephantiasis neuromatosa is frequently noted in the eyelid.
3. A proliferation inside the nerve sheaths, resulting in marked thickening and tortuosity of the nerves. This is usually called plexiform neurofibroma; when occurring in the lid it may be associated with elephantiasis neuromatosa of the overlying skin.

Among the various secondary manifestations are the following:

1. Invasion of bone causing either destruction or hypertrophy. When bones of the orbit, spine, or extremities are involved, both complications may lead to deformity and other sequelae.
2. Characteristic café-au-lait pigmentation of the skin either adjacent to a lesion or elsewhere over the body. The light-colored, irregular, flat, diffuse pigmentation is due to melanin in the deeper epidermal layers. Pigmented nevi may be associated with the lesion.
3. Fibroma molluscum—a small, multiple, localized skin nodule which is sometimes pedunculated; it is due to a simple proliferation of the fibrous tissue.
4. Lipoma.
5. Sebaceous adenoma.

PATHOLOGY

Microscopically, neurofibromas show diffuse proliferation of the Schwann cells and, less markedly, of the axons permeating the lesions in a diffuse and haphazard fashion. They occur either inside or outside of the

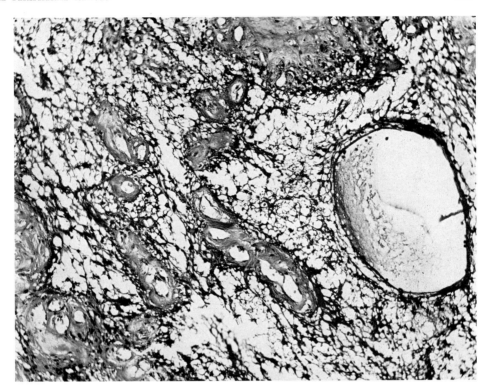

FIG. 6–1. Neurilemoma consisting of Antoni type-B tissue. Microcystic degeneration showing a degenerative cyst (at right) and blood vessels with thick collagen sheaths. (Courtesy of A. P. Stout.)

perineurium. Well-formed Wagner-Meissner tactile corpuscles are often present. Other structures that can sometimes be identified are melanoblasts, ganglion cells, and striated muscle cells.

Degeneration, which takes place in advanced stages of neurofibromatosis, results in a gelatinous or myxomatous tissue corresponding to Antoni's type-B growth seen in neurilemomas (Fig. 6–1).

The tumors associated with von Recklinghausen's disease (neurofibromas, gliomas, and meningiomas) have varied histologic characteristics and are widely disseminated throughout the central and peripheral nervous systems. It may therefore be assumed that the cause of the disease lies within the nerve cells and fibers, and that proliferation of the nerve tissue's supportive elements (the meninges, glia, endoneurium, perineurium, and neurilemma or sheath of Schwann) is merely a secondary process following degeneration of the affected nerve elements. Tumors in this disease appear to represent a reaction in the area of the nerve fibers rather than a neoplastic growth.[37]

CLINICAL COURSE

The lesions are first noted in the skin of children, sometimes as a patch of café-au-lait pigmentation or elephantiasis neuromatosa. It cannot be overemphasized that the manifestations are usually subtle. Awareness of the relationship of these changes to von Recklinghausen's disease was helpful in the diagnosis of the following cases:

1. A young boy with unilateral exophthalmos and a lesion in the scalp resembling elephantiasis neuromatosa. Glioma of the optic nerve was confirmed at operation.
2. A young girl with unilateral exophthalmos, café-au-lait pigmentation of the skin, and scoliosis. Glioma of the optic nerve was confirmed at operation.
3. A young girl with unilateral exophthalmos and an area of elephantiasis neuromatosa on the skin of the thigh. Glioma of the optic nerve was confirmed at operation.

4. Two young patients with unilateral exophthalmos, skin changes, and bony defects in the lateral wall of the orbit which proved to be neurofibromatoses with extension to the anterior cranial fossa.

5. An adult with papilledema of both eyes, multiple pedunculated neurofibromas of the skin, and deafness on the left side. Neuroma of the acoustic nerve was confirmed at operation.

Growth of the lesion may stop when the patient reaches maturity but may be resumed at any time later, sometimes in elderly patients with fatal results; e.g., extension of the lesion along nerves leading to the spinal roots may eventually involve the spinal cord, or a local malignant tumor such as a malignant schwannoma may arise at any site and metastasize via the bloodstream.

The cranial and sympathetic nerves, as well as the peripheral nerves, may be affected in von Recklinghausen's disease. Lesions such as gliosis or glioma or meningioma are at times found in the central nervous system, and solitary tumors of the neurilemoma group sometimes occur.

Mental retardation, psychic disorders, and epilepsy have been reported in association with neurofibromatosis.

Any of the cranial nerves may be affected, but most frequently the acoustic nerve. The olfactory and optic nerves are said to be spared because they are structurally different from the peripheral nerves. The optic nerve is not a true nerve but a fiber tract comparable with the intracerebral pathways of the brain (see Ch. 4, Glioma of the Optic Nerve, Retina, and Orbit). Its supportive tissues and enveloping sheaths also differ from those of the peripheral nerves. Still there is no doubt that the optic nerve is involved in neurofibromatosis.

EYE MANIFESTATIONS

Eye involvement in neurofibromatosis is much more common than indicated by clinical examination; any part of the eye or adnexa may be affected. In some reported cases involving the choroid, few or no clinical signs of the disease were detected. One patient had a cornea 1 mm larger in diameter on the involved side, with normal intraocular pressure. However, microscopic examination revealed extensive involvement of the choroid, ciliary body, iris, orbital nerves, and optic nerve.[10]

The most common radiologic findings in neurofibromatosis are enlargement of the orbit and partial loss of the walls; the roof and the apex are most often affected.

Homolateral facial hemihypertrophy involves the bones and soft tissues. Malformations of the sphenoid may lead to meningocele with pulsating exophthalmos.

Hydrophthalmos and intraocular hypertension are commonly detected at birth or soon after. Patients with glaucoma usually have homolateral plexiform neuroma of the upper lid or facial hemihypertrophy with or without bony changes.

Attention has been called to an arching upward of the inner portion of the lid border, with the outer half assuming a downward convexity. The extreme elasticity of the skin of the lid in this event provides an important physical sign contributing to correct diagnosis of neurofibromatosis of the orbit.[45]

Buphthalmos

Glaucoma with buphthalmos is not uncommon in ocular neurofibromatosis (Fig. 6–2).

FIG. 6–2. Neurofibromatosis of the choroid and ciliary body. A 9-year-old girl had an enlarged left eye with increased intraocular pressure, protrusion of the forehead, and a depression in the temporal region due to neurofibromatosis. The eye was enucleated because of intractable glaucoma. Microscopic examination confirmed the diagnosis.

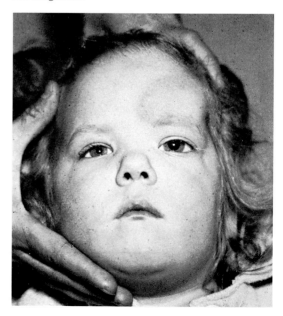

Eyelids

The lids, as well as adjacent skin of the face and temporal region, may show elephantiasis neuromatosa, localized single or multiple neurofibromas, fibroma molluscum, and café-au-lait pigmentation, alone or in various combinations (Fig. 6–3). In some instances diffuse thickening and hypertrophy of the skin, due to elephantiasis neuromatosa, causes ptosis. However, facial asymmetry noted soon after birth, rather than abnormality of any particular structure, may be the first manifestation of the disease.

The skin of the upper lid, even if it appears relatively normal, is unusually lax when the orbit is involved in neurofibromatosis. Thus, when comparison of the two upper lids reveals a greater elasticity in one, the disease may be suspected in the orbit on that side.

Orbit

Changes in the bony orbit, frequent manifestations of the disease (see Ch. 17, Fig. 17–10F and G), usually consist of bone destruction or, less often, bone hypertrophy.

The bone defect in the roof of the orbit may permit the transmission of intracranial pulsation to the orbital contents, producing pulsation of the globe (Fig. 6–4) which is synchronous with the pulse, unaccompanied by a bruit, and causes no discomfort. Some degree of exophthalmos may be present, due to brain herniation through the bone defect or to neurofibromas in the orbit or to both.

A 4-year-old girl who had had a slowly progressing proptosis of the left eye since the age of 2 subsequently developed poor vision and papilledema in the right eye. Proptosis spontaneously regressed in the left eye, then developed in the right eye over a period of a few weeks. Café-au-lait spots were scattered over the trunk. This was an unusual case of neurofibroma of the orbit with extension to the cranium (Fig. 6–5). Spontaneous regression of proptosis of the left eye was attributed to erosion of bone, permitting the contents of the decompressed orbit to enter the cranium. A 7-year-old sibling with more extensive café-au-lait spots had no overt manifestations of von Recklinghausen's disease.

An advanced case of neurofibroma of the orbit is shown in Figure 6–6.

Gliomas or meningiomas of the optic nerve or both may be manifestations of neurofibromatosis.

Hypertrophy may affect any of the orbital bones but is noted most often around the superior orbital margin, giving it a full round shape.

In cases where neurofibromatosis involves the ocular adnexa, I have frequently noted in the temporal fossa a marked depression (Fig. 6–3C) which seems to be due to atrophy of the temporal muscle.

Diffuse and often with systemic effects, orbital neurofibromas may invade the contiguous bone, reaching the cranial cavity and other vital areas. It is difficult to give any rule-of-thumb treatment plan. In view of the steadily progressive process, an exenteration and resection of any involved bone is sometimes advisable. If the tumor has extended toward or into the cranial cavity, a neurosurgeon's services are required.

Five of our patients with neurofibromatosis showed a striking enlargement of the optic foramen, indicating involvement of the optic nerve or its sheaths. Sometimes the entire optic canal is obliterated, owing to neurofibromatous erosion.

A type of neurofibromatosis has been described whose salient features are a plexiform neurofibroma of the orbit (and often the globe, optic nerve, and eyelids as well), with defects in the bony orbital wall, and intracranial growth in the middle cranial fossa which involves the sella turcica.[41]

In summary, exophthalmos may be a feature of neurofibromatosis because of neurofibromatous tissue in the orbit, erosion of orbital bone which allows herniation of the brain, glioma of the optic nerve, or meningioma of the optic nerve sheaths.

Conjunctiva

Many reports have appeared on involvement of the bulbar and palpebral conjunctiva. In one patient with buphthalmos the anterior ciliary nerves were affected with neurofibromatosis.[50,51] The appearance was that of numerous worms beneath the conjunctiva and attached to the sclera near the cornea. Another patient with bilateral plexiform neuroma of the conjunctiva also showed medullated corneal nerves.[24]

Uvea

Neurofibromatosis in this area is usually diffuse, involving the choroid, ciliary body, and iris (Fig. 6–7). Microscopically, ovoid

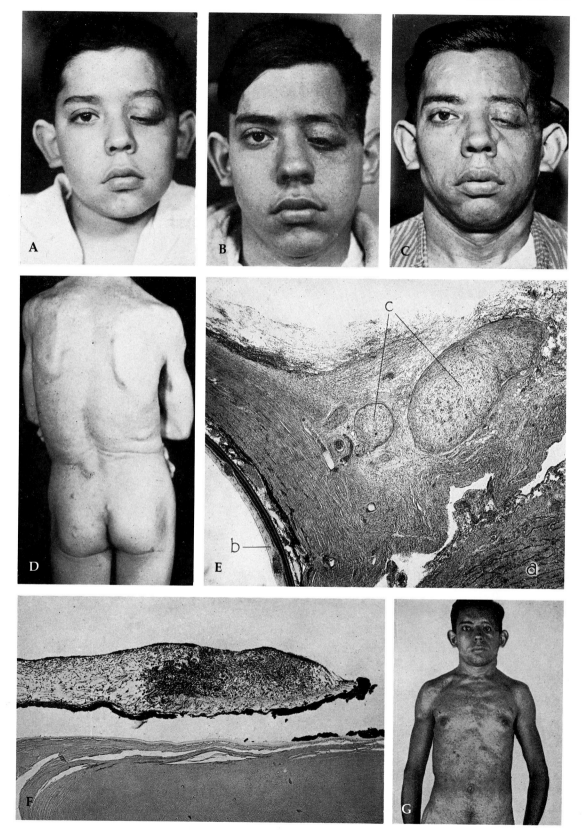

FIG. 6–3. Neurofibromatosis. **A.** Involvement of the left eyelids at age 12. **B.** At age 17. **C.** At age 22, by which time the temporal fossa had become depressed, and the skin showed elephantiasis neuromatosa and café-au-lait spots. **D.** Kyphosis, scoliosis, café-au-lait spots, and multiple fibromata mollusca on the buttocks. **E.** The eye was enucleated to permit elevation of the lid and use of a prosthesis for cosmetic effect. Sections of the globe showed neurofibromatosis of the large ciliary nerves (*c*). The retina is seen at *b* and the optic nerve at *a*. **F.** Melanoma of the iris discovered after enucleation. **G.** The patient wearing a prosthesis. The skin over the chest and abdomen shows numerous café-au-lait spots, pigmented nevi or neurofibromas, and fibromata mollusca.

FIG. 6–4. Neurofibromatosis. **A.** The right lids, cheek, and temporal region are involved in neurofibromatosis. The patient shows extensive elephantiasis neuromatosa, café-au-lait spots, hirsutism, and pulsation of the globe due to bony defects in the orbital roof. (An x ray showing the bony defects appears in Fig. 17–10F). **B.** Elephantiasis neuromatosa and café-au-lait spots of the skin in the buttock and sacral areas.

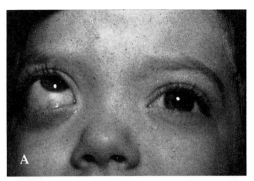

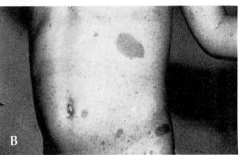

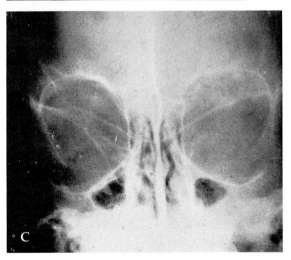

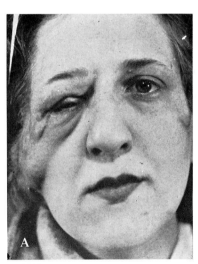

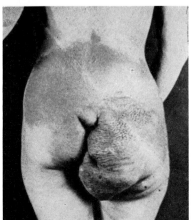

FIG. 6–5. Neurofibroma of the orbit with extension to the cranium. **A.** The markedly proptosed right eye was found to be due to a smooth firm mass palpable in the lower outer quadrant of the orbit. The optic disc was pale, and faint pulsations of the left eye were noted. **B.** Café-au-lait spots of various sizes were scattered over the trunk. **C.** In x rays the right orbit was smaller than the left and had a 6 mm optic canal. The left optic canal was poorly visualized because of bone dehiscence of the posterior part of the orbit. Neurofibromatosis as part of von Recklinghausen's disease was diagnosed after microscopic examination of biopsy tissue from the right orbit.

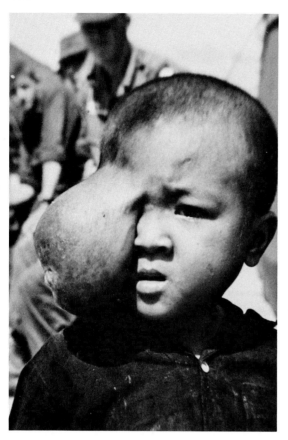

FIG. 6–6. Neurofibroma of the orbit. Advanced tumor in a 4-year-old Vietnamese boy. U.S. Army photo by 101st Airborne Brigade 10.)

bodies or Wagner-Meissner corpuscles are often found in addition to the usual characteristic changes of neurofibromatosis. There may be an increase in the number of ganglionlike cells (Fig. 6–7C) and frequently melanin in the tumor's fibrous cells.

The iris often shows changes of various kinds in uveal neurofibromatosis. Nodules over the iris surface consisting of proliferated stroma melanocytes have been mentioned;[6,35] also noted have been heterochromia and melanosis of the iris (Fig. 6–3F), a generalized thickening of the iris, partial iris coloboma, and excentric pupil with ectropion of the pigment epithelium.[19] These manifestations may simulate early malignant melanoma of the iris, particularly the tapioca type.

A patient with uveal neurofibromatosis and a malignant melanoma of the choroid of the left eye as well as a neurinoma of the

right orbit was described,[47] and several cases of neurofibromatosis associated with malignant choroidal melanoma.

To support the view that a benign or malignant uveal melanoma may be composed of apparently pure Schwann cells,[14] the author presented specimens showing nerves fanning out into tissue of the tumor, indicating its origin in the Schwann sheath.

Retina

Medullated nerve fibers in the retinal fiber layer have been often noted in patients with neurofibromatosis. Four of 12 patients with generalized neurofibromatosis in one series showed medullated nerve fibers of the retina. Routine ophthalmologic examinations revealed this finding in 4 of 130 inmates of a mental institution, but in only 1 among 3250 subjects in the general population.[27] Medullated nerve fibers of the retina were reported in both eyes of a patient with neurofibromatosis and bilateral optic nerve tumors.[20] A massive glioma of the retina was seen in a case of neurofibromatosis.[30]

Oligodendroglia of the optic nerve has been compared with Schwann cells of the peripheral nerves since both supply myelin for the axons.[11,12] In this event, the presence of medullated retinal nerve fibers in patients with neurofibromatosis supports the theory that gliomas of the optic nerve are oligodendrocytomas.

Retinal tumors have been noted in patients with neurofibromatosis, and in some instances the tumor clinically resembled those associated with tuberous sclerosis (see Ch. 4, Fig. 4–7).

There is considerable evidence of the relationship between von Recklinghausen's disease (neurofibromatosis), Bourneville's disease (tuberous sclerosis), von Hippel's disease (angiomatosis retinae), and Sturge-Weber-Dimitri disease.

Optic Nerve

Gliomas and, much less frequently, meningiomas may occur in conjunction with neurofibromatosis. In young patients with these associated lesions of the optic nerve, café-au-lait pigmentation of the skin may be the first and only other detectable sign of neurofibromatosis. Among 46 reported cases of neurofibromatosis in children under 12 years

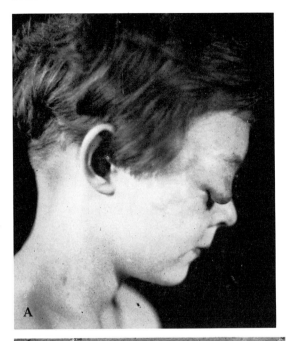

FIG. 6–7. Neurofibromatosis of the right upper lid, orbit, orbital nerves, and eyeball. **A.** Skin shows elephantiasis neuromatosa and café-au-lait spots. Corneal edema prevented examination of the interior of the buphthalmic eye. **B.** Under low power the choroidal tissue shows marked thickening due to the neurofibromatosis. **C.** High-power view of the section outlined in **B** showing (*a*) nerve and (*b*) ganglion cells. **D.** Section from the ciliary body showing similar thickening and ganglion cells. **E.** Section from the choroid showing a large, well-formed Wagner-Meissner corpuscle. (Courtesy of J. M. Wheeler.)

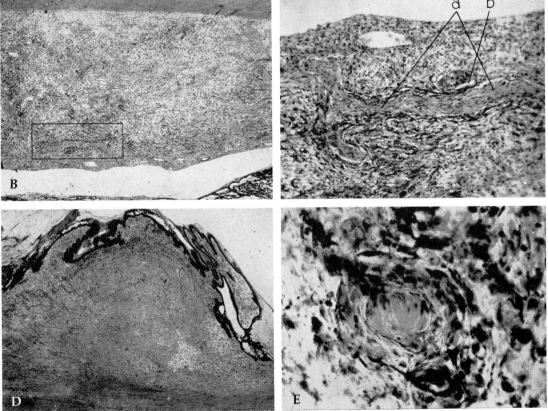

of age, 4 had glioma of the optic nerve and 2 of these had megalocornea and glaucoma.[16]

Treatment of neurofibromatosis is limited; the lesion does not respond to radiation. Sometimes the patient's appearance can be improved by excising tumor tissue and carrying out plastic repair. Operations to relieve the ptosis are unsatisfactory; if the lid is properly elevated it will not function well enough to protect the eye. When the eye is enucleated, the lid can be raised in a more or less fixed position, improving the patient's appearance considerably (Fig. 6-3G). The tumor, usually incompletely excised, recurs slowly and ultimately negates the effect of plastic surgery.

NEURILEMOMA (SCHWANNOMA)

The term *schwannoma* has been suggested for tumors developing from Schwann cells of the neural sheath[52] instead of the older terms *neurilemoma* and *neurinoma,* which designate tumors containing connective tissue elements.

Neurilemoma, a term proposed by Stout[46] and now widely accepted, denotes a cohesive, localized, well-encapsulated nerve-sheath tumor occurring anywhere along the course of a peripheral, cranial, or sympathetic nerve. Although usually benign, one case reported in the orbit manifested a sarcomatous transformation.[42] Neurilemomas develop in about 10% of patients with neurofibromatosis. These tumors (neurinoma, perineural fibroblastoma, peripheral glioma, schwannoglioma, schwannoma, and specific nerve-sheath tumor) show two types of growth, referred to as Antoni type A and type B. They are usually admixed, with one type predominating. Antoni type-A tissue (Fig. 6–8) is the solid portion, consisting of Schwann cells arranged in interlacing cords and of delicate connective tissue fibers with a high reticulum content. The nuclei tend to palisade or form in rows with clear intervening spaces. The cells and fibers may be arranged in organoid units called Verocay bodies, which resemble exaggerated tactile corpuscles (Fig. 6–9). The type-B tissue consists of a loose areolar arrangement of the Schwann cells with many microcysts which coalesce to form cystic spaces. As the tumor grows, these areas of cystic degeneration form cavities large enough to be quite conspicuous, and the blood vessels show thick collagen sheaths

FIG. 6–8. Early neurilemoma consisting of Antoni type-A tissue. (Courtesy of A. P. Stout.)

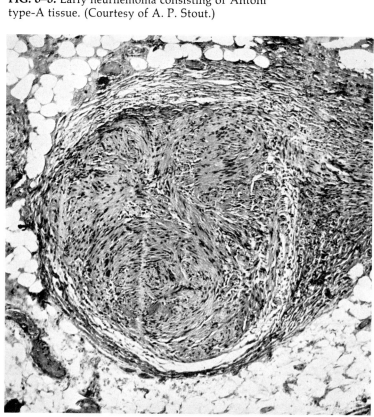

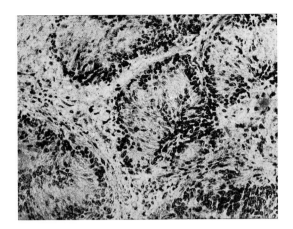

FIG. 6–9. Verocay bodies in a neurilemoma showing palisaded nuclei resembling grotesque tactile corpuscles. (Courtesy of A. P. Stout.)

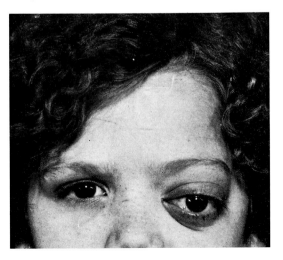

FIG. 6–10. Neurilemoma of the orbit. Exophthalmos in a 7-year-old girl was caused by a neurilemoma which, when excised, was well encapsulated.

(Fig. 6–1). Although axons are not typically found, they may sprout at the periphery of the tumor when the fibers of the involved nerve are injured by growth within the epineural sheath. Phagocytes loaded with lipoid material are at times a striking feature.

Orbital neurilemoma usually causes exophthalmos (Fig. 6–10) but no other distinctive clinical features (see Ch. 17, Orbital Neoplasms and Lesions Simulating Them). It tends to progress slowly and sometimes intermittently over a period of years. One such tumor first noted in a 2-year-old remained unchanged for 16 years and then resumed growth,[37] and another presented as retrobulbar neuritis.[32]

The well-encapsulated tumors can be easily shelled out by blunt dissection in the same way as a hemangioma. The Krönlein procedure is often the operation of choice. Although usually solitary, the tumors may be multiple. Thorough palpation of the orbit before closing the incision may reveal one or more other tumor sites. The tumors rarely recur after local excision, and the prognosis is excellent.

Neurilemomas may occur in the lid, the conjunctiva, or at the limbus.

Some choroidal tumors composed of Schwann cells have the histologic characteristics of neurilemomas, with typical palisading of the nuclei (see Ch. 7, Fig. 7–26). These choroidal tumors are usually grouped as melanomas without pigment.

MALIGNANT SCHWANNOMAS

Malignant tumors of peripheral nerves which arise from the Schwann cells include neurogenic or neurogenous sarcomas, malignant neurilemomas, malignant neurinomas, and fibrosarcomas of the nerve sheaths. They are characterized by the cells' tendency to grow in interlacing bundles associated with palisading nuclei and intercellular connective tissue containing long, straight reticulum fibers paralleling the long axes of the cells. Approximately half the lesions arise in patients with von Recklinghausen's disease. Various metaplastic tissues, *e.g.,* cartilage, bone, rhabdomyoblasts, and fat, are sometimes found.

In the majority of our cases the tumor has proved fatal. Malignant schwannoma has been reported in the epibulbar area and invading the orbit,[40] arising at the limbus and invading the orbit,[39] and a solitary lesion of the orbit causing proptosis.[33] In one instance[39] three recurrences after local excision finally made exenteration necessary. Malignant schwannomas that develop in the choroid are considered a type of malignant melanoma (see Ch. 7).

AMPUTATION NEUROMA

When a nerve is severed, a proliferation of Schwann cells and to a lesser degree of connective tissue cells is noted on the proximal end. New axons emerge and tend to follow the potential sheaths formed by the Schwann cells, accounting for the exuberant growth of Schwann cells. Some of the sheathed axons are embedded in scar tissue and course in all directions. This mass is often large and globular and may assume tumorlike proportions. If there is tugging, pain may ensue.

So-called amputation neuromas do not give rise to true neoplasms; they represent merely a proliferative and hyperplastic reaction to severance of a nerve. This may be any nerve, including a sympathetic nerve, anywhere in the body. The reaction is particularly likely to develop after a limb is amputated.

Since orbital nerves are often severed during surgery, it is surprising that there have been so few reports of amputation neuromas in this area. Many ciliary nerves are cut during enucleation or exenteration, particularly, but neuromas arising from them apparently seldom cause symptoms, probably because they are small and not subject to mechanical factors.

Since histologic examination of the orbit is rare after enucleation or exenteration, there is no way of determining the incidence of amputation neuromas.

Orbital amputation neuromas have been encountered during a study of nerve regeneration after opticociliary neurectomy, after opticociliary resection to relieve pain and to prevent sympathetic ophthalmia, and after enucleation. They are probably more common than has been generally supposed. Implants inserted after enucleation make it difficult to detect them.

An orbital amputation neuroma was described in a 3-year-old black boy.[3] The right eye was enucleated because of retinoblastoma; no implant was inserted. An indefinite resistance was palpable at the apex of the orbit two months postoperatively. A recurrence was not suspected as microscopic examination of the enucleated globe showed no extraocular extension of the tumor, and the operative section was beyond any tumor invasion of the optic nerve. Four months after enucleation a large, firm, sharply demarcated, freely movable mass 30–35 mm in diameter was palpable in the central portion of the orbit. It was in the muscle funnel and not attached to the bone. Since the choroid of the enucleated eye showed tumor invasion near the disc, and some tumor cells had extended beyond the lamina cribrosa, the diagnosis was recurrent retinoblastoma. The right orbit was exenterated, and microscopic examination showed an amputation neuroma. This patient's age and the keloid tendency of his race may have been partially responsible for the rapid regenerative process after enucleation. The time interval between severance of a nerve and appearance of an amputation neuroma varies from several months to over 50 years.

An amputation neuroma after excision of a pterygium was thought to have originated from a severed intrascleral nerve loop.[23]

NEUROGLIOGENIC TUMORS

Neurogliogenic tumors arise from the peripheral nerves as well as the central nervous system. In the central nervous system, including the retina, they are called glioneuromas when benign (composed essentially of mature glial and neuronal elements) and spongioneuroblastomas when malignant (composed of spongioblastic elements and neuronal cells in various immature stages) (see Ch. 2). Comparable tumors of the peripheral nerves are called ganglioneuromas when benign and neuroblastomas or sympathicoblastomas when malignant. The neoplastic elements stem from the spinal or sympathetic ganglion cells. All transitional stages are seen between a) glioneuromas and spongioneuroblastomas of the central nervous system and b) ganglioneuromas and neuroblastomas of the peripheral nerves.

GANGLIONEUROMAS

Ganglioneuromas are composed of more or less mature ganglion cells in a dense stroma of sheathed axons running haphazardly in all directions. They are localized and do not metastasize. Characteristically, they arise anywhere along the chain of sympathetic ganglia (which extend from the base of the skull to the coccyx) or in the suprarenal medulla.

If a ganglioneuroma is incompletely differentiated so that part or all resembles an undifferentiated neuroblastoma, it may have a malignant tendency. Although it has been stated that fully differentiated ganglioneuromas do not metastasize,[46] in a series here at the Eye Institute metastasis occurred in 18% of partially differentiated tumors and in 65% of those composed of both fully differentiated ganglion cells and completely undifferentiated sympathoblasts.

Theoretically, these tumors can arise from the ciliary ganglion within the muscle funnel of the orbit. Although such unrecognized tumors have undoubtedly occurred, I have never seen any case or any reports in the literature.

To my knowledge, there have been no reports of a tumor arising from the ganglion cells of the retina.

neuroblasts may be observed in bone marrow specimens.

According to Stout,[46] tumors in most of the reported cures of so-called neuroblastoma in children were partly differentiated ganglioneuromas rather than pure sympathicoblastomas.

These tumors are highly malignant and metastasize freely, especially through the bloodstream. Skeletal metastasis, particularly to the cranium, has been reported in 74% of cases.[38] When the orbital bones are involved (see Ch. 17, Fig. 17–10D), the tumor quickly gains access to the orbit and causes exophthalmos (Fig. 6–11). Bone metastases and exophthalmos commonly appear long before the primary focus is manifest. In fact, sometimes it is not detected before the postmortem examination.

When the orbit is affected it is usually on the same side as the primary tumor. In one case there was radiologic evidence of calcification above the kidney.[43] I know of no instance of a neuroblastoma metastasizing to

NEUROBLASTOMA (SYMPATHICOBLASTOMA)

Neuroblastoma, the second most common malignant tumor in children, arises from the same sites as ganglioneuromas, but tends to occur primarily in the adrenal medulla and in the retroperitoneal ganglia. However, a reported case associated with orbital metastasis had originated high in the cervical sympathetic chain.[43]

Neuroblastomas contain embryonal neuroblasts or sympathoblasts—undifferentiated, small, round cells arranged in groups without connective tissue stroma between the individual cells. A fibrous framework supports the separate groups. Fibrils and a few imperfect ganglion cells are often found. The fibrils, a distinctive feature, are part of the nerve cells and are arranged in either rounded masses or longitudinal bundles. The tumor cells are grouped around them in rosette formation.

Differential diagnosis depends on demonstrating axons by either tissue culture or special fixation of the tissue followed by silver impregnation. Electron microscopy is also very helpful. Another diagnostic aid is demonstration of catecholamines and their degradation products in the urine.[53] Also,

FIG. 6–11. Metastasis of a neuroblastoma to the left orbit. The primary site of the neuroblastoma in an 8-month-old boy was thought to be the suprarenal medulla. The left eye was exophthalmic, with considerable ecchymosis of the lids and conjunctiva from orbital inflammation due to necrosis of the tumor tissue.

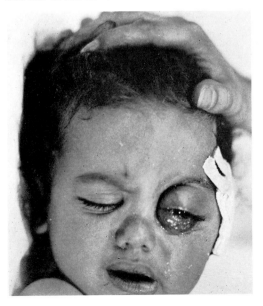

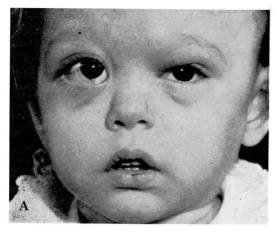

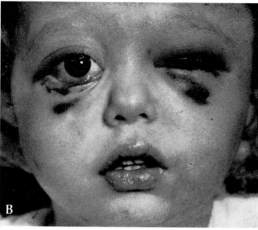

FIG. 6–12. Metastasis of a neuroblastoma to both orbits. **A.** Marked ecchymosis of the lids of both eyes, exophthalmos of the right eye, and partial closure of the palpebral aperture of the left eye, due to a neuroblastoma in the upper nasal quadrant of the orbit. **B.** The patient eight days later.

the eye instead of the orbit, although metastatic tumor cells have been demonstrated histologically in the choroidal vessels.

Two types of the disease are sometimes designated: a) the Pepper type, which appears as a uniform enlargement of the liver associated with a primary tumor of the right adrenal gland, and b) the Hutchison type, characterized by bone metastasis in the skull, particularly in the orbit, with the first sign of the disease being a lesion around the eye.

Unilateral or even bilateral exophthalmos in a child from 9 months to 9 years may be due to a neuroblastoma metastasizing to the orbit (Fig. 6–12). Half the patients are under age 2 when the condition is discovered.[2]

It is important for ophthalmologists to recognize the ocular manifestations of neuroblastoma which they often encounter in its early stages. Ocular involvement was reported in over 54% of 53 verified cases of this tumor;[2] the author considered Horner's syndrome one of the early signs. The spontaneous remission rate may reach 15%.[15] Remissions and spontaneous cures follow necrosis of the tumor and dedifferentiation of the cytology to that of a benign ganglioneuroma.

Since the first report that a malignant neuroblastoma might dedifferentiate into a benign ganglioneuroma,[8] spontaneous maturation of neuroblastoma has been described from time to time. It has been speculated that in neuroblastoma a major surgical procedure such as incomplete removal or x-ray therapy might increase the survival rate by stimulating an immunologic response to the tumor. The consensus now seems to be that surgery, irradiation and chemotherapy may cause tumor regression without effecting a cure. There remain, however, a few well-documented cases in which a proved neuroblastoma has undergone spontaneous maturation to a "cured" benign glioneuroma.

Two reported cases of histologically verified malignant neuroblastoma on subsequent biopsy turned out to be merely mature ganglioneuromas; and two other patients with histologically verified hepatic metastasis of neuroblastoma later showed no evidence of tumor.[22] Disseminated neuroblastoma in two sisters which spontaneously regressed to benign ganglioneuroma or to calcified residues has been described.[21]

Exophthalmos may appear long before the primary tumor is detected. The tumor tends to become necrotic and thus produce in the orbit inflammatory signs, ecchymosis, and hemorrhage (Fig. 6–12B). Ecchymosis of the lids is especially characteristic.

Theoretically, a neuroblastoma could arise primarily in the orbit from the ciliary ganglion; one such case was reported[26] and I believe I have seen two cases, but since no autopsy was performed a latent primary site elsewhere could not be ruled out.

In view of the tendency toward spontaneous remission, surgery, chemotherapy, or radiation during the acutely malignant phase may delay progress of the tumor until a less aggressive course sets in, preventing a fatal outcome.[38]

A reported case of bilateral neuroblastoma thought to be primary in the orbit was treated by chemotherapy and radiation. There was no evidence of disease two years later.[17]

PARAGANGLIOMAS

Paragangliomas arise from the paraganglion cells of the autonomic nervous system. They therefore originate in the adrenal medulla, the chain of ganglia extending from the base of the skull to the coccyx, the carotid body, the glomus jugulare, glomus caroticum, and glomus aorticum. A number of reports of both benign and malignant cases have been published.[1,13,18,25,31,34,48]

A nonchromaffin paraganglionic structure found in the orbit of a chimpanzee was described as a small oval nodule near the ciliary ganglion.[4] Although this finding has not been reported in human orbital tissue, theoretically a paraganglioma could arise in the muscle cone of the orbit.

Paragangliomas may be functioning (hormonally active) or nonfunctioning. A pheochromocytoma is a hormonally active paraganglioma arising from or near the suprarenal medulla. The paraganglionic cells in the suprarenal medulla, and less prominently in the adjacent retroperitoneal ganglia, show granules in the cytoplasm which have an affinity for chrome salts. For this reason these cells are usually called chromaffin cells, and their function is secreting catecholamines. When a tumor arises from them, an excessive amount of epinephrine is produced which raises the blood pressure and frequently causes retinal changes. The affected patients have paroxysmal or continuous hypertension, either of which is at times associated with hyperinsulinism and hyperthyroidism. These tumors are of interest to the ophthalmologist because they may manifest themselves through the retinal changes resulting from hypertension.

The granules are best demonstrated by fixing the tissue in Orth's fluid; they become brown with hematoxylin and eosin stain, and green with Schmorl's stain.

Tumors that are not hormonally active have the same histologic characteristics as those that are hormonally active except that they have no chromaffin granules. Hormonally inactive paragangliomas may develop wherever parasympathetic ganglia are found.

Paragangliomas are frequently confused with granular-cell myoblastomas.

NEUROEPITHELIAL TUMORS

When the peripheral nerves develop from the neural crest there may be cell rests from which neuroepithelial tumors sometimes arise. These tumors have morphologic characteristics similar to those of central nervous system cells. Thus, rare malignant neoplasms of the peripheral nerves may be composed of cells imitating CNS cells. Despite the histologic resemblance, however, the two types of tumors differ biologically in one important respect: neuroepithelial tumors in the peripheral nervous system can metastasize via the bloodstream and result in fatality.[46]

To my knowledge, no such tumors have been reported in the eye or adnexa although they could occur there.

A neuroectodermal tumor of the iris (anterior lip of the optic cup), which was present at birth, was excised at age 6 months.[28] Death resulted from cardiac arrest. Histologically the tumor resembled a glioneuroma with transition to a teratoid medulloepithelioma.

Two cases of glioneuroma which appeared to arise within congenital colobomatous defects in the ciliary body, iris, and retina have been described.[45] The authors considered them choristomatous malformations from divergent differentiation of the neuroepithelial cells at the advancing margin of the invaginated optic cup.

INTRASCLERAL NERVE LOOP

An intrascleral nerve loop may be mistaken clinically for an epibulbar tumor (Fig. 6–13). The long ciliary nerves normally loop into the sclera 4 to 7 mm from the limbus and then progress forward into the ciliary body. Instead of the nerve loop being confined to the innermost layers of the sclera, it sometimes extends to the external scleral surface and is seen clinically under the conjunctiva as a localized, elevated grayish-white nodule. Pigment may be noted around the nerve loop, representing the extension of uveal pigment cells accompanying the nerve through the sclera.

Such a nerve loop is sometimes excised, being mistaken for a conjunctival tumor. The pathologic report usually reads "fibroma,"

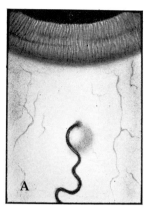

FIG. 6–13. Intrascleral nerve loop. A. At 6 o'clock, 4–5 mm from the limbus, is an elevated grayish lesion; in its margin an anterior ciliary artery enters the sclera at the site of an emissary dotted by uveal pigment. B. Section shows (a) an intrascleral nerve loop which extends just beyond the scleral surface, and (b) the ciliary body. C. Section shows (a) the cupola of a retroverted intrascleral nerve loop on the external scleral surface and covered only by conjunctiva and (b) the ciliary body.

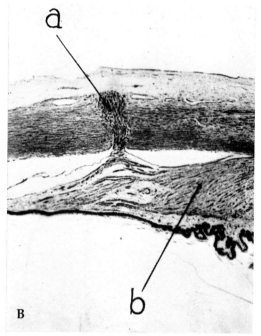

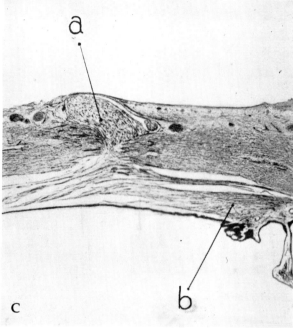

"neuroma," or "neurofibroma." The condition is unlikely to be correctly interpreted unless the ophthalmologist is aware of the possibility of such an anatomic variation. I know of three instances in which the loop of a long ciliary nerve was mistaken for a new-growth and excised.

MIXED NEUROGENIC TUMORS

A mixed neurogenic tumor of the orbit may arise from a congenital rest or malformation; an encephalocelelike protrusion of the brain during embryonic development becomes partially or entirely separated and develops independently. Such rests are also found at the base of the nose in the region of the lacrimal fossa.

At the 1957 meeting of the Verhoeff Society, I reported a case of congenital neurogenic rest of the orbit (posterior encephalocele) in a 14-month-old boy with proptosis of the right eye since birth. At surgery a large tumor mass surrounding the optic nerve proved to be a mixed neurogenic tumor. It was generally agreed that this came from congenital ectopic brain tissue—an encephalocele that reached the orbit through the sphenoidal fissure, which was shown by x rays to be enlarged. A bilateral case of anterior orbital meningoencephalocele has been reported.[7] The diagnosis can usually be established by x ray. The nature of encephalocele and meningocele is discussed in Chapter 17.

Tumors from these ectopic brain rests contain bipotential cells. They usually develop along the spongioblastic series and tend to resemble gliomas. If they develop along the neuroblastic series, the result may be a neuroepitheliomatous tumor or even a malignant lesion such as a neuroblastoma (retinoblastoma) or a medulloblastoma.

Some primary mixed tumors of the orbit have prominent ganglion cells, raising the question whether they could have originated in the ciliary ganglion. Although they are seen almost exclusively in children from 3 months to 6 years of age, one case occurred in a 58-year-old woman.[5]

REFERENCES

1. ABRAHAMS IW, FENTON RH, VIDONE R: Alveolar soft-part sarcoma of the orbit. Arch Ophthalmol 79:185–188, 1968
2. ALFANO JE: Ophthalmological aspects of neuroblastomatosis; a study of 53 verified cases. Trans Am Acad Ophthalmol Otolaryngol 72:830–848, 1968
3. BLODI FC: Amputation neuroma in the orbit. Am J Ophthalmol 32:929–932, 1949
4. BOTÁR J, PRIBÉK L: Corpuscule paraganglionnaire dans l'orbite (note préliminaire). Ann Anat Pathol 12:227–228, 1957
5. BOURQUET J, MAWAS J: Gliome encapsulé de l'orbite. Bull Soc Ophtalmol Fr, pp 224–246, 1931
6. CHODOS JB, MAEDER G: Neurofibromatose familiale de l'iris. Ophthalmologica 133:237–241, 1957
7. CHOHAN BS, PARMER IPS, BHATIA JN: Anterior orbital meningoencephalocele. Am J Ophthalmol 68:144–146, 1969
8. CUSHING H, WOLBACH SB: Transformation of malignant paravertebral sympathicoblastoma into benign ganglioneuroma. Am J Pathol 3:203–216, 1927
9. DAVIS FA: Plexiform neurofibromatosis (Recklinghausen's disease) of orbit and globe. Arch Ophthalmol 22:761–791, 1939
10. DAVIS FA: Primary tumors of the optic nerve (a phenomenon of Recklinghausen's disease). Arch Ophthalmol 23:735–821, 957–1022, 1940
11. DEL RÍO-HORTEGA P: Tercera aparición al concimiento morfológico e anterpretacion functional de la oligodendroglia. Mem Soc Espan Hist Nat 14:5, 1928
12. DEL RÍO-HORTEGA P: Anatomica Microscópia de los Tumores del Sistema Nervioso Central y Periferico. Madrid, SA Blass, 1934
13. DEUTSCH AR, DUCKWORTH JK: Nonchromaffin paraganglioma of the orbit. Am J Ophthalmol 68:659–663, 1969
14. DVORAK-THEOBALD G: Neourogenic origin of choroidal sarcoma. Arch Ophthalmol 18:971–997, 1937
15. ELLSWORTH RM: Discussion in Alfano JE, reference 2
16. FIENMAN NL, YAKOVAC WC: Neurofibromatosis in childhood. J Pediatr 76:339–346, 1970
17. FIRAT T: Cure of primary orbital neuroblastoma. Ann Ocul (Paris) 203:579–583, 1970

18. FISHER ER, HAZARD JB: Non-chromaffin paraganglioma of the orbit. Cancer 5:521–524, 1952
19. FRANCESCHETTI A: Discussion in Marshall D, reference 29
20. GOLDSMITH J: Neurofibromatosis associated with tumors of the optic papilla. Arch Ophthalmol 41:718–729, 1949
21. GRIFFIN MS, BOLANDE RP: Familial neuroblastoma with regression and maturation to ganglioneurofibroma. Pediatrics 43:377–382, 1969
22. HAMILTON JP, KOOP CE: Ganglioneuromas in children. Surg Gynecol Obstet 121:803–812, 1965
23. JOHNSON R, PRESTON R, NEWTON JC: Amputation neuroma following pterygium excision. Am J Ophthalmol 62:569–572, 1966
24. KOKE MP, BRALEY AE: Bilateral plexiform neuromata of the conjunctiva and medullated corneal nerves. Am J Ophthalmol 23:179–182, 1940
25. LATTES R, McDONALD JJ, SPROUL E: Non-chromaffin paraganglioma of carotid body and orbit. Ann Surg 139:382–384, 1954
26. LEVY WJ: Neuroblastoma: Br J Ophthalmol 41:48–53, 1957
27. MANZ HJ: Cited by Fischer H: Beitrag zur Recklinghausen Krankheit. Dermatol Z 42:143–168, 1924
28. MANZ HJ, ROSEN DA, MACKLIN RD, WILLIS WE: Neuroectodermal tumor of anterior lip of the optic cup; glioneuroma transitional to teratoid medullo-epithelioma. Arch Ophthalmol 89:382–386, 1973
29. MARSHALL D: Glioma of the optic nerve as a manifestation of von Recklinghausen's disease. Trans Am Ophthalmol Soc 51:117–155, 1953
30. MARTYN LJ, KNOX DL: Glial hamartoma of the retina in generalized neurofibromatosis, von Recklinghausen's disease. Br J Ophthalmol 56:487–491, 1972
31. MATHUR SP: Nonchromaffin paraganglioma of the orbit. Int Surg 50:336–339, 1968
32. MOHAN H, SEN DK: Orbital neurilemmoma presenting as retrobulbar neuritis. Br J Ophthalmol 54:206–207, 1970
33. MORTADA A: Solitary orbital malignant neurilemmoma. Br J Ophthalmol 52:188–190, 1968
34. NIRANKARI MS, GREER CH, CHADDAH MR: Malignant non-chromaffin paraganglioma in the orbit. Br J Ophthalmol 47:357–363, 1963
35. NORDMANN J, BRINI A: Von Recklinghausen's

disease and melanoma of the uvea. Br J Ophthalmol 54:641–648, 1970

36. PENFIELD W: Cytology and Cellular Pathology of the Nervous System, Vol 3. New York, Hoeber-Harper, 1932

37. PESCATORI F: Neurinomi solitari. Tumori 15:59–105, 1929

38. PHILLIPS R: Neuroblastoma. Ann R Coll Surg Engl 12:29–48, 1953

39. QUÉRÉ A, RICHIR C, DAVENNE C: Limbal schwannoma with malignant development. Arch Ophtalmol (Paris) 24:285–290, 1964

40. RADNÓT M: Malignes neurilemmom. Klin Monatsbl Augenheilkd 143:869–875, 1963

41. SABRI JA, DIAB A: Plexiform neurofibroma of orbit and lid with defects in walls of orbit and involvement of central nervous system. Arch Ophthalmol 52:598–602, 1954

42. SCHATZ H: Benign orbital neurilemoma; sarcomatous transformation in von Recklinghausen's disease. Arch Ophthalmol 86:268–273, 1971

43. SHAFFER RN: Neuroblastoma of the adrenal with orbital metastases. Am J Ophthalmol 30:733–740, 1947

44. SMITH B, ENGLISH FP: Classical eyelid border sign of neurofibromatosis. Br J Ophthalmol 54:134–135, 1970

45. SPENCER WH, JESBERG DO: Glioneuroma (choristomatous malformation of the optic cup margin); a report of two cases. Arch Ophthalmol 89:387–391, 1973

46. STOUT AP: Tumors of the Peripheral Nervous System. In Atlas of Tumor Pathology, Section 11, Fascicle 6, Armed Forces Institute of Pathology, published by the National Research Council, Washington DC, 1949

47. STRACHOV VP, SHEPKALOVA VM: Recklinghausen's disease, neurinoma of the right orbit and neoplasm of the left choroid. Vestn Oftalmol 18 (Pt 1):12, 1941

48. VARGHESE S, NAIR B, JOSEPH TA: Orbital malignant non-chromaffin paraganglioma; alveolar soft tissue sarcoma. Br J Ophthalmol 52:713–715, 1968

49. VERBECK B: Augenbeteiligung bei Neurofibromatose v. Recklinghausen. Klin Monatsbl Augenheilkd 155:751–764, 1969

50. VERHOEFF FH: Discussion of Snell S, Collins ET: Plexiform neuroma (elephantiasis neuromatosis) of temporal region, orbit, eyelid, and eyeball; notes of three cases. Trans Ophthalmol Soc UK 23:157–177, 1903

51. VERHOEFF FH: Discussion in Davis FA, reference 9

52. VINCENT NJ, Cleasby GW: Schwannoma of the bulbar conjunctiva. Arch Ophthalmol 80:641–642, 1968

53. WILLIAMS CM, GREER M: Homovanillic acid and vanilmandelic acid in diagnosis of neuroblastoma. JAMA 183:836–840, 1963

7

PIGMENTED TUMORS

Since tumors and other lesions involving melanocytes are encountered more frequently in ophthalmology than in other specialties, a discussion of the fundamentals of the subject seems justified.

Our imperfect knowledge of pigment cells has caused confusion in terminology. In different disciplines the same term may be used for quite different types of cells. For example, biologists use *melanophore* for certain branching cells with "contractile" properties, found in the skin of fish, amphibians, and reptiles. Medical investigators use *melanoblast* for a mature cell that is producing melanin, whereas to biologists it is an immature pigment cell during its migration from the neural crest.

The following definitions of pigment-bearing cells are based on terminology adopted in 1951 by the Subcommittee on Oncology of the Division of Medical Sciences of the National Research Council, with slight modifications:

Melanocyte	A mature melanin-producing cell with little or no growth potential (melanocytoma)
Melanoblast	An immature melanin-producing cell with growth potential (malignant melanoma or melanoblastoma)
Melanophage (macrophage)	A cell containing phagocytosed melanin
Melanophore	A "contractile" pigment effector cell found in lower animals
Incidentally pigmented cells (Lund-Kraus)	Basal cells of epithelium and tumor cells due to cytocrinia (Masson)

In general oncology, tumors in every category are designated as benign or malignant, but for some reason in the case of pigmented tumors *melanoma* implies tumor, obviating the usual adjective *benign* or *malignant*. In ophthalmology, however, it is essential to designate some melanomas as benign and others as malignant.

It is now common practice to refer to a benign uveal melanoma as a nevus. Nevus, as originally used clinically, usually refers to a congenital pigmented lesion of the skin, mucous membrane, and other sites. Although widely used by ophthalmologists, including myself, the more explicit term *benign melanoma* might be preferable.

The so-called nevus cell can be viewed as a variant of the pluripotential melanoblasts stemming from the neural crest. As such, it could theoretically be found in all melanomas except those from the retinal pigment epithelium.

Pathologists seem to agree that there is no typical nevus cell. Unless otherwise specified the term nevus refers to a pigmented lesion. Some eminent ocular pathologists do not identify nevus cells in melanomas of the choroid, ciliary body, and iris, while others believe these cells occur in melanomas throughout the uvea.

With full awareness of the limitations of a rigid classification based on our present knowledge of melanomas, I suggest the following categories:

1. Melanoma of the uvea—benign and malignant melanoma
2. Melanoma of the skin and mucous membrane—nevus and precancerous melanosis for the benign tumor; malignant melanoma and cancerous melanosis for the malignant tumor
3. Congenital melanoma—melanocytoma or blue nevus for the benign tumor, either of which may undergo malignant change; cellular blue nevus or malignant melanoma for the infiltrating tumor
4. Melanoma of the retinal pigment epithelium—hyperplasia and adenoma for the benign tumor; carcinoma for the malignant tumor

It is important to try to place melanomas in the proper category for better understanding of the natural history, clinical course, treatment, and prognosis for the different groups.

Clinically, the tumor can usually be established as a benign or a malignant melanoma but the type and its potential for infiltrating or metastasizing can merely be surmised.

A histopathologic examination often demonstrates that the tumor arises from the stroma, the pigment epithelium, the skin or conjunctiva (e.g., nevus, cancerous or precancerous melanosis), or that it is congenital (e.g., melanocytoma or blue nevus). The cytology may give some idea of the prognosis in such cases.

Certain epithelial lesions, neoplastic and otherwise, have cells containing melanin but should not be confused with melanomas. In this group are seborrheic keratosis, papilloma, basal-cell epithelioma, acanthosis nigricans, and scleroderma.

MELANIN IN GENERAL AND IN THE EYE

Melanin is a nonspecific term applied to almost all black, brown, or tan pigments—a heterogeneous group that absorb visible light in much the same way. In human embryos melanin usually appears in the protoplasm of the pigment epithelium of the retina at about the fifth week and in the protoplasm of the melanoblasts at about the fifth month.[125] Several morphologic types of melanin are found in the eye; for example, black and composed of large uniform discrete rods and spherules in the retinal pigment epithelium; light and in the form of smaller, different-sized, mainly ovoid granules in the melanocytes of the uvea.

Melanin is liberated from the protoplasm of melanocytes as a constant physiologic function of the epithelium of the skin or conjunctiva. It passes into the subcutaneous or submucosal tissues and is either absorbed or phagocytosed by the histiocytes of the dermis or submucosa. If a pigment-producing tumor develops somewhere in the body, enough melanin may be liberated to appear in abnormal amounts in the lymph nodes and urine. Melanin may also be liberated by pigment-producing cells as the result of hyperpigmented states, exposure to actinic rays, and cell necrosis. Even with a benign melanoma of the iris, liberated pigment dust is usually seen clinically in the lower portion of the anterior chamber. Free and phagocytosed melanin may sometimes be confused with hematogenous pigment histopathologically, but iron stains differentiate them.

CHEMISTRY AND FORMATION OF MELANIN

Melanin in the uvea has long been differentiated from lipofuscin and melanin in the pigment epithelium on the basis of their dissimilar chemical and physical properties. Tissue cultures also reveal a difference between the melanin in a conjunctival melanoma and in a uveal melanoma.[142] It may possibly be established eventually that melanins produced by various types of melanocytes differ in chemistry, staining reactions, spectral absorption, and in other ways.

The ophthalmoscopic appearance of the fundus depends largely on the degree of pigmentation in the pigment epithelium. When it is densely pigmented, no details of the choroid can be seen. If the choroid is also densely pigmented, the fundus is dark red as in blacks or other dark-skinned individuals; otherwise it has the relatively light red color seen in the average Caucasian. When the pigment is sparse, permitting observation of some details of the choroid, the fundus may be "tessellated" as a result of dense pigment in the choroidal melanocytes, or "albinotic" if there is little or no pigment in these melanocytes.

It has long been known that melanocytes contain a specific enzyme that oxidizes dopa into a black substance resembling melanin. *Dopa* is an abbreviation for the compound dihydroxyphenylalanine, which is extracted from a bean. The so-called dopa reaction distinguishes cells that produce melanin (melanocytes) from cells that merely harbor melanin (histiocytes, chromatophores, or melanophores). The melanocytes, which contain the specific oxidase, turn black in the dopa solution—called a positive dopa reaction. This oxidase was believed to be the agent responsible for the manufacture of natural melanin in melanocytes. The dopa reaction is specific for only one other type of cell—the myelogenous leukocyte which contains a polyphenol oxidase. Paper chromatography of the excretion of catechol derivatives by malignant melanoma patients revealed a substance resembling dopa in 22 of 28 patients examined.[159]

The dopa reaction is unrelated to the silver reaction of melanin. Silver blackens melanin wherever found—in melanocytes, in histiocytes, and free in lymph spaces; it blackens dopa-positive cells only if they happen to contain melanin. The dopa solution stains active melanocytes, which contain the specific oxidase, but does not affect the melanin in an inactive cell.

Some light was thrown on the problem by demonstrating that melanin is formed by the oxidation of tyrosine to dopa in the presence of the enzyme tyrosinase[104] which is present in normal mammalian skin[53] and in the enzyme that catalyzes dopa to dopa quinone. The latter compound goes through several intermediate nonenzymatic stages to produce a polymer that becomes linked to a protein (melanoprotein or melanin).

The initial cellular site of this activity has not been specifically identified, but it is very probably the cytoplasm. Active sites of protein synthesis most likely come together to produce filamentary structures variably enclosed within a membrane. When tyrosinase activity is noted but melanin has not yet been synthetized, the structure is a premelanosome.[125,160,161] The initial deposition of melanin on the protein filaments produces an immature melanosome with thickening of the rodlike filaments. Tyrosinase activity is still apparent. When enough melanin has been deposited to obliterate the lamellar pattern, the result is a nearly amorphous structure, the mature melanosome or melanin granule. In this final stage, there is no tyrosine activity; thus melanin concentration and tyrosinase activity are inversely related.

The cells around the growing margin of a malignant melanoma are more likely to contain oxidase (tyrosinase) than the presumably less active cells in the center.

Melanocytes, in addition to staining with silver, gold, and methylene blue, can be identified histochemically after incubation in solutions of tyrosine or dopa.[10] It has been proposed that tyrosine be used to detect neoplastic changes in melanocytes, but there is no evidence that tyrosinase is abnormally active in malignant cells.[53] Pigment production seems to depend on the amount of available tyrosinase (absent in albinos) or on factors favoring or inhibiting tyrosinase activity.[103]

The widespread dissemination of melanoma cells can result in remarkable clinical and pathologic conditions in which much of the body—including the parenchymal organs, the reticuloendothelial system, and the connective tissues—become heavily pigmented. Phagocytosis by these multiple cell types, rather than their conversion into melanocytes, is the likely basis for these changes. Free melanin in the bloodstream may also find its way into the urine, resulting in melanuria.

It has been suggested that uveal melanomas produce a growth substance that stimulates normal choroidal cells to abnormal growth.[32] Clinically, the elaboration of an enzyme or other substance by the tumor could explain the melanosis of tissue adjacent to or in contact with it. Cytocrinia (Masson) may also explain some of these cases of incidental pigmentation.

The conversion-by-oxidation of a melanogenic substance in the protoplasm into black visible melanin may be rapid and is apparently reversible; that is, after the melanin has formed, it may be reduced to an invisible premelanin. This explains how the pigment content of a nevus may increase rapidly and the change can be mistaken for active growth, and conversely how the pigment content may decrease with the lesion apparently disappearing spontaneously and then reappearing.

HORMONAL INFLUENCE ON PIGMENTATION

There is evidence of hormonal influence on pigmentation in lower animals and in man. The sex hormones in particular have been implicated. Some observers noting the low incidence of malignancy in melanomas in young people have suggested that the changes of puberty may have an activating effect. The pigment in the skin, in congenital nevi, and in the iris is also more marked at this time. It is important to remember that a so-called juvenile melanoma may resemble a malignant melanoma histologically but take a benign course. (See section Melanoma in Prepuberal and Puberal Age Groups.)

MELANOMA IN PREGNANCY

During pregnancy there may be increased pigmentation of the skin in various body areas, and existing nevi may darken. I have heard of a case in which a previously unrecognized flat nonpigmented nevus adjacent to the lower punctum became pigmented with each of the patient's five pregnancies within four years. In fact the pigment heralded the pregnancy, obviating any confirming test.

Although such changes cannot be considered predisposing to the development of melanoma, some investigators believe that an existing lesion is particularly likely to be activated during pregnancy,[167] whereas others do not consider pregnancy a threat to survival in women with melanoma.[12] The discovery of two cases of malignant choroidal melanoma during pregnancy suggested a possible relationship between the growth of these tumors and the increased secretion of pituitary and adrenal steroid hormones during gestation.[61] Pregnancy occasionally appears to induce a malignant change in a melanoma. I have seen several women with a malignant melanoma of the uvea during pregnancy. One patient, aged 21, had had a supposedly benign melanoma of the iris since birth. It increased in size during her first pregnancy, after which it resumed its original size. During her second pregnancy, the tumor again became activated and continued to grow steadily. The eye was enucleated, and malignant melanoma was confirmed microscopically.

Increased amount of the melanocyte-stimulating hormones (alpha-MSH and beta-MSH) are excreted by the pituitary gland during pregnancy.[39,54] When MSH is injected into human volunteers, the melanin in the skin increases and previously unnoticed nevi appear. Increased MSH excretion has been observed in patients with malignant melanoma, and human melanomas transplanted to animals have grown after crude pituitary preparations were administered, particularly MSH. All of this suggests that the activation of pigmented nevi and melanomas during pregnancy may be related to increased secretion of MSH, but whether this is a primary or secondary factor is unknown.

Other indications of hormonal influence on melanin are as follows: a) There is evidence that adrenocorticotropic hormone (ACTH) and cortisone may produce junctional nevi that progress to malignant melanomas. b) The pituitary gland has an effect on the movement of pigment in the melanophores in amphibians. c) The adrenal cortex influences the metabolism of melanin. d) A melanocyte-stimulating hormone whose amino acid sequence has been synthesized[82] darkens the skins of animals and man.[102]

The sex of a patient with melanoma plays a role in the prognosis. The disease favors female survival, which may be related to cyclical ovarian function since the disease is less apparent after the menopause.

TRAUMA

Proper evaluation of the role played by contusions and other injuries in the causation of cancer is difficult, although they are known to have preceded a certain percentage of neoplasms. In a review of 507 cases in the literature,[99] injury was mentioned as a possible factor in 66 (13%). There is no scientific proof that the relationship is more than coincidental, however.

An investigator who suggested the term *traumatic determinism*, to describe an organ's or a tissue's predisposition to injury because of an existing tumor, believed that traumas reveal more malignant tumors than they cause.[48] A person with a "silent" tumor may be more likely to sustain injury, even from a slight blow, at the tumor site than elsewhere. Such an injury may in fact lead to discovery of a tumor while a cure is still possible.

Whether a junctional nevus can be transformed into a malignant lesion by trauma is questionable, but x rays, ultraviolet light, xeroderma pigmentosum, and old burn scars —all known to be linked to epithelial carcinomas—may also be factors in initiating another form of epidermogenic carcinoma, the melanocarcinoma. In one series, three malignant melanomas developed in old burn scars; three developed in skin that had been irradiated for acne, basal-cell carcinoma, and a breast tumor, respectively; and one developed in a pigmented area of skin resulting from a severe sunburn. The latent period ranged from 5 to 40 years. Three cases of xeroderma pigmentosum, a hereditary disease characterized by sensitivity to ultraviolet and x rays, were complicated by melanocarcinoma, and in a fourth case the patient had three separate primary melanocarcinomas along with several basal-cell carcinomas.[1]

GENETIC FACTOR IN MELANOMA

There is some evidence of a familial tendency to develop ocular melanomas. A report described five cases in three generations of one family.[36] I have observed a malignant melanoma of the ciliary body in two sisters, and cases involving a mother and daughter have been reported.[22] A study of malignant melanoma in 22 families revealed 15 members affected in one family.[3] Salient features were the early age of onset and multiple lesions occurring mainly in persons with light hair and eyes and a light-to-sandy complexion.

A review of 45 patients with intraocular malignant melanoma revealed only one instance of familial involvement, and two familial instances were uncovered by a questionnaire-survey of 185 physicians.[111] This report cited two other patients with intraocular malignant melanoma: a man whose son had a cutaneous malignant melanoma of a big toe, and a woman whose sister had a cutaneous lesion of the same type, necessitating removal of two toes. All four of these cases were histologically confirmed. Another report cited choroidal malignant melanoma in a mother and daughter. The author had studied 13 relatives of 30 patients with proved malignant melanoma; 3 of the 13 (23%) had a choroidal nevus in the same eye as the relatives melanoma.[180]

Results of studies of benign choroidal melanoma in families indicate an autosomal dominant inheritance.[22,111,80]

According to some observers, the diffuse overabundance of uveal ganglion cells noted in five eyes with malignant melanoma, all in relatively young patients, suggests a possible congenital predisposition of some eyes to the development of melanomas.[196]

IMMUNITY

As cancer cells enter the bloodstream in many cases of malignant uveal melanoma, inherent growth-restraint or immunity is a very important and as yet indeterminate factor in the prognosis of these lesions as well as cancers elsewhere. Some authors believe the body has inherent restraints, and when these are ultimately understood, uveal melanomas and other malignant tumors may be controlled by means other than surgery.[2]

Cancer cells are frequently massed in the lumina of the blood channels in sections of eyes with malignant uveal melanoma. It is not surprising that they may be implanted distally over the body from these sites. One observer found tumor cells in the venous blood draining cancer areas in 75 of 123 different malignancies (60%) and in the peripheral blood of 12% of patients following operation for malignancies, as well as in 50 of those with inoperable lesions.[47] These findings were confirmed by demonstrating cancer cells in the peripheral blood of some patients during surgical manipulation.[147] A drop in the cancer cell count in the peripheral blood during chemotherapy was also noted.

There is thus no longer a question of whether cancer cells metastasize to distal sites but whether they can survive and grow there. Unknown forces may keep them dormant for a long time or even inhibit their growth completely. These forces are probably immunologic. When the implanted cells grow, the tumor's aggressive biologic activity overcomes the host's immunity.

This concept raises the question of the role of the primary site in the immunologic process, and whether the site may favor immunity at some stages of some tumors. One report, for example, casts doubt on what is being accomplished by enucleation for malignant uveal melanomas.[192] Only 3 of 23 patients over 60 years of age who had undergone enucleation for this disease had a normal life-span; 19 died of metastasis and 1 of intercurrent disease.

An exciting possibility is that a way may be found to stimulate the resisting forces as comparable forces can now be stimulated in the bacterial field. The present great interest in cancer immunology promises an important therapeutic breakthrough in this direction.

Patients with ocular malignant melanomas were found to have cell-mediated immunity against an antigen common to systemic malignant melanoma.[27]

Spontaneous regression certainly occurs in retinoblastoma and in cancerous melanosis of the skin and mucous membranes. There is also evidence that malignant choroidal melanoma undergoes spontaneous necrosis and regresses as an immunologic response.[141]

MELANOMA IN PREPUBERAL AND PUBERAL AGE GROUPS

So-called juvenile melanomas usually occur in the skin of the lids and lid margins and less frequently in the conjunctiva. They appear as flesh-colored tumors with little or no pigment and are frequently misdiagnosed both clinically and microscopically. They are really junctional nevi in which the subepithelial cells resemble malignant cells but the tumors do not metastasize or infiltrate. The fact that these tumors are often mistaken for malignant melanomas no doubt accounts in some measure for the belief that prepuberal and puberal melanomas follow a benign course (Fig. 7–1). The same lesion also occurs in adults, in whom it is no more likely to undergo cancerous changes than any other compound nevus.[1]

In a review of 27 cases of juvenile melanoma not one was found to have been correctly diagnosed clinically. An incorrect diagnosis of malignant melanoma had been made in 4 of the 6 adults in the series.[91] These findings advance a strong case for replacing the term *juvenile melanoma* by *spindle-cell nevus* or *epithelioid-cell nevus*. Experience indicates that conservative local excision is adequate for treating these tumors.

Most melanomas of the uvea in children are congenital melanomas, which have a better prognosis than the usual uveal melanomas of adults. In children they tend, like other congenital melanomas, to be associated with some degree of ocular melanocytosis. This was the case in the affected eye of 4 out of 7 patients under age 20 with malignant melanoma of the choroid.[186] The difference in pigmentation of the two eyes may be slight enough to be overlooked. Association of the melanoma with hyperpigmentation of the eye places it in the group of congenital melanomas. This is another reason for considering melanomas in children less malignant than in adults. However, except for the juvenile melanoma and congenital melanoma groups, the prognosis is just as grave as in adults. In a series of 5 cases[121] only 2 of the patients lived more than 5 years; all were age 12 or younger.

In the prepuberal and puberal age groups, malignant melanoma occurs almost as commonly in the iris as in the choroid, but this is not true in adults.

TYPES OF MELANOCYTES

There are three types of melanocytes and melanomas derived from them: a) those of the choroid, ciliary body, and iris; b) those of the skin and mucous membrane; and c) those of the stroma.

All melanin-bearing tumors or melanomas are neurogenic, and essentially all derive from the neural crest. An extremely rare group arising in the pigment epithelium of the retina, ciliary body, and iris may not stem from the neural crest, but they are neurogenic, arising from a layer of the optic vesicle or neural ectoderm.

MELANOCYTES OF THE CHOROID, CILIARY BODY, AND IRIS

The normal uveal melanocyte is long, narrow, branching, and pigment-bearing; when the pigment content is high it assumes a relatively plump polygonal shape with few or no

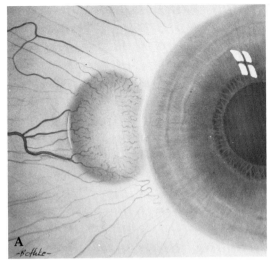

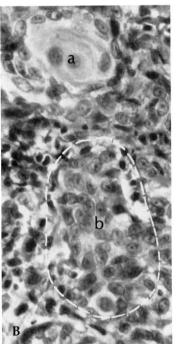

FIG. 7–1. Juvenile melanoma of the limbus. **A.** This salmon-colored, vascularized mass of unknown duration lay temporally on the right eye of a 12-year-old boy. **B.** Histologic examination showed proliferated basal epithelial cells expected in nevi. An epithelial dropping (*eintröpfein*) (*a*) is seen near the conjunctival surface of the tumor. At (*b*) is an area indicating how such migrated epithelial cells can suggest malignancy.

processes. Between these two extremes are transitional stages referable in part to the pigment content. Some tumors are composed largely of epithelioid cells, others of branching polygonal cells, and still others of spindle-shaped cells. Often the lesion shows a mixture of all three, suggesting the possibility of more than one type of uveal melanoma. The uveal melanocytes are dopa-negative in the adult and dopa-positive in the embryo. This fact, together with the cell's histologic characteristics in the normal state, in the pathologic state, and in cultures, places it definitely as a true pigment-producing melanocyte rather than merely a pigment-harboring cell. There is ample evidence that these cells are derived from the neural crest.

When uveal melanomas were cultured, the growing cells varied from branching, polygonal, pigment-bearing cells to long, bipolar, spindle-shaped cells, with or without pigment and resembling Schwann cells. All gradations between these two extremes were found, and regardless of the cell type of the tumor, in culture there was a transition from one type of cell to the other.[142]

It seems logical to assume that these different pigment-bearing cells of the uvea are actually various stages in the differentiation of a single cell type. Arising embryologically from the neural crest, they can be regarded as specialized nerve cells. One reason for their true nature remaining so long in doubt is that they do not begin to differentiate, i.e., to form melanin granules, until late in embryonic life when they are quite remote from their site of origin.[70]

Experiments involving amphibians, birds, and mammals revealed an early and extensive migration of precursor (colorless) pigment cells in the embryo. Some of these potential melanoblasts may be unfavorably situated for melanin synthesis, and may be stimulated to form melanin only under pathologic conditions. The cells at the crest are pluripotential only at the beginning and differentiate according to their subsequent location. The presence of more than one cell type in the same tumor may be detected in other neoplasms, but pluripotential cells are a special characteristic of those derived from the neuroectoderm.

The association of uveal melanomas with von Recklinghausen's disease has been clearly established not only clinically but also histologically, through their kinship to the ubiquitous Schwann cells.[129]

MELANOCYTES OF THE SKIN AND MUCOUS MEMBRANE

The junctional melanoblasts of epithelium can be identified at the twelfth week of embryonic life. They are located at the juncture of the epithelium and the stroma; in post-embryonic life they are referred to as junctional melanocytes. They are dendritic-shaped, secretory cells which supply melanin to the basal epithelium by pinocytosis (cytocrinia).

The black and the Caucasian have the same number of junctional melanocytes, but the black's cells are larger and produce more melanin.

The junctional melanocytes, the sole producers of melanin in epithelium, are distinct from the epithelium. Electron microscopy reveals that they have no tonofibrils but have the structure of secretory cells. The melanin is present as melanosomes, which are pigmented in relation to the amount of tyrosinase they contain. Fully melanized melanosomes lose their tyrosinase activity and become inert granules. The melanosomes seem to originate in nonmelanized inclusions.

These melanocytes can be demonstrated by vital staining, can be isolated from epithelial cells, can be grown in tissue culture, and can be transplanted and selectively destroyed in intact epithelium.

In infancy, melanin is produced by the junctional cells; production stops normally in about the second decade but may be activated by the onset of cancerous changes, by pregnancy, at puberty, and also by ultraviolet light, ionizing radiation, and ACTH.

The junctional melanocytes may manifest focal sites of proliferation and pigment formation even into early adult life. Accumulations of atypical epithelioid melanocytes are called junctional nevi when confined largely to the basal epithelium; dermal nevi, when activity of the basal epithelium ceases and the nevus cells are confined to the stroma; and compound nevi, when junctional activity is combined with the accumulation of nevus cells in the stroma.

After the nevi reach maturity they normally remain static throughout life until involution sets in, when they gradually begin to diminish in size and ultimately disappear.

The dendritic functional melanocytes have been interpreted as elaborating or excreting melanin in the same way that glandular cells excrete their products. On this basis it was concluded that they should really be considered glandular cells, the protoplasmic processes inoculating or injecting the pigment into the cells of the epidermis and dermis with which they come in contact.[116]

Nevus cells, in addition to growing diffusely in the epidermis and dermis, may grow in small clusters and nests beneath the epithelium. They are then viewed as abortive forms of specialized tactile organs such as Meissner's or pacinian corpuscles. These nests of nevus cells have been considered caricatures of Meissner's corpuscles which, when well formed, are undoubtedly identifiable in neurofibromatosis of the uvea.

The structure of a nevus in general has been described as follows: trunks of sensory nerves approach the deeper layers of the dermis beneath the site of the nevus; as they become increasingly superficial they lose their myelin; their Schwann sheath then becomes continuous with a syncytium of nevus cells along the nerve branches, like flowers on a stem with many branches. Nerve axons can be traced down the center of these branches (neuroid tubes), and the axons arborize around the nevus cells in the same way that they surround the tactile cells of Merkel and Ranvier.[116] Although some authors believe nevus cells are of Schwann cell origin, many others view them as altered melanocytes. Electron microscopy has shown that the morphology of the junctional melanocytes differs from that of contiguous epithelial cells and also Schwann cells.

The nevus cells, interpreted as basically Schwann cells, may thus sheathe the terminal branches of the sensory nerves, which act as a scaffolding or may appear at the nerve terminal as modified tactile cells. Both types may be present in the same tumor, with one or the other predominating.

It is not surprising that various combinations of malignant melanomas, neurilemomas, and neurofibromatoses have been reported in the ophthalmic literature. A patient with the general manifestations of von Recklinghausen's disease, neurilemoma of the right orbit, and a malignant choroidal melanoma in the left eye has been reported.[175] In one case, malignant choroidal melanoma was associated with multiple skin nodules of von Recklinghausen's disease.[66] In another case the choroidal tumor resembled a malignant melanoma but was diagnosed microscopically as a neurofibroma; subsequent general examination established a diagnosis of von Recklinghausen's disease.[123] A malignant choroidal melanoma has been reported with an acoustic neurofibroma.[9] Two patients had a malignant melanoma of the brain associated with neurofibromatosis.[14,18] Meningiomal and other neurogenic characteristics were found in a series of uveal melanomas.[191]

An interesting theory of the relationship of nevi to the evolution of hair follicles has been offered.[98] Since many lesions in man, including pigmented nevi, are considered to represent the imperfect survival of structures normal in lower animals, the term *progonoblastoma* has been applied to a pigmented nevus of the conjunctiva.[88,117]

What appear to be nevus cells are seen in some melanomas of the uvea, where true nevi have also been noted. Demonstration of the prevalence of nevus cells in uveal melanomas led one group to conclude that malignant uveal melanomas arise in benign uveal melanomas.[200] I believe that nevuslike cells occur in iris melanomas, but I have not found them in choroidal melanomas. Linking these observations with Masson's theory of neurogenesis is the fact that sensory nerve terminals are numerous in the anterior uvea. In any event, the identification of nevi in the uvea is consistent with the neurogenetic theory of their origin.

Another interpretation of the dendritic cell is that it represents only a morphologic variation of the basal cell, appearing in a wide range of transitional forms, from the typically dendritic to the typically basal cell. It is widely believed that the dendritic cell is a well defined functioning form of a normal pigment-producing basal cell.

A melanocyte in the retinal pigment epithelium is phototaxic, as shown by the protoplasmic extensions between the rods and cones noted under exposure to light. These extensions have been demonstrated in both animals and man. This phototaxic property in skin and mucous membrane might be an attribute of the basal layer of the epithelium, with the dendritic processes merely basal-cell alterations resulting from it. This theory is supported by several findings:

1. Dendritic cells increase in number after exposure to radiation, and later change back to normal-appearing basal cells. After human skin had been exposed to thorium-X, approximately 40% of all the basal epithelial cells became dendritic, indicating that dendritic cells were probably a func-

tional modification of ordinary basal cells.

2. Pigment in the basal cells is frequently located as a cap at the superficial pole of the cell. This is the pole toward the light.

3. On exposure to sunlight, pigment migrates through the epithelium, depleting the basal layer. Even cadaver skin darkens on exposure to ultraviolet light because of this migration of melanin to more superficial layers.

Dendritic melanocytes are present even in a state of rest and appear in their true form whenever there is an influx of pigment into the preformed protoplasmic channels. Such a flow of pigment has been demonstrated in amphibians and fish but not in higher animals.

CONGENITAL MELANOMA

Some melanomas seem to deserve a special category because of common features: natural history, clinical course, treatment, and prognosis. This group, to be referred to as congenital melanomas, includes melanocytoma—localized form—and ocular melanocytosis (melanosis oculi)—diffuse form, blue nevus and cellular blue nevus, congenital dermal melanosis (nevus of Ota and Ito), and congenital oculodermal melanosis. They tend to occur in brunettes. Most of the manifestations of hyperpigmentation that characterize ocular melanocytosis are seen normally in the eyes of blacks and orientals.

Spencer has suggested the following classification for "hyperpigmented melanocytic lesions"[172]:

I. Epithelial melanocytic lesions
  1. Focal
    a. Skin of eyelid
      1) Nevus
      2) Malignant melanoma
      3) Others (ephelis, lentigo)
    b. Conjunctiva
      1) Nevus
      2) Malignant melanoma
  2. Diffuse
    a. Skin of eyelid
      1) Acquired melanosis (Hutchinson's freckle)
        a) Benign
        b) Malignant
    b. Conjunctiva
      1) Acquired melanosis
        a) Benign
        b) Malignant
II. Subepithelial hyperpigmented melanocytic lesions
  1. Focal
    a. Eye "melanocytoma"
      1) Benign
      2) Malignant
    b. Skin + mucous membranes
      Blue nevus + cellular blue nevus
      1) Benign
      2) Malignant
  2. Diffuse
    a. Eye
      1) Uveal and scleral melanosis ("melanosis oculi")
      2) Conjunctival (subepithelial melanosis)
    b. Skin
      1) Dermal melanosis (nevus of Ota)
    c. Combined skin, eye, mucous membranes, and orbit
III. Uveal melanocytic lesions
  1. Benign melanoma (nevus)
  2. Malignant melanoma

Melanocytes normally occur in the dermis of skin and substantia propria of mucous membranes in adult animals. All congenital melanomas are believed to be phylogenetic or atavistic remains of a pigment system in animals. In the human embryo their precursors can be identified at the tenth week of embryonic life. Mongolian spot, a type of blue nevus, is found regularly over the sacrum, at least microscopically, in all races in the first year of life and may disappear after the fourth year. These atavistic remains may proliferate before or after birth, forming a tumefaction or progonoma. The cytologic spectrum ranges from densely pigmented polyhedral cells through densely pigmented spindle cells.

Clinically, blue nevi are so called because they are often bluish-black, due to the Dayleigh effect in which the light is scattered by particles smaller than 0.1% of the wavelength of light.[25]

The term *nevus*, without the type specified, merely designates some sort of congenital tumefaction. Blue nevus (clinical diagnosis) and melanocytoma (histologic diagnosis) are used interchangeably in this discussion.

The unilateral increase in pigment of the potentially pigment-bearing cells may occur throughout the eye, including the sclera (Fig. 7–2, see p. 10), the lids, and even the extra-ocular muscles. Sometimes, the difference in pigmentation of the two irides is so slight as to be detected only after careful comparison. These tumors, congenital melanomas, are frequently associated with uveal, conjunctival, and dermal melanoses. In fact, the majority of clinically diagnosed malignant melanomas of the uvea in young people show this association, which may be easily overlooked.

Ota[131] described dermal melanosis of the lower lid and sometimes the upper lid associated with ocular melanosis in about half the cases (Fig. 7–3). Ito[85] reported the dermal melanosis at sites distal to the eye, especially on dorsal surfaces in the neck and thoracic regions and at times associated with ocular melanosis. It has been estimated that about 80% of the oculodermal melanoses occur in females.

Melanocytosis may be confined to a sector of the eyeball. As a rule it is manifested primarily in the iris (Figs. 7–4, 7–5) as a sharply demarcated pigmented zone, sometimes with pigmentation of the adjacent conjunctiva and increased pigment in the corresponding area of the choroid. The hyperpigmented sector of the iris may appear relatively normal except

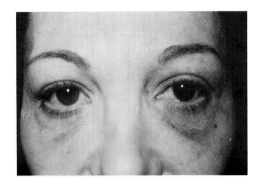

FIG. 7–3. Congenital ocular melanocytosis with nevus of Ota. In this case the nevus of Ota below the left eye was associated with a darker iris, choroid, and sclera than in the fellow eye.

FIG. 7–4. Congenital segmental ocular melanocytosis. A sector showing excessive pigmentation in an otherwise normal-appearing iris. **Inset:** Episcleral pigmentation corresponds to the sector of the iris lesion.

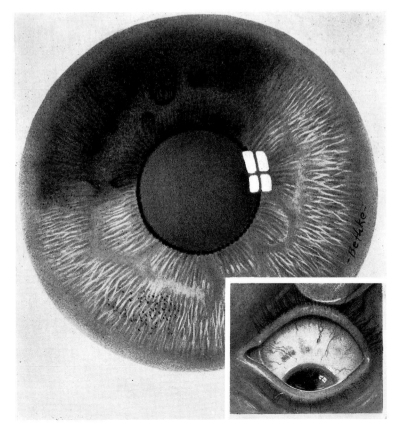

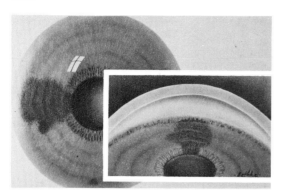

FIG. 7–5. Congenital segmental melanosis of the iris. Viewed with the gonioscope, the angle shows the pigmented iris processes usually present in congenital ocular melanocytosis.

FIG. 7–6. Congenital segmental melanosis of the iris. *A*. Segment of normal-appearing iris comparable with that of the fellow eye. *B.* Congenital melanosis of the conjunctiva. The choroid corresponding to the area of iris melanosis is darker than that of the fellow eye.

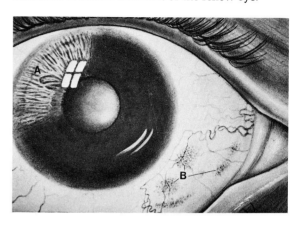

for a thicker anterior limiting layer and fewer crypts than usually characterize a highly pigmented iris (Fig. 7–6). In some instances the iris surface has pigmented nodules and papules instead of normal markings.

The group of congenital melanomas is well exemplified in a classical report on a type of benign melanoma of the optic nerve head, for which the authors proposed the term *melanocytoma*.[204] They felt, with justification, that it should be distinguished from a melanoma arising from the uvea proper. The cells closely resemble the normal stromal melanocytes of the uvea, in contrast to marked cellular pleomorphism of the usual uveal melanomas.[202] These melanocytomas show some local invasiveness but no orbital extension or metastasis. A melanocytoma of the iris, previously described,[140] appears in Figure 7–7 and a lesion originating in the sclera in Figure 7–8.

In a report of 34 cases of melanocytoma of the optic disc,[204] 20 with enucleation of the eye and 14 with no enucleation, 23 cases were followed over 5 years. The findings in these and similar published cases, and evaluation of the lesion's histopathologic characteristics, make it clear that the tumor has a negligible lethal potential and that enucleation is not indicated.

The differential diagnosis between a juxtapapillary malignant melanoma of the choroid and a primary melanocytoma of the disc rests on four factors:

1. A melanocytoma is almost always discovered during a routine examination,

FIG. 7–7. Melanocytoma of the iris. **A.** This black globular mass, in a 10-year-old girl, is supplied by nutrient vessels on each side. **B.** Gonioscopic examination of the lower portion of the anterior chamber reveals marked dispersement of pigment granules. **C.** Cytology of the tumor. (A. B. Reese.[140])

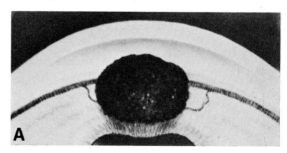

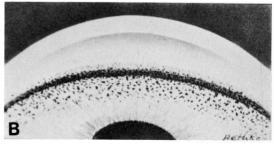

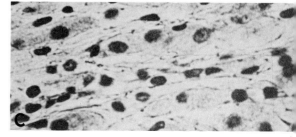

since it causes no subjective or objective visual difficulty, whereas a choroidal melanoma that has extended secondarily into the disc is likely to produce symptoms.

2. A melanocytoma is characteristically smaller, rarely occupying an area larger than the disc itself (Fig. 7-9); it is elevated several diopters toward the vitreous, is uniformly black, typically eccentric, and tends to involve the lower temporal sector where infiltration of the adjacent retina can be observed. A uveal melanoma that has extended onto the disc shows a much more varied pattern, with some degree of flat or bullous retinal detachment around the disc.

3. A melanocytoma is stationary, whereas a malignant uveal melanoma invading the nerve head can be expected to progress. Follow-up examinations with successive drawings or photographs of the disc and serial visual field studies are therefore important.

4. A melanocytoma is associated with racial hyperpigmentation, a high incidence being reported in blacks, Asiatics, Semites, and Mediterranean peoples, who rarely develop malignant uveal melanomas.

A melanocytoma is hamartomatous or progonomatous rather than neoplastic and can probably be regarded as atavistic, comparable with the tumorlike pigment formation in the optic nerve of certain reptiles.

With the gonioscope, pigmented iris processes are sometimes seen in the angle opposite the hyperpigmented area of the iris. Partial ocular melanocytosis in a sector of the iris may be mistaken for a melanoma. I do not believe that such an area ever becomes malignant.

Hyperpigmentation is encountered much oftener in the episclera than in the bulbar conjunctiva. It is slate blue, mottled, and has a predilection for the region of the anterior emissary where a black dot may mark the passage of the ciliary artery through the sclera. Similarly, hyperpigmentation of the skin—also slate blue—is located in the subepithelial stromal cells rather than in the epithelium.

Although the condition is congenital, increased pigmentation of the iris may not be noticed before puberty, when the first sign is increased subconjunctival pigmentation that does not become evident in the uveal tract until later. I have seen a case of ocular mela-

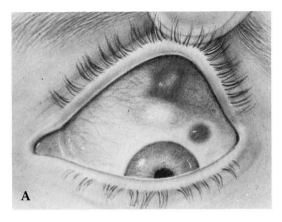

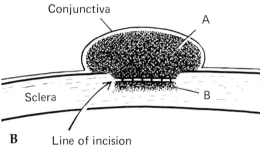

FIG. 7–8. Melanocytoma originating in the sclera. **A.** This dark subconjunctival mass had been present in the upper outer quadrant of the left eye of a 6-year-old girl since birth. When excision was attempted it proved to be mushroom-shaped, with the base replacing half the sclera. **B.** Schema shows (*A*) top of the tumor, sclera, and line of incision; (*B*) portion of tumor base left *in situ*. (A. B. Reese.[140])

nocytosis in which the iris was highly pigmented and, unlike the fellow iris, had no crypts. Scleral pigmentation was also marked.

Since an appreciable number of eyes with congenital ocular melanocytosis develop malignant tumors, it must be considered a potentially precancerous condition.

Ocular melanocytosis is not to be confused with a flat malignant melanoma, although such a lesion may be present, either the usual localized globular type or very diffuse. This association is more likely to be found in Caucasians than in blacks and orientals.

My impression is that the usual benign melanoma of the uvea found in about 6% of otherwise normal eyes is a congenital melanoma. The tumors are not apparent at birth but are usually first detected by ophthalmoscopy in a routine eye examination of children

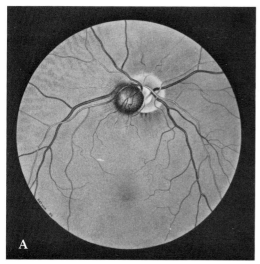 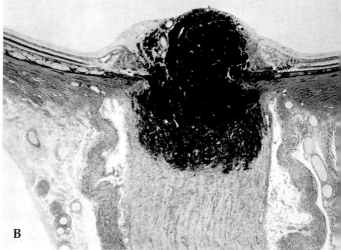

FIG. 7–9. Melanocytoma of the optic disc. **A.** This tumor, first diagnosed in a 52-year-old woman, remained unchanged during more than 25 years of observation. (Courtesy of G. M. Bruce.) **B.** A similar tumor in a 29-year-old black woman overlapped one-third of the upper temporal quadrant of the disc and also involved the optic nerve. It was discovered in a routine examination. The patient had 20/20 vision and no symptoms. No change was observed during five years of follow-up. (Courtesy of the Armed Forces Institute of Pathology.)

between the ages of 8 and 12. Some may not develop pigment and therefore go unrecognized.

A choroidal melanocytoma is sometimes diagnosed clinically as a malignant melanoma, leading to enucleation because the tumor is elevated and produces a field defect. Fluorescein angiograms may resemble those seen in cases of malignant melanoma.[89,164] In rare instances, the malignant change does not occur until late in life (Fig. 7–10).

In general pathology, blue nevi from various body sites have been observed for many years. About 25% of blue nevi show a syncytial fibrous element of sparsely pigmented Schwann cells. These so-called cellular blue nevi have a growth potential and are therefore viewed as an aggressive variant of the blue nevus.

There is no reason to believe that the blue nevi encountered elsewhere on the body differ from those in the eye and its adnexa. However, an apparent discrepancy seems to be the higher mortality of these tumors in

and around the eye in infants and adolescents than in the adult group.

Fatal cases of ocular melanomas, presumably of the congenital type, have been reported.[50,186]

In a series of 46 cases, 6 deaths were reported in patients under 20 years of age, and 2 in 15 patients with prepuberal melanomas.[4]

We have encountered one death in an 11-year-old patient and probably another in a 15-year-old lost to follow-up.

Since blue nevi can be viewed as congenital aberrations, evidence of other associated anomalies is not surprising. The following anomalies have been noted in eyes with congenital melanomas:

1. Remains of the hyaloid system at the disc in three cases, two of these with associated medullated nerve fibers. They can be attributed to the presence of oligodendroglia which fabricates myelin.
2. Remains of a pupillary membrane in two cases.
3. An anterior chamber cleavage syndrome in two cases—a 3-month-old infant[97] and a child of 2 years and 9 months in our series, both with a melanocytoma of the iris and ciliary body as well as buphthalmos.
4. Some degree of microphthalmos.
5. Ectopic lacrimal gland associated with a congenital melanoma of the conjunctiva.[185]

Congenital melanomas and the malignant melanomas that arise from them have a greater tendency to be familial than other

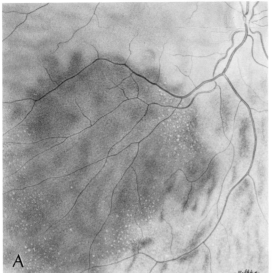

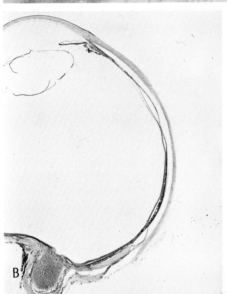

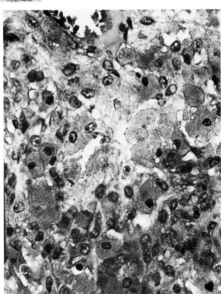

FIG. 7–10. Malignant melanocytoma of the choroid. **A.** Fundus of the right eye in a 62-year-old woman shows a flat, dark, diffuse tumor in the choroid below the macula; numerous light puncta at the periphery of the lesion were interpreted as drusen. **B.** Under low power the tumor is seen extending from the equator to the disc. **C.** High-power cytologic view confirmed the diagnosis of malignant melanocytoma.

melanomas. We have seen two instances in which a mother and daughter had malignant congenital melanomas of the choroid and two sisters had malignant congenital melanoma of the ciliary body. Other familial occurrences have been reported.[50,73]

MELANOMA OF THE DISC

Most melanomas that appear clinically in the disc arise primarily in the adjacent choroid and involve the nerve secondarily. However, they are at times primary in the disc, since

some of the lamina cribrosa stems from the choroid and is potentially pigment-bearing, especially in heavily pigmented individuals. The external laminae (lamina scleralis) are continuations of the scleral elements adjacent to the nerve, whereas the internal laminae (lamina choroidalis) are continuations of the choroidal elements. Although the internal laminae usually contain no pigment, melanocytes are sometimes seen in a heavily pigmented uveal tract (Fig. 7–11).

In the human eye the melanocytes are present in the peripheral portion of the lamina cribrosa but are not seen by ophthal-

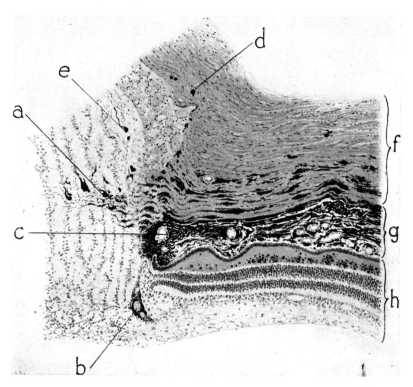

FIG. 7–11. Melanocytes in the lamina cribrosa.
Pigmentation of the lamina cribrosa (*a*) in an eye
with congenital ocular melanocytosis. A
pigmented cilioretinal artery (*b* and *c*) courses
from the choroid (*g*) to the retina (*h*).
Melanocytes are also seen in the pia (*e*), the dura
(*d*), and the inner layers of the sclera (*f*).

moscopy because of the surrounding thick,
relatively opaque nerve-fiber layer. They tend
to thin out or disappear in the central portion, but when present they may be seen with
the ophthalmoscope at the base of the physiologic cup (Fig. 7–12). This finding has been
reported in Japanese with otherwise normal
eyes.[130]

Benign melanomas in and around the disc
produce a corresponding enlargement of the
blind spot, whereas comparable lesions of the
choroid normally do not.

Many melanomas of the optic nerve and
disc that had been verified microscopically
proved to be primary malignant melanomas
of the papilla that arose in the region of the
lamina cribrosa.

A diagnosis of melanoma of the disc based
on clinical appearance alone is unreliable,
since the far more common juxtapapillary

choroidal malignant melanoma, viewed by
ophthalmoscopy, may appear to arise from
the disc. In juxtapapillary cases the lesion
arising in the choroid adjacent to the disc
takes the course of least resistance around
the termination of the lamina vitrea, through
the intermediary tissue of Kuhnt, and lobu-
lates over the internal surface of the optic
nerve head. The bulk of the tumor at its
farthest extension into the vitreous is over
the disc, making it seem clinically to arise
there. The question of whether primary
malignant melanoma of the disc occurs as an
entity has been raised.[40]

Pigment may also appear in the optic nerve
under the following conditions:

1. Extension of the pigment epithelium a
   short distance into the disc adjacent to a
   temporal conus. When it extends into the
   nerve it accompanies the lamina vitrea,
   which sometimes terminates a short distance into the nerve instead of at its margin. The pigment in the disc is more apparent than real in such cases because of
   the oblique angle of nerve insertion into
   the sclera.

2. The occasional presence of small, isolated, clearly demarcated foci of jet-black pigment located superficially in the nerve-fiber layer of the disc. They are assumed to originate from the adjacent pigment epithelium, which is often thicker and denser at its termination around the disc than elsewhere. This proliferation of the pigment epithelium at its termination around the disc may be due to a tug on the optic nerve around its insertion into the globe, induced by movement of the eyeball. On this basis the pigment spots on the disc are interpreted as excrescences of pigment epithelium that have migrated into the fiber layer of the disc.

3. Hemorrhage in the vaginal space around the optic nerve, in the orbit, or even in the globe which may undergo hemolysis, with deposition into the nerve of the resulting pigment granules. In such instances the pigment is found not in the stroma of the nerve but in the interstices of the nerve-fiber bundles where vascularity and absorption are minimal. This form of acquired pigmentation is in contrast to congenital pigmentation of the lamina cribrosa in which the pigment is found in the stroma. Sometimes this hematogenous pigmentation of the optic nerve is visible by opthalmoscopy.

4. Accumulation in the physiologic cup of the disc of freed granules from the pigment epithelium following an operation for serous detachment of the retina.

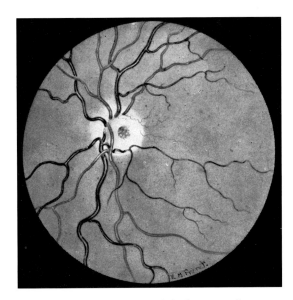

FIG. 7–12. Pigmentation of the lamina cribrosa in the physiologic cup of the optic disc. This was noted in an otherwise normal-appearing eye of a 72-year-old dark-complexioned man.

MELANOMA OF THE ORBIT

A benign or malignant melanoma of the orbit must arise at a site where there are melanocytes. In some instances they accumulate along the sheath of a ciliary nerve as it courses through the sclera or orbit. A melanoma arising from a site on the nerve where it passed through the sclera may be located partly in the choroid and partly in the orbit, resulting in an hourglass arrangement (Fig. 7–13, see p. 10).

Uveal melanocytes usually extend partly through the sclera via the emissaria and, particularly in highly pigmented individuals, may reach the external scleral surface or even the orbital structures in this way. In a case of congenital ocular melanocytosis I have found melanocytes in the extraocular muscles. These cells are normally found in the pia covering the optic nerve.

It is possible that instead of being primary in the orbit a melanoma may extend from a tumor in a neighboring structure. Such primary foci include the adjacent conjunctiva, caruncle, semilunar fold, or skin; a small or flat lesion in the uvea with early extension to the orbit; a necrotic melanoma in the uvea with orbital extension; a tumor in the nasal sinus; or a malignant melanoma at a distal site that has metastasized to the orbit.

I have reported a malignant melanocytoma of the orbit (Fig. 7–14).

A progressive, infiltrating blue nevus may be primary in the orbit (Fig. 7–15) as well as extending to it from beneath the skin and conjunctiva. Primary malignant melanomas of the leptomeninges have been reported, some of which extended along the optic nerve.

MELANOMA OF THE CORNEA

A melanoma is very rarely primary in the cornea (Fig. 7–16). It can originate from the Schwann cells of the corneal nerves or from

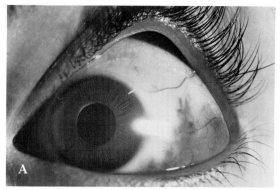

FIG. 7–14. Malignant melanocytoma of the orbit. **A.** The right eye of a 12-year-old girl showed progressive exophthalmos and a bluish-black subconjunctival tumor temporally, extending into the fornix with diffuse melanosis of the adjacent skin of the lid. The iris was darker than that of the fellow eye. The presence of papilledema indicated orbital extension. Total exenteration was carried out. The tumor recurred and the patient died. **B.** Gross specimen. **C.** Malignant cytology of the tumor.

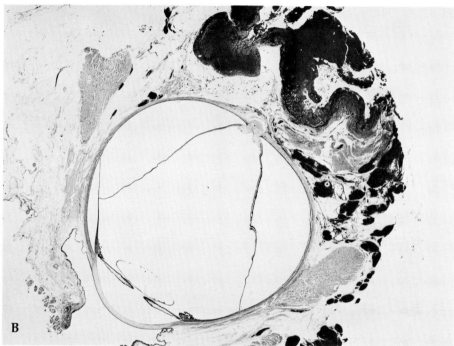

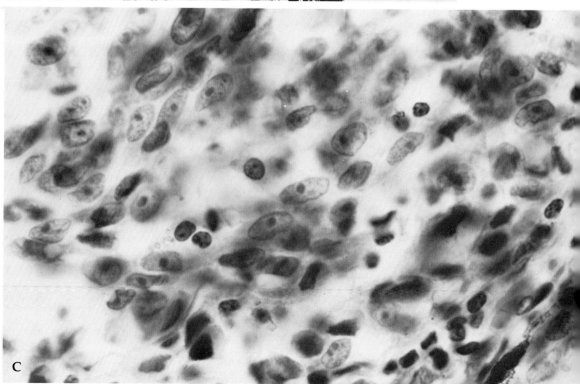

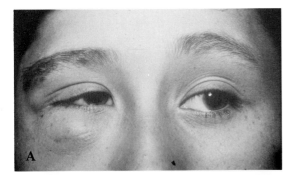

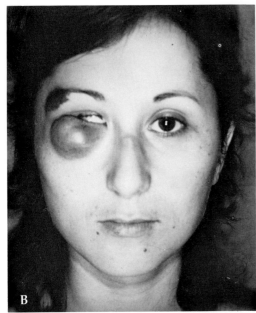

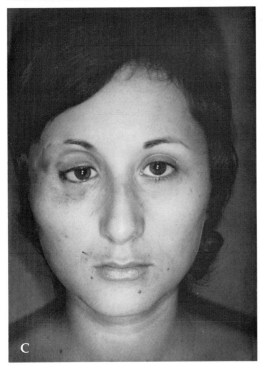

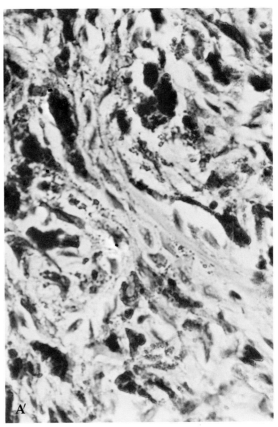

FIG. 7–15. Progressive blue nevus of the brow, lids, and orbit. Clinical appearance. **A.** At age 15 with cytology **(A′)**; **B.** At age 23. **C.** At age 27 one year after excision in Jerusalem of what was considered an encapsulated nevus of Ota. Since that time another lesion was removed from the temporal region, with the same diagnosis. (Courtesy of Y. R. Barishak, M. R. Wexler, and Z. Neuman of Jerusalem; and the Armed Forces Institute of Pathology.)

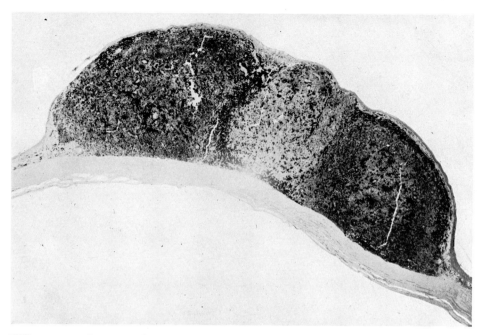

FIG. 7–16. Malignant melanoma of the cornea. Serial sections showed no connection with the limbus. The patient, an 89-year-old man, had noted this progressively enlarging lesion for two years. (Courtesy of W. A. McCormick and S. R. Irvine, Jr.)

FIG. 7–17. Malignant melanoma arising from a benign melanoma. The base of a malignant melanoma of the choroid (*a*) arising from a flat, heavily pigmented benign melanoma (*b*).

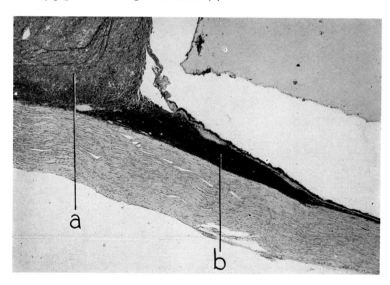

the basal cells of the corneal epithelium. That the basal cells are potential melanocytes is apparent from the melanin they display occasionally following irradiation or inflammation.

MELANOMAS OF THE UVEA

Malignant Melanomas Arising from Benign Melanomas

Histologically verified malignant melanomas of the uvea have arisen from preexisting benign melanomas (nevi) that were followed up to 25 years before they suddenly started to grow. On the other hand, no evidence of malignant transformation was found in 42 benign choroidal melanomas followed for several years.[179] In an additional follow-up averaging 9½ years on 28 of these 42 patients, no change was found in the size of the choroidal nevus.[178]

The change from a benign to a malignant choroidal melanoma is rare. One observer reported such a change after 7 years.[169] The finding of benign-appearing cells (nevus cells) along the edges of or within 73 of 100 malignant melanomas led to the conclusion that most and perhaps all such lesions originate in preexisting nevi.[200]

A study of 124 choroidal nevi in 112 patients showed no change during a follow-up averaging 2 years.[127] Among 22 patients with choroidal nevi situated in the macular area, 13 showed diminished visual acuity, 3 had serous detachment of the macula, and 3 had related macular degeneration. Fluorescein angiography revealed drusen in 35 cases and focal absence of retinal pigment epithelium in 10.

A relatively flat base extending into the adjacent uvea is often more pigmented and composed of more mature cells than the globular portion of the tumor (Fig. 7–17). Moreover, examination of early malignant melanomas (either found accidentally or arising in the macular region where they are recognized early) shows that they began to develop in the outer layers of the choroid or even in the suprachoroidea—additional evidence of possible change since these areas are the usual location of benign melanomas.

A flat, diffuse malignant melanoma of the choroid, iris, and ciliary body appears in Figure 7–18.

There are indications that a benign melanoma may become malignant as the result of

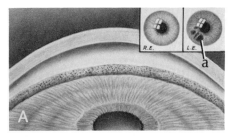
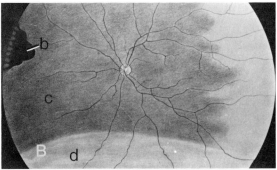

FIG. 7–18. Flat, diffuse malignant melanoma of the choroid, iris, and ciliary body. **A.** Gonioscopic view of the iris of the left eye in a 58-year-old woman which was slightly darker than that of the fellow eye (*a*) **inset.** The angle showed extensive pigment deposits, and the intraocular pressure was 36 mm Hg. **B.** View through the dilated pupil shows a melanoma of the ciliary body with ciliary processes (*b*), a flat melanoma of the choroid (*c*), and a detachment of the retina (*d*).

irritation from inflammation and perhaps from trauma. A malignant melanoma is sometimes found unexpectedly in microscopic sections of eyes long blind from some inflammatory process. These eyes, frequently atrophic, are the seat of long-standing and at times seemingly inactive disease, the original condition having been endogenous or exogenous inflammation.

The following cases show the possible role played by inflammation in precipitating the change from a benign to a malignant growth:

Case 1: A 72-year-old woman was referred to determine whether her blind right eye could be harboring a primary malignant melanoma, with her large nodular liver a secondary manifestation. The eye had been blind for 25 years, and in the preceding 24 hours had become painful and inflamed. The report of an examination 10 years after the onset of blindness revealed no light perception in the eye, posterior synechiae and iris bombé, old exudate in the pupillary area, and a complicated cataract which prevented a view of the interior.

At the time of referral the right eye was congested, with an intraocular pressure of 80 mm Hg. A diagnosis of uveitis and secondary glaucoma was made, and enucleation was performed because the eye was useless, disfiguring, and uncomfortable; also there was the remote possibility of a neoplasm, although there was no reason to suspect one. A small malignant choroidal melanoma in the macular region and the sequelae of extensive uveitis with complete union between choroid and retina (chorioretinitis) were found. The long-standing pathologic process appeared to have resulted from an earlier rather than a recent inflammation. All those who studied the sections agreed that the malignant melanoma had arisen from a preexisting benign melanoma and had probably been activated by the choroiditis.

Case 2: A 45-year-old woman had an area of old chorioretinitis in the fundus of the left eye. Some activity was indicated by several hemorrhages over the lesion. Several ophthalmologists agreed that it was of inflammatory origin. The macula appeared gray compared with its fellow eye. Her vision was 20/20. After 2½ years the macular area was grayer and elevated 2 to 3 diopters; vision was reduced to 20/200, and a central scotoma was noted in connection with the peripheral scotoma produced by the old peripheral chorioretinitis.

Six months later a solid-appearing gray elevation, in the macular area as well as above and temporally, had extended into the area of peripheral chorioretinitis. The diagnosis was malignant melanoma, believed to have arisen from a benign melanoma in the macular region which was activated by choroiditis. The eye was enucleated and the microscopic sections corroborated the clinical interpretation. There was evidence of choroiditis with a malignant melanoma stemming from the adjacent tissue.

Case 3: A 42-year-old woman was known to have a benign melanoma of the iris which began to grow actively after a bilateral iridocyclitis of four years' duration. She was a patient of M. J. Hogan's, who had seen a similar case earlier, and I know of one other.

A perforating ulcer or a lacerating injury to the eye that incites inflammation, either by damaging the intraocular structures or by exogenous infection, may also change a benign growth into a malignant one. This may occur even in an atrophic or phthisical globe, as shown by the following case:

A patient with atrophy of the globe following perforation of a corneal ulcer had sporadic attacks of acute inflammation in the eye for the next ten years. Twenty-six years after the per-

foration, exophthalmos developed and the eye was enucleated. The globe contained a malignant melanoma with extraocular extension; there was histologic evidence that it arose from a preexisting benign lesion.

Inflammation provoked by a necrotic malignant melanoma may also lead to atrophy or even phthisis of the globe, with partial arrest of tumor growth, which is resumed later. Such a case could be confused with the above-described type in which an old or active pathologic process seemingly causes a benign melanoma to undergo malignant change. But from whatever cause, malignant melanoma in long-blind eyes is sufficiently common to consider enucleation of a useless disfiguring eye.

PROGNOSIS

Mortality

On the basis of a five-year follow-up, the mortality rate for choroidal and ciliary body malignant melanomas is about 50%. But since it rises to about 65% after ten or more years, the usual five-year follow-up is inadequate. Such lesions arising elsewhere have a mortality rate of 80%–90%. Since melanomas of the iris have a different prognosis from those of the choroid and ciliary body, they will be discussed separately. The presence of malignant cells in the blood of patients with eye melanoma has little prognostic significance with one exception: when a shower of cells is isolated during surgery. In this circumstance, the five-year survival rate was reduced by half.[173]

In fatal cases of malignant melanoma, the average survival after enucleation is 46 months. Over 75% of these patients succumb within five years.[188]

Orbital Recurrence

The prognosis is graver when there is extraocular extension of the tumor. An extension in the form of a nodule through an emissary, without tumor necrosis, is usually encapsulated. If this capsule remains intact at the time of enucleation, the prognosis is probably not appreciably worsened. A diffuse extraocular extension associated with necrosis of the tumor and adjacent sclera is especially dangerous. A review of 1350 malignant melanoma cases recorded at the Armed Forces Institute of Pathology revealed extraocular extension in 81, approximately 6%. Of the 81, 67% died from metastasis—a mortality rate about 20% higher than for patients with no extraocular extension.

In an analysis of 95 cases of uveal melanoma with extraocular extension, it was found that one out of four patients had an orbital recurrence and four out of five died of metastatic disease.[43] In one of my patients who had an enucleation because of a malignant choroidal melanoma, sections of the globe showed extension into the optic nerve, with some residual tumor proximal to the operative section. An orbital recurrence ten years later necessitated an exenteration. After two and a half years there was no evidence of recurrence.

It is important to distinguish between residual malignant melanoma (left in the orbit at the time of surgery) and recurrent malignant melanoma after surgery. If proper measures are taken immediately after surgery, the prognosis is good in cases of the residual cancer but extremely poor in cases of the recurrent disease.

It is extremely rare for a patient to survive the recurrence of a malignant melanoma of the orbit. The average survival in cases I have seen is 15 months. Other reports showed that 6 of 8 patients died within a year,[126] only 1 in 9 lived over 5 years after exenteration,[43] and 1 lived 13 years.[113]

Metastasis

The tendency of these tumors to metastasize is due to tumor-cell invasion of the blood vessel walls. Free tumor cells are sometimes seen in large vascular channels within the tumor and in the dilated choroidal vessels adjacent to it (Fig. 7–19). Tumor cells were found in the blood vessels of the tumor in 20 of 27 eyes cut in serial sections.[190] Examination of 15 eyes serially sectioned revealed tumor cells infiltrating or replacing the blood vessel walls and breaking into the lumen in every case.[189] Free cancer cells were found in the blood of 19 of 20 patients with malignant melanoma of the uvea.[83] There is no doubt that tumor cells reach the bloodstream, but their growth may be inhibited by host immunity, preventing metastatic lesions.

The tumor may metastasize to almost any organ; although the most common site is the liver, metastases are found in the stomach, subcutaneous tissue, spine, lungs, and other body sites including the lymph nodes. In very rare instances the cells may spread by the bloodstream to another site in the same eye. A patient with a choroidal lesion had a metastasis to the ciliary body opposite the pri-

FIG. 7–19. Tumor cells invading the lumen of a blood vessel. The margin of a malignant melanoma of the choroid showing masses of tumor cells (*a*) in the lumen of a dilated vessel of the adjacent choroid.

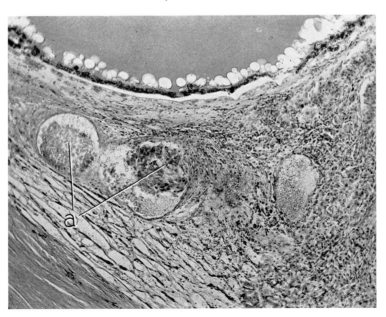

mary site. In a similar case the metastatic lesion attained a considerable size[184] and in another case involved the opposite eye and orbit.[59] The average interval between enucleation and the appearance of a metastatic focus is 37 months, but it may be 20 to 25 years, probably because of variable host immunity.

Factors of Prognostic Significance

Cytology. The type of cells composing the tumor is of prognostic importance. The spindle-cell tumor has the best prognosis and the predominantly epithelioid-cell tumor has the poorest. There are, of course, many gradations between these two extremes. In a report from the Armed Forces Institute of Pathology, the five-year mortality was 5%–10% for spindle-cell compared with 40%–50% for mixed and epithelioid tumors.[43] The ascending mortality rate from spindle-cell to epithelioid type follows a general principle: the more anaplastic the cell, the more malignant the neoplasm.

According to a report on small malignant melanomas, the two factors leading to a good prognosis are small size and spindle-cell type.[37] The authors pointed out, however, that a small melanoma may consist of mixed or epithelioid rather than spindle cells. Since the prognosis appeared to be about the same for both, small size appears to be more important than cell type.

Reticulum Content (Argyrophil Fibers). The tumor's argyrophil-fiber content, as well as its cell composition, may be a valid prognostic indicator. The intercellular elements of tissue in general are a structureless ground substance and three types of fibrils—collagen, elastin, and reticulum. Collagen, the most abundant, is readily stained by ordinary methods; elastin requires special stains, and reticulum cannot be stained by ordinary methods, but is the only one of the three stained with silver salts, hence the name *argyrophil fiber.*

Development of the Wilder silver stain gave impetus to the study of these fibers (Fig. 7–20). Reticulum, or argyrophil fiber, is a common constituent of benign and malignant tumors; it has been suggested that the prognosis may depend on the amount of fiber present in such tumors of the uveal tract.

In an analysis of 2535 cases of malignant melanoma of the choroid and ciliary body,[194] the argyrophil-fiber content was inversely proportional to the degree of anaplasticity. The spindle-cell tumor, the least anaplastic, lays down the most reticulum and has the best prognosis. The tumor composed predominantly of epithelioid cells, which are the most anaplastic, lays down the least reticulum and has the poorest prognosis.

Pigment Content. When the same 2535 cases were analyzed to determine the prognostic significance of the pigment content, survival was inversely proportional to the amount present. Only 4 patients with heavily pigmented lesions survived 10 years, compared to 83 with light, 91 with medium, and 48 with marked pigmentation.

Size. A study of 210 melanomas of the choroid and ciliary body led to the conclusion that the prognosis was significantly worse in the 50% with the largest tumors.[55] Tumor size gives some indication of cell type: small tumors are usually pure spindle-cell types, whereas large tumors contain a relatively high percentage of epithelioid cells.

If it is true that the smaller the malignant choroidal melanoma when detected the better the prognosis, it follows that a melanoma arising at a site where the patient's attention would be directed early to a visual defect would have the best prognosis. The preferred order should therefore be macula, periphery of the fundus above, periphery of the fundus nasally and temporally, and finally periphery of the fundus below.

Early or Late Enucleation. It is generally agreed that the earlier in the course of the disease enucleation is performed, the better the prognosis.

Operation for Retinal Detachment. The operation for retinal detachment due to a choroidal melanoma, on grounds that it is of the serous type, seems to accelerate tumor growth, promote extraocular extension, and often lead to metastasis and death.[28,120]

Diathermy. In cases of choroidal malignant melanoma misdiagnosed as serous detachment of the retina and treated accordingly with diathermy, the perforations may lead to orbital extension and seeding, with early death from metastatic tumor (Fig. 7–21).

See Diathermy, Light Coagulation and Cryotherapy in the Management of Intraocu-

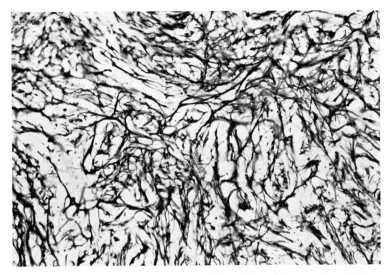

FIG. 7–20. Reticulum of a malignant choroidal melanoma (Wilder stain).

lar Tumors, by Robert M. Ellsworth, in Chapter 12.

BENIGN MELANOMA OF THE CHOROID

Benign melanomas (nevus, melanocytoma) of the uvea are congenital but are usually manifest clinically when they acquire pigment between the sixth and tenth years of life.

A histopathologic study of the characteristics of 102 benign melanomas of the choroid and ciliary body revealed that in 8 of 10 cases in which the lesion was discovered clinically it was mistaken for malignant melanoma and the eye was enucleated.[128] Large balloon cells with abundant foamy cytoplasm were noted in four cases. In another review of 200 cases of malignant choroidal melanoma, a 10% incidence of balloon cells was found, particularly in the spindle-cell type of tumor.[144]

These tumors range in shape from oval to round with smooth borders and little or no elevation (Fig. 7–22), in size from one to several disc diameters, and in color from brown to slate gray. They are usually located behind the equator, particularly around the posterior pole. A hyperpigmented eye is most likely to be involved, or perhaps the tumor is easier to detect in such an eye. Since the advent of indirect ophthalmoscopy, benign melanomas of the choroid are more readily seen. The incidence of about 1% quoted in the early literature is undoubtedly low; it is probably in the 6%–10% range.

Characteristic light puncta over the tumor

FIG. 7–21. Extraocular extension of a malignant choroidal melanoma following diathermy treatment. The patient, treated for supposedly serous detachment of the retina, died of systemic metastases several months after enucleation. (Courtesy of the Armed Forces Institute of Pathology.)

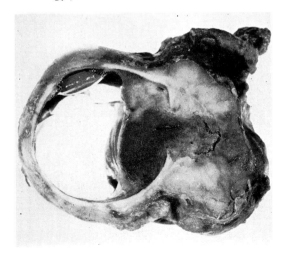

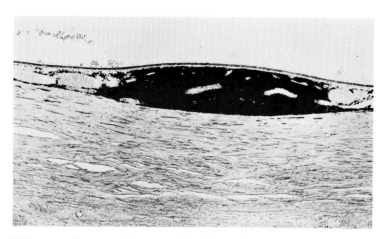

FIG. 7–22. Benign melanoma of the choroid. The tumor is slightly elevated, and the choriocapillaris is spared.

surface are caused by drusen of the overlying lamina vitrea, the amount varying from a few scattered dots to a solidly covered surface (Fig. 7–23, see p. 11). In other cases, the drusen are seen as a localized white plaque of tissue accentuated by degeneration of the overlying pigment epithelium.

Although a field defect corresponding to the tumor site is not common, scotomas have been reported when the melanoma involves the overlying choriocapillaris, when drusen changes of the lamina vitrea are particularly marked, or when the overlying retina is slightly elevated.[128] Using small targets, other observers found a field defect in 38% of 42 patients with benign melanomas.[179] Occasionally, a flat benign choroidal melanoma covers a whole sector of the fundus.

When a small melanoma is noted in the macular region with some reduction in vision, active growth may be suspected. However, the patient's blurred vision may be related to the melanoma without indicating active growth. It may be due to a refractional scotoma, to drusen changes, to a small focus of tumor necrosis giving rise to a mild inflammatory reaction, or to a vitreomacular traction syndrome promoted by a congenital adhesion between the hyaloid and a congenital melanocytoma.

Since benign choroidal melanomas rarely undergo malignant changes, frequent follow-ups of such patients are impractical. Efforts should be concentrated on identifying features suggesting the high-risk group—size of

tumor, elevation, pigment epithelium mottling or drusen formation,[65] particularly in fair-complexioned individuals.

MALIGNANT MELANOMA OF THE CHOROID

GROSS APPEARANCE

A malignant choroidal melanoma usually grows as a localized globular mass protruding toward the vitreous cavity. Its central portion tends to be more elevated and less pigmented than the periphery. If the tumor grows through the elastic lamina vitrea, a constriction or neck often develops between the head and the base, producing a mushroom shape (Fig. 7–24). Because of the constriction the head is likely to show sinusoid blood spaces from passive congestion. The head may be markedly congested, with constriction by the lamina vitrea causing greatly dilated vessels (Fig. 7–25). Sometimes the mushroom shape results from malignant growth at the site of a preexisting, more or less flat, benign melanoma (Fig. 7–17).

The tumor may become embedded in the underlying sclera, particularly in the macular region. This causes thinning and perhaps slight ectasia of the sclera but no actual tumor invasion. In this event, the growth may attain an appreciable size with minimal elevation.

CYTOLOGY

The histologic structure varies widely not only from tumor to tumor but from one part

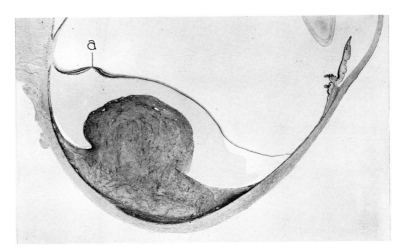

FIG. 7–24. Malignant melanoma of the choroid. The tumor is mushroom-shaped, and there is a detached retina. The fovea is shown at *a*.

to another of the same tumor (Fig. 7–26). Basically, these lesions are composed of spindle cells or epithelioid cells, or a mixture of the two. The spindle cells have a narrow, oval nucleus and an indistinguishable or ill-defined nucleolus. Epithelioid cells are round or polygonal and vary considerably in size and shape but are usually rather large. The nucleus is large, round and nucleolated, and multinucleated forms may be present. The abundant cytoplasm is usually homogeneous and acidophilic. In some instances the tumor is too necrotic for its cell composition to be determined.

The arrangement of the cells is fascicular, tubular, funicular, alveolar, or the growth pattern may be nondescript. In fascicular or "rhythmic" growth, the spindle cells appear in palisaded rows. This arrangement is believed to result from cellular amitosis rather than mitosis, the cells dividing directly one after another until rows are formed.

Tubular growth, due to a perithelial arrangement of the cells, seems to occur when the tumor nutrition is poor; cells around the blood vessels remain viable and grow, but elsewhere there is necrosis. In funicular growth, the tumor appears as solid cords that seem to be intertwined. Alveolar growth characterizes the more malignant, rapidly growing melanomas whose predominantly epithelioid, highly anaplastic cells have few or no fibrillar processes; the protoplasm is round to octahedral. They resemble carcinoma cells and are arranged in nests or alveolar masses surrounded by spindle-shaped, often pigmented tumor cells which form the stroma.

FIG. 7–25. Mushroom-shaped malignant choroidal melanoma with marked congestion of the tumor head. (*a*) The relatively avascular base of the tumor. (*b*) The congested head. (*c–c′*) Constriction by the lamina vitrea causing the greatly dilated vessels in *b*. (*d′–d*) The detached retina. (Courtesy of the Armed Forces Institute of Pathology)

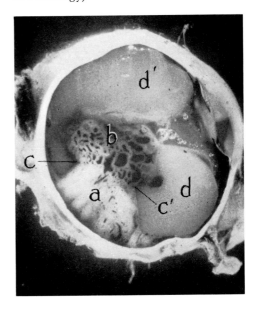

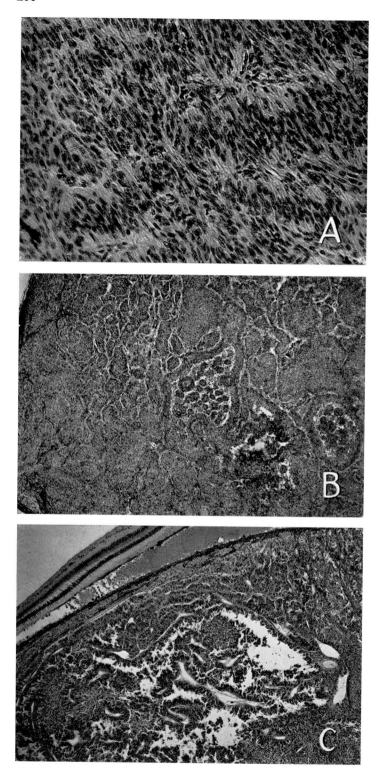

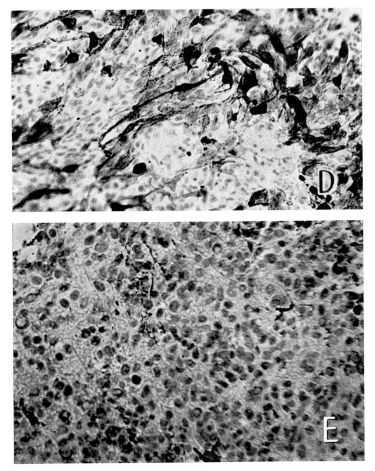

FIG. 7–26. Variations in the histologic structure of malignant melanoma of the choroid. **A.** Palisading of the nuclei. **B.** Fascicular growth. **C.** Epithelioid cells and alveolar arrangement resembling carcinoma. **D.** Branching cells. **E.** Nevus cells comprising most of the tumor.

FIG. 7–27. Flat malignant melanoma of the choroid. The diffuse lesion extended from *a* to *a₁*; an extraocular extension is seen at *b*. Other findings were detachment of the retina and secondary glaucoma.

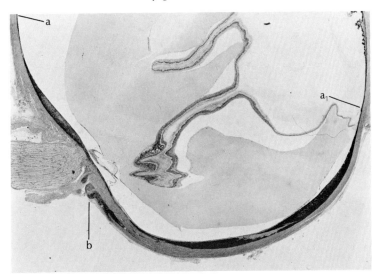

The pigmentation varies from none to very heavy, and is often most dense around necrotic areas. The melanin may be found in the tumor cells, free in the interstices of the tumor, or phagocytosed by leukocytes or tumor cells.

There may be connective tissue septa in which blood vessels course or areas of connective tissue that result from organized hemorrhage or necrotic tissue. The stroma, however, is composed largely of the tumor tissue itself. The new tissue seems to grow rapidly in, around, and through the older tissue which exhibits a slower growth. Thus, the tumor appears to contain three or four varieties of tissue, each developing at a different rate, and the stroma appears to be composed of spindle-shaped, pigmented tumor cells.

An overabundance of uveal ganglion cells has been noted in the choroid and ciliary body in cases of choroidal malignant melanoma, suggesting a congenital predisposition of some eyes to develop melanomas.[196]

DIFFUSE FLAT GROWTH

Although malignant uveal melanoma usually appears as a localized tumor mass, it occasionally occurs as a diffuse flat lesion (Fig. 7–27) which may involve a wide portion of the uvea or even the entire uvea (Fig. 7–18). A review of 844 globes with a diagnosis of malignant choroidal melanoma, from our pathology files, revealed 38 (4.6%) with a flat or diffuse type of growth involving at least one-fourth of the choroid in cross section and remaining external to the lamina vitrea. In the early stages such growths produce minimal symptoms, and they can be easily overlooked with the ophthalmoscope.

The cytologic range of these flat lesions is the same as for other uveal melanomas. Spindle cells predominate but even early cases may show epithelioid cells, and some flat lesions are composed of polyhedral cells characteristic of melanocytoma.

Whereas the usual benign choroidal melanomas are small and round to oval with a smooth border, flat melanomas are more extensive with an irregular growth pattern and with tonguelike projections into the adjacent choroid. The flat gray-to-brown lesions often show little contrast to the surrounding uninvolved fundus, particularly by direct ophthalmoscopic examination. The indirect ophthalmoscope, giving a less magnified image and more illumination, offers much greater contrast and is, in fact, essential for a full appraisal of this tumor.

The clinical picture of an unrecognized diffuse uveal malignant melanoma may be unusual, such as a ring-shaped limbal tumor or one with perilimbal and episcleral extensions.[170] A bilateral flat uveal melanoma was interpreted as a systemic disease of the uveal pigment cells allied to neurofibromatosis.[112]

Preoperative histories were available for patients with 28 of the 38 flat malanomas in one of our series. The presence of retinal detachment in 15 of the 28 eyes, and an associated retinal break in 6 of the 15, complicated the diagnosis. As there is little elevation of the tumor mass under the detached retina, the lesion may be considered a rhegmatogenous retinal detachment and be operated on for that condition.

A clinicopathologic study of 54 cases of diffuse malignant uveal melanoma revealed some interesting statistics:[56] an interval of over one year from onset to enucleation in 29 patients (59%) with two to seven years in 18 of the 29 (36.5%). Even at the time of enucleation the lesion was clinically unsuspected in 21 eyes (40%). Also, 19 of the 43 patients who could be followed had died of metastases; the tumor death rate was 73%. Glaucoma was associated with 59% of the flat choroidal melanomas reviewed. Two of our cases were treated as unilateral primary glaucoma. Because of the therapeutic miosis, the fundus was not adequately examined through the dilated pupil until the tumor was far advanced.

Another feature confusing the clinical picture is that some flat choroidal melanomas manifest inflammatory changes such as an active or regressive choroiditis, episcleritis, iridocyclitis, and even endophthalmitis and panophthalmitis. This inflammation seems to result from foci of necrosis in the tumor. Necrotizing scars were noted histologically in 44% of the cases of flat melanoma previously cited.[56] Even in the absence of these masking complications, flat choroidal melanomas may be hard to diagnose. In two instances in our series the fundus was initially pronounced normal although the patient had noted visual and field changes.

The difficulty in making an early diagnosis in 60% of patients, up to nine years in our cases and up to seven years in another series,[56] inevitably led to delayed surgical treatment. Late recognition of such tumors is particularly tragic because they are prone to infiltrate progressively both within and outside of the eye. The tumor had extended beyond the globe in 53% of our 38 cases at the time of enucleation. It may disseminate throughout the orbit, into the optic nerve and reach the subarachnoid space. Sometimes the orbital bones are invaded and even the adjacent sinuses and cranium.

MULTIPLE ORIGIN

Melanomas of the uvea may be multiple, a malignant lesion at times being found at one site and one or more benign lesions elsewhere. The benign lesions are composed of more mature cells than the malignant lesions and should not be confused with implantation growths, which are composed of implanted cancer cells from another site. Of 222 eyes enucleated for malignant uveal melanoma reviewed at our institution, a benign melanoma was also present in 23—in the iris in 15 (Fig. 7–28, p. 12), in the choroid in 7 (Fig. 7–29), and in the ciliary body in 1. Among the 189 eyes with a malignant choroidal lesion, a benign lesion was found in the iris in 11, elsewhere in the choroid in 6, and in the ciliary body in 1. Among 33 eyes with malignant melanoma of the iris or the ciliary body or both, a benign lesion was found in the iris in 4 and in the choroid in 1.

Among 50 eyes with malignant choroidal melanoma in another series,[157] 5 harbored one benign melanoma elsewhere in the uvea, and 1 harbored two. Although it is possible that all were originally benign melanomas of which only one became malignant, it is extremely rare for multiple malignant foci to develop in the same eye; very few cases have been reported.[150] Of two malignant choroidal melanomas, one was probably the result of metastasis.[184] Another patient had multiple melanomas in one eye: a benign melanoma in the sphincter muscle area, a malignant melanoma of the iris which involved the angle and ciliary body, and a large choroidal mixed-cell malignant melanoma. There was no evidence of continuity or spread from one to the other.[33]

One patient had multiple neurofibromas of the skin, multiple pigmented skin lesions, fibrosarcoma of the back, and multiple benign melanomas of both irides. There were also stigmata of acromegaly and other indications that the tumor involved the central nervous system.[69] Sometimes the multiple manifestations of neurofibromatosis, including the pigmented lesions, tend to follow the distribution of nerves.

Another possibility is that a cancerogenic agent acting on the entire uveal tract causes malignant melanoma to develop at one site and more or less benign lesions at other sites. Among analogous developments elsewhere are hereditary polyposes of the intestinal tract, multiple basal-cell carcinomas of the skin due to actinic rays, tumors of the mouth and lungs due to tobacco smoking, and hereditary bilateral retinoblastoma.

Breast carcinoma and uveal melanoma have been noted concurrently.[81]

FIG. 7–29. Multiple foci of melanomas. A densely pigmented malignant melanoma of the choroid and a small benign melanoma at *a*.

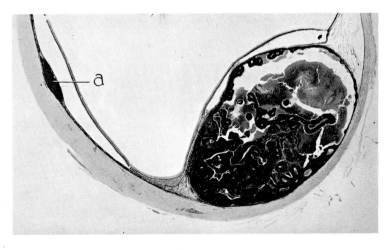

IMPLANTATION GROWTHS

Viable tumor cells may disseminate from the primary lesion, become implanted at distal sites in the eye and start to grow. Such implants usually appear on some vascular structure, ensuring nutrition. Cells from a primary choroidal tumor may pass into the subretinal fluid surrounding it and remain viable there, or they may be deposited and grow as discrete foci along the internal surface of the choroid or in the retina, particularly at the ora serrata or disc. Occasionally the cells enter the vitreous cavity and grow along the inner surface of the retina. I have seen only one instance of an implantation lesion on the iris from a malignant choroidal melanoma (Fig. 7–30).

NECROSIS

Necrosis and its sequelae (Fig. 7–31) may be prominent features of melanoma of the uvea. This complication was noted in some degree in 84 of 106 such tumors examined microscopically.[156] The necrosis is believed by some to begin when the tumor outgrows its blood supply—a possible explanation inasmuch as the blood supply often depends on large, thin-walled blood vessels with little display of capillaries. Once it has begun, a vicious circle may be established by virtue of the lethal toxicity of the necrotic tissue itself. Necrosis is unrelated to tumor size; even small benign melanomas may develop foci, and necrotizing scars are common histologic findings in most uveal melanomas.

On the other hand, pigmented tumors may undergo spontaneous necrosis and even regression, without perceptible deficiency of blood supply.[141] It may be that hitherto undetermined autoimmune factors are responsible for these phenomena. The large cystic spaces sometimes seen in these lesions probably result from necrosis and absorption instead of necrosis and organization by scar tissue (Fig. 7–32). Large cystic spaces may permit good transillumination of the tumor which can be misleading;[90] in some instances these are viewed as a Schwann-cell Antoni type-B growth.

A malignant choroidal melanoma regressed spontaneously over a seven-year period (Fig. 7–33).

In my opinion, necrosis of uveal melanoma is usually an autoimmune response which causes atresia of the blood vessels supplying the tumor. Our studies revealed histologic evidence of cellular and lytic necrosis in 18% of 100 uveal melanomas. Choroiditis or uveitis was noted clinically in all the eyes in this series. Because of the inflammatory manifestation, malignant melanoma was correctly diagnosed only after periods ranging from 4 months to 17 years.[141]

Coagulation or infarct necrosis of uveal melanoma was noted histologically in 5% of the aforementioned 100 eyes. Adding 12 more cases of coagulation or infarct necrosis from various sources gave a total of 17 eyes for statistical purposes. The cellular and lytic necrosis and the infarct necrosis were unrelated to tumor size, occurring in both small and large globular tumors as well as in flat diffuse tumors.

The patients with infarct necrosis had a clinical history of inflammation in the eye for weeks to years, masquerading as active or inactive choroiditis, scleritis, uveitis, and secondary glaucoma. Suddenly an acute phase ensued with pain, reduction in vision, and marked inflammation. Histologic sections of these eyes showed a coagulation or infarct necrosis of the tumor, due to an occlusive vascular process. It is postulated that the lytic and infarct necroses of the tumors were immunologic responses to the tumor antigen, causing involutional changes in the tumor even to complete regression.

FIG. 7–30. Implantation growth on the iris. This growth extended along the anterior surface of the iris in an eye harboring a malignant melanoma of the choroid.

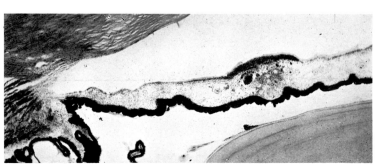

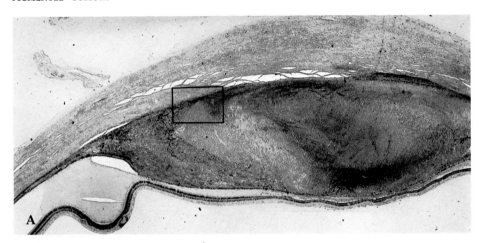

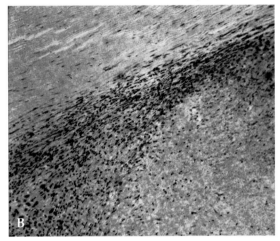

FIG. 7–31. Necrosis of a malignant melanoma of the choroid which caused an abrupt inflammatory episode. A 47-year-old woman complained of pain and redness in the right eye of three days' duration. Examination revealed moderate edema of both lids and marked edema of the conjunctiva which ballooned out of the palpebral aperture. Some cells in the aqueous and many in the vitreous produced sufficient cloudiness to prevent an accurate view of the fundus. Findings were a retinal detachment with some hemorrhage in the upper temporal quadrant and dilated episcleral vessels over the area corresponding to the detachment. **A.** Under low-power magnification the tumor shows necrosis of the central part and an inflammatory reaction in and around the tumor including the adjacent sclera. **B.** Under higher magnification the portion outlined in **A** shows sharp demarcation between necrotic and viable tumor with inflammatory reaction. (Courtesy of R. Collins.)

FIG. 7–32. Cystic malignant melanoma of the ciliary body. A large cyst occupies the central portion of the tumor.

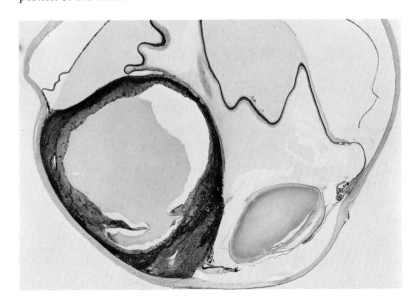

I believe the following statements are true, based on published information[141] supported by personal experience:

Malignant melanoma of the uvea may spontaneously and permanently regress to a scar. The lesion may also progress for a period and then become static, without regressing to the scar stage.

In certain instances, malignant melanomas of the choroid have permanently regressed and are not interpreted as such later by the clinician. These lesions are usually found either in the periphery or in the lower fundus where the field defect was not noted by the patient.

The sera of over one-third of 103 patients

FIG. 7–33. Spontaneous regression of a malignant choroidal melanoma. **A.** Pigmented mass in the right fundus of a 30-year-old woman. Although no biopsy was taken, it was diagnosed by several ophthalmologists as a malignant choroidal melanoma. Around the base was a zone of atrophy and secondary pigmentation. The lesion was observed regularly and regressed steadily. **B.** Seven years and two months after the first examination, a flat, atrophic scar with surrounding pigment disturbance was considered an instance of spontaneous cure. (A. B. Reese et al.[141])

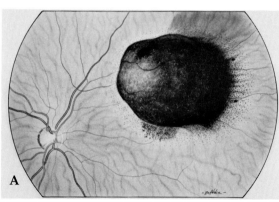

A

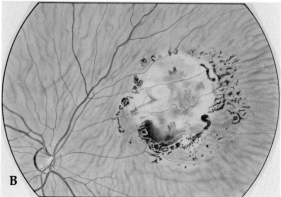

B

with malignant melanoma had antibodies to autologous melanoma cells.[107] According to another report, antibodies against the patient's own melanoma cells could be demonstrated in 7 cases of uveal melanoma.[136]

The necrotic tissue of a melanoma can produce as severe an inflammatory reaction as bacterial toxins do; cytotoxins permeate the globe and in severe cases affect all the eye structures. The iris, ciliary body, choroid, and retina may all become necrotic. When the sclera becomes necrotic, the tumor may extend diffusely in the orbit. The cells of the cornea lose their nuclei and the cornea becomes cloudy. Cataractous changes in the lens and hypopyon or a hyphema may develop. In some cases a vascularized fibrous membrane forms along the anterior surface of the iris. Glaucoma almost always ensues. The condition is difficult to diagnose correctly if glaucoma or inflammation or other anterior changes have occurred, preventing a view of the interior. These globes are sometimes enucleated because of a diagnosis of absolute glaucoma secondary to iridocyclitis or of endophthalmitis or panophthalmitis.

The tumor necrosis may set up a reaction severe enough to produce collateral inflammation and cellulitis in the orbit and some degree of exophthalmos. Disseminated tumor cells may even extend into the adjacent nasal sinuses. Necrotic malignant choroidal melanomas were diagnosed in one case by examination of biopsy tissue from the antrum, and in another by examination of tissue from the ethmoid (Cases 1 and 2 to follow). An analysis of eight of our cases with orbital recurrence showed that necrosis of the tumor played an important role in six, summarized briefly here:

Case 1 (Fig. 7-34): Endophthalmitis followed within a few weeks by panophthalmitis and exophthalmos made it impossible to view the interior of the eye. A comprehensive examination including x rays indicated a pathologic condition in the antrum which was explored. The orbital floor was necrotic, and tissue removed from the antrum showed malignant melanoma. Examination of the enucleated globe revealed a completely necrotic malignant melanoma and necrosis of most of the eye structures. Necrotic tumor tissue was seen outside of the necrotic sclera and in the orbit. Viable tumor extended through the floor into the antrum where it was actively growing. Treatment consisted of exenteration and radiation. The patient died.

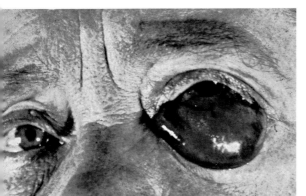

FIG. 7–34. Panophthalmitis from a necrotic malignant melanoma of the choroid. **A.** Exophthalmos and a markedly swollen bulbar conjunctiva give the clinical appearance of a severe panophthalmitis. **B.** The enucleated globe shows a necrotic melanoma of the choroid which gave rise to the inflammation.

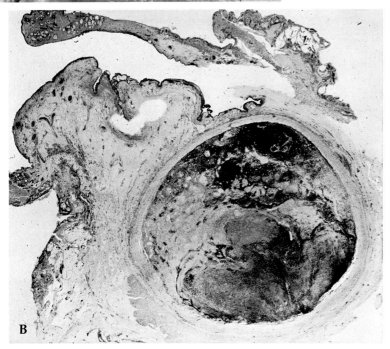

Case 2: An eye with poor vision for four years became inflamed. Symptoms, signs, and x rays implicated the sinuses, and an external ethmoid-frontal operation was performed. Necrotic tissue found in an opening into the orbit was removed and showed malignant melanoma. The sequence of events paralleled that in Case 1; the treatment and outcome were the same.

Case 3: Poor vision was noted in the eye for one year, with inflammation and exophthalmos during the eight months before enucleation. The globe showed a necrotic melanoma with marked inflammatory signs in and around it, and extension of the tumor through partly necrotic sclera. The treatment and outcome were the same as in the two previously cited cases.

Case 4: The patient's vision had become progressively worse, with recent onset of inflammation and pain. A trephine operation was performed for supposedly primary glaucoma, followed shortly by enucleation. A necrotic intraocular melanoma had extended through the sclera at several sites. One month after enucleation, inflammation and swelling developed in the orbital tissues. The diagnosis was abscess of the orbit which was treated by making an incision and establishing drainage. The same diagnosis was made a month later, and the treatment was repeated. Three weeks later the correct diagnosis of orbital recurrence was made. Treatment consisted of exenteration and radiation; the patient died.

Case 5: A necrotic intraocular melanoma gave rise to inflammation, extension beyond the globe, enucleation, orbital recurrence, and intracranial extension with temporal hemianopsia in the remaining eye. Radiation therapy was unavailing, and the patient died.

Case 6: The sequence of events was the same as in Case 5 except that there was no intracranial extension. Therapy included exenteration and radiation. The patient died.

Extension of an intraocular melanoma to the orbit in these six cases was largely due to necrosis of the tumor and sclera, with extra-ocular dissemination of tumor cells. In two cases the tumor cells reached the adjacent sinuses where they grew actively, and biopsy of these tissues led to the diagnosis. In one case the tumor extended intracranially and produced a hemianopsia.

An extraocular extension resulting from necrosis of the tumor and adjacent sclera is more diffuse and disseminated, and carries a poorer prognosis, than the usually localized and often encapsulated extension via an emissary.

Tumor necrosis seems to be a common cause of hemorrhage, which may be quite large, spreading to the vitreous and even reaching the anterior chamber. In some instances hemorrhage is the first observed manifestation of the tumor, either as such or because it has caused glaucoma. A neoplasm should always be suspected when there is an unexplained spontaneous intraocular hemorrhage. Another cause of hemorrhage is passive congestion of the blood vessels in the mushrooming head of the tumor from constriction of the neck of the tumor by the lamina vitrea (Fig. 7–25).

Lymphocytic infiltration is frequently seen not only in and around the necrosis of the uveal melanoma but also throughout the uvea harboring the melanoma. This inflammatory reaction, associated with tumor necrosis, is usually attributed to cytotoxic agents of degenerating melanocytes.

The tumor's necrotic areas usually contain more pigment than the viable areas. They may, in fact, contain virtually all the pigment in 'an otherwise slightly pigmented melanoma. A probable explanation is that the necrotic tissue is phagocytosed by lymphocytes or tumor cells, and the oxidase in the protoplasm of the phagocytosing cells converts the premelanin to melanin.

Necrosis of uveal melanomas may be characterized by a) minimal detectable changes associated with tumor cell death principally in the nuclei as pyknosis, karyorrhexis, or karyolysis, or in the cytoplasm as swelling and hydropic degeneration, or b) lytic or coagulation necrosis associated with inflammation or its sequelae. The patient may present with various symptoms such as blurred vision, swelling of the lids and conjunctiva, pain, and proptosis. The usual clinical picture in our 100 cases[141] was chemosis and congestion of the eyelids and conjunctiva at times associated with uveitis, localized scleritis, glaucoma, or detachment of the retina. Others found postnecrotic scars in 40% of flat malignant melanomas studied histologically[56] and concluded that this type of tumor is particularly prone to develop necrosis and inflammatory changes.

A malignant choroidal melanoma may cause so much inflammation that the eye becomes phthisical. Three such eyes were found among 24 globes in which histologic examination revealed an unsuspected choroidal melanoma.[92] Theoretically, the process that causes the phthisis may lead to complete sterilization of the tumor. However, these eyes often show activation of the growth after a quiescent period.

BEHAVIOR OF THE RETINA OVER THE TUMOR

Cystoid degeneration of the overlying retina has been noted in most early choroidal melanomas.[148] The retina seems to become detached when the tumor presses against a vortex vein or one of its branches, thus interfering with the return flow of blood and raising the pressure in the thin-walled veins. Fluid then diffuses into the choroid and subretinal space (Fig. 7–24). Detachment is occasionally secondary to the inflammation caused by necrosis or to disinsertion at the ora serrata. Holes, noted in the detached retina in the region of the ora serrata, have been attributed to the pull of the retina, which is thinnest in this area[181] but they may have occurred independently. The detachment, with the usual eosin-staining fluid underneath, may occur over the tumor site, around the base, or in the lower portion of the fundus.

Breaks in the retina, like those seen in the usual rhegmatogenous detachment, sometimes occur away from the tumor site.[15] This is particularly likely in cases of flat, diffuse malignant choroidal melanomas. We observed retinal breaks in 6 of 15 cases of retinal detachment associated with such lesions.

The risk of retinal detachment over the tumor site is reduced by adhesion between the retina and the tumor's inner surface. The rods and cones and varying amounts of nuclear elements of the retina disappear, leaving mostly glial tissue into which the underlying pigment epithelium proliferates; it sometimes proliferates into a thick, metaplastic, fibrous plaque which interposes itself between the retinal remains and the tumor's inner surface. The lamina vitrea, when intact, may show thickening and drusen changes. In rare instances the tumor grows into or even through the retina, its head protruding into the vitreous cavity beyond the level of the surrounding retina (Fig. 7–35, see p. 12).

GLAUCOMA

About one-third of the eyes removed for malignant choroidal melanoma are glaucomatous, for reasons not always clear. Glaucoma is a much more likely finding in large tumors than in small ones. Encroachment on the vitreous cavity seems to be one cause but not the only one. The tumor size seems less important than its position in relation to the vortex veins. A small tumor located near a vortex vein can apparently produce secondary glaucoma by interfering with the return of venous blood, thus promoting stasis and transudate.

More important factors in other cases seem to be hemorrhage in the vitreous or elsewhere, tumor necrosis followed by an inflammatory reaction, and lens swelling from dissemination of the cytotoxins in the eye. Plugging of the trabecular spaces by disseminated melanoma cells (melanomalytic glaucoma) is another possible mechanism.[198a] Glaucoma due to inflammation is characterized by a deep anterior chamber. When the glaucoma persists, peripheral synechiae eventually form, and the anterior chamber becomes shallow. If the tumor perforates the sclera, the intraocular pressure may become subnormal rather than elevated.

The tendency to develop glaucoma is probably modified by a toxin that emanates from the tumor and inhibits the production of aqueous by the ciliary body. This toxin may be produced by a histaminelike substance liberated by the necrotic tumor tissue. Its tendency to lower intraocular pressure may also be a factor in the subnormal pressure often encountered in eyes with malignant melanoma.

In a series of 96 eyes with malignant melanoma 19 presented clinically with glaucoma: 11 with a secondary angle-closure type and 8 with a secondary open-angle type.[198] Glaucoma was particularly prevalent in patients with a lesion of the iris alone, of the iris and ciliary body, or with a large posterior tumor associated with total retinal detachment. When malignant melanoma and glaucoma were present in the same eye, the diagnosis of tumor was missed ten times more often than when there was no glaucoma. This was probably due to the ophthalmologist's reluctance to dilate the pupil in such cases.

SYMPATHETIC INFLAMMATION

Most instances of so-called sympathetic inflammation associated with an intraocular tumor are reported in patients blind for years in one eye.[146] The eye is enucleated in the hope of favorably affecting the fellow eye which has an active uveitis. An unexpected melanoma revealed by the microscopic examination leads to the assumption that the inflammation in the fellow eye is sympathetic. Also, it is possible that a benign melanoma may be activated to malignant growth in the course of a bilateral endogenous uveitis, and the sequence erroneously attributed to sympathetic inflammation.

In a study of six cases of malignant melanoma thought to be associated with sympathetic uveitis, the site of a penetrating wound of the eye was found in five and could not be ruled out in the other, leading to the conclusion that intraocular malignant melanoma is yet to be proved a primary cause of sympathetic ophthalmia.[44] It is not certain from available evidence that sympathetic inflammation can be provoked by a uveal melanoma.

EXTRAOCULAR EXTENSION

Flat, diffuse melanomas are most likely to develop extraocular extensions (Fig. 7–27), usually by way of the emissaria. If not too far advanced, they are localized and encapsulated. These extensions are occasionally as large as, or even larger than, the primary intraocular growth. Some melanomas have an hourglass shape, being partly intraocular and partly extraocular (Fig. 7–13, see p. 10). This may be the natural contour when the tumor arises from a ciliary nerve coursing through an emissary.

A tumor may also reach the orbit by direct extension through the sclera; as previously mentioned this is usually facilitated by necrosis of the tumor and adjacent sclera. Such an extraocular extension is accompanied by inflammation of the orbital tissue and by dissemination of tumor cells that have little or no tendency toward encapsulation.

According to reports in the literature, the incidence of extraocular extension of choroidal malignant melanoma ranges from 15% to 40%. We have noted extension of the tumor into the optic nerve posterior to the lamina cribrosa in over 3% of our cases, which included some that were advanced, some with extraocular extensions, and some juxtapapillary cases. In only a few instances was the intraocular growth of average size. In the juxtapapillary cases the lesion may reach the optic nerve either by direct extension from the choroid via the border tissue or by extension in or along the retina. When the tumor reaches the cranium via the nerve, increased intracranial pressure usually ensues. I have seen a resulting defect in the temporal visual field of the fellow eye which led to blindness.

Malignant melanoma of the iris, ciliary body, and choroid may invade the optic nerve,[194] although much less frequently than does retinoblastoma. The nerve is more likely to be invaded in an eye with glaucoma and no light perception. In a patient suspected of harboring a necrotic malignant melanoma, a generous resection of the optic nerve at the time of enucleation is advisable.[171]

Melanoma may recur in the orbit months to many years after enucleation of the eye for malignant choroidal melanoma. I have seen an ipsilateral recurrence in the orbit 30 years after enucleation of an eye that showed two extensions through the sclera. Host resistance to residual tumor is probably the basic reason for such late recurrences. The same phenomenon is manifested in regard to metastatic foci of uveal melanoma which may appear many years after enucleation.

DIAGNOSIS

A histopathologic study of 7877 enucleated eyes from the files of the Armed Forces Institute of Pathology showed no malignant melanoma in 100 (19%) of 529 that were removed with a clinical diagnosis of malignant melanoma of the ciliary body or choroid, on the basis of a lesion visible by the ophthalmoscope.[51] This study was updated by adding 5889 more eyes. Applying the same criteria, the authors found simulating lesions responsible for 20% of enucleations for suspected malignant melanoma.[165]

In a review of 1398 consecutive enucleations at the Wills Eye Hospital, Philadelphia,

it was found that a visible fundal lesion had led to suspected malignant melanoma in 188 cases. The incidence of incorrect diagnosis was 3.7% for the ten-year period and only 1.9% for the final six years. The authors believe this much lower incidence of incorrect diagnosis compared with that for cases submitted to the Armed Forces Institute of Pathology can be explained by the fact that more cases of suspected melanoma are seen at large clinical centers where various diagnostic adjuncts are available.[166]

Subjective Manifestations

A malignant melanoma arising adjacent to the macular region is usually diagnosed earlier than a similar lesion arising elsewhere in the choroid. Among early signs are a relative or absolute scotoma, metamorphopsia, macropsia due to slight retinal separation, or an acquired hyperopia. In one reported case acquired hyperopia, an increase from 0.75 to 3.0 diopters, was the first sign of a malignant melanoma in the macular region. The vision was normal, and no fundal changes were noted. When the hyperopia reached 3.7 diopters, some fine pigmentary changes were observed. Two years later the eye was enucleated because of a detached retina, and the tumor was discovered.[74] A choroidal melanoma located away from the macula is usually not detected until the patient is aware of a field defect.

Pain from secondary glaucoma or, in rare cases, from involvement of a ciliary nerve may be the presenting symptom, or the patient may seek treatment for inflammation of the eye (iridocyclitis, uveitis, or endophthalmitis) caused by tumor necrosis. A scleritis may indicate a necrotic choroidal melanoma, even a very small one. In one patient, an abrupt inflammatory episode suggested an infarct necrosis (Fig. 7–31). The initial symptoms in a similar case were sudden pain, blurred vision, and inflammation with scleritis and marked ecchymosis of the bulbar conjunctiva.[79] In still another patient with necrosis the clinical picture was intepreted as a vitreous abscess. An evisceration was performed. The patient returned 11 years later with an orbital mass. It proved to be a recurrence of the necrotic choroidal melanoma which had been incorrectly diagnosed. Occasionally a severe panophthalmitis is found in association with exophthalmos or phthisis bulbi, following a partial spontaneous regression induced by tumor necrosis. Another manifestation may be a hemorrhage in the vitreous or, very infrequently, in the anterior chamber with or without glaucoma.

Objective Manifestations

The following characteristics may be helpful in diagnosing choroidal melanomas:

1. *Shape of the lesion.* The tumor's rather broad base, the constriction, and the mushroom-shaped head are often recognized. However, the retina may be tented by the head, in which case the mushroom effect is apparent only when the light of the ophthalmoscope passes through the translucent retina around the neck.

2. *Solid detachment of the retina associated with serous detachment.* The lesion appears solid and globular, with few folds and wrinkles, unless the retina is detached over the tumor site. Secondary or dependent serous detachments that are undulating or wrinkled, tremulous, and translucent may be noted (Fig. 7–36, see p. 13).

In a microscopic study of 33 eyes with partial retinal detachment due to malignant choroidal melanoma, 9 showed the retina lying in simple apposition to the tumor surface, and 24 showed partial detachment around the tumor. In 9 of the 24 there was a peripheral, flat detachment on the side opposite the tumor in the region of the ora serrata. This was considered to be a diagnostic sign of detachment due to choroidal melanoma.[62] Detachment of the pars ciliaris retinae has also been considered diagnostically significant;[94] this author found the condition frequently in association with malignant melanoma but never in idiopathic detachment of the retina.

Flap holes, typical of rhegmatogenous detachment, may be present in the retina overlying malignant choroidal melanomas, and they especially tend to accompany flat diffuse uveal melanomas.

When the tumor extends through the retina into the vitreous, the striking picture is easily recognized as a newgrowth. On the other hand, when the retina adheres to the tumor surface and displays pigmentary changes secondary to proliferation of the pigment epithelium, the picture may reflect an old chorioretinitis. Cystic retinal degeneration is at times noted over the tumor.

3. *Abnormal vascular pattern.* The vascular pattern in 20% of choroidal melanomas is abnormal over the surface; *i.e.,* it shows wide vascular channels of a type foreign to the choroid or retina. These blood sinuses probably represent varicose veins from passive congestion due to constriction of the portion of the tumor that has extended through the elastic lamina vitrea (Fig. 7–35, see p. 12). This seems to be a plausible explanation for the occasional vitreous hemorrhage noted when the tumor mushrooms through the lamina vitrea.[201]

The hemangiomalike clinical appearance of a collar-button-shaped choroidal melanoma caused by the strangulating effect of Bruch's membrane has been described.[197]

When the tumor grows into and through the retina the blood supply may come from the retinal rather than from the choroidal circulation. This results in dilatation of retinal vessels coursing between the disc and the tumor. The clinical picture may resemble that seen in angiomatosis retinae (Fig. 7–37).

4. *Dilated episcleral vessels.* In about one-third of malignant choroidal melanomas, the episcleral vessels corresponding to the tumor site are dilated (Fig. 7–38). They are usually considered nutrient vessels but in some instances suggest mild scleritis secondary to necrosis of the underlying tumor.

FIG. 7–37. Malignant melanoma of the choroid. A relatively small tumor at the periphery of the fundus may derive sufficient blood supply from the retinal circulation to produce enlarged and tortuous vessels at the disc similar to those seen in von Hippel–Lindau disease.

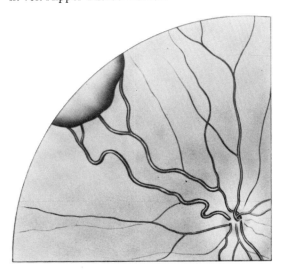

5. *Retinal striae.* Tenting of the retina, which produces radiating retinal striae, occurs in about one-third of malignant choroidal melanomas. Since it is also observed in inflammatory fundal lesions, in disciform degeneration of the macula, and in metastatic carcinoma, this phenomenon merely confirms the presence of a more or less solid expanding lesion.

6. *Hemorrhage.* Hemorrhage tends to play an inconspicuous role in choroidal melanomas. It is usually due to passive congestion from constriction by the lamina vitrea (Fig. 7–35, see p. 12) or to tumor necrosis. In inflammatory processes simulating melanoma, however, hemorrhage is common, particularly around the base of the lesion.

7. *Drusen.* Drusen bodies appear in early, relatively flat melanomas and over and around the base of mushroom-shaped lesions. They should not be confused with edema residues associated with simulating lesions (inflammation and macular degeneration) or with inflammation from necrosis of a melanoma.

8. *Role of inflammation.* Lesions that prove later to be choroidal malignant melanomas are sometimes misdiagnosed originally as inflammation. An inflammatory process arising from tumor necrosis may initially mask the tumor so that it escapes recognition; or as discussed earlier, an inflammatory process in the choroid may stimulate growth of a benign melanoma. I have seen two patients with proved malignant melanoma in one eye and evidence of an inactive choroiditis in the fellow eye. Malignant melanomas have developed after many years in a number of eyes with seemingly typical sequelae of choroiditis. They have sometimes developed in eyes long blind, with the same mechanism possibly involved; *i.e.*, a benign choroidal lesion has been stimulated to active growth by the pathologic process that caused the blindness.

9. *Extraocular extension.* The tumor's extraocular extension is seen as a vascularized mass on the sclera (Fig. 7–39, see p. 13) or as a small scleral nodule that may be overlooked unless the patient is told to direct the eye in extreme gazes with the lid retracted. If the growth has extended into the ciliary body, the extraocular nodule is sometimes observed at the external opening of the emissary of the anterior ciliary artery (Fig. 7–40, see p. 13).

10. *Associated benign melanoma of the iris.* Any malignant uveal melanoma, regardless of location, may be accompanied by one or many benign melanomas elsewhere in the uvea. They represent multiple origins of the tumor, the iris being a common site.

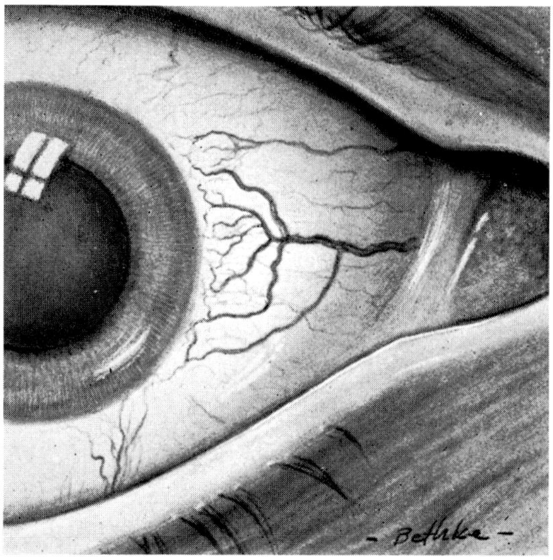

FIG. 7–38. Dilatation of episcleral vessels associated with melanoma of the uvea. Nutrient vessels over the sclera at the site corresponding to a malignant melanoma of the choroid and ciliary body.

11. *Juxtapapillary melanoma.* A choroidal tumor arising adjacent to the disc may bypass the termination of the lamina vitrea and extend over the disc, while growth of the remaining portion is restricted by the overlying lamina vitrea (Fig. 7–41). In such instances, the peripapillary melanoma may seem to arise from the disc (Fig. 7–42, see p. 14). I have heard of cases in which a melanoma arising at this site spreads around the nerve, clinically resembling a papilledema or optic neuritis.

The association of rubeosis iridis with uveal malignant melanoma has been emphasized in a report citing a 14.9% incidence in 308 cases.[26]

A yellowish-orange pigment over the surface of choroidal melanomas has been reported.[68a,168a] Histochemical and electron microscopic studies revealed that it is a lipofuscin contained in proliferated retinal pigment epithelial cells and in macrophages within and beneath the degenerated sensory retina.[57] Proliferated retinal pigment epithelial cells overlying the choroidal tumor have been shown to contain a greatly increased number of lipofuscin granules.[189a]

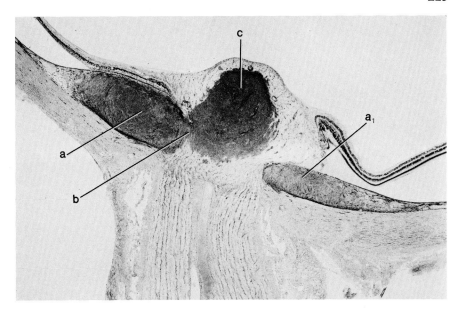

FIG. 7–41. Malignant melanoma of the choroid adjacent to the disc. The juxtapapillary tumor extends around the disc (*a* to *a₁*), circumvents the lamina vitrea at *b*, and grows forward into the disc (*c*).

TESTS

Scatter Illumination

This procedure consists essentially in viewing the lesion through a well-dilated pupil while a very bright direct ophthalmoscope light is cast below its lower margin. The examiner maneuvers the light and his head until the rays reflected from the choroid reach his eye (Fig. 7–43, see p. 14).

When a melanoma is present, the reflected rays do not penetrate it, and its border appears opaque or dark; the retinal blood vessels coursing over it seem to fluoresce—an effect never produced by simulating lesions.

Light is transmitted by scatter illumination in inflammatory processes, in macular degeneration, in metastatic carcinoma, in serous detachment of the retina, and in hemangioma of the choroid.

Contact Lens and Slit Lamp

Important information may be obtained by examination with the contact lens and slit lamp. The presence of a solid subretinal mass can often be established with this light beam directed on it. Also, when the beam is directed to one side of the suspected site, it may be possible to see the edge of a solid mass by scatter illumination even better than with the direct ophthalmoscope.

Transillumination

Although transillumination can provide valuable information, particularly when the retina is detached over the tumor, it can also give a misleading or even false impression. Subjective transillumination may be useful. A small point of bright light is passed across the anesthetized conjunctiva and sclera over the area of the tumor; if the tumor is opaque the light will not be readily transmitted to the rods and cones, and the patient will perceive no light or subdued light. When the point of light reaches an area away from the lesion, it is perceived as a bright glow even in the presence of a serous retinal detachment. The patient usually notes a sharp line of demarcation between the area of bright glow and the area where it either appears definitely diminished or disappears.

Among instruments for objective transillumination are those of Böke and Azarbaydjani and the Fiberoptic Transilluminator (Optical Technology, Inc., Palo Alto, Calif.). The usual procedure is to place a light source on the scleral surface behind the suspected lesion and then observe the red reflex or general illumination of the pupillary area. The point of light must be behind the transilluminated lesion; when it is situated posteriorly this may require an incision through the conjunctiva and Tenon's capsule. With too bright a light introducing considerable diffusion, a small or only slightly opaque area that transilluminates poorly might be obscured, or a false impression of clear transillumination might be gained.

In a variation of transscleral transillumination, the fundus may be examined with an ophthalmoscope, the source of illumination being the transilluminating instrument held over the sclera in the tumor area.

The transpupillary method of transillumination, which entails directing the light into the pupil and noting any interference with it over the sclera, is applied chiefly to lesions in the anterior segment. A beam of light may be introduced through the pupil by means of an indirect ophthalmoscope, while an assistant observes the amount of transillumination over the scleral surface. The conjunctiva may be incised to obtain a more posterior view of the transmitted light over the scleral surface than would otherwise be possible.

For lesions posterior to the ciliary region it has been suggested that the transilluminator be placed far back in the mouth and the transmitted light be observed through the pupillary area without opening the conjunctiva.

Retrobulbar diaphanoscopy has been advocated for diagnosing choroidal tumors. An incision is made in the conjunctiva in the region of the tumor. The assistant grasps the tendon of the nearest muscle and rotates the globe, then moves the diaphanoscope slowly toward the tumor. The surgeon observes the globe through an ophthalmoscope using only the light of the diaphanoscope. The tumor is seen as a black mass surrounded by the reddish glow of healthy transilluminated tissue.[21]

^{32}P Test for Intraocular Tumors

Introduction of the ^{32}P test into ophthalmology[183] was received enthusiastically. The test was used for several years at different centers, but then fell into disrepute. Its clinical effectiveness was generally agreed to be limited for several reasons: false positive readings in the case of inflammatory lesions; inaccessibility of lesions at the posterior pole; and misleading results due to inherent inaccuracies in the counting method.

However, with careful attention to basic principles and to improved techniques, it is now considered a reliable test for detecting intraocular tumors and for determining whether a melanoma is malignant. The neoplastic tissue incorporates the ^{32}P in its metabolic cycle, thus concentrating it in growing tumor tissue, in contrast to nonneoplastic tissue.

A recommended technique[78] is to administer 700 microcuries of ^{32}P intravenously and take a reading a minimum of 48 hours later for posteriorly located lesions. A solid-state, lithium drifted silicone detector is used instead of the original Geiger-Mueller detector, and a transistorized particle counter instead of the original rate meter. The 48-hour period allows enough time for the normal cells to be "flushed out" and the radioactive material to become concentrated in the tumor cells.

The conjunctiva is incised over the tumor site, and the rectus muscles that interfere with exposure are retracted. The tumor is accurately located with the indirect ophthalmoscope, as in the case of a retinal hole, and marks are made on the sclera with diathermy to outline the tumor.

Accurate location of a small lesion is extremely important because even a very slight error in placing the probe can result in a false low reading. Beta particles travel only 2.5–3 mm in tissue, making it necessary to place the probe exactly over the tumor. Experienced observers[78] take three readings over the tumor area and two or three over each of the other three control quadrants. The percentage difference between the tumor quadrant and the control quadrants gives the ^{32}P uptake. They have found a great difference, usually 150%–200%, in the case of a malignant lesion. A cutoff figure of 65% is their criterion for a positive test. They do not recommend the test for young patients or for pregnant women.

These workers[78] performed the test on 159 patients with suspected choroidal tumors over an eight-year period. Their results were as follows: 127 positives which included 124 primary malignant melanomas of the choroid, 2 metastatic carcinomas, and 1 false positive. None of the 32 patients with negative results has shown any evidence of malignant melanoma.

Other investigators administer 10 microcuries of ^{32}P orally per kilogram of body weight.[153] They believe the interval between dose and reading can be considerably longer than 45 hours, since very high radioactivity counts have been demonstrated in choroidal melanomas as long as two weeks after administration of ^{32}P. They also emphasize the necessity of accurately locating the lesion, especially small flat tumors for which the test is perhaps most valuable. In their opinion, the test should not be considered absolute but rather a means of comparing abnormal and normal tissue.

Since every effort should be made to control the variables and compare counts in similar areas, the control areas should be in the same eye. Errors due to factors such as previous ocular surgery, preexisting inflammatory conditions, and differences in blood supply to the two eyes are thereby minimized. They[153] obtained an average of 202% more counts per minute over malignant melanomas (confirmed by histologic study after enucleation) than over control areas in the same eye. A 100% increase in uptake over the lesion, rather than 65%, or twice that of the normal area, is their criterion for positive.

A detection probe and scaler unit for ^{32}P testing has been developed which has proved particularly useful for ocular tumors in the posterior segment.[152] Readings should be reproducible, with the average of multiple readings yielding the ultimate figure for areas of both normal and abnormal tissue. Readings in one area that vary widely might be due to malfunctioning equipment, voltage fluctuation, or other variables that could lead to errors. One-minute counting intervals are usual, but in the case of unduly low counts the accuracy of the test will be enhanced by lengthening the intervals to give higher counts.

Other authors have pointed out the need for further research into the effect of cell type, dosage, and interval between doses and testing, and stated that the ^{32}P test is effective only if the detecting device can be placed within 2 mm of the suspected tumor.[134]

Ultrasonography

See Section Ultrasonic Evaluation of Ocular and Orbital Tumors, by D. Jackson Coleman, in Chapter 12.

Palpation of the Sclera

The use of a blunt probe has been recommended to palpate the sclera over the region of a suspected malignant uveal melanoma located sufficiently anterior to be accessible; sclera is more resistant to palpation over the site of a tumor.

Withdrawal of Subretinal Fluid for Study

Tumor cells have been found in withdrawn subretinal fluid in five of six cases of choroidal melanoma[122] and in both cases in another report.[145] The Papanicolaou technique may be used.[64]

The diagnostic value of such examinations is questionable, however, in my opinion. Proliferated pigmented epithelial cells in the subretinal fluids are not uncommon, and it would be difficult indeed to diagnose cancer from individual isolated cells. Early growths are usually the most difficult to diagnose, and they are the ones that would probably not have broken through the lamina vitrea to gain access to the subretinal space. Since tumor tissue has been noted in the needle tract, the possibility of disseminating cancer cells by the puncture cannot be ignored. In fact, some surgeons do not recommend the procedure because of the danger of seeding, although they have identified tumor cells in the subretinal fluid.[28]

Melanin Test on Subretinal Fluid

In five cases of choroidal malignant melanoma, uniformly positive results were obtained with the melanin test, using iron chloride. The reaction was negative for the aqueous and vitreous, also for the subretinal fluid in idiopathic detachments. The test was therefore considered of diagnostic value.[29] A false negative result has been reported.[19]

Thermography

A measurable temperature elevation over the tumor has been demonstrated in patients with malignant breast cancer,[101] leading to the use of thermography diagnostically in various disciplines to detect hyperthermia and hypothermia. This modality has been applied in ophthalmology,[77] but an assessment of its value is awaiting further experience.

Biopsy

It is inadvisable to attempt diagnosis by biopsy.[16]

Other Recommendations

The presence of a retinal detachment over the tumor site may make the diagnosis difficult. In such cases it is often helpful to keep the patient flat in bed with the eyes masked for several days. The serous element of the retinal detachment may subside sufficiently to permit detection of the underlying solid mass. If the retina continues to be globular and smooth, rather than flat and folded, the detachment is probably solid.

Ektachrome infrared aero film has been recommended for use in fundal photography to reveal melanin, especially to differentiate choroidal melanomas from simulating lesions.[176]

Chloroquine and its analogues have an affinity for melanin. When they are tagged with ^{125}I, photoscanning shows subclinical metastases to nodes and lymphatics. Diagnostic use is not harmful to the lens or pigmented structure of the eye (retinal pigment epithelium), but a therapeutic trial is not yet indicated.[11]

Ultraviolet Light

Under ultraviolet light a seemingly unpigmented melanoma may appear to be loaded with rich brown pigment (Fig. 7–44, see p. 15).

DIFFERENTIAL DIAGNOSIS

In more than 10% of eyes containing advanced melanomas there has been a long delay in diagnosis and treatment. A malignant melanoma might be considered in the differential diagnosis of many lesions. Even where clear media afford a view of the lesion, there is one chance in five that the ophthalmologist will "overdiagnose" questionable lesions as malignant melanoma.[203] Small tumors, less than 5 dd in the largest dimension, carry a favorable prognosis.

Eyes with Clear Media

In eyes with media clear enough to visualize the interior, the following conditions may resemble a malignant choroidal melanoma:

1. *Benign choroidal melanoma.* Differentiation of benign and malignant choroidal melanomas was discussed earlier in this chapter. The most important factor is that in benign melanomas field defects corresponding to the site of the lesion are rare, difficult to find, and smaller than would be expected from the size of the lesion. Even in small malignant melanomas, scotomas are present, easy to find, and larger than would be expected from the size of the lesion.

2. *Hemangioma.* When hemangioma of the choroid is not accompanied by port-wine lesions of the skin on the face, head or neck, or by hemangiomatous lesions elsewhere in the eye, it may be misdiagnosed as malignant melanoma. The growth may be masked by opaque fibrous tissue resulting from metaplasia of the pigment epithelium between the choroidal lesion and the retina. Pigment changes in this tissue giving the lesion a dark color may contribute to the diagnostic error.

3. *Serous detachment of the retina.* Serous separations of the retina, particularly when long standing and associated with glaucoma, can be mistaken for malignant melanoma. Large cystic spaces tend to form in such detachments and may contain old hemorrhage with hemosiderin formation. These changes may make the detached retina bulky and dark, interfering with transillumination. In some cases brownish excrescences of the lamina vitrea, associated with marked proliferation of the overlying pigment epithelium, also interfere with transillumination.

During a diathermy operation for retinal detachment, if the points of the diathermy needle or the treatment sites cannot be seen by ophthalmoscopy in the fundus, the operator may suspect the presence of a flat choroidal tumor between the retina and the treatment sites. This impression is heightened if a scleral puncture yields no fluid or an unexpectedly small amount. Postoperatively, suspicion is reinforced if examination reveals reattachment of the retina and elevation of the area 7 to 8 diopters, with considerable pigmentation, due to the scleral buckle or to a silicone sponge. The elevation can be due to the diathermy treatments over the scleral surface causing it to shrink, not uncommonly causing an acquired hyperopia of as much as 8 diopters over the treated area. Moreover ^{32}P uptake may be significantly increased after a retinal detachment operation; hemorrhage produced in the choroid over the treated area adds to the confused clinical picture.

The presence of a retinal break or tear of

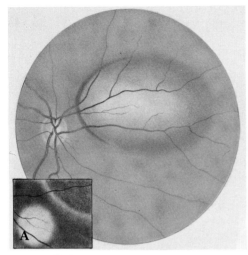

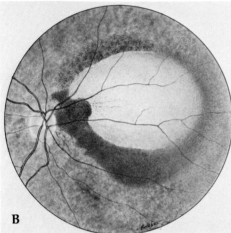

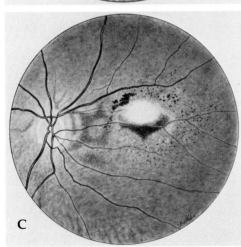

FIG. 7–45. Hematoma of the pigment epithelium simulating a melanoma. A 60-year-old woman suddenly noted disturbed vision in the left eye; a similar occurrence one year earlier in the right eye was diagnosed as malignant melanoma of the choroid, leading to enucleation of the eye. Sections of this eye showed a hematoma of the pigment epithelium. **A.** The lesion in the left eye at first examination resembled a melanoma except for a narrow collarette of hemorrhage at the nasal border. Inset shows the dark border by scatter illumination. **B.** Hemorrhage, pigment proliferation, and the general appearance made the diagnosis obvious 19 days later. **C.** After 13 months the lesion was reduced to a white fibrous scar surrounded by some proliferation of the retinal pigment. There was a suggestion of abnormal vascular channels between the lesion and the disc.

the type usually seen in rhegmatogenous detachment of the retina does not, of course, rule out a choroidal melanoma.[15,92]

4. *Hematoma under the pigment epithelium* (Fig. 7–45). This spontaneous hemorrhage occurs suddenly between the pigment epithelium and the lamina vitrea; although usually confined to the macular area, it may develop elsewhere. Clinically, the dark-colored hematoma has a sharply demarcated margin and an elevated surface. The hemorrhage arises from a vascular membrane that grows from the choroid around the end of the lamina vitrea at the disc and becomes interposed between the epithelium and the lamina vitrea (Fig. 7–46). Some ophthalmologists regard these hematomas as forerunners of disciform degeneration, but I have seen no evidence confirming this view.

The clinical picture changes quickly. Immediately after the hematoma appears it closely resembles a malignant melanoma, but within a few weeks its hemorrhagic nature is obvious. This condition may affect one eye only or both eyes usually years apart.

A sharply demarcated lesion in the macular area, seen clinically as dark-colored and elevated, may also be caused by serous detachment of the pigment epithelium from the underlying lamina vitrea.[118] Six such cases of subpigment-epithelial hematoma were erroneously interpreted as malignant melanoma and the eyes were enucleated.[12]

5. *Metastatic carcinoma.* In general, metastatic carcinomas of the choroid are flatter and lighter in color than melanomas. Lesions whose primary site is the breast are particu-

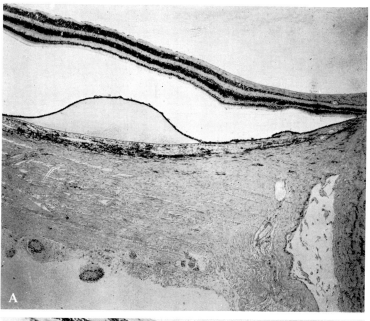

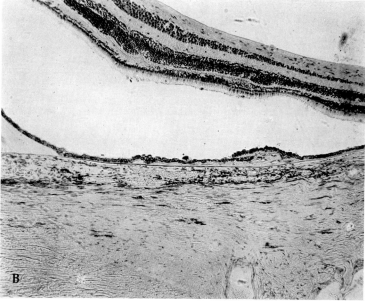

FIG. 7–46. Hematoma of the pigment epithelium
simulating a melanoma. **A.** Low magnification
reveals that the hematoma has dissected the
pigment epithelium from the lamina vitrea in the
macular area. **B.** Under higher magnification, a
vascularized membrane is seen extending from
the disc toward the hematoma between the
pigment epithelium and the lamina vitrea. The
hemorrhage seems to stem from this neovascularization. The patient complained of sudden loss
of vision, and the clinical picture resembled
that of a melanoma.

larly likely to be flat, whereas from other sites they tend to appear as localized masses. Ocular metastases from a primary carcinoma in the breast are usually correctly diagnosed, while other metastatic lesions are commonly mistaken for malignant melanoma. In most cases the ocular metastases occur late in the course of breast cancer when other manifestations are recognizable; with other tumors such as carcinoma of the bronchi, the gastrointestinal tract, or the thyroid, ocular symptoms may be the patient's presenting complaint. Indeed, cancer metastatic to the uveal tract may manifest itself before either the patient or the physician becomes aware of the primary site.

In some cases partial necrosis of a uveal metastasis causes proliferative changes in the overlying pigment epithelium. The resulting dark-colored lesion resembles a melanoma.

6. *Disciform degeneration.* The proliferative or disciform type of senile macular degeneration can be confused with a malignant melanoma arising in the macular region. The lesion is elevated and frequently dark in color (Fig. 7–47, see p. 15). However, the surface is less uniform than that of a malignant melanoma; it is frequently associated with old or fresh hemorrhage around the periphery or base or with whitish deposits due to residual edema in the adjacent retina. The deposits, which represent inspissated transudate, resemble the hard, white retinal deposits associated with vascular disease. Since hemorrhage and organization play an important part in the degenerative process, hemosiderin is partially responsible for the dark color. Drusen changes and pigment from epithelial proliferation are at times seen over the surface or around the periphery. Occasionally the degenerative changes are eccentric in relation to the fovea. The process in one eye may be so marked that it resembles a neoplasm, while the fellow eye may show slight or no changes. On the other hand, slight macular changes in the fellow eye, in the form of drusen or atrophy, are important confirmatory evidence of disciform degeneration.

7. *Hemorrhage in the vitreous, choroid, or subretinal space.* A hemorrhage in the vitreous sometimes makes it impossible to obtain a clear view of the involved area to determine the source. The difficulty may be compounded by hemosiderin changes. A choroidal or subretinal hemorrhage can be even more confusing; for example, when a large choroidal hemorrhage organizes, the picture

is made particularly obscure by the hemosiderin content and proliferation of the overlying pigment epithelium. Hemosiderin in the iris of the affected eye, however, strongly indicates intraocular hemorrhage, from whatever cause, and not melanoma.

The intraocular hemorrhage may result from sclerosed vessels associated with diabetes, hypertension, or other vascular disease, and may be precipitated by trauma or by sneezing, coughing, or vomiting. The condition of the retinal vessels in the uninvolved fellow eye may be significant. Hemorrhage from an occluded central retinal vein or one of its branches may break through the retina into the vitreous, and in some instances ushers in a serous detachment of the retina. Spontaneous intraocular hemorrhage at times occurs in very high myopia; when occurring in the choroid it could give rise to multiple dark globular elevations.

A hamartoma of children and young adults, described as simulating a malignant melanoma, was gray or black and slightly elevated.[67] I believe that this does not represent congenital maldevelopment, but rather is the sequela of massive hemorrhage at birth.

8. *Inflammation.* Over one-third of the conditions requiring differentiation from melanoma are inflammatory processes. They include active choroiditis (Fig. 7–48), se-

FIG. 7–48. Choroiditis simulating a small melanoma with necrosis. A dark gray, elevated lesion above the disc in a 45-year-old man showed some white deposits (residual edema) in the macular area. The lesion regressed, leaving the usual scar from choroiditis. (Courtesy of O. P. Perkins.)

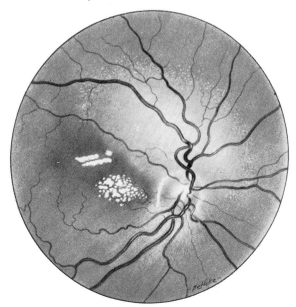

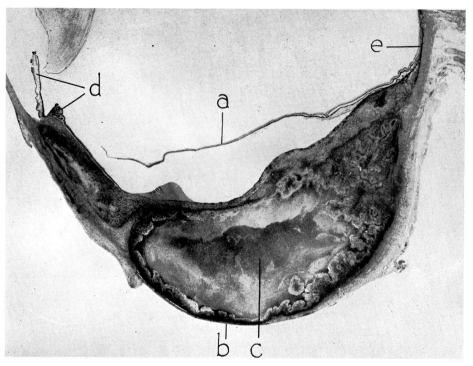

FIG. 7–49. Tuberculoma of the choroid. Involvement of the adjacent sclera resembled a newgrowth. (*a*) Detachment of the retina over the lesion is an artifact. The sclera at *b* is thinned and ectatic. (*c*) A large central area shows caseation. The iris and ciliary body at *d* and the choroid and retina at *e* appear essentially normal. Proliferation of the overlying pigment epithelium caused the lesion's dark color as seen with the ophthalmoscope. (Courtesy of J. S. McGavic.)

quelae of choroiditis, active effusive choroiditis with large, bullous elevations of the retina, scleritis with secondary choroidal detachment, and granulomas. These lesions are confused with melanomas because of their dark color, which may be due to stimulation of the pigment epithelium to proliferate or at times apparently to deep-lying hemorrhage that has been partially converted into hemosiderin.

Edema residues or inspissated edema is found at some sites in or around the inflammatory lesion in about half the cases, but seldom accompanies a melanoma. Hemorrhage is demonstrable in about half of these inflammatory lesions, typically as a collarette around them. Hemorrhage plays a negligible part in melanomas, especially the smaller ones. Vitreous hemorrhages from melanoma are very rare and associated only with large

lesions that either are necrotic or have broken through the lamina vitrea which constricts the neck of the veins.[43]

The lesion's inflammatory nature may be evidenced by a vitreous exudate over the site and by exudate from the lesion that dulls its surface markings. If the transudate or organization of the exudate leads to some retinal detachment, the clinical picture may be obscured.

A large tuberculoma of the choroid (Fig. 7–49) may produce little inflammatory reaction in the adjacent tissue or in the anterior of the eye. In such instances it may be confused with a melanoma, particularly if there is proliferation of the pigment epithelium. A gumma may also be well localized and produce little inflammation.

9. Hyperplasia of the pigment epithelium. Congenital hyperplasia of the retinal pigment epithelium is discussed in Chapter 2. Reactive hyperplasia of the pigment epithelium arises from inflammation of the choroid from any cause. An active proliferation may produce a localized, massive, pigmented lesion of metaplastic fibrous tissue which may be difficult, even microscopically, to differentiate from a true tumor.

10. Detachment of the choroid and ciliary body. Choroidal detachment may occur with hypotony after surgery or a perforating injury, or after inflammation of either the choroid or the adjacent sclera. Vogt-Koyanagi syndrome (Harada's disease) belongs in this category. Choroidal attachment may also be associated with retinal detachment and a deep anterior chamber, or with a transient hypotony due to sclerosis of choroidal vessels.

Choroidal detachment after an intraocular operation does not last long except in the event of a persistent leaking wound and hypotony, when it may continue indefinitely.

Choroidal detachment is usually seen as multilobular elevations, sometimes with a dependent serous detachment of the retina. A reported case of nonrhegmatogenous retinal separation associated with choroidal detachment resembled an annular ring melanoma.[119] There is no interference with transillumination; in fact, in my experience, light is transilluminated more brilliantly over the area of choroidal detachment than elsewhere over the fundus. Subjective transillumination is good, and light projection is accurate in the visual field corresponding to the detachment.

A delayed type of choroidal detachment may appear months to years after an operation or perforating injury, due to rupture of an epithelial inclusion cyst between the wound edges.

The eye of an elderly patient with swelling of the lids, proptosis, and a dark brown mass in the choroid and ciliary body on the nasal side has been described.[43] Melanoma with extraocular extension was suspected and the eye was enucleated. Histologic examination revealed that severe choroidal vascular disease had produced hypotony, which had in turn led to choroidal detachment.

11. *Cysts.* (a) *Cysts of the retina and retinoschisis.* Retinal cysts or schisis may be dark in color and transilluminate poorly because of hemorrhage with hemosiderin changes (Figs. 7–50, 7–51, see p. 16). A case of hemorrhagic macrocyst of the retina was mistakenly diagnosed as malignant choroidal melanoma, leading to enucleation of the eye.[151] The hemorrhage probably results from stretching of the cyst wall. The cyst may be congenital but enlarge during adult life. When congenital it is found in the lower portion of the fundus. The adult type of retinoschisis, in particular, is likely to simulate a melanoma.[163] Multiple large cysts also at times complicate a long-standing serous detachment of the retina.

(b) *Parasitic cysts.* When located in the subretinal space, a cysticercus cyst may produce uveitis. An intraocular tumor, including a melanoma, is then sometimes suspected. Intraocular infestation by echinococcus can cause the same problem in differential diagnosis.

12. *Staphyloma* (Fig. 7–52). A localized staphyloma in the anterior or posterior seg-

FIG. 7–50. Retinoschisis. The detached retina shows a large cyst (*a*) with some old blood along its inner surface at *a'*. This blood with hemosiderin gave the cyst a dark color and interfered with transillumination.

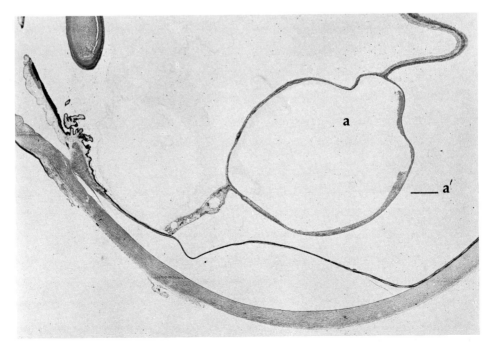

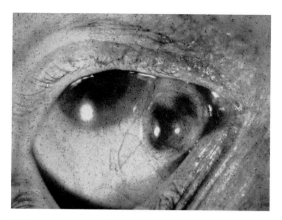

FIG. 7–52. A staphyloma suggesting a melanoma. This localized ciliary staphyloma developed after trauma and secondary glaucoma.

ment of the eye may be mistaken for a melanoma with extraocular extension.

13. *Carcinoma of the pigment epithelium.* This lesion often defies accurate clinical diagnosis. The rarest of eye tumors, it may be primary or arise from hyperplasia induced by an old intraocular pathologic process.

Diagnostic Importance of the Fellow Eye

The importance of examining the fellow eye cannot be overemphasized in the differential diagnosis of choroidal malignant melanoma. This is very often either ignored or done cursorily through a contracted pupil, yet pathologic changes may be revealed which point to the correct diagnosis. For example, it has been estimated that 25% of inflammatory lesions, 33% of macular lesions, and almost 50% of hemorrhagic lesions show some indication of a related process in the fellow eye.

Eyes with Opaque Media

In a small but significant group of essentially blind eyes, the interior cannot be seen satisfactorily because of opaque media. Various disorders are therefore at times confused with malignant choroidal melanoma. Iridocyclitis, endophthalmitis, glaucoma, or cataract may complicate the picture, making diagnosis more difficult. The glaucoma may cause corneal edema, pannus, or a bullous keratitis, any of which can prevent an adequate view of the fundus. Some of these changes are, of course, due to tumor necrosis, which in itself can diminish the transparency of the media.

Strong suspicion of a tumor in such an eye at times leads to enucleation, particularly since vision is irretrievably lost and the eye is often painful from secondary glaucoma. Enucleation is justified in view of the risk of preserving a useless and perhaps disfiguring eye that might contain a lethal tumor. The diagnosis of "possible intraocular tumor" is added to other clinical diagnoses when these eyes are sent to the laboratory for examination. Malignant melanoma is often strongly suspected from the sequence of events, from the fact that dilated episcleral vessels are confined to one quadrant or sector of the globe, and from results of the ^{32}P uptake test. Ultrasonograms are sometimes helpful in establishing the diagnosis in these eyes. (See section Ultrasonic Evaluation of Ocular and Orbital Tumors, by D. Jackson Coleman, in Chapter 12.)

In a series of 1000 eyes with malignant melanoma, 212 had opaque media that prevented visualization of the fundus.[114] A tumor was suspected in 99 but not even considered in the remaining 113. In another series, 24 of 228 eyes contained a clinically unsuspected choroidal melanoma; 18 of the 24 showed glaucoma with cloudy media, 3 showed phthisis bulbi and 3 retinal detachment. A melanoma was suspected, but not found, in 81 eyes of which 24 had glaucoma with hazy media, 11 had subretinal or choroidal hemorrhage, 3 had disciform degeneration of the macula, 15 had uveitis or endophthalmitis. Eight of the 16 eyes with serous detachment of the retina had glaucoma.[92]

A study of 15 patients with choroidal melanoma by dynamic tonometry showed definitely more pulse-synchronous oscillations in eyes with a tumor than in unaffected eyes; the method was considered particularly useful in examining eyes with opaque media.[84]

TREATMENT

Since numerous intraocular lesions simulate malignant melanoma and the possibility of a biopsy is usually ruled out, the treatment scale is tipped in favor of enucleation rather than temporization or therapeutic measures short of enucleation, including radiation, light coagulation, diathermy, and use of the laser beam. Otherwise, the uncertainty of the diagnosis may be difficult or even impossible for some patients to bear without serious psychologic trauma.

Full-thickness scleral resection for local excision of a choroidal melanoma[135] was attempted in a human eye with a malignant choroidal melanoma after experimental surgery in animals. According to the authors, the final visual acuity following surgery was "less than desirable."

Temporizing is in order when the lesion is small and relatively flat. If growth can be definitely established after repeated observations, enucleation can be carried out. Such melanomas are expected to have a spindle-cell cytology or to be melanocytomas (see Congenital Melanoma) with a good prognosis. Other factors to be considered in regard to temporization are the patient's advanced years, life expectancy, and emotional pattern as mentioned previously.

Before planning definitive treatment for melanoma, every effort should be made to ascertain whether metastasis has occurred. Besides x rays and the usual physical examination, the blood phosphatase level should be determined.

Surgery

Enucleation is the treatment of choice for choroidal malignant melanoma and for blind eyes when a melanoma cannot be ruled out. Care should be taken during the operation to avoid incising the capsule around an extraocular extension of the tumor. As mentioned earlier, such extensions occurring through the emissaries are usually encapsulated, and disturbance of the capsule may implant tumor seeds in the orbit.

Since malignant choroidal melanomas do not generally extend into the optic nerve, a long nerve stump is not imperative. An implant into the muscle funnel is indicated if, after delivery of the eye, there is no evidence of extraocular extension of the tumor. A rare exception is when an extension is encapsulated and undisturbed during the dissection. If the dissection is accidentally carried into the extraocular extension, immediate exenteration should be considered. Even if it is not done, however, an implant should not be used. An implant in the muscle funnel when there is residual tumor in the orbit may mask a recurrence, delaying detection. Prophylactic irradiation is not indicated even if residual tumor cells are thought to remain in the orbit.

When a tumor has spread extraocularly and is not encapsulated, presumably cancer cells have been disseminated into the orbital tissue, and exenteration is mandatory. Diffuse extraocular extension should be suspected if the melanoma has been necrotic and given rise to a diffuse inflammation around the eyeball. Recurrent melanoma in the orbit is an indication for exenteration.

In recent years the successful surgical excision of malignant melanoma of the iris and ciliary body has been added to our surgical repertoire.

Chemotherapy

Chemotherapy of malignant melanoma is unsatisfactory. The most promising agent is dimethyltriazenoimidazole (DTIC), which gives a 20% to 30% response with a median duration of eight months and a number of reported cures. The alkylating drugs (PAM, HN_2, Thio-TEPA, chlorambucil), the antimetabolites, and antibiotics are less successful. Immunotherapy, in the form of nonspecific immunostimulants and the inoculation of irradiated melanoma cells, is still under investigation.

Three cases of what appeared to be choroidal malignant melanoma were treated successfully with the cobalt plaque technique.[109] The radiation factors (fractionated dosage and duration of therapy) were computed on the basis of the tumor's size and mass. Dose fractionation permits the delivery of higher maximal levels with less damage to collateral tissue, and use of the computer with ultrasonic measurements minimizes the risk of excessive radiation. The authors recommended a total dose of 30,000 rads to the apex of a 5mm tumor, and 10,000 rads to the periphery at each fractional application. The tumor seems to have been arrested five and a half and four and a half years, respectively, after completion of treatment in two of the three cases reported. In the third case the patient was lost to follow-up after nine months.

BENIGN AND MALIGNANT MELANOMA OF THE CILIARY BODY

A malignant melanoma of the ciliary body often involves the choroid and iris in varying degree. In our series of 626 cases in the uveal tract, only 22 lesions were confined to the ciliary body. Both the choroid and ciliary body were involved in 37 cases, and the iris and ciliary body in 21 cases.

Among means for inferring ciliary body involvement are the following:

1. From the circumference of the tumor that is visible. When approximately three-quarters of the circumference is visible, the ciliary body is not likely to be involved or only slightly so. When half the circumference is visible, the ciliary body is probably involved. When only one-quarter is visible, the ciliary body is certainly involved.
2. From the presence of dilated episcleral vessels in the sector corresponding to the tumor site, noted in about 80% of our cases.
3. From the presence of cataractous changes in the sector corresponding to the tumor site, even when the tumor cannot be seen.
4. From the presence of a subconjunctival tumor nodule at the site of the scleral emissary of the anterior ciliary artery. Although this may connote acquired growth of a ciliary body tumor, a benign congenital hourglass melanoma of the ciliary body may extend through the scleral emissary. I have seen two such melanomas known to have been present since birth.

In the case of a melanoma at the periphery of the iris, it may be impossible to say preoperatively that the ciliary body is not involved. Inspection of the region through the dilated pupil, with the aid of the ophthalmoscope and the gonioscope, and also use of transillumination, may reveal evidence of ciliary body involvement and perhaps give an idea of the extent. A surgical exploration with direct inspection will determine the full extent and therefore the surgical treatment necessary.

PATHOLOGY

Benign and malignant melanomas in the ciliary body or in the choroid have the same cytologic characteristics except that there are fewer epithelioid cells in ciliary body tumors. Since a malignant melanoma of the ciliary body faces either the posterior chamber or the anterior chamber (via the root of the iris), it is not surprising that the aqueous may disseminate desquamated cancer cells and produce implantation growths wherever the nutrition is adequate. The cells or resulting growths may appear as discrete lesions or as extensions from the angle. They are found at or near the filtration angle, in the interstices of the trabeculae, and along the anterior surface of the iris (Fig. 7–53, see p. 16).

The implantations have a marked tendency to appear in the lower part of the anterior chamber and even along the posterior surface of the cornea, where they may remain viable. As the tumor is almost in direct contact with the vitreous, seeds are often seen floating therein or deposited along the surface of the retina and the disc (Fig. 7–54).

In addition to the primary malignant focus, patients with melanoma of the ciliary body may have one or more benign foci elsewhere in the uvea. These foci represent multiple origins and occur more often in the iris than in the choroid.

When the tumor spreads around the globe within the ciliary body, or around the angle of the anterior chamber, or diffusely over the surface of the iris, it is called a ring melanoma (Fig. 7–53, see p. 16). Two factors influence this type of growth: a) the area around the major arterial circle offers a good blood supply and the potential perivascular space offers little resistance, and b) the ciliary body acts as a confined space in pathologic processes. This is probably due to tissue cleavages which conform circumferentially to the smooth muscle; hemorrhage as well as tumor cells and inflammatory cells in the ciliary body tend to remain within the confines of this space.

As the tumor in the ciliary body grows forward, it sometimes extends through the root of the iris directly into the angle of the anterior chamber, producing an iridodialysis (Fig. 7–55, see p. 17) or the tumor may indent the equator of the lens, producing partial or complete cataractous changes.

When the tumor extends forward through the root of the iris and involves the angle, glaucoma may develop. Hypotony may ensue when a wide area of the ciliary body is impaired by the growth.

DIAGNOSIS

Early malignant melanomas of the ciliary body are usually occult, so that the diagnosis must be made from suspicious symptoms and signs. An early and consistent symptom is progressive uncorrectable visual loss. This may be due to cataractous changes usually in the periphery of the lens adjacent to the tumor site, to refractive aberrations caused by tumor-induced alterations in the noncataractous lens such as localized changes in lens shape, or to changes in lens position related to decentration or tilting.[58] Among the signs

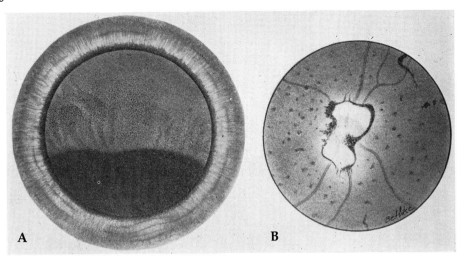

FIG. 7–54. Melanocytoma of the ciliary body with pigment and tumor seeds throughout the eye. **A.** Marked dispersion of tumor cells and melanin in the vitreous. **B.** Dispersed pigment around the optic disc and over the surface of the retina.

are prominent episcleral vessels corresponding to the tumor site, slight hyperpigmentation of the iris in comparison with its fellow, and iris freckles or seeds.

Both benign and malignant melanomas occur less frequently in the ciliary body than in the choroid. In our series the ratio was 1:6 for benign and 1:10 for malignant lesions.

Thirty-four of our cases in which the tumors involved the ciliary body—either alone or with the adjacent choroid or iris—were analyzed to determine the patient's presenting symptoms. Poor vision, the complaint of 20 patients, was due to retinal detachment in 10, cataract in 5 (one of whom had a dislocated lens), and apparently to glaucoma in 5. Pain, the presenting symptom in 10 patients, was attributed to glaucoma, although in several instances it may have resulted from involvement of the long ciliary nerve. Three patients who had no symptoms actually saw the tumor in their own eyes. In 2 other symptomless cases, friends saw the lesion, and in 3 a doctor discovered it during a routine examination. Two patients first noted acquired refractive changes. In another group of 13 patients with growths confined to the ciliary body, 3 had retinal detachments.

Implantation growths have been occasionally noted on the iris or cornea months before detection of the primary site. In such instances the patient may notice a color difference between the two irides.

In using transillumination as a diagnostic aid, the light source can be placed back of the suspected site, or it may be directed through the entire globe from the side opposite the suspected site. Either method permits observation of the amount of light transmitted by the lesion.

The growth is often best visualized by direct focal illumination through the dilated pupil. It appears as a dark mass arising from the ciliary region and extending toward the posterior chamber. The ora serrata, the orbiculus ciliaris, and the corona ciliaris, including the ciliary processes, can sometimes be identified. The ^{32}P test may be of special value because the tumor site is accessible to the probe.

Melanomas of the ciliary body seem less prone to necrosis than choroidal melanomas, but when necrosis occurs the ensuing inflammatory reaction—often the first manifestation of the tumor—may complicate the clinical picture. The tumor may develop one or more large cysts from necrosis. Light may be transmitted through the cysts when the eye is transilluminated, further confusing the diagnosis.

DIFFERENTIAL DIAGNOSIS

A malignant melanoma of the ciliary body is usually more easily diagnosed than its counterpart in the choroid because it can be inspected directly and is not obscured by changes in the overlying retina and pigment

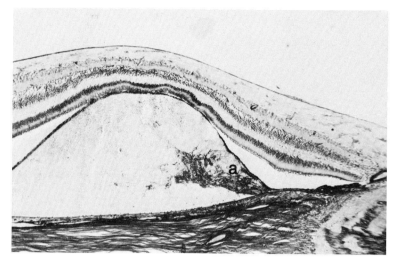

FIG. 7–56. Hematoma in the macular area clinically simulating a melanoma. The hemorrhage, which fans out in the subretinal space (*a*), apparently originated from a vascular membrane between the choroid and the pigment epithelium.

epithelium. The following conditions may enter into the differential diagnosis:

1. *Cysts*. Single or multiple intraepithelial cysts frequently occur in the ciliary body. When small they are undetected and clinically unimportant, being noted only in routine microscopic examination of the globe. A large cyst, however, is sometimes confused with a melanoma of the ciliary body and iris.

2. *Epitheliomas*. A benign epithelioma (adenoma) of the ciliary body is usually small and without clinical significance. A malignant epithelioma that arises from an adenoma is sometimes confused with a ciliary body melanoma.

3. *Other Conditions*. Also to be considered in the differential diagnosis are a) inflammatory lesions of a granulomatous nature such as gumma, tuberculoma, Boeck's sarcoid, and larval granuloma as well as nonspecific granulomas;[154] b) detachment of the ciliary body and choroid following an inflammation, operation, or perforating injury; c) hyperplasia of the pigment epithelium; d) leiomyoma; e) metastatic carcinoma; f) hemorrhage (Fig. 7–56); and g) diktyoma. An iridodialysis and recession of the ciliary body from a contusion received some time previously may simulate a ciliary body melanoma. Pigment dispersion and proliferation of pig-

ment epithelium around the dialysis, with or without incarceration of the ciliary processes, may add to the confusion.

BENIGN AND MALIGNANT MELANOMA OF THE IRIS

Assuming that any accumulation of tumor cells producing melanin constitutes a melanoma, the subject of iris melanomas becomes a complicated one. A study of 145 primary tumors of the iris led two authors[7] to conclude that it is rarely possible to distinguish sharply between a benign and a malignant melanoma or leiomyoma of the iris solely on cytologic grounds, because of their common neuroectodermal ancestry and overlapping histologic features.

The following types are seen:

Melanomas stemming from the optic vesicle composed of cells from the pigment epithelium of the iris a) that give rise to benign lesions seeming to be essentially hyperplastic and to malignant lesions (medulloepithelioma, diktyoma) either acquired or congenital, or b) that undergo metaplasia through all transitions from epithelium to well-formed smooth muscle (Ch. 2).

Melanomas stemming from the neural crest, comparable with choroidal and ciliary body melanomas, are discussed below.

BENIGN MELANOMA OF THE IRIS

Broadly speaking, a benign melanoma of the iris may be a true growth, a hyperplasia (Fig.

7–57), or a physiologic freckle. The present discussion will be confined mainly to true neoplasms.

Relation to Freckles

Pigmented freckles commonly occur on the anterior surface of the iris. Since they do not appear before the sixth year of life and seldom before the twelfth year, statistical data are based on findings in adult eyes. In a series of 300 of our adult patients with supposedly normal eyes, 145 or 48% had freckles on one or both irides. In 93 of these (64%) the freckles were on both irides—about equally in 82—and in 52 eyes (35%) they were unilateral.

Microscopically, freckles appear as clusters of pigmented melanocytes only a few cells thick along the anterior surface of the iris (Fig. 7–58). They can, in fact, be considered a localized thickening of the anterior limiting layer. In a study of sections of 100 eyes with normal irides and no malignant melanomas, I found such iris "melanomas" in 26. The term *freckle* should perhaps be used for the physiologic lesion and the term *benign melanoma* for the pathologic lesion, although such a distinction is not always possible clinically.

Some authors feel that the iris stroma often tends to become atrophic and relatively depigmented in old age; accumulations of melanocytes, present during most of the patient's life but masked by pigment in the surrounding stroma, become sharply outlined against the light gray, depigmented surrounding tissue. The result is an acquired type of freckle in older people.[23] I have not been aware of this process.

In my opinion, there is another type of freckle due to the migration and proliferation of pigment epithelial cells through the stroma to the anterior surface. This may happen without obvious reason but is associated particularly with eyes affected by primary glaucoma. Sometimes such epithelial hyperplasia is localized and assumes the proportions of a melanoma. A similar diffuse lesion may occur with a cuticular product across the angle and iris, causing glaucoma.[31]

A true benign melanoma of the iris is more extensive than a freckle, tends to be elevated above the iris surface, to extend more deeply into the iris stroma, and occasionally to increase the thickness of the iris. An ectropion of the pigment epithelium may occur opposite the melanoma. No endothelial layer has

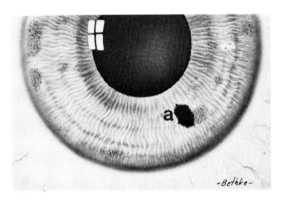

FIG. 7–57. Hyperplasia of the pigment epithelium of the iris, shown at *a*.

FIG. 7–58. Iris freckle. Freckle (*a*) on the anterior surface of the iris. The pigment epithelium is shown at *b*, the sphincter muscle at *c* with black clump cells, and the anterior capsule of the lens at *d*.

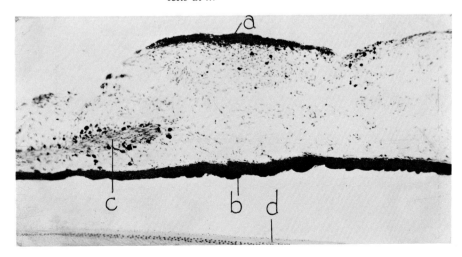

been identified over the surface of a benign melanoma.

The cytologic characteristics of benign iris melanomas are the same as for other uveal melanomas.

Incidence

An analysis of 43 cases of primary tumors of the iris showed 15 to be benign and 28 to be malignant melanomas.[42] These figures and those in our own records indicate a higher incidence of benign melanomas in the iris than elsewhere in the uvea, and higher than the 1% to 2% estimated by others. In view of the difficulty or even impossibility of diagnosing such lesions clinically or microscopically, an accurate estimate is out of the question. A given accumulation of melanocytes in the iris seen clinically may represent a true benign melanoma, a large physiologic freckle, or a hyperplasia.

Association with Malignant Melanoma of the Choroid

We have mentioned the finding of benign melanoma of the iris in microscopic sections of eyes with malignant melanoma of the choroid. This association was noted in 8.4% of cases.

Association with Malignant Melanoma of the Iris

A primary malignant melanoma in the iris or ciliary body was associated with benign melanoma of the iris in 12% of the cases. A malignant melanoma of the iris may also be associated with a benign melanoma of the choroid, rarely involving the long ciliary nerve (Fig. 7–59).

Association with Ipsilateral Skin Nevi

At times I have observed an iris melanoma associated with ipsilateral skin nevi, a finding that may help to indicate the true nature of a pigmented lesion of the iris.

Klien's Iris Tumors

Two types of benign melanotic tumors of the iris have been described, both ectodermal in origin and arising at the periphery of the dilator muscle. One type was composed of

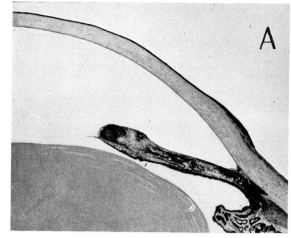
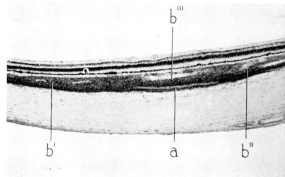
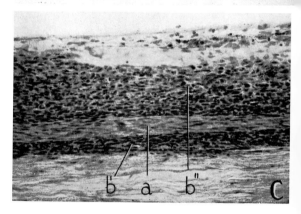

FIG. 7–59. Flat malignant melanoma of the iris with a benign melanoma of the long ciliary nerve. **A.** Low-power view of the diffuse tumor. **B.** Under higher power the long ciliary nerve (*a*) supplying the iris tumor shows a fusiform, pigmented enlargement (*b'*, *b''*, *b'''*). **C.** Under still higher power, the long ciliary nerve (*a*) is seen with its fusiform pigmented overgrowth of Schwann cells (*b'* to *b''*).

pigmented spindle cells associated with fibrils and the other, more common type was characterized by a group of deeply pigmented epithelial-type cells, usually in an alveolar arrangement.[93] In my opinion, these small tumorlike lesions at the periphery of the iris are probably hamartomas representing excess anlagen that stopped differentiating or underwent abnormal differentiation. They appear to be congenital developmental aberrations at the site where the pigment epithelium and the dilator muscle merge, and therefore should not be considered neoplastic. To my knowledge they are not clinically significant.

Relation to Leiomyoma and Neurinoma

See Chapters 6 and 9.

MALIGNANT MELANOMA OF THE IRIS

Relation to Preexisting Benign Melanomas

Most malignant melanomas of the iris develop from benign melanomas. Many investigators have reported cases delineating a clear history of a pigmented lesion observed since the patient's early years which developed into a malignant melanoma, and I have also seen such metamorphoses.

Incidence

In a report covering 125 cases of malignant melanoma of the iris treated by iridectomy, 48 of the lesions were discovered immediately prior to surgery, 30 were observed from 1 to 5 years earlier, 9 from 5 to 10 years earlier, 13 from 10 to 40 years earlier, and only 13 during childhood. No information was available on 12 cases.[149] These authors found a 15:1 ratio of choroidal and ciliary body tumors to iris tumors. Our records indicate an 8:1 ratio, but 13% of the iris lesions also involved the ciliary body.

Age

Patients with malignant melanoma of the iris are on the average one to two decades younger than those having such lesions elsewhere in the uvea. The average age of our patients has been 46 years, as compared with 40.8 years in the aforementioned series.[149]

In a review[30] of 21 cases there was one 8-year-old and the next youngest patient was 28. In another report[42] a 12-year-old was the youngest of 3 patients under 20. In an analysis of 46 cases from the AFIP Registry of Ophthalmic Pathology,[4] it was found that malignant melanoma involved the iris in 41% of the juvenile cases as compared with 6%–8% of the adult cases. Five patients were under 10, and 19 were under 20. Other cases in an infant[187] and two 9-year-olds[106,110] have been recorded. In one series of children the mortality rate was 4.8% for malignant melanoma of the iris;[42] in another series the overall mortality was 5.3% but 18% for such tumors of the posterior uveal tract.[4]

Pathology

The pluripotentiality of iris tissue makes it particularly difficult to interpret iris melanomas clinically. The cell content of tumors from the pigment epithelium may vary from mother cells to smooth muscle cells, or the tumor may resemble a medulloepithelioma (diktyoma). The typical iris melanomas, however, are cytologically comparable with melanomas of the choroid and ciliary body.

An analysis of 125 iris melanomas treated by iridectomy revealed that 87 contained apparently benign cells unlikely to produce distant metastasis.[149] Despite their inert appearance, however, these cells may infiltrate the anterior chamber angle, ciliary body, and outflow channels. They are occasionally dispersed by the aqueous and seed into the angle or onto other portions of the iris. The other 38 cases resembled choroidal melanomas and harbored cells considered capable of metastasis, although distant metastases were believed to have occurred in only 3 of the cases.

The explanation of the ring phenomenon in primary melanomas of the ciliary body also applies to primary melanomas of the iris (Fig. 7–60, see p. 17). The iris melanomas may involve the anterior portion of the ciliary body and thus come in contact with the major arterial circle, spreading through and around it.

As in the ciliary body, cancer cells from a primary tumor site in the iris may desquamate into the aqueous and become implantation growths on its anterior surface or at the filtration angle (Fig. 7–60B, see p. 17). Seeds implanted in this angle may extend as flat growths along the iris surface or the posterior surface of the cornea. They may appear at one or many sites around the circumference of the angle, but occur most often in the lower portion. Flat growths also extend by direct continuity from the primary site along the anterior surface of the iris.

A pseudoangioma of the iris was associated with a melanoma in a reported case.[8] When the eye was enucleated, microscopic examination revealed that the melanoma's vascular component overshadowed its neoplastic nature. In another case, an aggregation of vessels at the tumor border was found to be due to vascular proliferation.[80]

Particular attention is called to the type of iris melanoma with a uniformly diffuse growth that replaces the iris stroma, altering it very little in contour and thickness (Fig. 7–61). The mortality is relatively high since it is often incorrectly diagnosed or unrecognized until quite advanced.

DIAGNOSIS

A benign or malignant iris melanoma is usually symptomless and is detected by the physician in the course of a routine examination or by the patient himself or by a friend. This was the case in approximately 50% of our patients, but about one-third of them had sought medical advice because of blurred vision and pain due to glaucoma.

When an iris melanoma is recognized, its nature must be determined. A diagnosis of malignant melanoma is justified if growth can be definitely established by a) repeated observation and measurement, b) implantation growths or seeds on the iris, c) acquired freckles on the iris, d) disseminated cells in the filtration angle demonstrable by gonioscopic examination, e) blood vessels in the tumor, or nutrient vessels coursing through the iris to the tumor, or dilated episcleral vessels opposite the tumor site, or f) the onset of glaucoma.

The site most frequently favored by iris tumors is the periphery, especially the inferior and inferotemporal quadrants,[149] although the portion affected does not seem to have diagnostic significance.

Biopsy of an iris or a ciliary body melanoma is generally contraindicated because of the great possibility of seeding. This risk is minimized if the incision is made in the cornea by transfixion instead of at the limbus.

The distinction between iris seeds and freckles is important and may be difficult to make. In general, the seeds or implantation

growths are larger, darker, and more elevated; also they show no sharp tissue markings by slit-lamp examination. The tissue structure of freckles is similar in texture to that of the iris stroma. Both acquired freckles and seeds indicate active growth.

The following cases illustrate acquired iris freckles:

A flat melanoma, 1 by 3 mm, detected in the periphery of the iris during a routine examination, had apparently been present for a long time. It was observed every three to six months. Gonioscopic examinations, drawings, and photographs were made at varying intervals. After an eight-year period without change, the angle of the anterior chamber could no longer be seen over the tumor site with aid of the gonioscope, indicating an increase in elevation of the lesion (Fig. 7–62, see p. 18). At the same time two freckles, which had not been there six months earlier, were noted on the iris above the main lesion. A third freckle appeared above the others about two and one-half months later. The size of the main lesion was unchanged.

The eye was enucleated and microscopy revealed a malignant melanoma arising apparently from the site of a benign melanoma. Mature cells were more numerous in the freckles than in the main lesion and represented multiple origins of the tumor. The timing of their appearance suggested active or malignant growth of the main lesion.

The next case involves benign freckles:

A patient with malignant melanoma of the iris had four acquired freckles elsewhere on the same iris but none of the fellow iris. The tumor, which was excised locally, proved microscopically to be a malignant melanoma. After over 14 years there was no recurrence, and the pigmented freckles had not grown. This case offers further evidence that freckles are composed of mature cells that have little or no power of growth.

Transillumination is of little value in appraising suspected melanomatous lesions confined to the iris. An intraepithelial cyst of the iris has pigment epithelium on its posterior wall and so it does not transmit light. An intraepithelial cyst in the ciliary body at the base of the iris, pushing the root forward, transilluminates well because the posterior wall is composed of nonpigmented epithelium. The transscleral method of transillumination is usually more useful than the transpupillary method. If it is important to find out whether an iris melanoma extends into the ciliary body, the dark-adapted observer in a dark room should transilluminate across the eye with a strong light. The eye lights up like

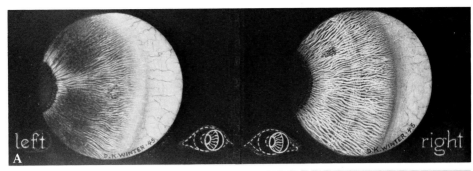

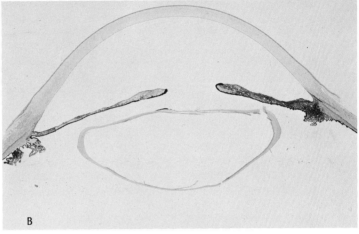

FIG. 7–61. Diffuse malignant melanoma of the iris. **A.** Sector of the left iris showing diffuse pigmentation with no actual tumor elevation, as was true of the remainder of the iris. Comparison with a corresponding sector of the normal iris of the right eye revealed the difference in pigmentation, the principal clinical feature of the lesion. With the gonioscope, however, tumor cells could be seen in the angle. **B.** Microscopic section shows diffuse infiltration of the iris and part of the ciliary body by cancer cells. (Courtesy of S. Richardson.)

a lantern; a light ring can be seen in the angle and a dark ring back of it. A melanoma involving the ciliary body stands out as a darker area in the dark ring.

The ^{32}P test is not helpful for a suspected lesion confined to the iris, but when the tumor extends into the ciliary body a significant amount of radioactive phosphorus may be taken up.

The gonioscope may help determine whether an iris melanoma extends into the ciliary body by revealing a widening of the ciliary body ring on each side of the iris tumor. Dilatation of the episcleral vessels corresponding to the suspected site would offer confirmation. It can also be helpful to examine the posterior chamber through a dilated pupil.[158]

For a reason unknown to me, the filtration angle as viewed with the gonioscope is usually deeper opposite the base of the tumor than elsewhere.

It is important to recognize the diffuse type of iris lesion that is frequently not diagnosed until late in its development.[149] The combination of increasing pigmentation of one iris

with ipsilateral glaucoma should arouse suspicion. This type of heterochromia is not to be confused with melanosis oculi. Tumor seeding in the filtration angle and over the iris surface is particularly marked in diffuse lesions and may be of diagnostic aid in early cases.

When the melanoma is in the periphery of the iris, it may be difficult to decide whether the ciliary body is involved. The presence of episcleral vessels corresponding to the location of the iris tumor, or localized cataractous changes in that area, may indicate involvement of the ciliary body. A clinical examination even with the gonioscope may not confirm this suspicion; confirmation sometimes must await direct inspection of the lesion at the time of operation.

Evidence of active growth must be evaluated either by very accurate measurements and drawings or by photographs. In connection with a slight change, the clinical impressions of both patients and relatives are often unreliable. Moreover, an iris lesion frequently shows accentuated pigmentation, e.g., at puberty or during pregnancy, but this does not necessarily imply active growth.

The appearance of nutrient vessels in the tumor or coursing to it in the iris stroma may be a significant factor in establishing activity of a lesion. Incomplete dilatation or "splinting" in the area signifies stromal invasion. In addition, the pupil may appear to be elongated toward the lesion, a distortion at times accentuated by ectropion uveae.

Tumor seeds or satellites may be seen as implantations over the iris surface or in the lower angle of the anterior chamber. A tumor seed and an iris freckle can be difficult to differentiate. The decision is made easier if the fellow iris has comparable freckles. Local excision is permissible if all extraneous pigmented lesions appear to be freckles rather than seeds.

Granular pigment in the lower part of the filtration angle is virtually a constant finding in the presence of even a benign melanoma. This fine pigment dust over the trabecula is unlikely to be confused with the larger tumor seeds which tend to grow over the iris surface, and does not constitute a contraindication to excisional iridectomy.

Elevated intraocular pressure in the involved eye suggests that the filtration angle is involved and that the lesion is too extensive for local excision. This can almost always be verified by gonioscopy. In diffuse lesions where the first manifestation is an iris darker than its fellow, glaucoma develops early. Again, gonioscopy may be the only means of verification. Needless to say, local excision is contraindicated in such instances.

If a suspected lesion is located near the pupillary area, it may safely be kept under observation, but iridectomy is probably in order when a similar lesion is in the periphery of the iris near the angle area. Any additional growth in the periphery would involve extension into the angle, ciliary body, or cornea. In this event, a timely iridectomy might well obviate more extensive surgery later. A peripheral lesion may be successfully excised, even if in apposition to the cornea, if the cornea or angle structures are not actually invaded.

Tapioca Melanoma

The usual iris melanoma is seen as a localized, elevated, pigmented mass replacing the normal iris. An atypical growth pattern shows single or multiple foci of nodules resembling tapioca.[143] The clusters of nodules, usually pale to translucent, may lie over part or all of the iris (Fig. 7–63). In some instances the nodules are pigmented. The clusters may be concentrated in one segment of the iris (Fig. 7–64). Although the tapioca type behaves much like a typical iris melanoma, it tends to occur at an earlier age. About one-third of the patients develop glaucoma.

Follow-up of our cases, from 2 months to 11 years, revealed no local recurrence in those undergoing surgery, and no local or distant extension of the tumor. In one case the melanoma was exacerbated during the patient's two pregnancies.

Tapioca melanoma seems to be a clinical variant of the protean disease of neurofibromatosis (von Recklinghausen's disease). Iris nodules that must be differentiated from tapioca nodules are found in sarcoidosis, congenital ocular melanocytosis, and a punctate iris pigmentation whose nature is unknown.[31]

Electron microscopic studies[86] have confirmed the low-grade malignancy of the tumor cells resembling those in spindle-cell type choroidal melanoma.

DIFFERENTIAL DIAGNOSIS

Of 7877 enucleated eyes examined at the Armed Forces Institute of Pathology, 529 had been clinically diagnosed as malignant melanoma of the ciliary body or choroid, on the basis of an ophthalmoscopically visible lesion. On pathologic examination, however, no malignant melanoma was found in 100 of the 529, or 19%.[51]

In a subsequent report, no tumor was found in 24 (35%) of the 69 eyes with a preoperative diagnosis of malignant melanoma of the iris.[52]

The following conditions may confuse the diagnosis:

1. *Alterations in the pigment epithelium.* Many assorted conditions that may resemble iris melanoma are due to various nonneoplastic changes in the iris pigment epithelium.

2. *Atrophy of the iris stroma.* When the pigment epithelium is bared and appears as a black localized area, due to atrophy or necrosis of the overlying stroma, it may simulate a melanoma. This may happen when a peripheral anterior synechia is quite broad (Fig. 7–65) and localized. Also, in the early stages of so-called essential atrophy of the iris, the pigment epithelium may be bared over a localized and sharply demarcated area of the iris and thus simulate a melanoma. In such instances the pupil is drawn to the opposite side of the lesion, whereas in iris melanoma it is drawn toward the tumor site.

3. *Staphyloma.* In staphyloma the localized thinning of the cornea or sclera, with uveal tissue lining the interior, may resemble a dark globular tumor.

4. *Tumors of the pigment epithelium or its anlagen.* A tumor originating in the pigment epithelium of the iris or ciliary body, or in anlagen of this epithelium, may require differentiation from the usual melanoma. These tumors include leiomyoma, diktyoma (medulloepithelioma), adenoma or epithelioma of the ciliary epithelium, and carcinoma of the pigment epithelium.

5. *Granuloma.* Lesions of one of the granulomatous diseases such as syphilis (gumma), tuberculosis (tuberculoma), or sarcoid are usually vascularized and nonpigmented and show some inflammatory features. In recent years, it has been appreciated that xanthogranuloma may simulate a melanoma or angioma of the iris, particularly in young people.

An iris abscess has been confused with a malignant melanoma.[68,124]

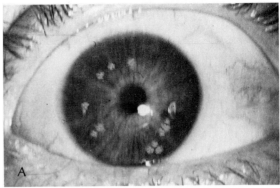
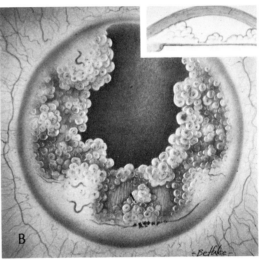

FIG. 7–63. Tapioca melanoma of the iris. **A.** Scattered gray nodules on the surface of the iris in a 48-year-old man. They progressed in number and size over a 13-year-period during which time he refused surgery. **B.** Before enucleation because of secondary glaucoma the multiple nodules, each with a central blood vessel, resembled tapioca. Inset shows the extent of the tumor in the anterior chamber. The histologic diagnosis was malignant melanoma. (A. B. Reese et al.[143])

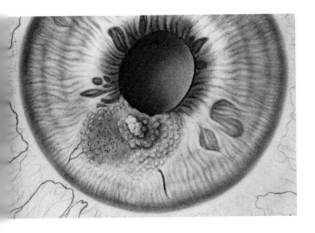

FIG. 7–64. Segmental type of tapioca melanoma. This iris tumor in a 36-year-old man was supplied by two nutrient vessels. (A. B. Reese et al.[143])

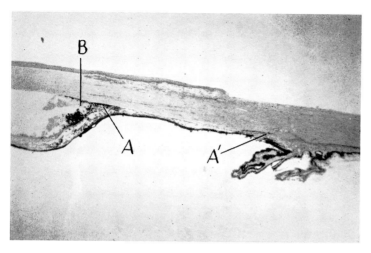

FIG. 7–65. Broad synechiae which may simulate a melanoma clinically. A 52-year-old woman was treated for glaucoma for two years. The eye was enucleated on suspicion of a melanoma of the iris. Section shows peripheral synechiae extending from A to A′, with atrophic iris stroma and intact pigment epithelium. Desquamated and hyperplastic pigment epithelium is seen in the angle at B.

FIG. 7–66. Xanthogranuloma of the iris (fibroxanthoma). A 5-month-old infant had a spontaneous hemorrhage in the anterior chamber. At 11 months, when the blood had absorbed, the lesion was noticed. The iris was darker (hemosiderosis) than that of the fellow eye.

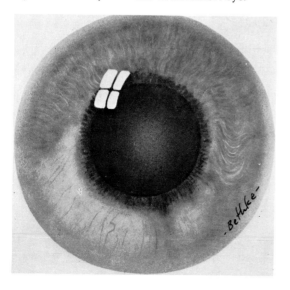

6. *Metastatic tumor of the iris.* In the few cases I have seen of this rare lesion, the metastatic focus was necrotic and gave rise to a severe iridocyclitis with secondary glaucoma. The metastatic focus may manifest itself before the primary focus.

7. *Malignant lymphoma.* This disease may appear as grayish-white, tumorlike mass in the iris and anterior chamber.

8. *Implantation cyst of the anterior or posterior chamber.* A history of trauma or previous surgery would ensure the correct diagnosis in these cases. In one unique case[199] an innocuous pigmented cyst in the angle of the anterior chamber, attached to the trabecular network, was mistaken for a malignant melanoma, leading to enucleation of the eye. The cyst appeared to have arisen from a villus of iridic pigment at the root of the iris.

9. *Congenital ocular melanocytosis.* See Congenital Melanoma.

10. *Leiomyoma.* See Chapter 9.

11. *Neurinoma.* See Chapter 6.

12. *Juvenile xanthogranuloma (nevoxanthoendothelioma, histiocytoma)* (Fig. 7–66). A juvenile xanthogranuloma may appear in the iris of infants 3 to 18 months old as a localized, yellowish-brown infiltration. It usually receives attention because of recurrent hyphema with or without glaucoma. If glaucoma develops, the condition may first be seen as a buphthalmos. Typical skin papules may be present, especially in the axilla.

13. *Encysted foreign body.* A more or less inert foreign body may penetrate the eye and rest in the iris or angle. If encapsulated by fibrous tissue, a localized mass may develop; the inflammatory reaction is sometimes negligible.

14. *Siderosis from a ferrous foreign body in the globe.* This condition is characterized by pigmentary and degenerative changes after a latent period of weeks to years. The extent of the changes varies with the size and chemical composition of the particle and also with its position in the eye (Fig. 7–67).

15. *Hemosiderosis from repeated intraocular hemorrhage.* Any condition that causes repeated hemorrhage in the anterior chamber may produce this heterochromia. One patient showed a pigmented retrocorneal membrane following occlusion of the central retinal vein.[162]

16. *Spontaneous semitransparent iris cyst.*[76] The clinical picture in all reported cases includes a slow-growing, semitransparent vesicle, pigmented or nonpigmented, usually localized in the pupillary area.

17. *Miscellaneous conditions.* These include aberrant lacrimal gland[24] and neurofibroma.

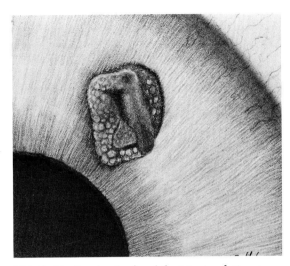

FIG. 7–67. Foreign body of the iris simulating a melanoma. A piece of steel, surrounded by siderosis, has become implanted on the anterior surface of the iris.

TREATMENT

Melanoma primary in the iris or the ciliary body so frequently involves the two structures that it seems practical to consider the treatment of both together. Five courses may be pursued in the treatment of iris–ciliary body melanomas:

1. *Temporization*—when there is no history of progression, the tumor shows no neovascularization and is not supplied by nutrient vessels.
2. *Basal iridectomy*—when the tumor appears to show growth but does not involve the angle. Neovascularization and nutrient vessels are usually evident.
3. *Enucleation*—when the tumor shows a diffuse, flat growth pattern, usually with evidence of desquamated tumor seeds on the iris and in the angle; when it shows a ring type of growth, usually accompanied by secondary glaucoma; and when it is too large for excision.
4. *Iridocyclectomy*—exploration with this procedure in mind when it is suspected or established that the tumor involves the ciliary body.
5. *Corneoscleroiridocyclectomy (goniectomy) with graft*—when the tumor involves the iris, ciliary body, and the angle.

Iridocyclectomy and corneoscleroiridocyclectomy will be discussed in a special section by Ira S. Jones.

Temporization

Since iris melanomas have a relatively low malignant potential and tend to grow slowly, observation is frequently the best course. Discrete pigmented iris lesions varying in size and elevation are relatively common and must often be observed for some time for evidence of malignant behavior. Many if not all malignant iris melanomas arise from benign lesions that are small and rather flat in the beginning but may achieve considerable size and elevation. In the absence of other clinical criteria of malignancy described previously, progression establishes the diagnosis.

According to our present knowledge of the behavior of iris melanomas, observation is the preferred course in some cases that would formerly have been treated surgically. This is particularly true of a localized tumor sufficiently far from the angle to be treated by iridectomy, instead of enucleation, if it should start to grow. The patient's age and life expectancy are factors to be considered in deciding on the best course of treatment for a given lesion, especially if enucleation of an eye with good vision is being considered.

Whether there is a special risk in continuing to observe iris melanomas in young women who are pregnant or in the child-bearing age is a question. Melanomas in general are believed to be occasionally activated by pregnancy.[17,132] Pregnancy seemed to affect the behavior of the lesion in three young women in our series. In one the melanoma gave rise to a hyphema; in another the lesion evident from childhood enlarged and then regressed but in a subsequent pregnancy grew rapidly and the eye had to be enucleated. In the third case a long-standing static melanoma of the iris enlarged and regressed during two pregnancies, but during the third grew so markedly that enucleation was required.

Puberty may also have an activating influence on melanomas. Four of our cases were in prepuberal children. One of them, 10 years of age when the tumor was discovered, was followed by the same observer during the next six years. Its clinical behavior then prompted an excisional biopsy. Histologic study indicated complete excision of a malignant melanoma.

Iridectomy

A patient at times becomes very apprehensive about a melanoma which he discovers or the ophthalmologist finds in a routine examination and keeps under continued observation. Regardless of whether the usual criteria for removal exist, excision by simple iridectomy may be indicated to relieve the patient's serious apprehension.

The object of excisional iridectomy is to remove the tumor entirely without causing tumor cells to disseminate in the eye or in the incision. To this end, the limbal incision must be large enough to permit removal of the lesion by basal iridectomy under direct observation. The following technique is recommended (Fig. 7–68). A conjunctival flap is dissected down to the limbus at the point where the tumor is located; pre- or postplaced sutures are inserted as in a cataract extraction. A small conjunctival flap is more easily manipulated. The anterior chamber is entered with a keratome, or by scratch incision, on one side of the lesion to avoid disturbing it. The incision should be as far back and as near the scleral spur as possible to avoid shelving of the cornea. This would con-

FIG. 7–68. Excision of a melanoma of the iris. **A.** A peripheral section is made with as little overhanging sclera as possible. The cornea is retracted by a traction suture to expose the tumor. Dotted lines indicate the two radial cuts to be made. Three sutures are preplaced. **B.** Traction is exerted centrally with forceps while radial cuts are made on each side of the tumor from the pupillary margin to the base of the iris. **C.** The freed portion of the iris containing the tumor is torn from its insertion in the ciliary body. **D.** The excised specimen is pinned flat on a wooden tongue depressor before fixation, to avoid distortion. The depressor should be saturated with saline or Ringer's solution or, preferably, covered with a rubber finger guard before pinning on the specimen.

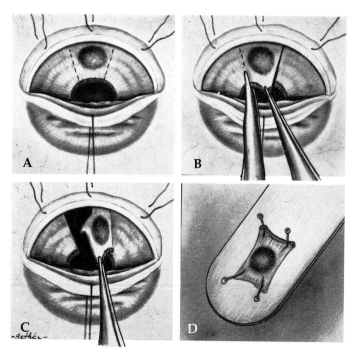

ceal the periphery of the iris, preventing an adequate view and increasing the difficulties of carrying out the basal iridectomy.

The section is enlarged on both sides of the lesion, somewhat less than a full 180° usually providing sufficient exposure. A silk traction suture placed through the corneal margin of the incision improves the view and allows wide separation of the wound lips when the tumor is withdrawn. Traction on the iris toward the pupillary area facilitates inspection of the iris peripheral to the tumor, to determine whether the ciliary body is involved.

The pupillary margin of the iris is grasped at one side of the tumor, and while traction is exerted centrally, a radial cut is made with scissors at the base of the iris. This cut is repeated on the opposite side of the tumor, and the included iris tissue containing the lesion is torn from its insertion into the ciliary body. The latter step can be successfully executed only if both radial cuts extend to the extreme periphery of the iris where it merges into the ciliary body; that is, the initial incision must be sufficiently far back to avoid a corneal shelf.

The excised iris and tumor tissue tends to curl and become distorted. Microscopic sections fixed from the specimen in such a state will be difficult to study, and indeed it may be impossible to determine whether the tumor has been completely removed (Fig. 7–69A).

Special care of the excised specimen helps the pathology laboratory, which in turn can obtain more accurate information for the surgeon. The specimen should be pinned carefully on the end of a tongue depressor prior to fixation. To prevent dehydration and shrinkage of a small specimen, the tongue depressor can be coated with a bland ointment, or the finger of a rubber glove can be slipped over it. This technique is suitable for radial sections showing the full extent of the excised iris and tumor (Fig. 7–69B).

Enucleation

Enucleation is indicated for the following types of tumors: those showing a diffuse flat growth pattern, usually with tumor seeds on the iris and in the angle; those showing a ring type of growth, usually involving the ciliary body and accompanied by secondary glaucoma; those invading the cornea; those with

FIG. 7–69. Excised melanoma of the iris. **A.** An iris tumor removed by iridectomy which was permitted to curl and become distorted before being placed in fixative. With such a specimen it is difficult to determine from microscopic sections the extent of the tumor and whether the excision is complete. **B.** In this section, handled as described in Figure 7–68, the relationship of iris and tumor tissue is clear, and the adequacy of the excision can be assessed.

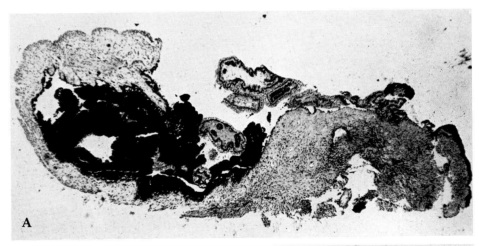

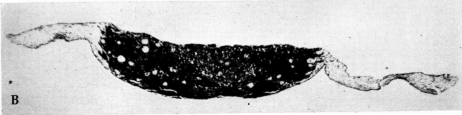

glaucoma present only in the involved eye; and those too large for excision.

Residual tumor tissue in the eye after iridectomy may be deduced from either microscopic or clinical evidence or both. Lacking histologic evidence that the tumor has been totally excised, the diagnosis of malignant melanoma itself is not sufficient grounds for enucleation unless there is clinical evidence of remaining tumor. In one series, there were apparently 11 such cases.[149] The pathologist should not be expected to bear the sole responsibility for this decision.

When, beginning about 1958 it was recognized that these iris-ciliary body melanomas seldom metastasize or seed, and that they are malignant only in the sense that they locally infiltrate, it became apparent that total excision should prove curative. Thus the interest in iridectomy, iridocyclectomy, and corneoscleroiridocyclectomy with graft.

Iridocyclectomy and Corneoscleroiridocyclectomy

IRA SNOW JONES

When the decision has been made that a growth involving the iris and ciliary body should be removed, and it has been judged small enough to remove by iridocyclectomy, careful planning by the surgeon becomes essential. An excellent review of iridocyclectomy[183a] covers the history and development of the various techniques.

Certain assumptions seem reasonable: first, that the scleral spur and adjacent sclera are involved when microscopic studies reveal numerous pigment cells, as is true in many cases; and second, that the tumor is usually larger than it appears to be clinically, so that surgery should be planned accordingly.

Preparation of the patient. Preoperative management may be the same as for a cataract extraction under general anesthesia except that the pupil is not dilated and greater attention is given to achieving low vitreous pressure.

Keeping the pupil contracted makes the limits of the tumor easier to define. Also, a greater portion of uninvolved iris may be spared, and sometimes a round pupil may be retained. In those cases where doubt exists as to whether the ciliary body is involved, the contracted pupil is an aid to easy inspection of the iris root since it puts the iris on a stretch.

Osmotic agents given before surgery lower the vitreous pressure and reduce the likelihood of vitreous loss when the ciliary body is separated from the base of the vitreous. Intravenous urea by the drip method is begun one hour before surgery, and general anesthesia should be used.

Choice of approach. The limbal incision with a perpendicular scleral cut (Fig. 7-70), referred to as the T incision, is chosen when no graft material is available or in the case of a slow-growing tumor. In a patient of advanced age, variations of the T incision may be elected to give greater exposure. These include two scleral perpendiculars, sometimes called the trapdoor (Fig. 7-71), and more than two, sometimes called the banana skin (Fig. 7-72).

By far the most satisfactory method for complete removal of these tumors is trephining and removing a corneoscleral button with the tumor attached. If, when centered, the posterior part of the button extends farther back than necessary, it may be altered by a chord cut across the posterior extension.

A refinement of the trephine technique consists in dissecting a half-thickness scleral flap and trephining in the uncovered thin bed. This may eliminate the necessity for a graft (Fig. 7-73).

Finally, in the rare instances when an attempt must be made to remove a large tumor, a strip or band may be outlined using curved lines concentric with the limbus and equidistant from each other (Fig. 7-74).

Of course, a suitable donor eye has to be available before the recipient eye is cut. The transplant must be identical in size and appearance with the removed button or strip.

Technique. A fornix-based flap should be used since it clears the operative field.

If a limbal incision is selected, it may be made to one side of the tumor site and enlarged with scissors. The *ab externo* incision is usually preferable to a keratome incision. The opening should be large enough to give good exposure.

At this point a gentle pull on the iris toward the pupil will serve to show whether the tumor is confined to the iris. If so, a simple excision with a margin of normal iris on all sides will suffice.

If the ciliary body must be exposed, a scleral perpendicular cut or cuts are made, the scleral spur is divided with a spatula, and the scleral flaps are folded back. The extent of ciliary body involvement is indicated by the darker color of the tumor compared with the normal tissue. A loupe or operating microscope is essential. If the exposure seems inadequate, the incision should be enlarged.

The next step is probably the most important one. On the opposite side of the globe a conjunctival and scleral incision is made over the pars plana and an 18-gauge needle introduced into the posterior part of the vitreous cavity. Vitreous (1.0 to 1.5 ml) is withdrawn and set aside.

Scissor cuts are then made around the iris part of the tumor. The tumor is lifted and dissected from the uninvolved portion of the ciliary body so that the specimen is removed in one piece.

Special caution should be used to avoid plunging the scissor point into the vitreous, which is stroked away from attachments to the specimen with cellulose sponges.

Diathermy applications may be made directly to the ciliary body if bleeding is a problem, but usually transscleral applications after closure will suffice.

Closure is made in a standard manner using absorbable sutures. Care should be taken to close the scleral incision snugly and accurately to prevent vitreous from inserting itself between the wound edges as intraocular pressure rises. Air is placed in the anterior chamber to hold back the vitreous. The flap is used to cover the entire closure.

The vitreous that earlier was set aside is now reintroduced through the needle opening into the vitreous cavity, taking care not to raise the vitreous pressure abnormally. Usually, all of the removed vitreous cannot be reintroduced. The needle hole is circled with diathermy applications.

The technique when a graft is to be used varies somewhat (Fig. 7–75A–D). The corneoscleral cuts are begun with a trephine and completed with scissors. The vitreous withdrawal is done. Using the corneoscleral button as a handle, the tumor is lifted up, iris cuts and ciliary body cuts are made, and the vitreous is stroked off as the tumor is delivered. It sometimes happens that a tumor will prove to be slightly larger than the exit hole and will mold itself to go through. The donor button, properly oriented, is then placed and sutured. Here again, numerous, accurate, snug sutures are indicated. The remainder of the procedure is as previously described.

Postoperative care. Because of the exposure of the vitreous to possible contamination, systemic antibiotics should be administered for three days after surgery. The patient is kept supine for 24 hours, and bed rest is required for the first week. These measures help to maintain the air in the anterior chamber.

Complications. Hypotony, either from ciliary body dysfunction or wound leakage, may account for some oozing of blood into the globe. This need cause little concern unless it invades the vitreous. Usually the hypotony is temporary, but occasionally it goes on to phthisis.

The graft may become opaque, but since it is not in the line of sight the effect is negligible.

The vitreous in contact with the wound may allow ingrowth of fibroblasts with late detachment of the retina.

I. S. Jones

PROGNOSIS

The low overall mortality in our series of 140 patients with iris melanoma on whom follow-up information was available agrees with reports by others. Four deaths due to metastatic spread are known to have occurred in this group (3% mortality). It is significant that no deaths occurred among patients for whom excisional iridectomy was the definitive therapy.

Analysis of the four fatal cases reveals that enucleation was ultimately performed. Microscopic examination showed spread of the tumor beyond the reach of local excision. Interestingly, three of the four patients had the diffuse type of melanoma in which treatment is likely to be delayed because of failure to recognize the true nature of the lesion. It cannot be definitely proved, of course, that surgical interference before enucleation in three of the four cases contributed to the fatal outcome. It seems obvious, however, that the surgeon should immediately resort to enucleation if there is clear-cut evidence that local excision will not remove the entire tumor.

An unusual reported case shows the unpredictability of these tumors.[95] A large melanoma involving the iris and ciliary body in an only remaining eye, diagnosed by many ophthalmologists as malignant, was followed over a 20-year period. The patient's medical history indicated that a smaller lesion had been present for at least 30 years before the observation period. The eye was obtained for sectioning after this patient's death from an unrelated disease, and the diagnosis of malignant melanoma was confirmed.

In a series of 105 cases of malignant melanoma of the iris,[6] no deaths occurred even after prolonged periods and despite extraocular extension at the time of enucleation, indicating that these tumors are for the most part locally invasive and rarely metastasize.

Four factors have been suggested as influencing the relatively good prognosis in cases of iris melanoma compared with similar lesions elsewhere in the uveal tract. Iris melanomas are detected earlier because of their location; their cell type appears to be less malignant; the collagen-cuffed iris vessels help to resist invasion; and the tumors may benefit from a growth-inhibiting factor in the aqueous humor.[96]

Investigators who studied 125 cases treated by iridectomy concluded that if an iris tumor was small enough to be removed by iridectomy, the prognosis was excellent, regardless of the histologic picture.[149] A tumor that was not excised completely might lead to

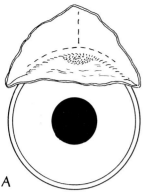
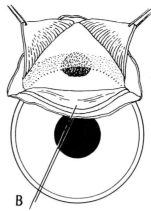

FIG. 7–70. **A.** Limbal incision with single perpendicular scleral cut. **B.** Exposure by folding back sclera.

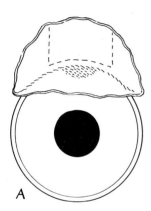
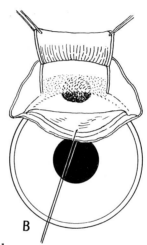

FIG. 7–71. **A.** Limbal incision and two scleral trapdoor cuts. **B.** Exposure by folding back trapdoor.

FIG. 7–72. **A.** Limbal incision and cuts making more than one scleral flap (banana skin). **B.** Exposure by folding back flaps.

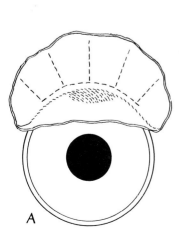
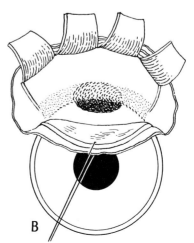

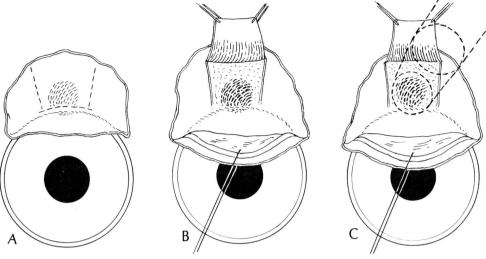

A   B   C

FIG. 7–73. Trephination under a half-thickness scleral flap. **A.** Outlined. **B.** Flap folded back. **C.** Trephine in the thin bed.

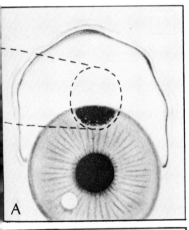

FIG. 7–74. Technique for outlining a corneoscleral band.

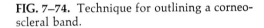

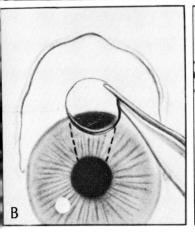

A

FIG. 7–75. A. In full-thickness corneoscleral trephination, the corneal part is perforated first. **B.** The trephine cut is completed with scissors, leaving the button attached to the underlying tumor. **C.** The button is lifted; iris and ciliary body cuts are made, and the vitreous is stroked free. **D.** The wound is closed with a corneal or corneoscleral matching button graft. (A. B. Reese et al.[142a])

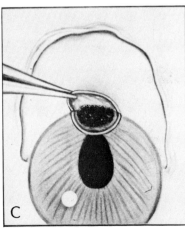

B   C

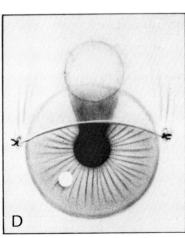

D

ultimate enucleation of the eye because of recurrence or secondary glaucoma. Even with such a delayed intraocular recurrence, however, the prognosis was relatively good as only 2 of the 6 patients in this group developed distant metastases. The prognosis for the diffuse type of malignant melanoma of the iris was poorer than for the usual localized type; among 67 cases, 4 patients died of metastases, 4 died without obvious metastases or recurrence; no data were available on 20; and 39 were living without tumor. The follow-up periods were as follows: 16 patients—0 to 5 years; 19 patients—5 to 10 years; 4 patients—10 to 15 years. As mentioned earlier, 3 of our 4 patients who died had the diffuse type.

MELANOMA OF THE SKIN AND MUCOUS MEMBRANE

Benign pigmented tumors of the conjunctiva and skin of the lids are generally called nevi (Fig. 7–76). Masson suggested that nevi of the skin and mucous membrane have a dual origin: superficial, from proliferation of the melanoblasts at the epidermal junction, and deep, from the schwannian elements of the dermal nerves. The nevi may increase in number and size with advancing years, but tend to gradually flatten and fade after middle age and to disappear entirely. Therefore, any new pigmented lesion developing in persons past middle age should be viewed with concern.

The triad of multiple-cell nevoid tumors, mandibular bone cysts, and skeletal abnormalities constitutes the basal-cell nevus syndrome.[115] Although ophthalmic abnormalities have been noted in over 30% of these patients,[13,71] they have seldom been described, as the entity is generally unfamiliar to ophthalmologists.[49]

It is often difficult to decide whether a nevus is junctional, compound, subepithelial, or the type referred to as juvenile melanoma. In general, a flat lesion is a junctional nevus with changes largely confined to the basal layer of epithelium. There may be some elevation due to accumulated nevus cells under the epithelium, in which case we are probably dealing with a compound lesion. A subepithelial nevus may be suspected if the growth is markedly elevated and the epithelium displays a papillomatous pattern. The pure junctional nevus present in youth is either con-

genital or appears early in life, often at puberty. In time, more and more nevus cells accumulate under the epithelium, and with advancing years the lesion tends to become compound or subepithelial.

In analyzing sections of over 100 conjunctival nevi and nevi of the skin of the lids, I found that 95% of both groups retained junctional activity.

Junctional changes may be acquired in adult life, in which case the condition will be referred to here as *precancerous melanosis*, a separate term that seems warranted in view of its distinctive clinical characteristics. The malignant phase is referred to as *cancerous melanosis*. Since all these tumors are assumed to arise from junctional changes in the basal layer, the types may be combined or merge one into another. In general, however, the following clinical entities are clear-cut: the nevus and the malignant melanoma arising from it, and the precancerous melanosis and the malignant melanoma or cancerous melanosis arising from it.

The incidence of malignant melanoma arising from a nevus of the conjunctiva or skin of the lids is considered to be higher than that of similar tumors elsewhere, which do not have as much junctional activity. Less than 25% of malignant melanomas of the skin arise from nevi, and skin nevi have only a 1:100,000 to 1:250,000 chance of becoming malignant.[174]

About one-fourth of conjunctival malignant melanomas arise from a preexisting congenital nevus, one-half from acquired precancerous melanosis, and one-fourth arise *de novo* or the origin cannot be identified. The last-named group is understandable since the malignant lesion can develop from a pure junctional nevus, a compound nevus, or a combination of the two, or may appear spontaneously without going through a precancerous stage.

A cholinesterase-positive, flesh-colored juvenile melanoma has been described which does not arise from the melanocytes at the epidermal-dermal junction but from Schwann's cells in the dermis.[195]

A divided nevus (kissing nevus) refers to the simultaneous occurrence of nevi on opposing sites of the upper and lower lids. The two nevi form a unit with the lids closed and are divided when the eye is open. In a series of 8 divided nevi, one became malignant following cosmetic surgery.[63] Ten cases were reported in Denmark, and the author had

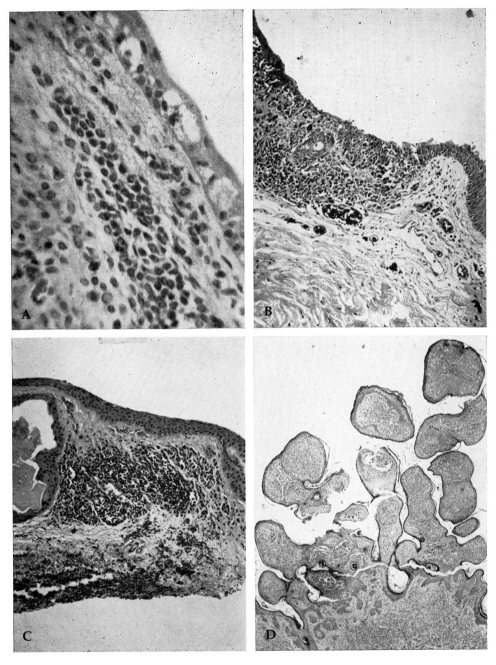

FIG. 7–76. Types of conjunctival nevi. A. Junctional nevus with a few nevus cells in the submucosal stroma. B. Compound nevus. C. Subepithelial nevus with normal-appearing conjunctiva covering the surface and a layer of connective tissue between the conjunctiva and the nest of nevus cells. At left, a conjunctival cyst and at right a downgrowth of conjunctiva. D. Papillary nevus of the skin of the lid. (Courtesy of the Armed Forces Institute of Pathology.)

noted only 25 in the world literature.[45] This lesion suggests that some nevi are formed at least by the fourth month of embryonic life, at which time the palpebral fissure separates.[174]

NEVUS

FREQUENCY

Nevus is the most common tumor of the conjunctiva, accounting for about one-third of tumors excised from this structure. The conjunctival nevus will be discussed since it most concerns the ophthalmologist; in general, what is said applies equally to nevi of the skin of the lid margin.

PATHOLOGY

Sections of 50 nevi from the conjunctiva, limbus, semilunar fold, and caruncle were examined microscopically. The following histologic features were identified: The tumor, though never encapsulated, was well localized and showed little tendency to infiltrate. In four-fifths of the cases it was in direct apposition to the overlying epithelium; in the others, there was a definite stromal layer between the tumor and the basal layer of the epithelium.

The nevus cells tended to assume a nestlike formation. The nucleus was characteristically round to oval, but occasionally polygonal or spindle-shaped. The chromatin was fine, rather densely and evenly distributed, and often contained a refractile vacuole. Sometimes there was a nucleolus. Mitoses were extremely rare. The protoplasm stained faintly with eosin, was usually somewhat granular, and the polyhedral cells had a limiting border to their protoplasm.

In about two-thirds of the cases, pigment could be demonstrated in the protoplasm of nevus cells, either with the usual hematoxylin and eosin stain or with a special silver stain. The pigment was frequently seen in the upper zone of the nevus where the cells were strongly dopa-positive. Passing downward, less and less melanin was encountered and the cells showed a correspondingly fainter dopa reaction until in the deepest layers none was usually obtained.

Pigment was also found in the stromal cells (histiocytes) disseminated throughout the tumor in about two-thirds of the cases. Four percent of the tumors were composed of long, branching, pigmented cells and were believed to be blue nevi.

The epithelium over the tumor manifested downgrowths or pseudoepitheliomatous changes in two-thirds of the cases. In at least half the cases these epithelial downgrowths formed multiple cysts, some of considerable size. The downgrowths might appear as isolated islands of epithelium; sometimes they were arranged in whorls or formed "pearls." A papillomatous formation is at times found in such tumors, particularly if the caruncle is involved. In half the lesions, the tumor cells extended into the overlying epithelium and partially or wholly replaced it. In about 20% of the cases, lymphocytes or plasma cells accumulated in the stroma under the tumor or were present in the tumor itself. In 10% of the cases, a stratum of degenerated connective tissue was seen in conjunction with hyalin formation and faint traces of calcium in the stroma under the tumor site.

Stages of transition from the basal layer of the epithelium to the nevus cells could be recognized in some nevi, particularly if they were flat and diffuse (junctional) and tended to invade and replace the overlying epithelium.

CLINICAL CHARACTERISTICS

A conjunctival nevus is most commonly seen at or near the limbus, especially in the interpalpebral region (Fig. 7–77, see p. 18). The growth may also involve the adjacent cornea, but even without a corneal extension it may, like any other limbal growth, produce secondary, superficial opacification of the adjacent cornea. One report described two cases of primary nevi of the cornea.[182] A lesion is at times situated on the lid margin (Fig. 7–78) and may involve the adjacent conjunctiva and skin (Fig. 7–79). The semilunar fold and caruncle are also common sites.

The nevus is characteristically elevated, sharply demarcated and pigmented. It may be any shape and varies in size from a mere speck to a large tumor that may include the skin, lid margin, semilunar fold and caruncle, as well as the palpebral and bulbar conjunctiva. Although its pigmented portion is obvious, an unpigmented flat area may be overlooked. Tumor tissue remaining after excision accounts for some so-called recurrences.

The lesion is usually light brown to jet black, but in about one-third of the cases it is salmon-colored. Lesions seen before puberty often show no dark pigmentation (Fig. 7–80, see p. 18). When small and flat such lightly pigmented lesions are inconspicuous. There may also be spotty pigmentation or dark pigmented cysts over a salmon-colored background (Fig. 7–81, see p. 19).

The lesion's pigment content may change rather rapidly at puberty or in adult life; some formerly nonpigmented lesions become pigmented, or partially pigmented tumors become increasingly pigmented. In the latter case, both the patient and the doctor can mistake the change for tumor growth. Pigment can apparently increase without any increase in tumor cells; invisible premelanin is converted into visible melanin. The pigment content of a nevus also tends to increase during pregnancy, when there is a malignant melanoma elsewhere, or from stimulation of the melanocyte-stimulating hormone (MSH) by ACTH.

The pigment content of a nevus may decrease, rather than the number of tumor cells, accounting for an apparent clinical regression. There is then no change in the size or volume of the lesion. On the other hand, the decrease in pigment may coincide with a diminution in the size and volume of the tumor and an actual reduction in the number of tumor cells. The nevus may, in fact, completely disappear, owing to spontaneous necrosis of the cells from an unknown cause (Fig. 7–82).

A subepithelial nevus lying in the deeper layers of the skin may appear blue.

Skin nevi containing hairs are subepithelial with no junctional activity and therefore with little or no growth potential (Fig. 7–83). Although such nevi are generally considered innocuous, malignant transformation has been reported.[41]

Nevi of the plica semilunaris and caruncle sometimes become pedunculated and protrude beyond the lid margin. Diffuse junctional nevi may be flat, mottled brown, and have an uneven undulating conjunctival surface. The presence of an active junctional component implies growth, particularly when the conjunctival cells are replaced by intraepithelial extension of tumor cells; the normal conjunctival luster is impaired and the surface has a dull, stippled appearance. In contrast, the conjunctiva over a nevus with no junctional activity looks normal.

Conjunctival nevi may be associated with multiple cysts. When the cysts are small,

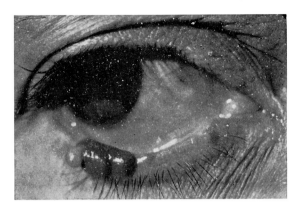

FIG. 7–78. Nevus of the lid. A darkly pigmented, elevated, sharply demarcated nevus of the lid margin, and a cyst at the temporal margin.

FIG. 7–79. Nevus of the upper and lower lids, face, and conjunctiva. The diffuse, flat, pigmented nevus involved the skin (A) as well as the bulbar conjunctiva (B).

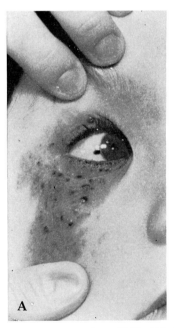

A

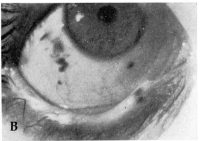

B

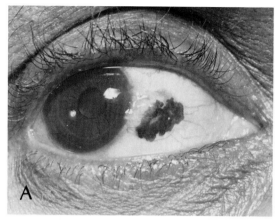

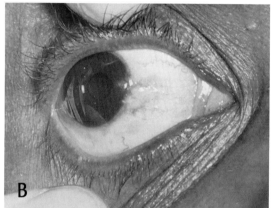

FIG. 7–82. Spontaneous regression of a conjunctival nevus. A 40-year-old black woman noted an increase in size of a dark spot first observed in the right eye six months earlier. **A.** Examination showed an elevated, sharply demarcated, jet-black lesion of the bulbar conjunctiva with a nonpigmented part extending to the limbus. Within seven weeks the tumor had regressed spontaneously to about one-fourth its former size. **B.** Three weeks later all pigment had disappeared, leaving a dull granular nonelevated site. **C.** After two months without change, a biopsy was taken from the site. Microscopic examination showed structureless, amorphous, degenerated tissue with no visible nuclei under the conjunctiva. Coagulation necrosis is seen at *a* and *b,* with calcium deposition in *a.* The necrosis was interpreted as a spontaneously regressed congenital nevus of the conjunctiva. (Courtesy of D. Tinkess.)

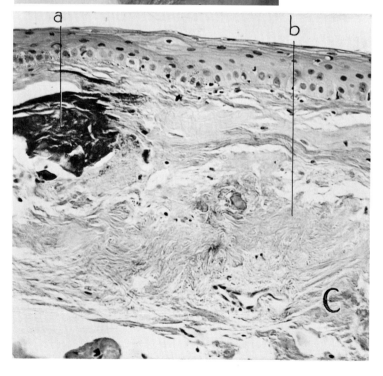

diffuse and numerous, the growth has a peculiar translucency which has led to the term *gelatinous nevus* (Fig. 7–84, see p. 19). The cysts can become large, multilocular and numerous, dominating and confusing the clinical picture.

Some nevi also manifest a papillomatous type of growth.

The growth of nevi seems commensurate with body growth during the first decade (Fig. 7–85), the pigment becoming prominent between the ages of 4 and 14, and particularly at puberty. In some instances the nevi are congenital and manifest pigment in infancy.

In the early years junctional and compound nevi prevail, and in the later years the subepithelial type predominates. The common so-called mole (each adult averages eight to ten over the body) is a subepithelial nevus with no junctional activity and therefore harmless. The exceptions are nevi on the soles of the feet, palms of the hands, and external genitalia of adults, a high percentage of which are junctional or compound with sufficient growth potential to warrant prophylactic excision. Nevi of the conjunctiva and skin of the lids, which also have a high incidence of junctional activity, are in the same category.

The natural history of nevi indicates a cyclic change from the active period (junctional changes) in youngsters, through the quiescent period in young adults, to the final stage of complete involution in older patients, as shown by the fact that patients over 50 have few or no nevi.

DIFFERENTIAL DIAGNOSIS

A nevus is usually easily diagnosed. When pigmented it may be confused with pigmented papilloma, early pigmented basal-cell epithelioma, or pigmented seborrheic papilloma. When nonpigmented, it may be confused with lymphoma, neurofibroma, fibroma, xanthoma, senile keratosis, papilloma, intraepithelial epithelioma (Bowen's disease), and histiocytoma (xanthogranuloma).

TREATMENT

Excision

The only treatment indicated for a nevus of the conjunctiva, skin of the lids or lid margins is excision. In my opinion, partial exci-

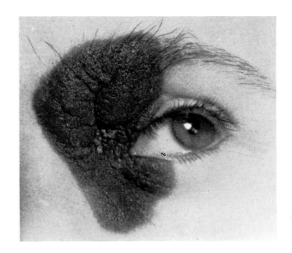

FIG. 7–83. Hairy nevus of the skin and lids. A jet-black, sharply demarcated, elevated nevus involving the lid margins and skin around the inner canthus.

FIG. 7–85. Enlargement of a nevus of the brow over a 33-month period. The increase in size is considered commensurate with growth and normal acquisition of pigment with age, rather than tumor activation. **A.** Age 3½ months. **B.** Age 2 years. **C.** Age 3 years.

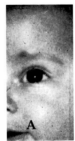 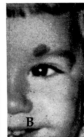 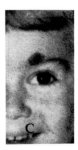

sion or biopsy of a nevus in no way predisposes to active growth. If the diagnosis is uncertain, tissue should be removed for microscopic examination.

Even though nevi seldom become malignant, conjunctival nevi and skin nevi around the eye are more likely to do so than similar lesions elsewhere. There is no reason for the patient to take any such risk when the lesion can be completely excised without jeopardizing the eye or its function. About 95% of conjunctival nevi and 90% of nevi of the skin and lid margin have junctional activity. Excision can be deferred until puberty or until it can be done under local anesthesia.

When there is doubt about the advisability of excision, because of the position of the lesion, it should be undertaken when the following conditions obtain:

1. Suspicion or indication that the nevus is enlarging and undergoing malignant transition as evidenced by neovascularization of the tumor and nutrient vessels coursing to it.
2. Location of the lesion where it is chronically irritated, particularly true of the caruncle, semilunar fold, and margin of the lower lid.
3. Inflammatory signs appearing spontaneously in or around the tumor.
4. Undue apprehension on the part of the patient or his family as to the potential seriousness of the lesion; simple excision may allay their anxiety.
5. Unsightly appearance of the lesion.

Conjunctival Nevus. Excision is usually a simple procedure (Fig. 7–86). A traction suture passed through the lesion obviates handling it with forceps and expedites the operation. If an appreciable amount of bulbar conjunctiva must be removed, it is helpful when closing the wound to pass a double-arm suture through the superficial scleral layers, and pass each arm through the conjunctival edges. Such anchorage in the sclera divides the pull on the conjunctiva necessary to complete the wound closure with interrupted sutures.

For a limbal tumor encroaching on the cornea (Fig. 7–87), the corneal portion must be included in the excision. This is facilitated by first performing a superficial lamellar keratectomy. The incision line can be made with a large trephine, which straddles the lesion at the appropriate distance from it, or the line can be outlined by a scalpel. When the proper depth in the cornea is reached by one of these means, the superficial lamellae, including the tumor, can be reflected as far as the limbus with a sharp spatula.

At the proper distance around the tumor, the bulbar conjunctiva is incised and dissected back, keeping as close as possible to the scleral surface as far as the limbus. The entire mass can then be freed by cutting with a cataract knife, first from one side and then from the other. Excision by transfixion with a cataract knife is preferable to excision with

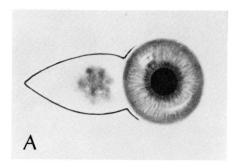

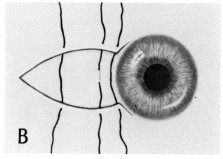

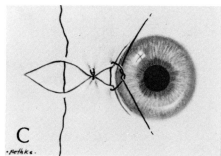

FIG. 7–86. Excision of a conjunctival tumor. **A.** Outline of the incision. **B.** Placement of sutures. The middle suture is anchored in the sclera. **C.** Tying of the anchored suture, with the other interrupted conjunctival sutures in place.

scissors. The denuded area is repaired as shown in Figure 7–86C.

When the nevus is flat and only partially pigmented, it may have nonpigmented extensions that are not readily discernible. The extent of the excision indicated may be difficult to estimate. The ultraviolet light (Wood or Hague light) is useful for the purpose. It outlines the tumor area as a dark zone even where there is no clinically visible pigment.

In the event of very extensive corneal involvement, the superficial lamellar keratectomy may be followed by a lamellar graft in the denuded corneal area. This is usually un-

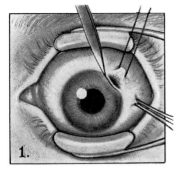
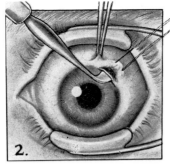
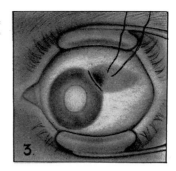
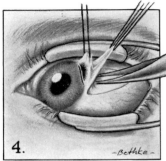
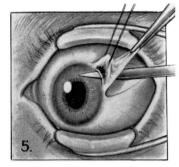

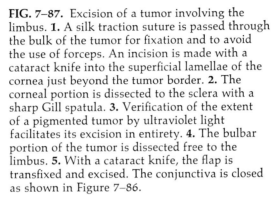

FIG. 7–87. Excision of a tumor involving the limbus. **1.** A silk traction suture is passed through the bulk of the tumor for fixation and to avoid the use of forceps. An incision is made with a cataract knife into the superficial lamellae of the cornea just beyond the tumor border. **2.** The corneal portion is dissected to the sclera with a sharp Gill spatula. **3.** Verification of the extent of a pigmented tumor by ultraviolet light facilitates its excision in entirety. **4.** The bulbar portion of the tumor is dissected free to the limbus. **5.** With a cataract knife, the flap is transfixed and excised. The conjunctiva is closed as shown in Figure 7–86.

necessary, as the denuded corneal area epithelializes with very little scarring.

As discussed earlier, there may be some melanosis of the epithelium adjacent to or in the vicinity of a nevus. Sometimes it is scattered over such a wide area that excision would seriously deplete the conjunctiva. When the lesion's nature is in doubt, a biopsy specimen should be taken from the sites in question before widespread excision is attempted. If there are junctional changes or indications of a precancerous melanosis, the pigmented area should be included in the excision.

Nevus of the Lid. A nevus of the lid margin may require a block excision and plastic repair similar to that required for an epithelioma of the lid margin.

Nevus of the Semilunar Fold and Caruncle. No special problems are encountered in excising a nevus in this area. There are usually no functional or cosmetic sequelae. Although the canaliculi should be avoided if possible, they can be sacrificed if necessary, particularly the upper one, without causing a disturbing epiphora. If the lower canaliculus must be excised, epiphora usually results but tends to become annoying only when the eye is irritated by wind, cold, or smoke.

Radiation

Nevi are radioresistant. Moreover, radiation can free some of the lesion's pigment in which case granules can be deposited in the underlying connective tissue. Observation of the deeply deposited pigment after excision may lead to the mistaken belief that the lesion has not been completely removed.

MALIGNANT MELANOMA OF NEVUS ORIGIN

When a nevus develops into a malignant tumor, it is a localized, elevated or even pedunculated, single or multiple tumor mass with varying amounts of pigment (Figs. 7–88, 7–89, see p. 19). Vascularization and large nutrient episcleral vessels coursing into the tumor are constant and important clinical features. Histologically, this malignant tumor is usually composed of large epithelioid cells with nucleolated nuclei (Fig. 7–89B, see p. 19).

Exenteration of the orbit is the treatment for malignant conjunctival melanoma arising from a nevus. Irradiation is not indicated, and enucleation is inadequate since it is necessary to remove a wide margin around the primary lesion as well as the conjunctiva and adjacent tissue. Some malignant melanomas of the limbal region have been treated by radical excision followed by a corneoscleral graft.[108]

Resection of the regional lymph nodes and lymphatics is indicated in most cases on the same grounds as for cases of cancerous melanosis.

PROGNOSIS

Series of cases of malignant conjunctival melanoma reported thus far yield too few data to draw conclusions as to the prognosis. The mortality rate is certainly high, however, perhaps comparable with that of some of the more malignant forms of skin melanoma. Almost all 1190 cases of malignant melanoma in one series involved the skin and mucous

FIG. 7–88. Malignant melanoma of the conjunctiva arising from a congenital nevus. The mass indents the adjacent sclera.

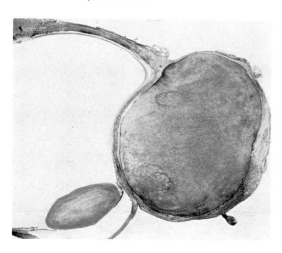

membrane.[133] There was an overall 21.4% five-year cure rate: 25.7% for the 47 ocular tumors and 18% for the 173 tumors of the head and neck. The cure rate was only 17% when definitive surgery was delayed more than one month after local excision, compared with 39.9% when such surgery was done immediately. According to another report, the mortality rate drops sharply after age 70, and the survival time is significantly longer for women than for men.[1]

PRECANCEROUS AND CANCEROUS MELANOSIS

Proliferation and pigment formation by the junctional melanocytes of the conjunctiva and skin normally stop during the second decade of life. The terms *precancerous* and *cancerous melanosis* refer to such proliferation and pigmentation occurring in adults. These tumors of the mucous membrane and skin have been variously designated as benign and malignant lentigo, senile freckle, lentigo melanosis, lentigo malin des vieillards, la mélanose circonscrite précancereuse, präecancerose Melänöse, extramammary pagetoid melanoma, intraepithelial melanoma, acquired junctional nevus, and superficial melanocarcinoma.

Precancerous and cancerous melanoses develop principally in mucous membranes. The conjunctiva of the eye is exposed while other mucous membranes are concealed, giving ophthalmologists an unusual opportunity to detect these tumors early and to follow their course under favorable conditions of examination.

The tumors are flat, produce no symptoms, and in the usual concealed mucous membrane can lurk undetected for an indefinite period of time. This last characteristic probably accounts for the fact that in a series of 337 cases of malignant melanoma studied histologically there was a mortality of 94% among the 50 patients whose lesions occurred in mucous membranes other than the conjunctiva.[1] These hidden symptomless tumors seem to account for the relatively common finding of metastatic melanoma with no demonstrable primary site.

Precancerous melanosis of mucous membranes appears subtly in middle age; it may remain essentially stationary, alternately progress and regress, disappear completely, or advance steadily over months or years to the cancerous phase. In rare instances the tumor progresses extensively, leading to the clinical suspicion that the cancerous phase has been reached, but it then regresses spontaneously. In one such case (Fig. 7–90) the bulbar conjunctiva and fornix became extensively involved. Another distinctive feature is progression not only at the original site but also at distal sites, with no clinical evidence of continuity between them.

The extent of the fluorescent melanin on the conjunctiva can be more fully appreciated when viewed by ultraviolet light, which reveals affected areas not seen with the usual light source (Fig. 7–91). Pigment changes on the facial skin in some patients with cancerous melanosis of the conjunctiva are revealed only by ultraviolet light, showing up as a mottled freckling.

Even a lesion that progresses to the cancerous stage tends to remain essentially a flat melanosis. However, there is usually some degree of thickening or a tumefaction at one or more sites, from which the biopsy should be taken. When biopsy material is taken merely from a melanotic site, the cytologic picture is usually nonmalignant. Since at least 90% of the tumor may consist of benign cells, it is important to obtain sections from the cancerous area.

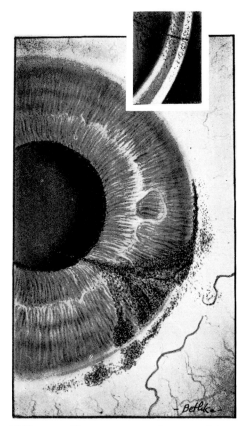

FIG. 7–90. Precancerous melanosis of the cornea and limbus. The tumor area in a 60-year-old woman regressed without treatment, although the bulbar conjunctiva and fornix had become extensively involved. Slit-lamp view (inset) shows location of the pigment in the epithelium.

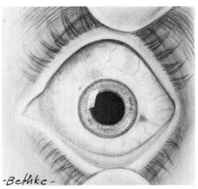

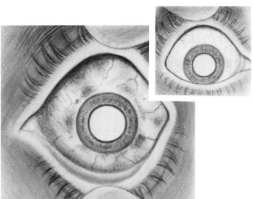

FIG. 7–91. Early precancerous melanosis of the conjunctiva. Above: Eye examined by usual illumination. Below: Ultraviolet light shows the extent of the tumor and (inset) appearance of the normal fellow eye. The white pupils represent fluorescence of the normal lens.

NATURE, FREQUENCY, AND CLINICAL COURSE

I believe that only half as many malignant melanomas arise from nevi as from precancerous melanosis. Malignant melanomas that seem to arise from normal conjunctiva (instead of from a known preexisting melanosis or nevus) often have the clinical and histologic picture of cancerous melanosis. They are therefore interpreted as instances of this lesion without the long transitional stage from precancerous to cancerous melanosis.

It is difficult to estimate the percentage of malignant melanomas of the conjunctiva that arise *de novo*, for several reasons:

1. About 10% of normal eyes have some localized melanosis of the conjunctiva, which the person rarely notices. I have usually interpreted such lesions as congenital melanoses, but some may be acquired. In any event, since many people are unaware of harboring melanosis, it is difficult to say that a malignant melanoma arises *de novo* rather than from an unrecognized preexisting melanosis or flat nonpigmented nevus.
2. A malignant melanoma of the conjunctiva may be of the cancerous melanosis type, presumably occurring without a transitional period from precancerous melanosis.
3. The ophthalmologist may have failed to question the patient specifically regarding a preexisting melanosis or nevus before histopathologic study of the biopsy material.

PATHOLOGY

The earliest changes, which seem to be the same as those we associate with a junctional nevus, appear in the cells of the basal layer (Fig. 7–92). These cells increase in number and become pigmented, swollen, hydropic, and separated from one another by clear spaces. The swelling gives a large protoplasmic element to the cells, which may be either clear or interspersed with pigment granules. Some cells show an enormous globular distention associated with degeneration of the nucleus, which stains poorly and looks granular. Several or many adjacent cells may become confluent, leaving clear spaces containing the degenerated products of the involved cells. The protoplasm of the less swollen cells may be finely granular or honeycombed like foam cells; the chromatin may be rarefied and the nucleolus rather large.

As the disease progresses it enters a transitional or active precancerous stage; the hydropic cells extend toward the free surface of the epithelium, show anaplastic tendencies, and occasionally incite an inflammatory cell infiltration. Cancerous melanosis is established when the cells penetrate the epithelium to its free surface and invade the subepithelial tissue. The cells may also invade regional lymph vessels (Fig. 7–93), nodes, and remote organs.

In some places these altered melanocytes in the basal layer proliferate to form a layer only two or three cells thick; in other places they segregate into clumps or nests that invade the submucosa. These nests may also invade the overlying mucosa (intraepithelial growth); here, by virtue of their pigment content or clear hydropic protoplasm, they contrast sharply with the normal mucosal cells (Fig. 7–94, see p. 20). Single heavily pigmented cells or lightly pigmented cells with clear protoplasm may be seen in the superficial layers of the mucosa, sharply demarcated from their surroundings.

In the usual flat areas of cancerous melanosis there may be hyperpigmented nodules with the benign cytologic characteristics of a melanocytoma.[46]

At some sites the altered melanocytes in the basal layer invade and entirely replace the overlying mucosa. Occasionally, small epithelial whorls with slight cyst formation may be seen beneath the mucosa. In the submucosa there are also cells containing phagocytosed pigment. Sometimes areas containing a considerable number of pigment-bearing phagocytes are seen beneath a relatively normal-appearing nonpigmented mucosa, beneath a thin atrophic mucosa, or at a site where there is little or no mucosa on the surface.

At the limit of the extension into the submucosa, there is frequently a chronic inflammatory reaction of plasma cells and other types of lymphocytes. In conformity with the diffuse nature of the lesion, these precancerous changes may appear over wide areas throughout the basal layer. As the tumor becomes increasingly malignant (Fig. 7–94B, see p. 20) the cells become more anaplastic and more difficult to identify.

Cancerous melanosis of the conjunctiva tends to be intraepithelial in its growth. It has

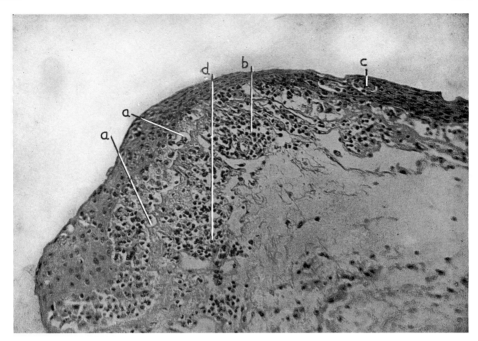

been referred to as intraepithelial melanoma and as a pagetoid form of melanocarcinoma.

In general this tumor infiltrates but does not metastasize in its early phase. Eventually, however, unless completely eradicated, it becomes aggressive and metastatic. Cancerous melanosis of the conjunctiva may extend into the globe.[72]

FIG. 7-92. Cancerous melanosis developing from precancerous melanosis. Section of the conjunctiva showing early stage of cancerous melanosis. The changes have occurred principally in the basal layer of the epithelium: (a) swelling and hydrops of the proliferated basal cells, (b) tumor invasion of the submucosa, (c) intraepithelial growth, and (d) mild lymphocytic infiltration.

DIAGNOSIS

Precancerous melanosis of the conjunctiva (Fig. 7–95) and adjacent skin of the lids manifests itself as a diffuse, nonelevated pigmentation with a granular appearance; sometimes the involved conjunctival surface shows a slight loss of luster. In the typical case, it first appears between the fourth and fifth decades, and malignant change does not occur for five to ten years, although this interval may be much longer or shorter. (In some instances the melanosis is malignant from the beginning.)

A most important characteristic of the lesion is its diffuseness. It may be so diffuse as to involve the entire conjunctiva (bulbar and palpebral) and adjacent skin, and may even terminate fatally by metastasis, without ever having formed an elevated tumor mass (Fig. 7–96, see p. 21). Malignant areas may appear at any site and often at many sites, either simultaneously or at irregular inter-

FIG. 7–93. Cancerous melanosis of the conjunctiva. Cells from the tumor mass (A) have spread to and engorged the adjacent lymphatics at a, b, and c. (A. B. Reese.[139])

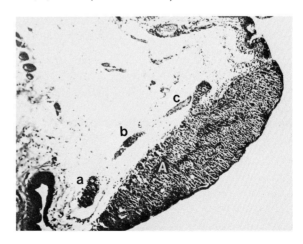

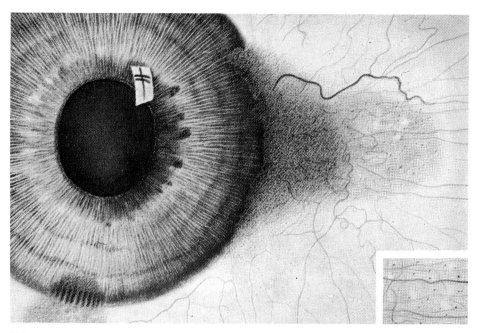

FIG. 7–95. Precancerous melanosis of the bulbar conjunctiva. **Inset:** High magnification of a section from the less pigmented portion of the temporal area reveals the pigmented dots that represent intraepithelial extensions from the basal layer into the overlying epithelium.

vals, usually remaining flat as in the precancerous stage, but at times becoming somewhat elevated. The extensive flat diffuse growth pattern of these tumors seems to be due largely to two factors: a) their tendency to invade the lymphatics and b) their multiple sites of origin—both of which are important considerations in the treatment.

Extensive involvement of the conjunctiva and skin distal to the site of origin, by multiple and seemingly independent foci, is probably due to spread by continuity or by emboli in the lymphatics or to independent areas of junctional activity.

Signs of inflammation may accompany the onset of malignant growth in an area of melanosis. One patient sought medical advice because the lesion was painful and inflamed. Another had a marked inflammation of the conjunctiva with a mucopurulent discharge.

The lesion may regress spontaneously in some areas while progressing in others (Fig. 7–97, see p. 21) or may regress until it has completely and permanently disappeared (Fig. 7–98).

A malignant melanoma of the conjunctiva arising from clinically unrecognized acquired melanosis has been described.[75] The diagnosis of this type of cancerous melanosis *sine pigmento* can usually be verified by employing ultraviolet light (Fig. 7–44, see p. 15) and then confirmed by biopsy.

SPONTANEOUS REGRESSION

The varied clinical course of these melanomas, sometimes to complete regression, suggests an autoimmune factor, although a glandular or a hormonal factor has also been considered. A patient with actively growing cancerous melanosis was reported to have been cured by the serum of a patient whose cancerous melanosis had undergone spontaneous regression.[177] In another case, a histologically confirmed cancerous melanosis treated with pituitary extract disappeared and had not recurred after eight months.[166a]

Hutchinson or Senile Freckle

The so-called Hutchinson or senile freckle (precancerous melanosis) occurs in exposed areas of the skin. It arises from the basal epithelium, grows slowly, and tends to become malignant although it is less aggressive than melanomas arising from a junctional nevus.[174] Histologically, the lesion shows diffuse involvement of the basal layer of the epithelium without invasion of the dermis.[20]

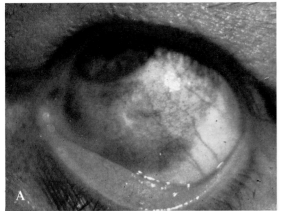
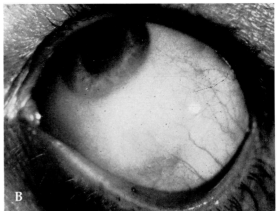
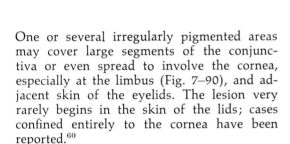

FIG. 7–98. Regression of precancerous melanosis following radiotherapy. **A.** Precancerous melanosis of the bulbar conjunctiva which had developed over a 2-year period in a woman 44 years of age. The diagnosis was established by biopsy. **B.** Complete disappearance of the lesion one and a half years after completion of the treatment. (Courtesy of A. Sherman.)

One or several irregularly pigmented areas may cover large segments of the conjunctiva or even spread to involve the cornea, especially at the limbus (Fig. 7–90), and adjacent skin of the eyelids. The lesion very rarely begins in the skin of the lids; cases confined entirely to the cornea have been reported.[60]

DIFFERENTIAL DIAGNOSIS

Nevus. The nevus is congenital, circumscribed, elevated, and often contains multiple small cysts. It rarely becomes malignant. If it does, the result is a localized, elevated or sometimes even pedunculated, single or multiple tumor mass. In both its benign and malignant phases it is radioresistant. A very flat diffuse nevus can simulate precancerous melanosis, especially when it is virtually nonpigmented and later acquires pigment. Such local or diffuse pigment may be observed in a nevus at puberty, during pregnancy, after exposure to ultraviolet light and ionizing radiation, and following ACTH therapy. If a lesion has been present throughout the patient's living memory, is somewhat elevated, shows microcysts, and has a rather undulating, irregular surface with normal luster, it could be reliably identified as a nevus.

In contrast, precancerous melanosis is acquired during middle age, is flat, diffuse, and has a dull, stippled surface without luster. In this stage and to a lesser extent in its cancerous stage, the melanosis may show clinical regression (Fig. 7–98).

Congenital melanosis. One type occurs in the conjunctiva and the other in the episclera under the conjunctiva:

1. The conjunctival type is localized, flat, brown to black, and usually adjacent to the limbus. Present from birth or shortly thereafter, it undergoes little or no change throughout life, and is due to pigment in the basal layer of an otherwise normal conjunctiva. The conjunctival basal layer adjacent to the limbus is a potentially pigment-bearing tissue; a diffuse form of this melanosis is normally seen in members of highly pigmented races.
2. The subconjunctival type is mottled, slate blue to black, and localized in the episclera. It is particularly marked in cases of complete or partial congenital ocular melanocytosis or in darkly pigmented individuals. It is most likely to be seen in the sclera between 10 and 1 o'clock and to a lesser extent between 4 and 8 o'clock, and to be concentrated at the site of an emissary of the anterior ciliary artery. When not too dense, it can be resolved with the slit lamp into branching, spider-shaped cells.

To my knowledge neither of these two types of congenital melanosis has ever led to malignant growth. They occur in about 10% of otherwise normal eyes. The subconjunctival type is closely related to the degree of pigmentation elsewhere over the body, the incidence being definitely higher in hyperpigmented individuals and races.

Congenital ocular melanocytosis. Both congenital conjunctival and episcleral melanoses are noted constantly as a feature of congenital ocular melanocytosis.

Ochronosis. Exogenous or endogenous ochronosis is characterized by the pigmentation of cartilage anywhere in the body, particularly noticeable in the ears and in tissues that have undergone arthritic changes. Dark urine may be a diagnostic sign. In a reported case, pigmentation in the sclera of a patient's only eye because of ochronosis was erroneously diagnosed as a malignant melanoma leading to enucleation.[168]

Subconjunctival extension of an intraocular benign melanoma. A benign congenital melanoma of the ciliary body may extend through an emissary of the anterior ciliary artery and appear as a pigmented lesion under the conjunctiva.

Acanthosis nigricans. This diffuse pigmentation of the skin and mucous membranes is caused by release of the pituitary melanocyte-stimulating hormone (MSH) due to adrenal cortical deficiency (Addison's disease). Since it sometimes affects the conjunctiva, cornea, and skin of the lids, differentiation from a neoplastic type of melanosis may be required. The lesion is occasionally a sign of a fatal carcinoma of the adrenal gland.

Pigmentation from mascara. Symmetrical and bilateral punctate pigmentation of the palpebral conjunctiva from mascara, when very marked, may bear some resemblance to precancerous melanosis.[137]

Miscellaneous conditions. The sudden appearance of an abnormal amount and distribution of melanotic pigment in rare cases indicates a systemic disease such as arsenical intoxication, Addison's disease, and hemochromatosis. In hemochromatosis, pigmentation of the conjunctiva or lid margin was found in 13 of 44 patients.[38] This pigmentation was noted in 3 of 5 untreated patients with secondary hemochromatosis. On the other hand, only 8 of 37 patients who had previously completed venesection therapy showed pigmentation. Histopathologic examination of three eyes removed at autopsy revealed iron within the corneal epithelium and in the ciliary body—the first time this has been recorded.

The use of epinephrine in the conjunctiva may result in black dots which, when abundant, resemble early precancerous melanosis.

After excision of a melanoma of the conjunctiva, extensive cauterization of the sclera is sometimes carried out for bleeding and possible occult tumor sites. The resulting eschar may leave black spots over the sclera which later can be confused with residual or recurrent tumor.

TREATMENT

Ophthalmologists, reluctant to treat cancerous melanosis of the conjunctiva in its early and symptomless stage by adequate surgery, have too often carried out several local excisions over six to ten years or even longer. When total exenteration is finally done, it may be too late to expect a cure. To be sure, it takes courage to recommend a mutilating operation in such cases, even though it may be lifesaving.

Total Conjunctivectomy

It seems advisable to treat some cases of cancerous melanosis of the conjunctiva by total conjunctivectomy. This procedure consists of halving the entire upper and lower lids, beginning with an incision through the lid margin at the gray line. Each lid is divided with scissors into an anterior and a posterior half. The anterior half includes the cilia, skin, and orbicularis muscle; the posterior half includes the tarsus, the conjunctiva, and its substantia propria. In the upper and lower fornices where exposure is difficult, the dissection can be facilitated by traction sutures. After all the conjunctiva and substantia propria have been removed, the lids are sutured together over the cornea. In some cases a half-thickness mucous membrane graft has replaced the excised conjunctiva.

In-continuity lymphatic resection, which is in the province of the head and neck surgeon, is usually performed two weeks after the total conjunctivectomy. This procedure involves excision of the lymphatic channels, the regional lymph nodes, and part of the parotid gland, in an effort to remove any tumor cells in the nodes or in transit via the lymphatics. From 30 to 40 nodes are usually removed for microscopic study.

In cases of cancerous melanosis, lymphatic and nodal resection should be done with either local excision or exenteration.[35] Histologic sections of specimens show frequent extension of the tumor into the lymphatics, which is clinically evident from the appearance of tumor sites far from the primary lesion. Of 11 patients with cancerous melanosis of the conjunctiva who had lymphatic and nodal resection, 2 showed node metastasis. In one of them, 1 of 54 nodes was positive for cancer cells and in the other, 3 of 49 nodes. Although the pathology report was negative for the other 9 patients, the known false negative rate in such conditions is about 30%, suggesting that perhaps 3 of the 9 had positive nodes that were not detected by the pathologist. Three of the 11 patients with a negative report have had local recurrences. If a patient dies of distant metastasis but the local area is negative for cancer cells, surgery did all that could be expected, as the disease had already passed beyond the surgical field. On the contrary, local recurrence means inadequate local excision.

When patients with clinically negative nodes have had in-continuity node dissection, histologically positive nodes were found in 40% of the cases.[100] Among eight of our patients with cancerous melanosis who had total conjunctivectomy and lymphatic resection, two had unsuspected positive nodes.[35] It is generally agreed that node dissection after the involvement is clinically apparent is of little value, and that the cure rate is higher in patients who have had in-continuity dissection of clinically uninvolved nodes combined with wide local excision of the lesion.[34]

Discontinuous dissection of the nodes sometimes replaces in-continuity dissection.

Regional perfusion using radioactive isotopes is at times an adjunct to surgical excision and node dissection.[5]

Conjunctivectomy is advised only when the biopsy material unequivocally indicates cancer, never on clinical evidence alone even if the melanosis has progressed extensively. Because of the usual long period between melanosis and a confirmed diagnosis of cancer, wide excision of a localized cancerous tumefaction seems logical in some elderly patients; the diffuse areas of melanosis are left alone or treated with radiation.

The recommended treatment for cancerous melanosis of the skin is local excision of the primary lesion with a wide margin of normal-appearing skin, combined sometimes with in-continuity resection of lymphatics and regional lymph nodes even though there is no clinical evidence that they are involved in the disease process.

PROGNOSIS

In a series of 62 cases classified as cancerous melanosis, we could follow 36 for five years or more; there was microscopic confirmation in 32 patients, of whom 13 died of metastasis.[138] This 40% mortality rate is undoubtedly low for a number of reasons. The interval between recognition and outcome averaged 12 years, ranging from 3 to 25 years. Because of this long period of waxing and waning, patients were frequently lost to follow-up. Also, in any such group there are multiple recurrences with repeated local excisions, suspected metastases where the outcome is unknown, and deaths of undetermined cause.

It is very difficult, for obvious reasons, to quote meaningful figures on the incidence and prognosis of precancerous melanosis that progresses to cancerous melanosis. However, in our series of patients followed five years, we found a 17% incidence.

IMMUNOLOGIC ASPECTS OF OCULAR NEOPLASMS

It has long been known that tumor-associated antigens exist in patients with ocular tumors, and that these patients have immune reactions to them. Much promising work has been reported[26a] in cases of ocular melanoma, as well as retinoblastoma, resulting sometimes in determining the diagnosis and predicting the prognosis. The author notes that this assay is in the experimental stage and that follow-ups are not long enough to determine prognostic value. He points out that ocular melanoma is the best model in which to study immunotherapy because the associated antigens and immunologic response have been demonstrated, clinical monitoring of tumor growth is relatively easy, and at the time of enucleation the amount of tumor remaining in the body is low. However, he emphasizes the paucity of controlled studies, and estimates that it will take a large number of patients studied over a period of 5 years to determine the value of immunotherapy in ocular neoplasms.

REFERENCES

1. ALLEN AC, SPITZ S: Malignant melanoma; a clinicopathological analysis of the criteria for diagnosis and prognosis. Cancer 6:1–45, 1953

2. ANDERSON B, O'NEILL J: Malignant melanoma of the uvea; observations based on growth and behavior, enucleation refused or delayed. Arch Ophthalmol 58:337–347, 1957

3. ANDERSON DE, SMITH JL JR, McBRIDE CM: Hereditary aspects of malignant melanoma. JAMA 200:741–746, 1967

4. APT L: Uveal melanomas in children and adolescents. Int Ophthalmol Clin 2:402–410, 1962

5. ARIEL IM, OROPEZA R, PACK GT: Intracavitary administration of radioactive isotopes in the control of effusions due to cancer; results in 267 patients. Cancer 19:1096–1102, 1966

6. ASHTON N: Primary tumours of the iris. Br J Opthalmol 48:650–668, 1964

7. ASHTON N, WYBAR K: Primary tumours of the iris. Ophthalmologica 151:97–113, 1966

8. BAGHDASSARIAN SA, SPENCER WH: Pseudoangioma of the iris; its association with melanoma. Arch Ophthalmol 82:69–71, 1969

9. BAIR HL, LOVE JG: Acoustic neurofibroma associated with melanoepithelioma of the choroid: successful removal of both tumors. Mayo Clin Proc 12:481–485, 1937

10. BECKER SW JR, FITZPATRICK TB, MONTGOMERY H: Human melanogenesis: cytology and histology of pigment cells (melanodendrocytes). Arch Dermatol Syphilol 65:511–523, 1952

11. BEIERWALTES WH, LIEBERMAN LM, VARMA VM, COUNSELL RE: Visualizing human malignant melanoma and metastases: use of chloroquine analog tagged with iodine 125. JAMA 206:92–102, 1968

12. BERKOW JW, FONT RL: Disciform macular degeneration with subpigment epithelial hematoma. Arch Ophthalmol 82:51–56, 1969

13. BERLIN NI, VAN SCOTT EJ, CLENDENNING WE, ARCHARD HO, BLOCK JB, WITKOP CJ, HAYNES HA: Basal cell nevus syndrome. Ann Intern Med 64:403–421, 1966

14. BERLINGER W: Ein Beitrag zur epithelialen Genese des Melanins. Arch Pathol Anat 219:328–365, 1915

15. BERSON E, BIGGER JF, SMITH ME: Malignant melanoma, retinal hole, and retinal detachment. Arch Ophthalmol 77:223–225, 1967

16. BETTMAN JW, FELLOWS V: Differential diagnosis of dark lesions of the posterior fundus. Trans Pac Coast Otoophthalmol Soc 36:87–97, 1955

17. BIRD BF JR, McGANITY WJ: The effect of pregnancy on the clinical course of malignant melanoma. South Med J 47:196–200, 1954

18. BJÖRNEBOE M: Primäres Melanosarkom des Gehirns, massenhafte Naevi pigmentosi der Haut: ausgedehnte Neurofibromatose der Hautnerven. Frankfurt Z Pathol 46:363–373, 1934

19. BLODI FC: Personal communication

20. BLODI FC, WIDNER RR: The melanotic freckle (Hutchinson) of the lids. Survey Ophthalmol 13:23–30, 1968

21. BÖKE W, AZARBAYDJANI M: Retrobulbar diaphanoscopy in the diagnosis of choroidal tumors. Klin Monatsbl Augenheilkd 144:815–828, 1964

22. BOWEN SF JR, BRADY H, JONES VL: Malignant melanoma of eye occurring in two successive generations. Arch Ophthalmol 71:805–806, 1964

23. BROWNING CW, SWAN KC: Experiences with some tumors of the iris. Trans Pac Coast Otoophthalmol Soc 29:107–132, 1948

24. BRUCE GM: Aberrant glandular tissue in the iris. Trans Am Acad Ophthalmol Otolaryngol 56:47–51, 1952

25. CAMPBELL CJ: Personal communication

26. CAPPIN JM: Malignant melanoma and rubeosis iridis; histopathological and statistical study. Br J Ophthalmol 57:815–824, 1973

26a. CHAR DH: Immunologic aspects of intraocular neoplasms. In Peyman GA, Apple DJ, Sanders BR (eds): Symposium on Ocular Tumors. New York, Appleton, Century, Crofts, 1976 (in press)

27. CHAR DH, HOLLINSHEAD A, COGAN DG, BALLINTINE EJ, HOGAN MJ, HERBERMAN RG: Cutaneous delayed hypersensitivity reactions to soluble melanoma antigen in patients with ocular malignant melanoma. New Eng J Med 291:274–277, 1974

28. CHRISTENSEN L, ROWEN GE: Diagnosis of malignant melanoma by subretinal fluid studies. Arch Ophthalmol 54:477–480, 1955

29. CIBIS P: Ueber die subretinale Flüssigkeit bei Melanosarkom der Aderhaut (the subretinal fluid in melanosarcoma). Klin Monatsbl Augenheilkd 104:424–433, 1940

30. CLEASBY GW: Malignant melanoma of the iris. Arch Ophthalmol 60:403–417, 1958

31. COGAN DG, REESE AB: A syndrome of iris nodules; ectopic Descemet's membrane and unilateral glaucoma. Doc Ophthalmol 26:424–433, 1969

32. COLENBRANDER MC: Mathematical diffusion of choroidal sarcoma infiltration. Ned Tijdschr Geneeskd 96:1235–1237, 1952

33. CONDON RA, MULLANEY J: Multiple malignant melanomata of the uveal tract in one eye. Br J Ophthalmol 51:707–711, 1967

34. CONWAY H, HUGO NE, McKINNEY P: Excision of glands in continuity for malignant melanoma; review of end results following several techniques. Arch Surg 94:129–133, 1967

35. COSMAN B: Personal communication

36. DAVENPORT RC: A family history of choroidal sarcoma. Br J Ophthalmol 11:443–445, 1927

37. DAVIDORF FH, LANG JR: The natural history of malignant melanoma: small vs large tumors. Trans Am Acad Ophthalmol Otolaryngol 79:310–320, 1975

38. DAVIES G, DYMOCK I, HARRY J, WILLIAMS R: Deposition of melanin and iron in ocular structures in haemochromatosis. Br J Ophthalmol 56:338–342, 1972

39. DEUTSCH S, MESCON H: Melanin pigmentation and its endocrine control. New Eng J Med 257:222–226, 1957

40. DeVEER JA: Juxtapapillary malignant melanoma of the choroid and so-called malignant melanoma of the optic disc. Arch Ophthalmol 51:147–160, 1954

41. DOBSON L: Prepubertal malignant melanomas. Am J Surg 89:1128–1135, 1955

42. DUKE JR, DUNN SN: Primary tumors of the iris. Arch Ophthalmol 59:204–214, 1958

43. DUNPHY EB, FORREST AW, LEOPOLD IH, REESE AB, ZIMMERMAN LE: Symposium on the diagnosis and management of intraocular melanomas. Trans Am Acad Ophthalmol Otolaryngol 62: 517–555, 1958

44. EASOM HA: Sympathetic ophthalmia associated with malignant melanoma. Arch Ophthalmol 70:786–790, 1963

45. EHLERS N: Divided nevus. Acta Ophthalmol (Kbh) 47:1004–1011, 1969

46. ELSAS FJ, GREEN WR, RYAN SJ: Benign pigmented tumors arising in acquired conjunctival melanosis. Am J Ophthalmol 78:229–232, 1974

47. ENGLE HC: Cancer cells in the circulating blood. Acta Chir Scand (Suppl) 201, 1955

48. EWING J: Personal communication

49. FEMAN SS, APT L, ROTH AM: The basal cell nevus syndrome. Am J Ophthalmol 78:222–228, 1974

50. FENSKE HD, BURR SP: A lethal iris melanoma in a child. Survey Ophthalmol 9:1–4, 1964

51. FERRY AP: Lesions mistaken for malignant melanoma of the posterior uvea. Arch Ophthalmol 72:463–469, 1964

52. FERRY AP: Lesions mistaken for malignant melanoma of the iris. Arch Ophthalmol 74:9–18, 1965

53. FITZPATRICK TB: Human melanogenesis. Arch Dermatol Syphilol 65:379–391, 1952

54. FITZPATRICK TB, SEIJI M, McGUGAN AD: Melanin pigmentation. New Eng J Med 265:374–378, 1961

55. FLOCKS M, GERENDE JH, ZIMMERMAN LE: The size and shape of malignant melanomas of the choroid and ciliary body in relation to prognosis and histologic characteristics: a statistical study of 210 tumors. Trans Am Acad Ophthalmol Otolaryngol 59:740–758, 1955

56. FONT RL,, SPAULDING AG, ZIMMERMAN LE: Diffuse malignant melanoma of the uveal tract; a clinicopathologic report of 54 cases. Trans Am Acad Ophthalmol Otolaryngol 72:877–895, 1968

57. FONT RL, ZIMMERMAN LE, ARMALY MF: The nature of the orange pigment over a choroidal melanoma; histochemical and electron microscopical observations. Arch Ophthalmol 91:359–362, 1974

58. FOOS RY, HULL SN, STRAATSMA BR: Early diagnosis of ciliary body melanomas. Arch Ophthalmol 81:336–344, 1969

59. FOSTER J, HENDERSON W, COWIE JW, HARRIMAN DSF: Choroidal sarcoma with a metastasis in the opposite orbit. Br J Ophthalmol 41:42–47, 1957

60. FRANÇOIS J, GILDEMYN H, RABAEY M: Melanose cancereuse de la cornée. Ann Ocul 189:496–504, 1956

61. FRENKEL M, KLEIN HZ: Malignant melanoma of the choroid in pregnancy. Am J Ophthalmol 62: 910–913, 1966

62. FUCHS A: Zur Klinischen Bedeutung der umschriebenen Netzhautabhebung an der Ora serrata bei beginnendem Aderhautsarkom. Klin Monatsbl Augenheilkd 98:606–617, 1937

63. FUCHS A: Divided nevi of the lids. Urol Cutan Rev 54:88–90, 1950

64. GAIPA M: The Papanicolaou method in the diagnosis of tumors of the eye and adnexa. Boll Ocul 35:491–502, 1956

65. GANLEY JP, COMSTOCK GW: Benign nevi and malignant melanomas of the choroid. Am J Ophthalmol 76:19–25, 1973

66. GARTNER S: Malignant melanoma of the choroid in von Recklinghausen's disease. Am J Ophthalmol 23:73–78, 1940

67. GASS JD: An unusual hamartoma of the pigment epithelium and retina simulating choroidal melanoma and retinoblastoma. Trans Am Ophthalmol Soc 71:171–185, 1973

68. GASS JDM: Iris abscess simulating malignant melanoma. Arch Ophthalmol 90:300–302, 1973

68a. GASS JDM: Differential diagnosis of intraocular tumors. St. Louis, CV Mosby, 1974, p. 30

69. GOLDSTEIN I, WEXLER D: Melanosis uveae and melanoma of the iris in neurofibromatosis (Recklinghausen). Arch Ophthalmol 3:288–296, 1930

70. GORDON M: Pigment-Cell Growth. New York, Academic Press, 1953

71. GORLIN RJ, VICKERS RA, KELLEN E, WILLIAMSON JJ: Multiple basal cell nevi syndrome; an analysis of a syndrome consisting of multiple nevoid basal-cell carcinoma, jaw cysts, skeletal anomalies, medulloblastoma and hyporesponsiveness to parathormone. Cancer 18:89–104, 1965

72. GOW JA, SPENCER WH: Intraocular extension of an epibulbar malignant melanoma. Arch Ophthalmol 90:57–59, 1973

73. GREER CH: Congenital melanoma of the anterior uvea. Arch Ophthalmol 76:77–78, 1966

74. GREEVES RA: Choroidal sarcoma at the macula. Trans Ophthalmol Soc UK 61:123–127, 1941

75. GRIFFITH WR, GREEN WR, WEINSTEIN GW: Conjunctival malignant melanoma originating in acquired melanosis sine pigmento. Am J Ophthalmol 72:595–599, 1971

76. GUERRY D III, WIESINGER H: Spontaneous cyst of iris. Am J Ophthalmol 44:106–107, 1957

77. GUIBOR P, KEENEY AH: Thermography and ophthalmology. Trans Am Assoc Ophthalmol Otolaryngol 74:1032–1043, 1970

78. HAGLER WS, JARRETT WH II, HUMPHREY WT: The radioactive phosphorus uptake test in diagnosis of uveal melanoma. Arch Ophthalmol 83:548–557, 1970

79. HALLDEN U: Malignant melanoma of the choroid clinically simulating scleritis attended by amotio retinae. Acta Ophthalmol (Kbh) 33:489–491, 1955

80. HAMBURG A: Iris melanoma with vascular proliferation simulating a hemangioma. Arch Ophthalmol 82:72–76, 1969

81. HENKIND P, ROTH MS: Breast carcinoma and concurrent uveal melanoma. Am J Ophthalmol (Suppl) 71:198–203, 1971

82. HOFMANN K: Synthesis of melanocyte-stimulating hormone derivatives. Ann NY Acad Sci 8:689–707, 1960

83. HORODEŃSKI J: Investigations on the presence of free cells of malignant melanoma of the uvea in peripheral blood. Klin Oczna 39:407–412, 1969

84. HÖRVEN I: Dynamic tonometry and choroidal melanoma: a new diagnostic approach. Arch Ophthalmol 82:440–445, 1969

85. ITO M: Genesis of Mongolian spot and blue nevus. Part V in Studies on Melanin. Tohoku J Exp Med (Suppl) 55:21–39, 1952

86. IWAMOTO T, REESE AB, MUND ML: Tapioca melanoma of the iris. 2. Electron microscopy of the melanoma cells compared with normal iris melanocytes. Am J Ophthalmol 74:851–861, 1972

87. JACKSON R, WILLIAMSON GS, BEATTIE WG: Lentigo maligna and malignant melanoma. Can Med Assoc J 95:846, 1966

88. JENDRALSKI F: Der Naevus conjunctivae ein Progonoblastom. Arch Pathol Anat 233:226–234, 1921

89. KALIL RF: Personal communication

90. KENNEDY RE: Cystic malignant melanomas of the uveal tract. Am J Ophthalmol 31:159–167, 1948

91. KERNEN JA, ACKERMAN LV: Spindle-cell nevi and epithelioid-cell nevi (so-called juvenile melanomas) in children and adults. Cancer 13:612–625, 1960

92. KIRK HO, PETTY RW: Malignant melanoma of the choroid: a correlation of clinical and histological findings. Arch Ophthalmol 56:843–860, 1956

93. KLIEN BA: The ciliary margin of the dilator muscle of the pupil with reference to some melanomas of the iris of epithelial origin. Arch Ophthalmol 15:985–993, 1936

94. KLIEN BA: Detachment of pars ciliaris retinae (a contribution to the diagnosis of malignant intraocular tumors). Arch Ophthalmol 26:347–357, 1941

95. KOENIG IJ: Malignant melanoma of the iris and ciliary body of a one-eyed patient. Arch Ophthalmol 51:656–662, 1954

96. KORNBLUETH W, TENENBAUM E: The inhibitory effect of aqueous humor on the growth of cells in tissue culture. Am J Ophthalmol 42:70–80, 1956

97. KURZ GH: Melanocytoma of the anterior uvea; an unusual tumor associated with buphthalmos. Survey Ophthalmol 8:511–517, 1963

98. LAIDLAW GF, MURRAY MR: A theory of pigmented moles; their relation to the evolution of hair follicles. Am J Pathol 9:827–838, 1933

99. LANE LA: Discussion in Stieren E: Sarcoma of the uveal tract following trauma. Arch Ophthalmol 12:980–982, 1934

100. LANE N, LATTES R, MALM J: Clinicopathological correlations in a series of 117 malignant melanomas of the skin of adults. Cancer 11:1025–1043, 1958

101. LAWSON R: Implications of surface temperatures in the diagnosis of breast cancer. Can Med Assoc J 75:309–310, 1956

102. LEHMAN JA, CROSS FS, RICHEY WG: Clinical study of forty-nine patients with malignant melanoma. Cancer 19:611–618, 1966

103. LERNER AB: Melanin pigmentation. Am J Med 19:902–924, 1955

104. LERNER AB, FITZPATRICK TB: Biochemistry of melanin formation. Physiol Rev 30:91–126, 1950

105. LERNER AB, McGUIRE JS: Effect of alpha- and beta-melanocyte stimulating hormones on the skin colour of man. Nature (Lond) 189:176–179, 1961

106. LERNER HA: Malignant melanoma of the iris in children; a report of a case in a 9-year-old girl. Arch Ophthalmol 84:754–757, 1970

107. LEWIS MG, IKONOPISOV RL, NAIRN RC, PHILLIPS TM, FAIRLEY GH, BODENHAM DC, ALEXANDER P: Tumour-specific antibodies in human malignant melanoma and their relationship to the extent of the disease. Br Med J 3:547–552, 1969

108. LISTER A: The treatment of malignant pigmented tumors in the neighborhood of the limbus. Trans Ophthalmol Soc NZ 6:5–13, 1952

109. LONG RS, GALIN MA, ROTMAN M: Conservative treatment of intraocular melanomas. Trans Am Acad Ophthalmol Otolaryngol 75:84–93, 1971

110. LUDER P, LANDOLT E: A diffuse malignant melanoma of the iris; a case of a nine year old child. Ophthalmologica 141:363–369, 1961

111. LYNCH HT, ANDERSON DE, KRUSH AJ: Heredity and intraocular melanoma: study of two families and review of forty-five cases. Cancer 21:119–125, 1968

112. MACHEMER R: Zur Pathogenese des flächenhaften malignen Melanoms. Klin Monatsbl Augenheilkd 148:641–652, 1966

113. MacRAE A: Prognosis in malignant melanoma of choroid and ciliary body. Trans Ophthalmol Soc UK 73:1–30, 1953

114. MAKLEY TA JR, TEED RW: Unsuspected intraocular malignant melanomas. Arch Ophthalmol 60:475–478, 1958

115. MARKOVITS AS, QUICKERT MH: Basal cell nevus. Arch Ophthalmol 88:397–399, 1972

116. MASSON P: Pigment cells in man. In Gordon M et al (eds): Biology of Melanomas, Vol 4. New York, NY Academy of Sciences, 1948

117. MATHIAS E: Zur Lehre von den Progonoblastomen. Arch Pathol Anat 236: 424–445, 1922

118. MAUMENEE AE: Serous and hemorrhagic disciform detachment of the macula. Trans Pac Coast Otoophthalmol Soc 40:139–160, 1959

119. McDONALD PR, DE LA PAZ V, SARIN LK: Nonrhegmatogenous retinal separation associated with choroidal detachment. Trans Am Ophthalmol Soc 62:226–247, 1964

120. McLEAN JM: Case reported before the Verhoeff Society, Washington D.C., 1957

121. McWORTER HE, FIGI FA, WOOLNER LB: Treatment of juvenile melanomas and malignant melanomas in children. JAMA 156:695–698, 1954

122. MEISNER W: Zur Diagnose des Aderhautsarcoms. Klin Monatsbl Augenheilkd 70:722–732, 1923

123. MOORHOUSE JH: Case of neurofibroma of the choroid of acoustic nerve type. Trans Ophthalmol Soc UK 59:416–420, 1939

124. MORTADA A: Subacute and chronic inflammatory iris nodules due to pyrogenic bacteria. Br J Ophthalmol 46:669–673, 1962

125. MUND ML, RODRIGUES MM, FINE BS: Light and electron microscopic observation on the pigmented layers of the developing human eye. Am J Ophthalmol 73:167, 1972

126. NAQUIN HA: Orbital reconstruction (using temporal muscle). Am J Ophthalmol 41:519–521, 1956

127. NAUMANN GOH, HELLNER K, NAUMANN LR: Pigmented nevi of the choroid; clinical study of secondary changes in the overlying tissues. Trans Am Acad Ophthalmol Otolaryngol 75: 110–123, 1971

128. NAUMANN G, YANOFF M, ZIMMERMAN LE: Histogenesis of malignant melanoma of the uvea. I. Histopathologic characteristics of nevi of the choroid and ciliary body. Arch Ophthalmol 76:784–796, 1966

129. NORDMANN J, BRINI A: Von Recklinghausen's disease and melanoma of the uvea. Br J Ophthalmol 54:641–648, 1970

130. OGAWA K: Ueber Pigmentirung des Sehnerven. Arch Augenheilkd 52:437–454, 1905
131. OTA M: Nevus fusco-coeruleus ophthalmomaxillaris. Tokyo Med J 63:1243–1245, 1939
132. PACK GT, SCHARNAGEL IM: The prognosis for malignant melanoma in the pregnant woman. Cancer 4:324–334, 1951
133. PACK GT: The problem of malignant melanoma. Proc 2nd Nat Cancer Conf, Cincinnati, 1952, pp 55–70
134. PACKER S, LANGE R: Radioactive phosphorus for the detection of ocular melanomas: a critical evaluation. Arch Ophthalmol 90:17–20, 1973
135. PEYMAN GA, DODICH NA: Full-thickness eye wall resection: an experimental approach for treatment of choroidal melanoma. I. Dacrongraft. Invest Ophthalmol 11:115–121, 1972
136. RAHI AH: Autoimmune reactions in uveal melanoma. Br J Ophthalmol 55:793–807, 1971
137. REESE AB: Pigmentation of the palpebral conjunctiva resulting from mascara. Am J Ophthalmol 30:1352–1355, 1947
138. REESE AB: Precancerous and cancerous melanosis. Am J Ophthalmol 61:1272–1277, 1966
139. REESE AB: Expanding lesions of the orbit (Bowman Lecture). Trans Ophthalmol Soc UK 91:85–104, 1971
140. REESE AB: Congenital melanomas. Am J Ophthalmol 77:798–808, 1974
141. REESE AB, ARENAS-ARCHILA E, JONES IS, COOPER WS: Necrosis of malignant melanoma of the choroid. Am J Ophthalmol 69:91–104, 1970
142. REESE AB, EHRLICH G: The culture of uveal melanomas. Am J Ophthalmol 46:163–174, 1958
142a. REESE AB, JONES IS, COOPER WC: Surgery for tumors of the iris and ciliary body. Am J Ophthalmol 66:173–183, 1968
143. REESE AB, MUND ML, IWAMOTO T: Tapioca melanoma of the iris. Part 1. Clinical and light microscopy studies. Am J Ophthalmol 74:840–850, 1972
144. RILEY FC: Balloon cell melanoma of the choroid. Arch Ophthalmol 92:131–138, 1974
145. RINTELEN F: Zur Differentialdiagnose der Aderhautsarkome. Z Augenheilkd 94:320–324, 1938
146. RIWCHUN MH, DeCOURSEY E: Sympathetic ophthalmia caused by non-perforating intraocular sarcoma. Arch Ophthalmol 25:848–858, 1951
147. ROBERTS S, WATNE A, McGRATH R, McGREW E, COLE WT: Technique and results of isolation of cancer cells from the circulating blood. Arch Surg 76:334–346, 1958
148. RONES B, LI IGER HT: Early malignant melanoma of the choroid. Am J Ophthalmol 38:163–170, 1954
149. RONES B, ZIMMERMAN LE: The prognosis of primary tumors of the iris treated by iridectomy. Arch Ophthalmol 60:193–205, 1958
150. ROSEN DA, MOULTON GN: Multiple melanoma in one eye. Am J Ophthalmol 36:73–75, 1953
151. RUIZ RS: Hemorrhagic macrocyst of the retina mistaken for malignant melanoma of the retina. Arch Ophthalmol 83:588–590, 1970
152. RUIZ RS: New radioactivity detection probe and scaler for phosphorus 32 testing of ocular lesions. Trans Am Acad Ophthalmol Otolaryngol 76:535–536, 1972
153. RUIZ RS, McGEHEE FO JR, ALLEN HC: A new technique of ^{32}P testing of lesions of the posterior segment. South Med J 65:844–846, 1972
154. RYAN SJ, FRANK RN, GREEN WR: Bilateral inflammatory pseudotumors of the ciliary body. Am J Ophthalmol 72:586–591, 1971
155. SALVADOR AH, BEABOUT JW, DAHLIN DC: Mesenchymal chondrosarcoma: observations on 30 new cases. Cancer 28:605–615, 1971
156. SAMUELS B: Anatomic and clinical manifestations of necrosis in 84 cases of choroidal sarcoma. Arch Ophthalmol 11:998–1027, 1934
157. SCHAPPERT-KIMMYSER J: Die Frequenz der sogenannten Uvealmelanome in Augen mit und ohne Sarkom. Arch Augenheilkd 100/101:46–58, 1929
158. SCHEIE HG: Gonioscopy in the diagnosis of tumor of the iris and ciliary body with emphasis on intraepithelial cysts. Trans Am Ophthalmol Soc 51:313–331, 1953
159. SCOTT JA: 3,4-dihydroxyphenylalanine (DOPA) excretion in patients with malignant melanoma. Lancet 11:861–862, 1962
160. SEIJI M: Formation of mammalian melanin. Jap J Derm (ser B) 73:4–6, 1963
161. SEIJI M, FITZPATRICK TB, SIMPSON RT, BIRBECK MS: Chemical composition and terminology of specialized organelles (melanosomes and melanin granules) in mammalian melanocytes. Nature 197:1082–1084, 1963
162. SHAVER RP: Pigmented iris and retrocorneal membrane simulating an iris melanoma. Arch Ophthalmol 78:55–57, 1967
163. SHEA M, SCHEPENS CL, PIRQUET SR: Retinoschisis. I. Senile type: a clinical report of 107 cases. Arch Ophthalmol 63:1–9, 1960
164. SHIELDS JA, FONT RL: Melanocytoma of the choroid clinically simulating a malignant melanoma. Arch Ophthalmol 87:396–400, 1972
165. SHIELDS JA, ZIMMERMAN LE: Lesions simulating malignant melanoma of the posterior uvea. Arch Ophthalmol 89:466–471, 1973
166. SHIELDS JA, McDONALD PR: Improvements in the diagnosis of posterior uveal melanomas. Arch Ophthalmol 91:259–264, 1974
166a. SHUKLA BR, NATH K, AHUJA OP, NEMA HV: Intermittent melanophora. Br J Ophthalmol 48:452–454, 1964
167. SIEGEL R, AINSLIE WH: Malignant ocular melanoma during pregnancy. JAMA 185:542–543, 1963
168. SKINSNES OK: Generalized ochronosis. Arch Pathol 45:552–558, 1948
168a. SMITH LT, IRVINE AR: Diagnostic significance of orange pigment accumulation over choroidal tumors. Am J Ophthalmol 76:212–216, 1973
169. SMOLIN G: Malignant change of a benign melanoma; report of a case. Am J Ophthalmol 61:174–177, 1966
170. SPAULDING AG, GREEN WR, FONT RL: Ring-shaped limbal tumor; secondary to unrecognized diffuse malignant melanoma of the uvea. Arch Ophthalmol 77:76–80, 1967
171. SPENCER WH: Primary neoplasms of the optic nerve and its sheaths: clinical features and current concepts of pathogenetic mechanisms. Trans Am Ophthalmol Soc 70:490–582, 1972
172. SPENCER WH: Discussion in Reese AB: Congenital Melanomas. Trans Am Ophthalmol Soc 71:186–192, 1973

173. STANFORD GB, REESE AB: Malignant cells in the blood of eye patients. Trans Am Acad Ophthalmol Otolaryngol 75:102–109, 1971

174. STEGMAIER OC: Life cycle of nevus. Mod Med 31:79–91, 1965

175. STRACHOV VP, SHEPKALOVA VM: Recklinghausen's disease, neurinoma of the right orbit and melanosarcoma of the left choroid. Vestn Oftalmol 18:12–16, 1941

176. SUCKLING RD, DONALDSON KA: Detection of melanin in choroidal tumors; use of Ektachrome infrared aero film. Arch Ophthalmol 83:700–703, 1970

177. SUMNER WC, FORAKER AG: Spontaneous regression of human melanoma; clinical and experimental studies. Cancer 13:79–81, 1960

178. TAMLER E: A clinical study of choroidal nevi; a follow-up report. Arch Ophthalmol 84:29–32, 1970

179. TAMLER E, MAUMENEE AE: A clinical study of choroidal nevi. Arch Ophthalmol 62:196–202, 1959

180. TASMAN W: Familial intraocular melanoma. Trans Am Acad Ophthalmol Otolaryngol 74:955–958, 1970

181. TERRY TL, JOHNS JP: Uveal sarcoma—malignant melanoma; a statistical study of ninety-four cases. Am J Ophthalmol 18:903–913, 1935

182. THEODOSSIADIS G, LITSIOS B: Primary nevi of the cornea. Am J Ophthalmol 75:695–699, 1973

183. THOMAS CI, KROHMER JS, STORAASLI JP: Detection of intraocular tumors with radioactive phosphorus: a preliminary report with special reference to differentiation of the cause of retinal separation. Arch Ophthalmol 47:276–286, 1952

183a. VAIL DT: Iridocyclectomy: A review; gleanings from the literature. Am J Ophthalmol 71:161–168, 1971

184. VELHAGEN C: Ueber den Befund von zwei Choroidealsarkomen in einem Augapfel. Klin Monatsbl Augenheilkd 64:252–255, 1920

185. VERDAGUER J JR: Personal communication

186. VERDAGUER J JR: Prepuberal and puberal melanomas in ophthalmology. Am J Ophthalmol 60:1002–1010, 1965

187. VON BURKI E: Case report of a malignant melanoma of the iris in an infant. Ophthalmologica 142:487–499, 1961

188. VON HIPPEL E: Fortsetzung meiner Sarkom-Statistik. Graefes Arch Klin Ophthalmol 135:76–78, 1936

189. VON PAPOLCZY F: Zur Prognose des Uveasarkoms. Klin Monatsbl Augenheilkd 99:518–527, 1937

189a. WALLOW IHL, TS'O MOM: Proliferation of the retinal pigment epithelium over malignant choroidal tumors: A light and electron microscopic study. Am J Ophthalmol 73:914–926, 1972

190. WATZOLD GYOTOKU K: Zur Pathogenese des Aderhautsarkoms. Graefes Arch Klin Ophthalmol 120:209–228, 1928

191. WESTERVELD-BRANDON ER: The nature of choroidal tumors. Ned Tijdschr Geneeskd 96:3043–3044, 1952

192. WESTERVELD-BRANDON ER, ZEEMAN WP: The prognosis of melanoblastoma of the choroid. Ophthalmologica 134:20–29, 1957

193. WHITE LP, LINDEN G, BRESLOW L: Studies on melanoma; the effect of pregnancy on survival in human melanoma. JAMA 177:235–238, 1961

194. WILDER HC, PAUL EV: Malignant melanoma of the choroid and ciliary body; a study of 2535 cases. Milit Surg 109:370–378, 1951

195. WINKELMANN RK: Cholinesterase in the cutaneous nevus. Cancer 13:626–630, 1960

196. WOLTER JR, BRYSON JM: Overabundance of uveal ganglion cells in eyes with choroidal melanoma. Am J Ophthalmol 62:1034–1038, 1966

197. WOLTER JR, SCHUT AL, MARTONYI CL: Hemangioma-like clinical appearance of a collar-button melanoma caused by the strangulation effect of Bruch's membrane. Am J Ophthalmol 76:730–733, 1973

198. YANOFF M: Glaucoma mechanisms in ocular malignant melanomas. Am J Ophthalmol 70:898–904, 1970

198a. YANOFF M, FINE BS: Ocular Pathology: A text and atlas. Hagerstown, Harper & Row, 1975, pp 610–612

199. YANOFF M, ZIMMERMAN LE: Pseudomelanoma of anterior chamber caused by implantation of iris pigment epithelium. Arch Ophthalmol 74:302–305, 1965.

200. YANOFF M, ZIMMERMAN LE: Histogenesis of malignant melanomas of the uvea. III. The relationship of congenital ocular melanocytosis and neurofibromatosis to uveal melanomas. Arch Ophthalmol 77:331–336, 1967

201. ZIMMERMAN LE: Personal communication

202. ZIMMERMAN LE: Melanocytes, melanocytic nevi, and melanocytomas. Jonas S Friedenwald Memorial Lecture. Invest Ophthalmol 4:11–41, 1965

203. ZIMMERMAN LE: Problems in the diagnosis of malignant melanomas of the choroid and ciliary body. Am J Ophthalmol 75:917–929, 1973

204. ZIMMERMAN LE, GARRON LK: Melanocytoma of the optic disc. Int Ophthalmol Clin 2:431–440, 1962

8

ANGIOMATOUS TUMORS

Intraocular and extraocular hemangiomas are divided into two general groups: polymorphous and monomorphous. Polymorphous hemangiomas arise from the elements formed at one stage or another during embryonic development of the vascular bed (Fig. 8–1). They are therefore not sharply demarcated entities. Indeed, one type often merges into another, or much more commonly the same tumor has characteristics of more than one type.

Morphologically, the polymorphous tumors are classified according to the predominant growth pattern:

1. The angioblastic hemangioma (Fig. 8-2) is composed of primitive anaplastic endothelial cells similar to those found in the embryo before true vascular channels develop. They are appropriately called hypertrophic hemangiomas of infancy, as they occur principally during this period.
2. The capillary hemangioma has capillary spaces (Fig. 8–3) representing the next most primitive stage in blood vessel development. It also occurs most commonly in the young.
3. The cavernous hemangioma, which usually occurs in adults, has simple endothelium-lined spaces larger than those in capillary hemangiomas (Fig. 8–4). It is the most common tumor of the orbit, where progressive growth gives rise to exophthalmos. When removed from the orbit in its capsule, there is no bleeding from any recognizable afferent feeding vessel.
4. Two types of racemose hemangiomas are encountered: The first is a localized tumor mass in the orbit of an adult, composed of large tortuous vessels that may pulsate. This tumor is serious, for it tends to produce pressure atrophy and to infiltrate the surrounding structures. It is thought to result from arterialization of previously existing vascular channels (Fig. 8–5). The second type is the so-called arteriovenous aneurysm of the retina. Since venous hemangiomas of the retina have thick walls composed of smooth muscle, they may be confused with racemose hemangiomas.
5. The telangiectatic hemangioma consists of dilated thin-walled vessels separated by the parenchyma of the host tissue (Fig. 8–6). There are transitional forms between this type and a cavernous hemangioma.

Monomorphous hemangiomas, the rarer of the two types, arise from some specific element of the blood vessel (Fig. 8–1).

There is controversy over whether hemangiomas belong in the neoplastic family. I believe the polymorphous type is probably not

FIG. 8–1. Elements of blood vessels. Schema shows a capillary (*a*) and a small artery (*b*). The reticulum sheath is seen at *c*, the endothelial cells at *d*, the smooth muscles cells at *e*, and the pericytes at *f*. (Redrawn from Maksimov AA, Bloom W: *A Textbook of Histology*. Philadelphia, Saunders, 1944)

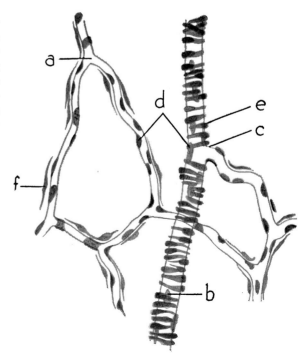

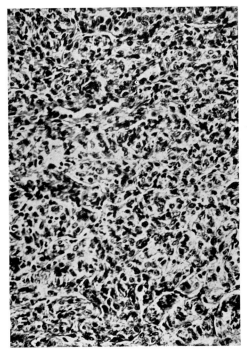

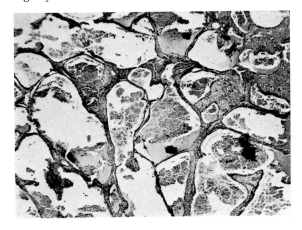

FIG. 8–2. Angioblastic hemangioma of the upper lid. Tissue from a small tumor noted for eight months in a one-year-old girl, with no appreciable change in size.

FIG. 8–4. Cavernous hemangioma of the orbit. Tissue from a tumor in a 65-year-old man who had progressive unilateral exophthalmos for eight years.

FIG. 8–3. Capillary hemangioma of the orbit. Tissue from a tumor in a 3-month-old boy which was noted at birth and had grown.

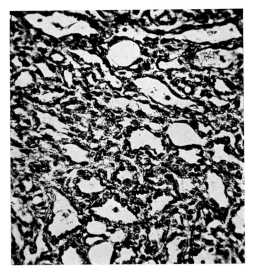

FIG. 8–5. Racemose hemangioma of the orbit. The tumor in a 6-year-old boy was removed by the Krönlein procedure, with no recurrence after three years.

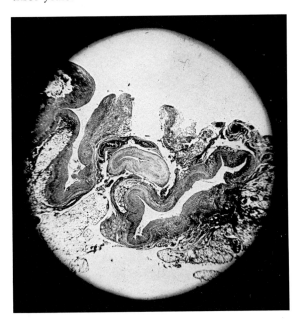

a true neoplasm as it does not have a common stem cell nor does it have the potential for unlimited growth, infiltration, or metastasis. However, the monomorphous type seems to be a true neoplasm in that each hemangioma arises from some specific element of the blood vessel and exhibits behavior associated with a neoplasm. In this group are the hemangiopericytomas, which stem from the pericytes; the hemangioendotheliomas, which stem from endothelial cells; and the leiomyomas or leiomyosarcomas, which stem from the smooth muscle cells. All three may be malignant and are sometimes referred to as angiosarcomas.

POLYMORPHOUS HEMANGIOMAS

Polymorphous hemangiomas frequently undergo changes, such as a spontaneous sclerosing process because the vascular spaces tend to become thrombosed. The blood within the large spaces participates in the general circulation, but since it flows very slowly it has a low oxygen content and can be regarded as venous blood. This sluggish anoxemic blood coagulates readily. The rapid development of thrombosis and fibrosis in some cases leads to increased volume of the orbital contents with the onset of acute symptoms.

The sclerosis can change both the clinical and histologic aspects of a hemangioma to the point where it is unrecognizable, causing confusion especially in the nomenclature. Sclerosing hemangiomas have been called angiofibromas, angiolipomas, xanthomas, etc., according to the predominant tissue. Calcium deposition and the formation of phleboliths and bone are among the regressive changes demonstrable by x rays. In some instances a hemangioma is completely ossified (Fig. 8–7). Despite varying final results, the basic lesion is a hemangioma, and it seems of doubtful value to coin new terms when such tumors can be grouped under sclerosing hemangiomas.

Angioblastic and capillary hemangiomas of early childhood may grow rapidly for a few months after their appearance, but they tend to regress spontaneously and disappear by the end of the fifth year.

The histologic substrate of the sclerosis is an overgrowth of supporting connective tissue which starts in the center of the tumor. It subsequently constricts the lumina of the vessels and finally occludes them. Foreign-body giant cells appear, and hemosiderin is deposited in the endothelial cells or left free in the tissue. If fat is deposited in the endothelial cells, the tumor may appear yellow because of these foam cells, simulating a xanthoma.

The pseudoxanthomatous cells and the glial proliferation in cerebellar hemangiomas have been considered to be signs of sclerosis,[4] which might explain the secondary changes in the retinal tumors of von Hippel's disease.

Cavernous angiomas of the orbit tend to undergo secondary sclerosis. Most cases reported as orbital angiofibromas can be interpreted as sclerosing cavernous angiomas. Also, the clinical and histologic picture of a sclerosed hemangioma in the orbit may be similar to that of an orbital granuloma or pseudotumor.

A peculiar form of sclerosis and regression is observed in juvenile angiofibroma of the nasopharynx in young males. The tumor regresses as sexual maturity advances. This tumor, like other nasopharyngeal lesions, may cause exophthalmos.

POLYMORPHOUS HEMANGIOMAS IN THE RETINA, DISC, AND OPTIC NERVE

Hemangiomas are comparatively rare in the retina. They represent mesoblastic tumors arising in tissue derived from the neuroectoderm. Angiomatous tumors of the retina are often associated with similar lesions in the central nervous system. In several diseases they occur simultaneously at both sites.

Confusion has arisen, however, because of the different terminology and classifications for angiomatous lesions of the central nervous system and the lack of uniformity in nomenclature for blood vessel growths that involve this system (including the retina) and comparable tumors elsewhere. For instance, a neuropathologist may use the term *hemangioblastoma* for a hemangioendothelioma and a hemangiopericytoma. When possible, I have adhered to the classification of angiomatous lesions of the retina and central nervous system commonly used by general pathologists.

ANGIOMATOSIS RETINAE

A complete vascular unit is composed of an afferent vessel supplying a capillary bed which is in turn drained by an efferent vessel. Therefore angiomatosis retinae—also known

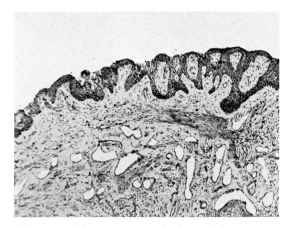

FIG. 8–6. Telangiectasis of the lower lid. A small port-wine stain in a 35-year-old woman was removed for cosmetic reasons. The histologic examination showed an area of telangiectasis just beneath the skin.

as von Hippel's disease, hemangioblastosis retinae, and hemangiogliomatosis—represents a developmental failure of complete vascular units. The basic lesion in its pure form (before any secondary changes) consists of aberrant vascular units which course to and from a localized, elevated, opaque tumor mass (Fig. 8–8, see p. 21).

The onset of retinal and cerebral lesions may be noted over a wide age range. They are often only local manifestations of extensive systemic disease.

The familial nature of retinal angiomatosis has long been recognized. The mode of inheritance is considered to be dominant; the disease is believed to be transmitted by females and to affect a slightly higher proportion of males. Genetic study of families of affected patients is recommended.[30] The history of four patients from three generations of one family with von Hippel–Lindau disease was reviewed.[44] The patients' ages at onset ranged from 17 to 39 years, and three had retinal involvement.

Pathology

This congenital mesodermal malformation with neoplastic traits, which occurs in the neuroectodermal tissue of the retina, may be multiple and in at least half the cases affects both eyes. Although the retina is characteristically involved, the tumor may also develop in the optic nerve (Fig. 8–9, see p. 22; Fig. 8–10).

The periphery of the retina is a preferred site for this tumor, which progresses slowly,

FIG. 8–7. Ossification of a choroidal hemangioma. **A.** Circumscribed tumor adjacent to the disc in an otherwise normal eye of a 19-year-old girl. The adjacent uveal vessels are large and numerous. **B.** High-power magnification reveals bone surrounded by many large vascular channels, suggesting the diagnosis.

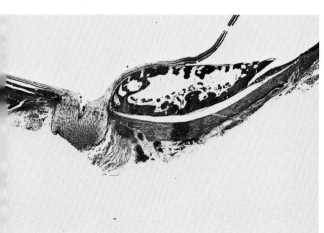

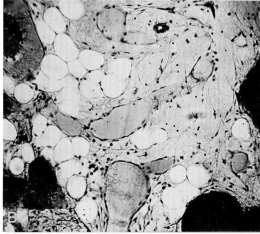

usually toward the vitreous cavity, but it has been known to invade the choroid, lens, and cornea and to perforate the globe.

The tumor's most characteristic feature is the formation of vascular channels representing capillary hyperplasia. Solid areas of angioblastic cells may have more growth potential than areas showing capillary spaces. The angioblastic nature of the more primitive cells is sometimes indicated by erythropoiesis in the newly formed capillaries.

An intravascular network of reticulum can be demonstrated. Swollen cells with foamy cytoplasm are interspersed with the vessels. They are regarded as endothelial or reticulum cells which contain phagocytosed fat, probably freed by the lymphostasis caused by the tumors in the nerve tissue, although some observers felt that the pseudoxanthomatous cells denoted a sclerosing process similar to that occurring in hemangiomas elsewhere in the body.

It has been suggested that von Hippel's disease should be reinterpreted as an instance of multicentric glomic neoplasia.[83] This author stressed the unquestionable carotid-bodylike picture in the cerebellum as well as in the retina.

Diagnosis

The tumor soon causes secondary changes in the retina. As viewed by the ophthalmoscope, the transudates invariably found around the vascular tumor are white, somewhat elevated, and may be extensive. Retinal detachment eventually occurs, caused by transudates, by hemorrhage, or by contracture. The retinal changes may dominate the clinical picture, masking the original lesion. In view of later complications including secondary glaucoma, cataract, and atrophy of the globe, the correct diagnosis may be made only after microscopic examination of the enucleated eye.

Von Hippel's disease may involve the disc instead of the retina, manifesting itself solely as a primary angiomatous tumor of one or both discs or the adjacent retina. This condition may be bilateral.[12] A case of juxtapapillary retinal angiomatosis in a 76-year-old man has been reported.[45] The possibility of von Hippel's disease may not be considered, since the tumor is on the disc and the characteristic afferent and efferent retinal vessels are absent.

Association with Lindau's Disease

The retinal lesion is often a local manifestation of extensive systemic disease.[40] Lindau's disease, which has a definite familial tendency, is characterized by combined retinal and cerebellar hemangiomas as well as by vascular malformations of somatic organs. These cerebellar and retinal hemangiomas may occur independently or concomitantly. They may also appear in the pons and in the medulla, where they may produce syringiomyelia. Choked disc is rare despite the presence of a cerebellar tumor.[60]

Cerebral hemangiomas are extremely rare. They may stem from the leptomeninges and really represent angioblastic meningiomas. The occurrence of concomitant lesions such as cysts in the pancreas, and the kidney, hypernephromas, and tumors of the epididymis points to a systemic disease of the mesenchyme.

A case of neurofibromatosis with acoustic nerve neuroma and retinal angiomatosis has been reported.[19]

Treatment

Small lesions in retinal angiomatosis have responded well to light coagulation[44,63] or cryotherapy, whereas the latter proved more effective for larger lesions or those associated with retinal detachment.[63] Electrosurgery has been used successfully for more than 30 years. One author reported cures in 70% of 47 patients treated by electrosurgery.[75] A case in which diathermy proved effective is shown in Figure 8–11, see p. 22. (See Diathermy, Light Coagulation, and Cryotherapy in the Management of Intraocular Tumors, by Robert M. Ellsworth, in Chapter 12.)

COATS'S DISEASE

Since Coats's original clinicopathologic description of the lesion later called by his name, its nature has been broadly interpreted, and even today the term is ambiguous. Some authorities use it for almost any unexplained acquired tissue in a child's eye, whereas it is specifically interpreted by others. It has been suggested that the term *Coats's disease* be reserved for an exudative retinitis in children associated with a congenital retinal telangiectasis,[46] and that the retinopathy in adults preceded by uveitis and

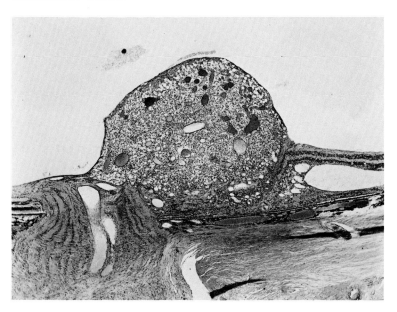

FIG. 8–10. Angiomatosis of the disc and adjacent retina (von Hippel's disease). The tumor in a 53-year-old man had shown slow progressive growth over a ten-year period.

FIG. 8–12. Coats's disease. The fundus in a 6-year-old boy shows a dark bluish bullous detachment of the retina; scattered red globules represent telangiectasis. (Courtesy of R. T. Paton.)

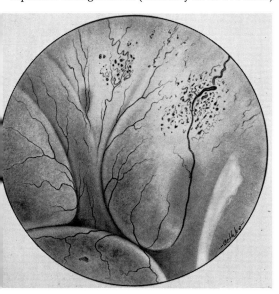

hyperlipemia (so-called adult Coats's disease) be called hyperlipemic retinitis to distinguish it from the usual Coats's disease.[28] Other authors[78] propose three groups of the retinal angiomatoses: the arteriovenous angioma of von Hippel–Lindau, the microaneurysmal retinitis of Leber, and the telangectasis of Reese,[57] all of which may finally lead to the accepted clinical picture of Coats's disease.

Duke-Elder gives the following classification:[15]

1. Cases seen usually in the young, starting with a number of congenital anomalies of the smaller vessels and progressing to massive exudates (the multiple miliary aneurysms of Leber or retinal aneurysms of Reese).
2. Cases seen usually in adults, in which inflammation plays a major role. He points out that in the two conditions the final appearance of the fundus may be the same, and that many authorities consider them a single clinical and pathologic entity arrested at different stages in its evolution.

An adult and a juvenile type of Coats's disease have been described,[16,81] the essential pathologic feature being deposition of free cholesterol and the cholesterol esters in the external layer of the retina and of these same lipids along with fatty acids in the subretinal space. Therefore, Coats's disease differs from the other ocular histiocytoses in which cholesterol is not the lipid involved. In adults, the trigger mechanism seems to be a previous uveal inflammation in the presence of hypercholesteremia. In young people with no evidence of uveal inflammation or abnormal plasma lipid levels, there must be some intermediary tissue factor. According to these investigators, there is highly suggestive evidence that this tissue factor is an acid mucopolysaccharide which probably combines with the lipoprotein complex. Hydrolysis of this complex would free the cholesterol for deposition in and under the retina while the fatty acids would be extravasated into the subretinal space.

In Coats's original description, the primary manifestation was hemorrhage from the capillaries of the outer plexiform layer of the retina, perhaps caused by a constitutional change in the blood vessels associated with an alteration of the blood.[10] But in his later report he considered the primary feature to be hemorrhage in the outer layers of the retina and thence into the subretinal space. Because of the exudative and inflammatory features, he suggested that the term *external hemorrhagic retinitis* be replaced by *external exudative retinitis*.[11] The cause of the hemorrhage that might be incidental and secondary is unknown.

The unilateral dark globular retinal detachment, a common feature of Coats's disease (Fig. 8–12), is usually detected in young male patients when a completely detached retina, or the reflected light from it, is seen in the pupillary area. The lesion's dark, sometimes greenish-brown color is due to hemorrhage and its secondary changes (hemosiderin). Its globular shape results from accumulated blood in the outer layers of the retina or the subretinal space. The hemorrhage usually does not reach the vitreous, which is relatively clear. A vascular process in the nature of a telangiectasis is almost invariably observed at one or more sites over the retina (Fig. 8–12; Fig. 8–13A and B, see p. 23). The process may be masked by the opaque detached retina.

Coats's disease was associated with deafness and mental retardation in four siblings with muscular dystrophy,[65] and bilateral cases were associated with massive glial proliferation in the retina of a 13-year-old girl[25] and with retinitis pigmentosa.[51]

Coats's disease and angiomatosis retinae (von Hippel's disease) may resemble each other in the advanced stages. Nondescript afferent and efferent vessels arise from one or more tumor masses found in von Hippel's disease. The passive congestion due to atresia and occluded vessels supposedly leads to edema, which explains the changing fundal picture and the hemorrhage typically extending externally toward the subretinal space. In progressive cases of both diseases the outcome is detachment of the retina. Angiomatosis retinae is most frequently seen in early life, although it may also appear in older age groups.[77a]

In a review[50] of 51 cases of Coats's disease seen in our tumor clinic up to 1965, the average age of patients at the time of diagnosis was 8 years, and 78% were male. Half the group showed a progressive course to retinal detachment and glaucoma over an average follow-up of 5 years; in the other half the disease remained stationary. Vascular changes, principally telangiectasis, were manifested in 88%.

Pathology

On microscopic examination, newly formed vascular channels are found in the inner layers of the retina (Fig. 8–13C and E, see pp. 23, 24). The material of their walls and lumina is similar to, and continuous with, the thick homogeneous basement membrane. In some places the channels appear completely occluded by this material. Retinal telangiectasis may progress to Coats's disease. A 13-year-old girl had noted increasingly blurred vision of the right eye for three months. Residual edema in the macula produced a star. A conspicuous feature revealed by the PAS stain (Schiff's periodic acid stain) is a thick, red, homogeneous basement membrane under the endothelium, seen in this case. The membrane is an acid mucopolysaccharide deposited in varying amounts, sometimes to an extent appearing to occlude the entire lumen. Formation of this membrane under the endothelium may possibly be a significant factor in atresia or even occlusion of the vessel lumina and in vascular ectasis and the formation of collateral channels.

The channels vary from congeries of capillaries to cavernous spaces; the caliber of their lumina also varies, in some places amounting to dilatations of aneurysmal proportions (Fig. 8–13D, see p. 24).

Hemorrhage from the blood sinuses accumulates in the retina and passes through the external layers of the retina to the subretinal space. Here it becomes organized or undergoes changes to form hemosiderin and crystals. Large blood cysts sometimes form and protrude from the external surface. They contain hematogenous debris and giant cells.

Hyaloid eosin-staining foci, representing residual edema, are conspicuous in the retina, tending to accumulate particularly in the external plexiform layer.

Diagnosis

The retinal vascular lesions in these cases should be viewed as telangiectases rather than hemangiomas because the abnormal vascular channels are dispersed throughout the retina instead of having their own stroma. The lesions are not essentially aneurysmal. The aneurysmal dilatations that occur involve the acquired channels, not the preexisting ones. These lesions seem to be venous rather than arterial in origin.

There is some evidence that the telangiectasis of the retina described here is related to Rendu-Osler-Weber disease or hereditary hemorrhagic telangiectasis. Telangiectatic lesions may develop in various body areas. One of our patients had telangiectasis of the skin of the upper lid of the affected eye; another had localized telangiectatic vessels of the conjunctiva of the affected eye. We have not noted any hereditary tendency. In a reported case,[80] the disease was associated with intermittent filamentary keratitis. The authors speculate about the possible relationship between vascular anomalies in the conjunctiva and filamentary keratitis.

Retinal capillary aneurysms have been reported with similar changes of skin.[22]

I believe the term *Coats's disease* should be reserved for the characteristic and rather consistent clinical picture of a unilateral, dark, perhaps greenish bullous detachment of the retina unilaterally in young children. The lesion's angiomatous nature is often recognized at some site where the retina is still more or less in place, particularly during an adequate examination under general anesthesia. Telangiectasis of the retina should be considered a possible, though not inevitable, precursor of Coats's disease. Such a telangiectasis may remain static, progress to complete retinal detachment (Coats's disease), or give rise to intermittent hemorrhages with no serious secondary changes.

Progressive fundal changes sometimes occur, followed by marked spontaneous regression which seems to be due to the transitory nature of the residual edema.

Treatment

The uncertain course of retinal telangiectases raises the question of whether any therapy can be beneficial even when they are detected early. I have not found radiation beneficial. If the process is localized and the retina not detached, light coagulation, diathermy, or cryotherapy may prove effective.

MULTIPLE RETINAL ANEURYSM

Leber described this condition in 13 patients, 11 from the literature and 2 of his own.[38] It is characterized by multiple aneurysms of the smaller arteries and usually affects young males. The lesions, which sometimes hang like berries on a stalk, are associated with retinal exudates similar to those found in retinitis circinata. Since macular changes, retinal hemorrhages, and retinal detachment ensue, the final clinical picture resembles that of Coats's disease. The underlying cause of the multiple retinal aneurysms has been considered to be a hereditary weakness of the vessel walls. In my opinion the retinal degeneration first described by Leber is identical with the retinal telangiectasis that I consider the forerunner of Coats's disease.

CAVERNOUS HEMANGIOMA

Retinal

The following features have been described as characteristic of cavernous hemangiomas: a) grapelike aneurysmal dilatation of vessels comprising a sessile tumor of the retina; b) frequently drainage of tumors by a major retinal vein usually of normal caliber; c) usually no association with intraretinal or subretinal exudation; d) occasionally hemorrhage into the vitreous; e) grayish tissue within the tumor in many instances; f) extremely slow filling of the tumor, as shown by fluorescein angiography, and little or no evidence of dye leakage from the vascular abnormalities; g) occasional association with cavernous hemangioma of the brain.[21] This author pointed out the association of such tumors with similar vascular anomalies of the central nervous system and the skin, together with a familial tendency (Gass syndrome). The major retinal vessels are unaffected, and angiography gives a characteristic slow perfusion of the tumor with fluorescein. A lesion of this kind occurs in the retina and optic nerve as a localized cluster of saccular aneurysms arising from the inner surface and filled with dark venous blood (Fig. 8–14, see p. 24).

The lesions have a negligible growth potential, but if they give rise to vitreous or subretinal hemorrhage, treatment by photocoagulation, cryotherapy, or diathermy may be indicated. Otherwise, they are static tumors that must be differentiated from other vascular malformations such as angiomatosis retinae, racemose hemangioma, and retinal telangiectasis. Retinal telangiectasis is a congenital anomaly affecting the arterioles, venules, and capillary bed of the retina, whereas cavernous hemangioma is a localized tumefaction isolated from the normal retinal tree. Angiomatosis retinae is easily differentiated, as well as racemose angioma of the retina.

Venous hemangiomas are benign tumors composed of thin-walled vessels with a relatively large lumen. The walls consist mainly of varying amounts of smooth muscle, whereas the walls of capillary and cavernous hemangiomas have a single endothelial layer with a reticulum sheath.

It is difficult to evaluate the ophthalmic literature on venous hemangioma because the term is unwisely used interchangeably with cavernous hemangioma. A syndrome of congenital venous malformation in the orbit may at times be associated with venous malformations elsewhere.[42] Hemangioma of the orbit is almost always of the cavernous type. Venous hemangiomas of the orbit are rare. I have treated only one histologically confirmed case. It occurred in a 64-year-old man whose progressive exophthalmos of the right eye was first noted at age 59. Excision and radiation resulted in complete regression, and there was no recurrence after 11 years.

Either cavernous or venous hemangioma of the retina and optic nerve may be bilateral, though much more marked in one eye than in the other.

Orbital

The most common primary orbital tumor is a cavernous hemangioma. It is seen in adults as a localized expanding lesion causing exophthalmos and in some instances secondary changes in the optic nerve due to pressure. It may also exert sufficient pressure on the sclera to cause hyperopia or retinal striae or both. The tumor is usually located in the muscle funnel and almost invariably manifests itself temporally as a mass eventually palpable through the upper or lower lid.

The proptosis may vary owing to variable stasis of the venous circulation or to movement that increases the congestion in the jugular area, e.g., compression of the vein, bending of the head, crying, or coughing. This proptosis may be reduced somewhat by pressure.

A type of so-called venous hemangioma has thick-walled veins, with smooth muscle in the walls and also in the stroma as independent foci. Such lesions are difficult to distinguish from vascular leiomyomas, hemangiopericytomas, and benign mesenchymomas.

In a series of 21 cases of deep orbital vascular malformations, 16 were treated surgically by the subfrontal and temporal approaches. Only one-third of these tumors were revealed by carotid angiography.[9] This is not surprising since no afferent feeding vessel is observed when an orbital hemangioma is excised. In one instance, unilateral exophthalmos which was first noted in puberty became more pronounced during the pregnancy of a 31-year-old woman. It proved to be due to an orbital cavernous hemangioma.[84]

I do not know of any recurrence after surgical removal of this type of tumor. The diagnosis and treatment are discussed in Chapter 17.

Conjunctival

Most conjunctival hemangiomas originate at the inner canthus near the caruncle and semilunar fold. When originating from the limbus, they encroach on the cornea. A subconjunctival hemangioma may arise from the scleral vessels or from the sclera itself. A hemangioma arising from the palpebral conjunctiva may be pedunculated and must be differentiated from a granuloma.

RACEMOSE HEMANGIOMA (ARTERIOVENOUS ANEURYSM)

Retinal

An angiomatous tumor of the retina, consisting of more or less fully developed vessels, occurs either in one specific area or over the entire retina. In some instances there is similar involvement of the midbrain. The vessels are nondescript and therefore difficult to differentiate, but both arteries and veins probably participate.

Racemose hemangiomas, which are congenital, are sometimes associated with facial hemangiomas. A familial tendency has been observed, with no symptoms of the lesion usually appearing before the age of 30.

Retinocephalic vascular malformations[7,73,82] have been referred to as racemose hemangiomas. Since the advent of angiography, their protean nature has been appreciated. The retinal lesion in a child with monocular amblyopia or esotropia may first lead to recognition of the disease by an ophthalmologist. Angiomatous features are at times noted in the face, lids, conjunctiva, jaws, nose, and throat. The characteristic fundal picture is an arteriovenous anastomosis adjacent to the disc. Autopsy findings are unilateral retinal arteriovenous malformation with ipsilateral involvement of the optic nerve, chiasm, optic tract, and basal ganglia.

Direct arteriovenous communication between enlarged and tortuous arteries and veins can usually be identified, and small aneurysmal dilatations of the affected arteries are not uncommon. In some cases there may be cilioretinal communications or small areas of degeneration and pigmentation over the involved areas of the retina. There is no pulsation of the vessels. Instead of, or in addition to, the arteriovenous communication, some patients show a marked increase in the number, size, and tortuosity of the retinal vessels (Fig. 8–15). Vision in the affected eye is often impaired. Sudden loss of vision was the first manifestation of the disease in some reported cases.

In one case, histologic examination of the eye showed blood vessels occupying the entire thickness of the retina and even extending for some distance into the vitreous cavity.[35] The optic nerve was involved in a mass of blood channels (Fig. 8–16). In another case, intermittent exophthalmos caused by an intracranial arteriovenous aneurysm and orbital varices was cured by excising the entire malformation via a frontotemporal approach.[13]

Orbital

Racemose hemangiomas seldom develop in the orbit. In three of our cases the orbital tumor consisted of fully developed hypertrophied vessels. Two other tumors I have seen were located nasally in the orbit and appeared subconjunctivally under the caruncle as conglomerate tortuous pulsating masses of large mature vessels. The tumor was first noted in one patient at age 35 (Fig. 8–17). It increased in size, particularly during the patient's pregnancy three years later. Progressing steadily, it invaded the surrounding structures resulting in exophthalmos and diplopia as well as several spontaneous hemorrhages.

Drastic surgical procedures, such as tying off large afferent vessels and in some instances the intracranial portion of the internal carotid artery, are often necessary to stay the progressive process. Large, dilated, mature vessels sometimes appear as a conglomerate mass under the conjunctiva, giving the impression that the resulting proptosis is due to a racemose hemangioma, whereas these may be nutrient vessels supplying an orbital tumor. In one case the orbital lesion proved to be a neurofibroma.

In some instances associated orbital lesions produce exophthalmos and pulsation of the eyeball. The pulsation probably results from

FIG. 8–15. Retinocephalic vascular malformation. A 30-year-old woman with poor vision in this eye throughout her life was free of symptoms suggesting intracranial involvement. She was seen before the advent of angiography.

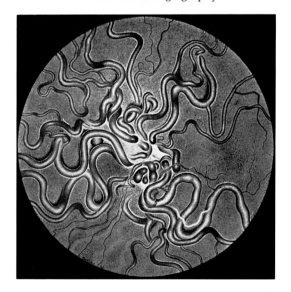

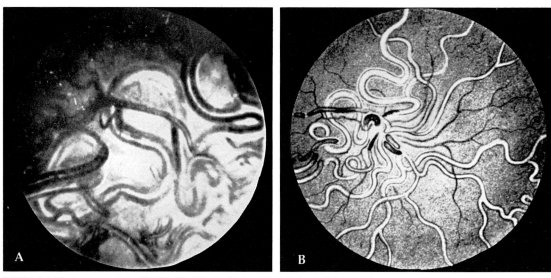

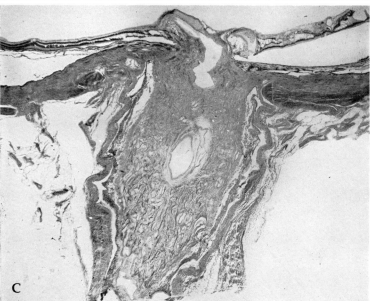

FIG. 8–16. Racemose hemangioma of the retina and optic nerve. Tortuous retinal vessels seen in photograph (A) and drawing (B) of the right fundus in a 21-year-old man who also had a facial hemangioma. C. Section from this eye shows tumor involvement of the retina, optic nerve, and chiasm; the cerebrum was also involved. (Courtesy of E. F. Krug and B. Samuels.[35])

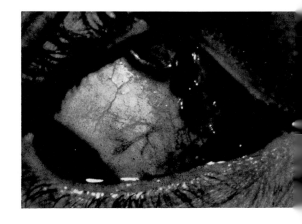

FIG. 8–17. Racemose hemangioma of the orbit. Large, tortuous, fully developed blood vessels were seen in the eye of a 35-year-old woman. Ten years later she had successive ligations of the common carotid artery, the external carotid artery, and the internal carotid artery intracranially, in an effort to stay the steady growth of the tumor.

arterialization of the venous tracts. Such orbital manifestations are attributed to occurrence of these racemose angiomatous lesions
near the optic nerve, where they form part
of the abnormal vascular tract leading to the
midbrain. The exophthalmos may be transient, especially if due to a thrombosis.

Conjunctival

Racemose hemangiomas rarely involve the
conjunctiva. Spontaneous bleeding from the
conjunctiva is usually due to the presence of
hemangiomas,[53,56,77] but malignant melanomas have been found to be the cause in
some cases.[74,76]

Differential Diagnosis

Among conditions to be considered in the
differential diagnosis are the following:

1. Intracranial arteriovenous aneurysm which
   in the late stages is often characterized by
   widening and tortuosity of the retinal vessels. The veins are less numerous than in
   racemose hemangioma, and there is no
   direct arteriovenous communication. The
   arteries appear normal, and both eyes are
   affected. The retinal vessels also become
   widened and tortuous as the result of
   acquired conditions such as arteriosclerosis, thrombosis of the central vein, and
   hyperviscosity states, e.g., polycythemia
   vera.
2. Sturge-Weber-Dimitri disease, in which
   the retinal veins may also become widened
   and tortuous, although the principal
   changes are found in the choroid.
3. Angiomatosis retinae (von Hippel–Lindau
   disease), in which the definite retinal tumor
   has large afferent and efferent vessels that
   show no evidence of anastomosis. The
   neurologic signs indicate a tumor of the
   cerebellum or fourth ventricle rather than
   of the midbrain. The clinical picture of
   angiomatosis retinae in the early stages,
   particularly if beginning at the periphery,
   may be confused with that of a racemose
   angioma of the retina. In fact, one of the
   first recorded cases of von Hippel's disease
   was initially reported as an arteriovenous
   aneurysm; the true nature of the lesion
   was revealed during the clinical course.[20]

Brain Lesions

Since racemose angiomas of the retina were
first reported, their possible association with
similar ipsilateral lesions of the brain has
been suspected. The association of retinal,
cerebral, and facial racemose angiomas, and
recognition of this syndrome as one of the
phakomatoses, has been widely accepted. Evidence of an arteriovenous aneurysm of the
midbrain was found in 22 of 27 cases of
retinal arteriovenous aneurysm culled from
the literature; the report did not specify
whether the other 5 patients had a neurologic
examination.[82] This author also found abnormalities of the retinal vessels in 14 of 20
cases of arteriovenous aneurysm of the midbrain in reported cases. Among 9 cases of his
own, 7 had both retinal and midbrain vascular lesions and the other 2 had only midbrain
lesions.

Pathology

The abnormal vessels usually form tracts
from the retina to the midbrain. They cover
and permeate the optic nerve and extend
through the chiasm and optic tract to the
dorsum of the midbrain. Histologic examination reveals many tortuous, dilated vessels in
affected portions of the brain, optic tract
and optic nerve, with the intervening nerve
tissue in various degrees of atrophy and
gliosis.

In some chronic cases the vessels constitut-
ing the lesions apparently become arterial-
ized. The consensus is that this occurs when
the symptoms appear. Some of the thin-
walled vessels may rupture, giving rise to
hemorrhage into the brain and subarachnoid
space. The encroachment of these abnormal
vessels on the aqueduct causes either a constant or an intermittent hydrocephalus with
dilatation of the lateral and third ventricles—
a feature noted in every case examined post
mortem.

Embryology

A lesion of the anterior plexus of primordial
cerebral blood vessels is likely to affect the
retinal blood vessels. Later this vascular
mesenchyme splits into three layers, and if
the superficial layer is affected, this could ac-

count for the simultaneous appearance of retinal and facial skin hemangiomas. It therefore seems logical to assume that a common lesion could be responsible for vascular anomalies of the midbrain, retina, and skin of the face.

Diagnosis

Sometimes the disease is symptomless and its presence is detected when vascular anomalies are discovered in the retina. Symptoms seem to depend on arterialization of the vascular channels or on thrombosis in, or hemorrhage from, the vessels. The nature of the symptoms is related to the location of the lesion. The patient may experience sudden or gradual visual failure. When sudden, it is usually accompanied by headache, vomiting, and exophthalmos—complications indicating either a hemorrhage or thrombosis. Gradual visual loss is doubtless due to secondary retinal atrophy and gliosis.

Symptoms first referable to the midbrain may be varied. In the event of hemorrhage, blood accumulates in the subarachnoid space eliciting the usual symptoms such as sudden headache, vomiting, and neck rigidity with or without loss of consciousness. After these acute manifestations have subsided, signs of a midbrain lesion are apparent. A thrombotic type of vascular lesion may result in unilateral third-nerve paralysis with contralateral hemiplegia (Weber's syndrome) or with contralateral tremor (Benedict's syndrome). Hemianopsia, epilepsy, and sometimes hypothalamic signs are noted in some cases. Associated mental and psychic disturbances may be either temporary or permanent.

X-ray films at times show thinning and erosion of bone, in some cases to such an extent that the inner table is completely absorbed and the diploë exposed. The various foramina in the base of the skull may enlarge, and bone erosion may extend to the apex of the petrous portion of the temporal bone. Encephalography, ventriculography, and arteriography sometimes yield diagnostic information.

Some patients develop angiomas of the face, usually in the trigeminal distribution and invariably on the side of the affected eye. Some of these skin angiomas show pulsation, and pigmented nevi have been found.

Treatment

Various types of treatment have been tried with discouraging results. These include deep x-ray therapy, ligation of the common and internal carotid arteries, exploration of the lateral ventricles in an attempt to ligate vessels on the affected side, and insertion of radon seeds into the retinal lesion.

Prognosis

In one series of seven cases[82] there were six deaths: one 5 years after the onset of symptoms, another 14 years, the other four from 6 to 11 years. Among patients with neurologic symptoms living at the time of the report, the lesion had been present from 7 months to 16 years with an average of 5 years. Some patients develop blindness early while others retain almost normal vision for years.

HEMANGIOMA OF THE OPTIC NERVE AND DISC

True angiomatous tumors of the optic nerve and disc are extremely rare. In making the diagnosis, one must exclude the formation of blood vessels on the disc occurring in conditions such as glaucoma, thrombosis of the central vein, and optic neuritis. The optic nerve may be involved in cases of racemose hemangioma of the retina, especially when the lesion is associated with cerebral hemangioma (Figs. 8–15, 8–16).

An angiomatous tumor found at autopsy in the intracranial part of the optic nerve, an angiomatous tumor of the intraorbital portion of the optic nerve consisting of capillaries and dilated vessels, an angioma of the disc consisting solely of capillaries and endothelial cells, and similar tumors with secondary glial proliferation have all been considered manifestations of von Hippel–Lindau disease. These lesions are not uncommon, but are often misinterpreted.

I have seen one case of cavernous hemangioma of the disc and adjacent retina (Fig. 8–18, see p. 25), and similar reported cases seem to belong to this group. When the fundal tumor in von Hippel's disease is located in the disc instead of the retina, it resembles angiomatous tissue clinically but lacks the usual identifying large afferent and efferent vessels (Fig. 8–9, see p. 22).

An angioblastic type of angioma of the papilla, with some areas of fully developed capillaries, was considered possibly to have arisen from a remnant of the hyaloid artery.[64] In a unique case, an angiomatous tumor of the disc increased markedly in size; histologic examination showed proliferation of the pericytes only.[62] I believe this should be classified as a glomus tumor (hemangiopericytoma).

POLYMORPHOUS HEMANGIOMAS IN THE UVEA

CHOROIDAL HEMANGIOMAS

Incidence

Of 130 patients with verified choroidal hemangiomas, 50% had the Sturge-Weber syndrome, and of 250 with verified Sturge-Weber syndrome, 100 had choroidal hemangiomas; relatively few of the remaining cases were diagnosed.[14] A 39-year-old woman was treated over nine months for edema of the left macula. The diagnosis veered between inflammation and a neoplasm, with metastatic tumor a possibility, for the next four years. The course and appearance finally suggested a choroidal hemangioma (Fig. 8–19, see p. 25).

Age

Since the tumors affect young people mainly, especially the 10–20 age group, they have been considered congenital even though not detected in the first few years of life. Among 28 cases of histologically proved choroidal hemangiomas,[32] the average age at the time of enucleation was 35 years, and the first symptom related to the lesion was noted at an average age of 19 years.

Pathology

Choroidal hemangiomas are usually classified as cavernous because they have wide, thin-walled vascular spaces containing practically no connective-tissue stroma. The majority are located at the posterior pole. About 25% are diffuse throughout the choroid and frequently associated with a facial hemangioma.[32]

Among numerous changes secondary to choroidal angioma, the most conspicuous is formation of a membrane over the tumor surface (Fig. 8–20). A proliferative reaction of the pigment epithelium results in a layer of tissue resembling the cuticular element of Bruch's membrane. Fibrous elements such as connective tissue and some pigment-bearing cells are also present. Degenerative changes such as calcification and ossification may be observed in this epichoroidal membrane. Interposed between the retina and the surface of the choroidal angioma, this membrane confuses the clinical picture and may make a correct diagnosis difficult.

Osteoblastic changes are not infrequently found by x ray in hemangiomas, at times leading to confusion of the lesion with an osteosarcoma.

In rare instances, a choroidal hemangioma undergoes ossification and may be mistaken for a primary osteoma of the choroid (Fig. 8–7). Proliferative changes of the pigment epithelium overlying the tumor are partially responsible for the fact that a choroidal

FIG. 8–20. Hemangioma of the choroid. The tumor (a), found in an eye removed because of a perforating injury, had an epichoroidal membrane (b) with pigment calcification and ossification.

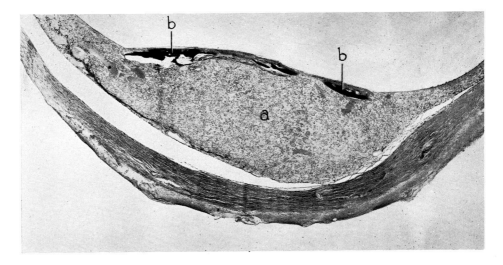

hemangioma sometimes simulates a melanoma (Fig. 8–21).

The retinal tissue adjacent to the hemangioma undergoes degenerative changes, becoming edematous, cystic, and atrophic. Secondary cystic degeneration of the macula is an early complication, even when the tumor lies on the nasal side of the disc.

Retinal detachment, seen in over 90% of the microscopic specimens, may be caused by transudation or by hemorrhage. Large transscleral blood vessels have been found under the tumor, suggesting a possible relationship between the tumor and the short posterior ciliary arteries acting as feeder vessels.[32]

Glaucoma is a late complication. Most globes in which a choroidal hemangioma is incidentally found after enucleation are removed because of absolute glaucoma.

It is of passing interest that the choroid in some fish is thicker and more vascularized than in man. At the posterior pole it is transformed into a vascular body surrounding the optic nerve like a horseshoe. This angiomalike body has been called the choroidal gland of Erdl. Because a choroidal hemangioma in man has a predilection for the posterior pole, it might be viewed as a progonoma.

FIG. 8–21. Isolated choroidal hemangioma compressing at its border a preexisting choroidal nevus. This represents an exaggeration of the normal tendency toward compression of choroidal melanocytes at the border of a hemangioma (*a*) where a nevus (*b*) was by chance located. The variably pigmented ring around the periphery of the hemangioma should be borne in mind in the differential diagnosis of a malignant melanoma. (Courtesy of H. Witschel and R. L. Font.[79])

Diagnosis

Clinical diagnosis of a choroidal hemangioma is difficult unless there is an associated facial hemangioma. Perhaps 75% of histologically confirmed choroidal hemangiomas are unsuspected, suggesting that they may lurk unrecognized. If small, they probably produce no symptoms and are overlooked in a routine examination.

A choroidal hemangioma tends to develop in young adults with a history of slowly decreasing visual acuity and perhaps progressive hyperopia. Ophthalmoscopic examination reveals a moderately elevated mass adjacent to the disc, more often on the temporal side, and perhaps with an inferior serous detachment of the retina. The overlying and adjacent retina may show some transudate, some white residual edema, and particularly some cystoid changes. Light is transmitted through the lesion by scatter illumination. Sometimes indirect ophthalmoscopy reveals the vascular channels or at least the tumor's vascular nature.

Hemangiomas belonging to this polymorphous group sometimes show progression during pregnancy (Fig. 8–22, see p. 26).

The primary diagnoses in a series of 28 cases[32] included malignant melanoma of the choroid (8 cases). Sturge-Weber syndrome (3 cases); "tumor" (2 cases); 2 cases each of blind painful eye and hemangioma of the choroid; and 1 case each of chronic inflammatory disease, phthisis bulbi, acute glaucoma, secondary glaucoma, buphthalmos, and absolute glaucoma. In the other 5 cases no clinical diagnosis could be made. Glaucoma was present in 11 of 20 cases in which tension was

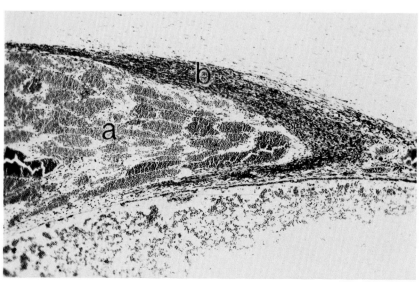

reported. In all but 3 cases, retinal detachment was demonstrated either clinically or by microscopic examination.

Secondary ocular changes (*e.g.,* uveitis, glaucoma, cataract, corneal clouding) are particularly likely to appear early in patients with the diffuse type of tumor usually seen in Sturge-Weber disease.

The following diagnostic tests may be of value:

1. Fluorescein angiography—see Stereofundus Photography and Fluorescein Angiography in the Diagnosis of Intraocular Tumors, by J. Donald M. Gass, in Chapter 12.
2. Radiodiagnostic tests—see Special Radiodiagnostic Studies of the Orbit, by Stephen L. Trokel, in Chapter 12.
3. Compression of the globe—use of this method during examination of the tumor may cause some blanching.[61]

Treatment

The specific treatment for choroidal hemangioma is enucleation, usually performed when secondary changes have resulted in blindness and pain. Results in occasional reports of attempts to destroy the tumor by diathermy have been generally discouraging, although in a reported case[61] perforating diathermy under constant ophthalmoscopic guidance led to improvement.

Cryosurgery may prove effective, as may various forms of radiotherapy in early cases (which are seldom diagnosed), though its value is still in question. Destruction by light coagulation, especially for sufficiently localized tumors, may be the treatment of choice in selected cases. (See Diathermy Light Coagulation and Cryotherapy in the Management of Intraocular Tumors, by Robert M. Ellsworth, in Chapter 12.)

MENINGOCUTANEOUS ANGIOMATOSIS (STURGE-WEBER DISEASE)

The complete syndrome includes an intracranial and a facial hemangioma with an ipsilateral choroidal hemangioma and congenital glaucoma.[82a] At least two of these lesions must be present to warrant the diagnosis. Incomplete forms of the syndrome are more frequently seen (Fig. 8–23, see p. 26).

Sturge-Weber disease, an ipsilateral angiomatosis which may involve simultaneously the nervous system, the skin, and the uvea, has not been well defined. Different conceptions of the pathologic features inevitably led to the association of four or five names with the syndrome. An attempt is made here to use descriptive terms, although it is difficult to find one comprehensive designation for a lesion affecting various organs.

Some French authors consider the disease to be a variety of the *neurocutaneous syndrome.* This term not only fails to differentiate the entity from some other phakomatoses, but also assumes that the syndrome is essentially a combination of neural and cutaneous lesions, which is not yet proved. The intracranial lesions probably involve the meninges and intracerebral vessels primarily, rather than the neural tissue. Other terms such as *encephalotrigeminal angiomatosis, encephalocutaneous angiomatosis,* and *meningocutaneous angiomatosis* are preferable because they at least indicate the lesion's angiomatous character.

Some neurologists both in this country and abroad prefer the term *encephalotrigeminal angiomatosis,* but *meningocutaneous angiomatosis* is most frequently used in ophthalmologic literature. Still many authors continue to use *Sturge-Weber syndrome,* named for the ones who first described its salient features.

The frequent association of unilateral glaucoma with ipsilateral facial and choroidal hemangioma has long been noted. An intracranial angioma has been suspected in patients with contralateral epileptic seizures of the jacksonian type; an autopsy on such a patient revealed a meningeal angioma which accounted for the neurologic symptoms. Demonstration of a characteristic x-ray picture for the intracranial angioma was of clinical importance, establishing it as an independent syndrome and confirming the diagnosis.

During extensive histologic studies on the brain of a patient with meningocutaneous angiomatosis, it was shown that the x-ray shadows were caused by intracranial calcifications rather than by calcium deposits in the pial angioma; the intracerebral changes were thought to represent the primary lesion.[34]

Since the facial component at least is noted at birth, the lesion must be congenital (Fig. 8–24). Other features appear in infancy or early childhood; the diagnosis is most often made within the first six months to year of life. A hereditary tendency has been assumed but supportive evidence is meager.

Incidence

Many cases of complete meningocutaneous angiomatosis have appeared in the literature. The combination of facial angioma and ipsilateral glaucoma is much more common than indicated by the reports, and would be described only if there were some unusual feature of the particular case.

Pathology

Ocular, dermal, and intracranial angiomas undoubtedly have a common genesis. The metameric distribution of angiomas is usually explained on a developmental basis. During development of the brain's blood supply, the primordial vascular system splits into an inner layer serving the brain and retina, and an outer layer serving the meninges, choroid, and face. A common derivation of the meningeal, choroidal, and facial vessels can explain malformations affecting all three vascular systems. The functional parallelism between the meninges and the choroid is noteworthy. Meningocutaneous angiomatosis is essentially a congenital malformation of this system of vascular mesoderm.

The occurrence of most facial angiomas along one or more branches of the trigeminal nerve has led some investigators to speculate about possible nerve influence, and others to consider meningocutaneous angiomatosis primarily a mesodermal malformation, but there is insufficient evidence to support either view.

Various theories have been advanced to explain the development of glaucoma in a patient with facial angioma. Since in rare instances no angiomatous changes could be found in the affected eye, the theories must not be based exclusively on a space-consuming lesion and attending changes.

Theories based on the presence of an angioma of the uvea include the following:

1. A choroidal angioma increases the bulk of the intraocular contents or compresses the vortex veins.
2. Angiomatous changes in the ciliary body result in increased production of aqueous humor, which has been called plethoric glaucoma. Increased permeability of the ciliary vessels has been demonstrated by the accelerated appearance of intravenous fluorescein in the anterior chamber and by the increased protein content of this aqueous in such a case.

3. Angiomatous changes in the iris may block the angle of the anterior chamber. The veins connected with Schlemm's canal may be involved in the process.
4. A simultaneous orbital or intracranial angioma produces mechanical interference.

Theories based on the absence of an angioma in the uvea include the following:

1. The tendency of facial angioma to follow branches of the trigeminal nerve may be of etiologic significance. Disturbances of the sympathetic system or the vasomotor nerves have been suggested, a view supported by the finding of decreased dilatation of the pupil of the affected eye in patients given epinephrine.
2. A primary congenital anomalous obstruction of the angle as seen in cases of hydrophthalmos.
3. Alteration in capillary permeability.

Intracranial Changes

The most characteristic intracranial manifestations are unilateral foci of calcification in the occipital and parietal lobes and, rarely, in the cerebellum. The calcium, located in the blood vessel walls, is associated with atrophy of the adjacent nerve tissue and loss of neural cells in the outer layers of the cortex with secondary calcareous deposits in these areas. The damage may be severe when the lesions develop in the cerebellum.

The majority of pial angiomas are found in the same area as the intracranial calcifications. These angiomas, usually of the racemose type, consist of dilated and hypertrophied vessels. Although there has been some question as to whether the brain calcifications are the primary intracranial lesions or secondary to the meningeal angiomas, it is now generally assumed that the pial angiomas are primary, precipitating the intracerebral calcifications. The enlarged pial veins may also calcify, and the pial angiomas may lead to localized thickening of the overlying bones. Similar angiomatous lesions of the pia have been found in the spinal cord associated with angiomas of the skin of the legs—regarded as a variation of the meningocutaneous syndrome.

The intracranial changes may cause manifold symptoms which arise early in life. They include a) epileptic seizures, either generalized or of the jacksonian type, at sites con-

tralateral to the intracranial lesion; b) hemiplegia, especially when there are calcifications
in the parietal lobe; c) hemianopsia when
there are calcifications in the occipital lobe;
and d) mental deterioration resulting from
the secondary cortical changes.

Treatment of the intracranial lesions presents difficulties. However, successes have
been reported with surgical extirpation of degenerated foci, radiotherapy, and electroco-
agulation.

Skin Lesions

The dark red facial hemangiomas of meningocutaneous angiomatosis, present at birth,
are disfiguring (Fig. 8–23, see p. 26). As indicated, they are distributed over one or more
branches of the trigeminal nerve and may
even cover a larger area than it innervates.
In rare cases these skin angiomas involve
the trunk or the extremities or both (Fig.
8–24). When bilateral, they may be associated with unilateral or bilateral glaucoma.
The eye seems to be affected when the facial
angioma involves the lid and the conjunctiva.

Nevus flammeus or *port-wine nevus*, terms
used by dermatologists for facial angiomas,
seem inappropriate. These angiomas may be
of the telangiectatic or cavernous type. They
are usually dark red and flat. Proliferation of
the skin, as a secondary change, may cause
facial asymmetry. In most cases these facial
angiomas are ipsilateral with the pial angiomas.

Ocular Manifestations

Hydrophthalmos. The majority of facial angiomas are associated with hydrophthalmos,
implying that the glaucoma results from ocular changes that are congenital. The clinical
appearance and pathogenesis of these congenital glaucomas are the same as for the
usual hydrophthalmos caused by maldevelopment of the filtration angles. The condition is
always ipsilateral with the facial angioma,
which may be bilateral. Contralateral chronic
glaucoma, in addition to ipsilateral hydrophthalmos and facial angiomas, has been reported. In several cases the cornea was definitely enlarged but not the globe, undoubtedly a minor manifestation of hydrophthalmos.

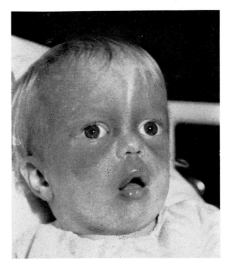

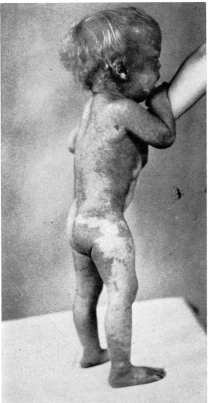

FIG. 8–24. Sturge-Weber disease involving most
of the face and body.

Chronic Glaucoma. In only about 12% of cases of facial angioma associated with glaucoma do the globes fail to enlarge.[6] These patients probably have a congenital predisposition toward glaucoma, but the increased intraocular pressure does not become manifest for some time after birth. In several instances the patient's intraocular pressure appeared to be consistently normal, but the affected eye showed deep cupping of the disc with typical defects of the visual field. The tension in the affected eye might be within normal limits but still higher than in the fellow eye.

Changes in the Uvea. The very dark-colored fundus sometimes seen in affected eyes is believed to indicate a choroidal telangiectasis or a uveal angioma. When the choroidal vessels can be seen they appear enlarged and tortuous. The iris of the affected eye is darker than that of the fellow eye; several cases of heterochromia have been associated with facial angioma.

Histologic Changes. In a review of histologic examinations of the affected globe, angioma of the choroid was the most frequent pathologic feature, not unexpected in view of the developmental relationship between the facial and choroidal vessels. A congenital anomaly of the angle found in one specimen was similar to that occurring in hydrophthalmos; there were no intraocular angiomatous changes.

Diagnosis

It is not difficult to diagnose the complete syndrome of meningocutaneous angiomatosis: cerebral symptoms, a facial angioma, and angiomatous lesions of the eye associated with glaucoma.

The facial angioma is obvious, and the ocular changes usually recognized readily. Skull x rays, the most valuable diagnostic aid toward establishing the presence of an intracranial angioma, reveal characteristic sinuous shadows in the form of double-contoured tortuous lines ("railroad tracks"). These shadows cannot be seen in infants who have not yet developed secondary calcareous degeneration, but have been observed in young children.

An intracranial angioma may be detected by angiography, by encephalography, and by electroencephalography.

HEMANGIOMA OF THE CILIARY BODY AND IRIS

Hemangioma of the ciliary body is extremely rare; many of the reported cases were probably granulomas or malignant melanomas. I have seen two hemangiomas of the iris, one of which could be verified microscopically. This patient had a hemangioma of the upper lid on the same side as the iris lesion. Angiomatous dilatation of the iris vessels has been noted in patients with Sturge-Weber disease. A unilateral cavernous hemangioma of the iris in a neonate was associated with bilateral abnormal retinal vasculature as well as generalized cutaneous and visceral hemangiomas.[52] An author who reviewed the literature also reported a case of hemangioma of the ciliary body associated with retinal detachment.[55] One report included a review of the literature and two further cases in which angiomas of the ciliary body were removed by cyclectomy.[8]

A case of pseudoangioma of the iris associated with a melanoma has been described.[3] On microscopic examination the melanoma's vascular component overshadowed its neoplastic component. In another case, an aggregation of vessels at the border of the tumor was found to be due to vascular proliferation.[26]

POLYMORPHOUS HEMANGIOMAS OF THE LID, CONJUNCTIVA, AND ORBIT

(Figs. 8–25, 8–26, 8–27, see p. 27; Fig. 8–28)

HEMANGIOMAS OF THE NEWBORN

Incidence

It is estimated that 1% to 2% of full-term infants have this type of angioblastic hemangioma somewhere on the skin (hypertrophic hemangioma, benign hemangioendothelioma, "strawberry hemangioma"). During the period when oxygen was being freely administered to premature infants, the incidence of such lesions was even higher. It seems to be in inverse proportion to the birth weight: 10% at the 3 to 4 pound weight, 20% at 2 to 3 pounds, and 45% at 1 to 2 pounds. Now that oxygen is either withheld from premature infants or used with more controls, the incidence has dropped below 5%. A parallel decline in the incidence of retrolental fibroplasia and skin hemangioma suggests a common etiologic factor.

Further evidence of a kinship between retrolental fibroplasia and skin hemangioma includes the following: a) The pathology of retrolental fibroplasia includes hemangiomatous tissue in the retina extending into the vitreous (Fig. 8–29). b) This tissue has the same histologic characteristics as skin hemangiomas of infants (Fig. 8–30). c) Skin hemangiomas and retrolental fibroplasia follow the same clinical course in infants; in the large majority of cases they appear within the first five weeks of life, and an active progressive phase is followed by a regressive or cicatricial stage. d) The incidence of both conditions is in inverse proportion to the birth weight. e) Infants developing retrolental fibroplasia have a higher incidence of skin hemangiomas than those who do not (25% and 11%, respectively).

Clinical Course

Hemangiomas in infants are frequently multiple and diffuse, occurring primarily in the skin, sometimes as a brilliant red mark. In iceberg fashion, they usually have a small skin component and an extensive subcutaneous component. In some cases, however, they are poorly demarcated subcutaneous tumors that involve not only the lid and brow area but also extend into the orbit, producing some degree of exophthalmos.

About 20% of hemangiomas of the newborn are recognized at birth, and the other 80% within five weeks. The tumor may progress for six to nine months, sometimes to an alarming degree. It gradually undergoes involution so that over a period of years there is partial or even complete regression.

As the tumor regresses its initial bright red color fades to a dull bronze, with wrinkling of the overlying skin. This sclerotic process, first and most markedly noted in the central portion, spreads gradually until the entire tumor disappears. Ulceration of the central portion may occur coincidentally with rapid regression.

Both infantile and adult hemangioma occur in the orbit, and their clinical behavior and treatment are entirely different. Infantile hemangioma may grow rapidly. In rare instances the eyeball is pushed forward between the lid margins, exposing the cornea and leading to corneal perforation. Surgery is

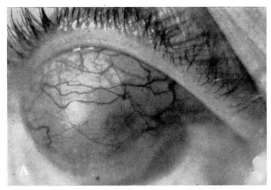
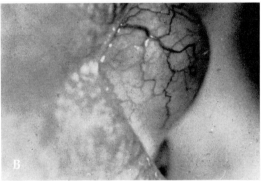
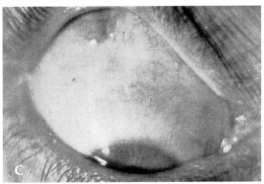

FIG. 8–28. Hemangioma between the upper lid and the globe. **A, B.** Anterior and lateral views of the tumor in a 50-year-old woman before treatment with sodium morrhuate injections. **C.** Anterior view one year after treatment. The tumor could not have been excised without damage to the levator muscle. The injections did not impair function of the levator or superior rectus muscle.

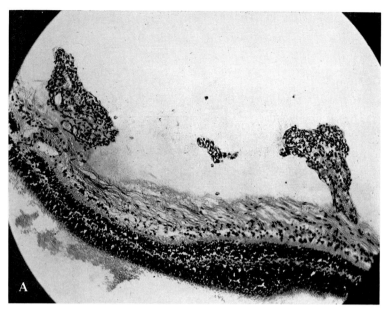

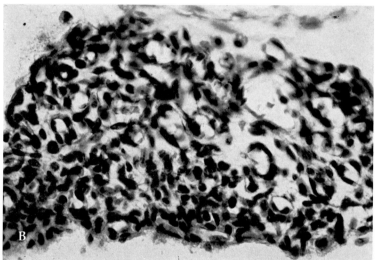

FIG. 8–29. Angiomatous tissue in retrolental fibroplasia. **A.** Section of the retina of a 1-pound 10-ounce premature infant with active retrolental fibroplasia. Angiomatous tissue extends from the internal retinal surface at two sites. **B.** High-power magnification of section from one of the angiomatous extensions.

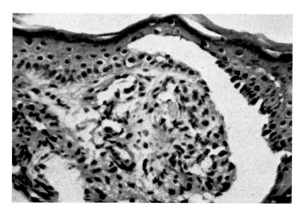

FIG. 8–30. Skin hemangioma of the newborn. Section removed from a buttock of a 2-pound 3-ounce premature infant, at the age of 42 days, is similar to that shown in Figure 8–29B.

indicated only to establish the diagnosis when it is not obvious. The tumor undergoes a natural regression, but to prevent complications, such as exposure of the cornea and amblyopia from obstruction of the pupil, x ray in small doses is effective.

In a review of 145 primary tumors of the iris, only 3 proved to be angiomas. They were successfully treated by simple iridectomy without recurrence six, five, and two years postoperatively.[1]

Unlike the infantile hemangioma, the adult type is well encapsulated and is the orbital tumor most satisfactorily removed by a Krönlein operation. There seem to be no sizable afferent vessels and the operation is therefore comparatively bloodless. The apparent absence of feeding vessels may explain the frequent failure of angiograms to reveal the nature of the tumor.

In one reported series[36] 61% of the lesions were present at birth; another 25% were either present at birth or developed within the first month of life. The remaining 14% developed after the first month. Regression was first observed before the sixth month in 16% of the cases, between 6 and 12 months in 65%. The involution process required several years; the lesion had disappeared in the majority of patients by age 5 whether treated or not. Lesions that enlarge during the first few months of life and stop growing before age one usually involute. From 7% to 10% of hypertrophic hemangiomas of this type persist beyond the seventh year.

A mucocele of the tear sac in an infant may have a bluish color and resemble a hemangioma.

Treatment

As these tumors tend to regress without treatment, no therapy is instigated in the majority of cases; the parents are told that the tumor is benign and the outcome in all probability will be successful. However, treatment is indicated when the lesion is so located around the eye that marked progression might alter and distort the lids and brow causing disfigurement, also when the tumor occludes the palpebral aperture sufficiently to obstruct vision and cause amblyopia ex anopsia. The purpose of intervention is to stay the process until the regressive phase begins.

Cryotherapy. A superficial lesion may be treated by some form of cryotherapy, applied weekly or every other week depending on the response. The effects extend to a surprising depth, often resulting in a satisfactory regression.

Sclerosing Solutions. It is often advisable to treat lesions involving subcutaneous structures with sclerosing solutions, commonly sodium morrhuate 5% or sodium psylliate 2%. The solution is injected into the body of the lesion, with care to avoid infiltrating the surrounding structures, especially the orbit and the tissue around the eyeball. The starting dose of 0.3–0.5 ml is increased every two to four weeks to 1.0 ml, as indicated by the reaction.

With some large lesions there may be a residual fibrous mass after completion of a series of injections (Fig. 8–31, see p. 27); it is well localized and can be excised surgically if indicated. Therefore, even though a diffuse lesion may not respond completely to the injection, it is at least reduced to a localized mass that can be excised (Fig. 8–32).

FIG. 8–32. Nonencapsulated hemangioma of the orbit. The lesion, in the upper anterior lateral aspect of the orbit of a 1-year-old girl was too diffuse for excision. **A.** Before treatment with sodium morrhuate injections, which resulted in a circumscribed, firm, encapsulated mass that could be easily excised. **B.** One year after completion of treatment.

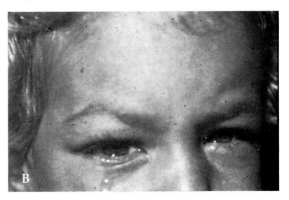

When afferent vessels supplying the tumor can be palpated over the rim of the orbit nasally or temporally, the injection should be made at the site where they enter the tumor. A suitable vasoconstrictor is an aqueous solution of Sotradecol 1% in two or three injections of 0.2 ml or 0.3 ml, or sodium morrhuate solution 5%. Figure 8–33 shows the usual site of palpable afferent vessels supplying hemangiomas in and around the lid.

Irradiation. (See also Radiotherapy of Ocular and Orbital Tumors, by Patricia Tretter, in Chapter 12.)

Radon seeds were used in the past, but this therapy should be avoided if possible as some of the gamma rays may reach the lens, with the seeds remaining active for many years even though the persisting radioactivity is weak. Large, progressive hemangiomas that do not respond to sclerosing solutions or to carbon dioxide snow, and for which surgery is not indicated, are the exception (Fig. 8–34). The radiosensitivity of these tumors permits the use of rather small doses of x ray. This, coupled with improved modern x-ray techniques for precise delivery of the x rays, minimizes the possibility of undesirable sequelae.

A single dose of 250–300 r in air may be sufficient to start regression of the hemangioma, although a second dose is sometimes required. The treatment factors are 80 kv, focal skin distance 15–20 cm, half value layer from 1–2 mm Al.

Surgery. Surgery is seldom indicated since these hemangiomas are usually diffuse with considerable skin involvement. Even if no skin is involved, when an attempt is made to excise a seemingly localized tumor it is usually found to be diffuse and void of a capsule. I believe that growth may even be accelerated after such an attempt.

Chemotherapy. In three described cases of infantile hemangioma of the orbit and ocular adnexa, the natural course toward involution was accelerated by systemic corticosteroid therapy.[27]

KAPOSI'S SARCOMA

This peculiar disease cannot be classified accurately. The basic pathologic changes are anastomosing capillaries (Fig. 8–35) with endothelial proliferation which is associated with interstitial spindle cells. These cells may dominate the picture, suggesting the structure of a fibrosarcoma. Conversely, the lesion may resemble a cavernous hemangioma.[17] One or more bluish to red skin nodules or a maculopapular eruption on the extremities heralds the onset of the disease. As it progresses, primarily affecting the face, such nodules sometimes occur on the lids.

In a review of Kaposi's sarcoma involving the eyelids and conjunctiva,[39] the palpebral conjunctiva was found to be the most commonly affected. The authors described a case involving only the bulbar conjunctiva.

Kaposi's sarcoma may be associated with lymphoma or leukemia[23,37,48,54,59] as well as anemia and thrombocytopenia.

PYOGENIC GRANULOMA

The term *pyogenic granuloma* is usually applied to excessive and often recurrent granulation tissue on cutaneous and mucous membrane surfaces, associated with inflammation (chalazion, hordeolum) or a sequela of surgical repair (squint operation) or trauma. It seems to be an abnormal response to the stimulus for repair, similar to the keloid tendency. "Proud flesh" is the lay term for this exuberant proliferation. The condition is

FIG. 8–33. Location of usual main afferent vessels supplying hemangiomas in and around the iris. Branches of the lacrimal, frontal, and facial arteries course over the rim of the orbit. If such an artery supplying a hemangioma is palpable, the sclerosing solution should be injected in and around it.

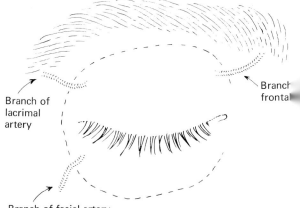

Branch of lacrimal artery

Branch frontal

Branch of facial artery

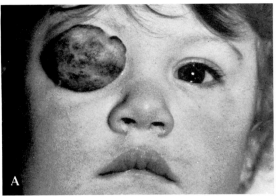

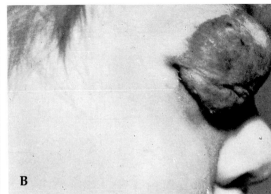

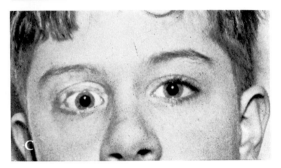

FIG. 8–34. Extensive hemangioma of the lids. **A.** The large diffuse lesion completely covers the eye. **B.** Profile view. **C.** Result after treatment consisting of radon seeds inserted in the tumor and later excision of the redundant skin.

FIG. 8–35. Kaposi's sarcoma. A 63-year-old man, known to have had the disease for 11 years, complained of persistent tearing of the left eye of one-year duration. A painless nodular mass over the left lacrimal sac was removed by dacryocystectomy. Histologic examination confirmed the diagnosis of Kaposi's sarcoma.

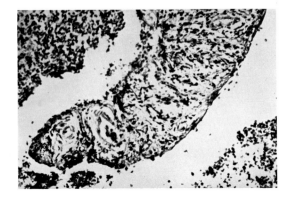

sometimes diagnosed clinically and histopathologically as a hemangioma. In one reported case[18] diagnosis of the lesion as a squamous-cell carcinoma led to enucleation.

Histologically, the granulation tissue is infiltrated with inflammatory cells. So rich is the capillary element that hemangioma is suggested.

TELANGIECTASES

Telangiectases of the skin of the lids, usually congenital, appear as purple discolorations caused by dilatation of the superficial dermal vessels. The condition is also known as nevus flammeus and port-wine stain. It may appear independently elsewhere but it is usually a feature of Sturge-Weber disease. Telangiectasis of the retina is described under Coats's disease.

Rendu-Osler-Weber Disease

Patients with this hereditary and familial condition have multiple telangiectatic tumors —in the skin, the mucous membranes of the nasal and oral cavities, and the intestinal tract. They have a history of repeated hemorrhages, usually epistaxis. Involvement of the conjunctiva and skin of the lids is comparatively rare. Eye signs of this disease include retinal hemorrhages associated with degeneration of the elastic fibers in the arterioles of the retina, choroid, and lamina vitrea. A possible relationship to Coats's disease and also to pseudoxanthoma and angioid streaks of the retina has been suggested.

Senile

Multiple small foci of acquired telangiectasis in the upper layers of the corium of the skin (sometimes called strawberry hemangiomas) or the conjunctiva are common senile manifestations. They usually consist of one or more very tortuous vessels of different caliber. Some authorities regard the lesions as real tumors, and others look on them as mere passive ectasia of the venous part of the capillaries.

HEMANGIOLYMPHANGIOMA

Coexistence of a hemangioma and a lymphangioma, sometimes called a hemangiolymphangioma, is not surprising in view of the common genesis of blood and lymph vessels.

VARICES

Varices of the orbit may produce intermittent exophthalmos. In two reported cases there was radiographic evidence of localized orbital varices, present at birth in one and not detected until the third decade in the other.[49] In one case the varix was demonstrated by orbital venogaphy, and in the other orbital phleboliths were conspicuous in the plain film. Other causes of intermittent exophthalmos include orbital varices with intracranial extension, and arteriovenous malformations. In a review of 133 cases of postural intermittent exophthalmos,[47] the abnormality in all but one was an orbital venous varix communicating with the cavernous sinus through the superior orbital fissure.

MONOMORPHOUS HEMANGIOMAS (ANGIOSARCOMAS)

The orbit may harbor hemangioendotheliomas and hemangiopericytomas as well as leiomyomas and leiomyosarcomas, all of which are grouped under angiosarcomas. To my knowledge no benign polymorphous hemangioma has ever become malignant.

HEMANGIOPERICYTOMA

A hemangiopericytoma is composed predominantly of cells derived from the pericytes—primitive mesenchymal cells which are found in the walls of small blood vessels. In the orbit, the tumors grow in a circumscribed fashion and metastasis is rare, although at other body sites they may be locally aggressive with a 20%–25% incidence of metastasis.

The pericytes are contractile but have no myofibrils, and are assumed to have some relationship to smooth muscle cells. In contrast, the proliferating endothelial cells in a hemangioendothelioma are inside the reticulum sheath of the vessel wall (Fig. 8–36). It is often necessary to employ silver reticulin

FIG. 8–36. Hemangioendothelioma of the lid demonstrating the intraluminal proliferation of endothelial cells.

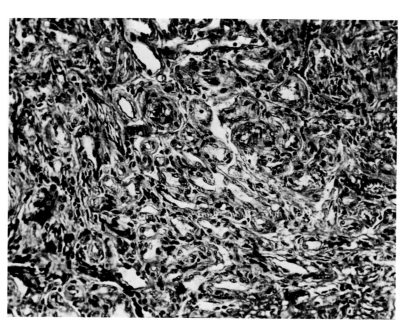

stains to appreciate the lesion's structure. Round or spindle-shaped cells are found around the proliferating capillaries (Fig. 8–37).

Hemangiopericytomas may be benign or malignant. The difficulty in differentiating them from vascular meningiomas, based on the histologic appearance and staining characteristics, has been stressed.[71] Six in a series of 285 such lesions occurring in soft tissues over the body were in the orbit; 14% of the 285 were known to have metastasized.[59] It is imperative to remove the tumor completely, without rupturing the capsule, at first surgery. Small remaining portions may cause a re-

currence[29] with the resulting growth infiltrating the orbital tissues, perhaps leading to exenteration. Invasion of the orbital bones[24] or the cranial cavity[67] can be fatal. A hemangiopericytoma of the right lid in a 68-year-old woman had invaded both orbits, the nose, the sinuses, and the anterior cranial fossa.[43]

FIG. 8–37. Hemangiopericytoma of the outer canthus. The tumor, noted for three months in a 50-year-old man, was excised. Histologic examination showed atypical hemangiopericytoma **(A)** especially well seen by the silver stain **(B)**.

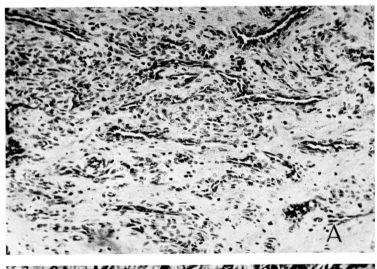

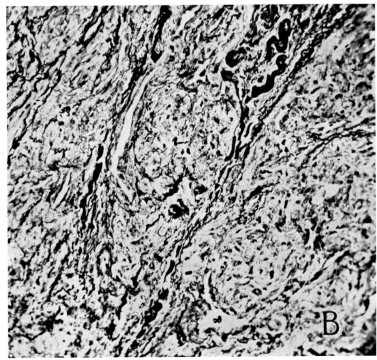

An interesting form is the neuromyoarterial glomus tumor with its congeries of blood vessels and nonmyelinated nerve fibers. The vessel walls are thick due to several layers of plump pericytes. In a reported case, a tumor of the choroid contained glomus cells and had some characteristics of a hemangiopericytoma.[5] Angiomatosis retinae (von Hippel–Lindau disease) has been considered a type of glomus tumor.

The glomus tumor is a caricature of the normal neuromyoarterial glomus found especially in the fingers and toes. This highly specialized structure shunts the arterial blood into the veins without passing it through the capillaries. It is an organoid growth which features pericytes, whereas most hemangiopericytomas are nonorganoid. Sometimes the two types are combined. Although usually sharply circumscribed, the glomus tumor can infiltrate but does not metastasize.

Since these cells have been identified in the uvea, glomus tumors can theoretically occur there. In one case such a tumor in the lid did not cause pain but was sensitive to touch; it recurred twice after excision.[33]

Hemangiopericytoma of the orbit is best treated by excision. As there is no capsule or surrounding cleavage plane, only a wide excision will extend beyond tumor tissue.

HEMANGIOENDOTHELIOMA

A hemangioendothelioma stems from endothelial cells. Its histologic characteristics are a) the formation of small anastomosing vascular channels outlined by a delicate framework of reticulin fibers, and b) growth of more atypical embryonic endothelial cells than are required to line the channels.

Silver reticulin stain helps to clarify the tumor's features: the tubes stand out in sharp relief because even in malignant lesions each one has a delicate fibrous supporting framework of reticulum. An aid to identification is the predominance of proliferating endothelial cells inside of the lumina, which are outlined by the reticulum sheaths. As previously mentioned, in a hemangiopericytoma the proliferation occurs outside the reticulum sheath.

In a series of 18 hemangioendotheliomas in soft tissues over the body, one was primary in the lid in a 17-year-old girl (Fig. 8–38, see p. 28), and another was primary in the orbit in a 40-year-old woman. Both tumors recurred repeatedly after excision. Of the other 16

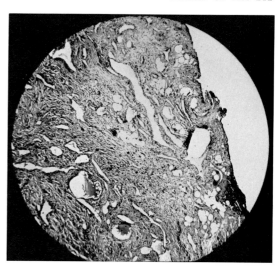

FIG. 8–39. Lymphangioma of the inner canthus. A mass on the right inner canthus and bridge of the nose in a 6-year-old boy was first noted at age 1. It had been removed twice, recurring each time.

patients, 10 were known to have died of metastases, 4 had no evidence of tumor 8, 12, 30, and 62 months after removal, and 2 were lost to follow-up.[68]

In a series of 181 hemangioendotheliomas, 111 were benign and 70 were malignant.[70] Of the malignant group, 11% metastasized. This investigator apparently included the hypertrophic hemangiomas of infants in the benign group.

A hemangioendothelioma of the choroid in a 3-year-old caused retinal detachment and led to enucleation of the eye for suspected retinoblastoma.[41]

Malignant hemangioendotheliomas are also best treated by complete and wide excision.

LEIOMYOMA AND LEIOMYOSARCOMA

Developing from the smooth muscle of large veins, these solitary tumors project either into the lumen or outside the vessel wall. Vascular leiomyomas may be difficult to distinguish from venous hemangiomas. The smooth muscle in venous hemangiomas thickens the vascular walls but maintains its proper relationship to the lumen. However, the smooth muscle predominates in vascular leiomyomas, and is often found paralleling the vessel's long axis.

LYMPHANGIOMAS OF THE CONJUNCTIVA, LID, AND ORBIT

(Fig. 8–39; Fig. 8–40, see p. 28)
Lymphangiomas are congenital benign vascular tumors that progress slowly. There seems to be no justification for classifying them into capillary, cavernous, and other types, as is done with hemangiomas. The clinical descriptive term *elephantiasis* should be avoided as it includes not only true lymphangiomas but also acquired conditions due to stasis in lymph vessels or to tissue edema. Hemorrhagic lymphangioma is some times used to designate lesions with prominent elements of hemorrhage into the lymphovascular spaces.

Incidence and Age of Onset

In a series of 62 cases of lymphangioma involving the ocular adnexa[31] 22 were in the conjunctiva (35%). Unlike such lesions elsewhere, they were first noted at the average age of 25 years. Some no doubt represented the rather common lymphangiectases and were therefore not true lymphangiomas.

Lid lesions, unquestionably true lymphangiomas, accounted for 11 cases in this series (18%) and were first noted at the average age of 2 years. In this category were cases involving the conjunctiva and face as well as the lid. Orbital lesions (29 cases or 47%) included those also affecting the lid, conjunctiva, and face. Although the average age of onset was slightly over 6 years, the tumor was first manifest in three patients from 27 to 44 years old. This author[31] suggested that an important factor in the sudden expansion of ocular lymphangiomas might be the dialyzing effect of the thin endothelial wall in the presence of blood; a similar effect is noted in the so-called subdural hematoma.

Orbital and lid lymphangiomas tend to be occult until the sudden onset of hemorrhage, usually in young people, leads to detection.[58] When the hemorrhage occurs in the orbit, the eye may protrude at an alarming rate. If the hemorrhage is relatively superficial, it appears almost black, due to static, nonaerated blood and hemosiderin. Because of this color, melanoma may be suspected (Fig. 8–41, 8–42).

Lymphangiectases are sometimes visible under the bulbar conjunctiva. When filled with blood they appear dark or even black, and show a linear pattern conforming to the direction of the lymph channels. Also, the slit lamp may reveal a fluid line separating the lymph from the blood. In five reported cases the conjunctival lymphatics were filled with blood.[2]

Sites

Thirteen of the tumors in the aforementioned 62 cases[31] were confined to the orbit. In 11 other orbital cases there was also involvement of the lids or conjunctiva. Five patients had a lymphangioma involving the orbit, lids, conjunctiva, and face; 3 of the 5 also had a lymphangioma of the palate. All 29 patients had exophthalmos, which in 6 of them was either intermittent or variable. In 2 of these 6 the increase was associated with coryza, in 1 with the menses, in 1 with crying, and another showed a postural increase. Of the 6 patients whose orbital lymphangioma was as-

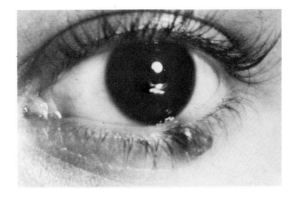

FIG. 8–41. Lymphangioma with dark blood cyst simulating a melanoma. The nature of the tumor on the lower lid of a 17-year-old girl was established on histologic examination after excision.

FIG. 8–42. Lymphangioma of the upper lid. A dark hemorrhage in the lesion makes it resemble a melanoma.

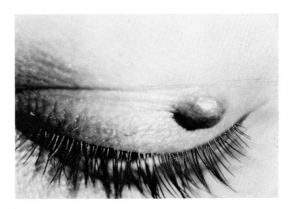

sociated with ecchymosis or hemorrhage, 1 had intermittent external hemorrhages from the conjunctiva.

Proptosis and muscle imbalance were the most common complications of orbital lymphangiomas, and ptosis of the upper lid was the next most common (Fig. 8–43, see p. 28). Two cases of lymphangioma of the limbus in children were neglected for several years, as their seriousness was not recognized.[72] The cystlike lesions grew slowly, gradually encircling the limbus and extending into the orbit. As the proptosis progressed, the patients had recurrent hemorrhages into the tumors.

Pathology

The orbital lymphangiomas in the aforementioned series[31] were difficult to delineate as to gross pathologic characteristics because the majority were cystic in some portion, and collapse of the cyst during surgery altered the gross appearance. If the cystic portion did not contain blood, the lesion was often not recognized until the cyst was inadvertently opened, with escape of clear or straw-colored fluid. When the lesions contained new blood or, more commonly, old degenerated blood, a blood cyst could be recognized very early but could seldom be removed intact. Most gross specimens therefore consisted only of a cyst wall. The lymphocytic element varied widely, but heavy infiltration with lymph follicles was common.

Lymphangiomas are most often confused with hemangiomas, especially if the previously described endothelium-lined spaces contain red blood cells. If the spaces are small and inconspicuous and there is a large lymphocytic element, the diagnosis may be nonspecific granuloma. When the endothelium has been lost from the lining of the spaces, and degenerated blood is found, the diagnosis of blood cyst or organized hematoma is often made. In general, lymphangioma is suggested in cases manifesting endothelium-lined spaces varying in size and containing lymphocytes in the stroma.

Diagnosis

Lymphangiomas of the conjunctiva, lid or orbit are usually easily diagnosed; their nature may be suggested by ipsilateral lymphangiomas of the face, nasal cavity, paranasal sinuses, or palate. Clinically, the lesion is usually marked by slow progression during the patient's growing years. Complications, chiefly repeated hemorrhages into the lesion, may provide valuable clues to the correct diagnosis. In the presence of an upper respiratory infection, the lymphoid tissue which is a common component of the lymphangioma becomes involved in the inflammatory process; the lesion is then more likely to become apparent to the patient or his family. This sequence is characteristic of lymphangioma cases.

Orbital lymphangiomas without lid or conjunctival involvement can be suspected but probably not diagnosed until the orbit is explored surgically. The presence of a blood cyst suggests a cystic orbital lymphangioma, usually confirmed by microscopic examination of the cyst wall.

Spontaneous hemorrhage into a lymphangioma causes sudden swelling and redness. Sometimes the hemorrhage is precipitated by trauma (Fig. 8–44). Its absorption may lead to neovascularization, eventually making the lesion resemble a hemangioma. The association of trauma with an orbital blood cyst may lead the surgeon to drain the cyst without removing the wall for study; in this way some cystic lymphangiomas go undiagnosed.

Treatment

Treatment of lymphangiomas is not satisfactory. They grow slowly so that repeated drainage of hematomas, with or without partial excisions and plastic repair, may be carried out over a period of years. Since the tumor is diffuse and nonencapsulated, it does not lend itself to clean excision. This is especially true of deep lymphangiomas in the lid and in the orbit; indeed, ill-advised attempts at complete surgical removal may greatly damage the orbital structures. When the orbit is explored by a Krönlein approach, the presence of blood cysts resembling a bunch of Concord grapes may lead to the suspicion of an orbital lymphangioma. The cysts should be drained of their dark blood and a pressure dressing applied. This type of drainage may have to be done two or even three times.

Recurrent exophthalmos with ecchymosis indicates hemorrhage into the lymphangiomatous spaces which sometimes absorbs spontaneously. Occasionally, however, the hemorrhage is followed by a slow, steadily progressing exophthalmos. This may result from the breakdown of blood and imbibition

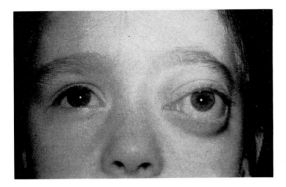

FIG. 8–44. Lymphangioma of the orbit with a blood cyst. An exophthalmos was noted following trauma to the left eye. At surgery a blood cyst was found to be part of a lymphangioma.

FIG. 8–45. Lymphangioma of the skin of the upper lid, conjunctiva and temple. A dark cystic birthmark in a 34-year-old man became much less noticeable after three desiccating treatments with electrocautery at four-month intervals.

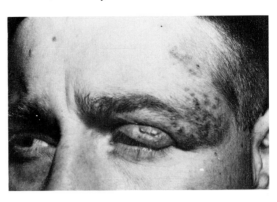

of fluid by dialysis, similar to that observed in chronic subdural hematoma. Such patients often do well after simple drainage of the blood cyst.

Treatment by radiation or sclerosing solutions is generally inadequate, although radiation might be effective for lesions with a heavy lymphocytic infiltration.

Electrocautery desiccating current has proved useful in treating superficial hemangiomas of the skin and conjunctiva, particularly the diffuse type containing black static blood (Fig. 8–45). The needle should be long enough to reach the tumor through multiple punctures 2 to 3 mm apart. When the lesion has shrunk, the electrocautery is stopped. One or two more treatments may be given at two- or three-month intervals if needed.

Prognosis

The literature holds scant information on the eventual outcome of lymphangiomas of the ocular adnexa. Some lesions show little or no change after the patients become adults.

REFERENCES

1. Ashton N: Primary tumours of the iris. Br J Ophthalmol 48:650–668, 1964
2. Awdry P: Lymphangiectasia haemorrhagica conjunctivae. Br J Ophthalmol 53:274–278, 1969
3. Baghdassarian SA, Spencer WH: Pseudoangioma of the iris—its association with melanoma. Arch Ophthalmol 82:69–71, 1969
4. Bailey OT, Ford R: Sclerosing hemangiomas of the central nervous system; progressive tissue changes in hemangioblastomas of brain and in so-called angioblastic meningiomas. Am J Pathol 18:1–27, 1942
5. Berard-Badier Mme, Laffargue P, Farnarier G: Tumeur choroidienne d'un type glomique particulier. Ann Ocul (Paris) 201:1005–1016, 1968
6. Blodi F: Naevus flammeus faciei und Glaukom ohne Vergrösserung des Bulbus. Ophthalmologica 117:82–89, 1949
7. Bonnet P, Dechaume J, Blanc E: L'anévrysme cirsoïde de la rétine (anévrysme racemeux); ses relations avec l'anévrysme cirsoïde de la face et avec l'anévrysme cirsoïde du cerveau. J Med Lyon 18:165–178, 1937
8. Bruck C: Rare tumors of the iris and ciliary body. II. Hemangioma simplex of the ciliary body. Klin Monatsbl Augenheilkd 154:49–51, 1969
9. Caron J-P, Le Besnerais Y, Comoy J, Careul N, Houdart, R: Discussion des voies d'abord de l'orbite, dans les cas d'exophtalmies neurochirurgicales. Neurochirurgie 14:843–854, 1968
10. Coats G: Forms of retinal disease with massive exudation. Roy Lond Ophthal Hosp Rep 17:440–525, 1907–1908
11. Coats G: Retinitis exudativa (retinitis haemorrhagica externa). Arch Ophthalmol 81:275–327, 1912
12. Darr JL, Hughes RP, McNair JN: Bilateral peripapillary retinal hemangiomas. Arch Ophthalmol 75:77–81, 1966
13. DeLima LJ, Penzholz H: A case of intermittent exophthalmos. J Neurol Neurosurg Psychiat 31:81–84, 1968
14. Duke-Elder S: System of Ophthalmology, Vol IX, Diseases of the uveal tract. St Louis, CV Mosby, 1966, p 808

15. DUKE-ELDER S: System of Ophthalmology, Vol X, Diseases of the retina. St Louis, CV Mosby, 1967, p 166

16. DUKE JR, WOODS AC: Coats's disease. II. Studies on the identity of the lipids concerned, and the probable role of mucopolysaccharides in its pathogenesis. Br J Opthalmol 47:413–434, 1963

17. DUTZ W, STOUT AP: Kaposi's sarcoma in infants and children. Cancer 13:684–694, 1960

18. FERRY AP, ZIMMERMAN LE: Granuloma pyogenicum of limbus. Arch Ophthalmol 74:229–230, 1965

19. FRENKEL M: Retinal angiomatosis in a patient with neurofibromatosis. Am J Ophthalmol 63:804–808, 1967

20. FUCHS E: Aneurysma arterio-venosum retinae. Arch Augenheilkd 11:440–444, 1882

21. GASS JDM: Cavernous hemangioma of the retina; a neuro-oculo-cutaneous syndrome. Am J Ophthalmol 71:799–814, 1971

22. GAUTIER-SMITH PC, SANDERS MD, SANDERSON KV: Ocular and nervous system involvement in angioma serpiginosum. Br J Ophthalmol 55:433–443, 1971

23. GELLIN GA: Kaposi's sarcoma: three cases of which two have unusual findings in association. Arch Dermatol 94:92–94, 1966

24. GOODMAN SA: Hemangiopericytoma of the orbit. Am J Ophthalmol 40:237–243, 1955

25. GREEN WR: Bilateral Coats's disease; massive gliosis of the retina. Arch Ophthalmol 77:378–383, 1967

26. HAMBURG A: Iris melanoma with vascular proliferation simulating a hemangioma. Arch Ophthalmol 82:72–76, 1969

27. HILES DA, PILCHARD WA: Corticosteroid control of neonatal hemangiomas of the orbit and ocular adnexa. Am J Ophthalmol 71:1003–1008, 1971

28. IMRE G: Coats's disease and hyperlipemic retinitis. Am J Ophthalmol 64:726–728, 1967

29. JAKOBIEC FA, HOWARD GM, JONES IS, WOLFF M: Hemangiopericytoma of the orbit. Am J Ophthalmol 78:816–834, 1974

30. JESBERG DO, SPENCER WH, HOYT WF: Incipient lesions of von Hippel–Lindau disease. Arch Ophthalmol 80:632–640, 1968

31. JONES IS: Lymphangiomas of the ocular adnexa; an analysis of 62 cases. Trans Am Ophthalmol Soc 57:602–665, 1959

32. JONES IS, CLEASBY GW: Hemangioma of the choroid: a clinicopathologic analysis. Am J Ophthalmol 48:612–628, 1959

33. KIRBY DB: Neuromyoarterial glomus tumor in the eyelid. Arch Ophthalmol 25:228–237, 1941

34. KRABBE KH: Facial and meningeal angiomatosis associated with calcifications of the brain cortex. Arch Neurol Psychiat 32:737–755, 1934

35. KRUG EF, SAMUELS B: Venous angioma of the retina, optic nerve, chiasm and brain. Arch Ophthalmol 8:871–879, 1932

36. LAMPE I, LATOURETTE HB: Management of cavernous hemangiomas in infants. Postgrad Med 19:262–270, 1956

37. LAW IP: Kaposi sarcoma and plasma cell dyscrasia. JAMA 229:1329–1331, 1974

38. LEBER T: Über eine durch Vorkommen multipler Miliaraneurysmen charakterisierte Form von Retinaldegeneration. Graefes Arch Klin Ophthalmol 81:1–14, 1912

39. LIEBERMAN PH, LLOVERA IN: Kaposi's sarcoma of the bulbar conjunctiva. Arch Ophthalmol 88:44–45, 1972

40. LINDAU A: Studien ueber die Kleinhirncysten. Acta Pathol Microbiol Scand (Suppl) 1:1–128, 1926

41. LISTER A, MORGAN G: Choroidal haemangio-endothelioma. Br J Ophthalmol 47:215–221, 1963

42. LLOYD GAS, WRIGHT JE, MORGAN G: Venous malformations in the orbit. Br J Ophthalmol 55:505–516, 1971

43. MACOUL KL: Hemangiopericytoma of the lid and orbit. Am J Ophthalmol 66:731–733, 1968

44. MACRAE HM, NEWBIGIN MB: Von Hippel Lindau disease; a family history. Can J Ophthalmol 3:28–34, 1968

45. MANSCHOT WA: Juxtapapillary retinal angiomatosis. Arch Ophthalmol 80:775–776, 1968

46. MANSCHOT WA, DEBRUIJN WC: Coats's disease: definition and pathogenesis. Br J Ophthalmol 51:145–157, 1967

47. MAYFIELD FH, WILSON CB: The pathological basis for postural exophthalmos; case report. J Neurosurg 26:619–623, 1967

48. MAZZAFERRI EL, PENN GM: Kaposi's sarcoma associated with multiple myeloma. Arch Intern Med 122:521–525, 1968

49. McCORD CD, SPITALNY LA: Localized orbital varices; two cases with radiographic findings. Arch Ophthalmol 80:455–460, 1968

50. MORALES AG: Coats's disease; natural history and results of treatment. Am J Ophthalmol 60:855–865, 1965

51. MORGAN WE III, CRAWFORD JB: Retinitis pigmentosa and Coats's disease. Arch Ophthalmol 79:146–149, 1968

52. NAIDOFF MA, KENYON KR, GREEN WR: Iris hemangioma and abnormal retinal vasculature in a case of diffuse congenital hemangiomatosis. Am J Ophthalmol 72:633–644, 1971

53. NIRANKARI MS, SINGH D: Pedunculated hemangiomas of conjunctiva; a report of two cases. Am J Ophthalmol 52:266–268, 1962

54. O'BRIEN PH, BRASFIELD RD: Kaposi's sarcoma. Cancer 19:1497–1502, 1966

55. OKSALA A, LINDGREN I, AHLAS A: Haemangioma of the ciliary body. Br J Ophthalmol 48:669–672, 1964

56. PRASAD GN, VERMA BB: Pedunculated hemangioma: report of a case. Ann Ophthalmol 3:1289–1290, 1971

57. REESE AB: Telangiectasis of the retina and Coats's disease. Am J Ophthalmol 42:1–8, 1956

58. REESE AB, HOWARD GM: Unusual manifestations of ocular lymphangioma and lymphangiectasis. Survey Ophthalmol 18:226–231, 1973

59. REYNOLDS WA, WINDELMANN RK, SOULE EH: Kaposi's sarcoma. Medicine 44:419–443, 1956

60. SAEBO JA: Von Hippel–Lindau's disease. Acta Ophthalmol (Kbh) 30:129–165, 1952

61. SCHEPENS CL, SCHWARTZ A: Intraocular tumors: bilateral hemangioma of the choroid. Arch Ophthalmol 58:477–482, 1958

62. SCHIECK F: Das Peritheliom der Netzhautzentralgefässe, ein bislang unbekanntes Krankheitsbild. Graefes Arch Klin Ophthalmol 81:328–339, 1912

63. SELLORS PJH, ARCHER D: The management of retinal angiomatosis. Trans Ophthalmol Soc UK 89:529–543, 1969

64. Sidler-Huguenin H: Ein Endotheliom am Sehnervenkopf. Graefes Arch Klin Ophthalmol 101: 113–122, 1919–1920

65. Small RG: Coats's disease and muscular dystrophy. Trans Am Acad Ophthalmol Otolaryngol 72:225–231, 1968

66. Souders BF: Juxtapapillary hemangioendothelioma of the retina. Arch Ophthalmol 41:178–182, 1949

67. Spaeth EB, Valdes-Dapena A: Hemangiopericytoma. Arch Ophthalmol 60:1070–1073, 1958

68. Stout AP: Hemangio-endothelioma; a tumor of blood vessels featuring vascular endothelial cells. Ann Surg 118:445–464, 1943

69. Stout AP: Hemangiopericytoma. Cancer 2:1027–1054, 1949

70. Stout AP: Tumors of the blood and lymphatic vessels. In Pack GT, Ariel IM (eds): Treatment of Cancer and Allied Diseases, Vol 8, Tumors of the soft somatic tissues and bone, 2nd ed. New York, Hoeber-Harper, 1964, Ch 9a, pp 130–178

71. Sugar HS, Fishman GR, Kobernick S, Goodman P: Orbital hemangiopericytoma or vascular meningioma. Am J. Ophthalmol 70:103–109, 1970

72. Swan KC, Emmens TH, Christensen L: Experiences with tumors of the limbus. Trans Am Acad Ophthalmol Otolaryngol 52:458–469, 1947–1948

73. Theron J, Newton TH, Hoyt WF: Unilateral retinocephalic vascular malformations. Neuroradiology 7:185–196, 1974

74. Tuovinen E: Pedunculated malignant melanoma of the conjunctiva with bloody tears. Acta Ophthalmol (Kbh) 40:149–152, 1962

75. Vail D: Angiomatosis retinae: 11 years after diathermy coagulation. Trans Am Ophthalmol Soc 55:217–238, 1957

76. Watson AG, Campbell JS, Tolnal G, Hill DP: Pedunculated malignant melanoma of conjunctiva. Can J Ophthalmol 5:386–391, 1970

77. White FP: Haemorrhage from the conjunctiva: notes on a case of capillary angioma. Br J Ophthalmol 29:635–637, 1945

77a. Wise GN, Dollery CT, Henkind P: Retinal Circulation. New York, Harper & Row, 1971, p 260

78. Witmer R, Verrey F, Speiser P: Retinal angiomatosis; atypical cases of retinal angiomatosis and telangiectases. Bibl Ophthalmol 76:113–123, 1968

79. Witschel H, Font RL: Survey Ophthalmol (in press)

80. Wolper J, Laibson PR: Hereditary hemorrhagic telangiectasis (Rendu-Osler-Weber disease) with filamentary keratitis. Arch Ophthalmol 81:272–277, 1969

81. Woods AC, Duke JR: Coats's disease. I. Review of the literature, diagnostic criteria, clinical findings, and plasma lipid studies. Br J Ophthalmol 47:385–412, 1963

82. Wyburn-Mason R: Arteriovenous aneurysm of midbrain and retina, facial naevi and mental changes. Brain 66:163–203, 1943

82a. Yanoff M, Fine BS: Ocular Pathology: A text and atlas. Hagerstown, Harper & Row, 1975, p 30

83. Zak FG: An expanded concept of tumors of glomic tissue. New York J Med 54:1153–1165, 1954

84. Zaubermann H, Feinsod M: Orbital hemangioma growth during pregnancy. Acta Ophthalmol (Kbh) 48:929–933, 1970

9

LEIOMYOMA

A leiomyoma or a leiomyosarcoma may arise from smooth muscle in the ciliary body, the iris, the orbit, and the media of blood vessels. This smooth muscle is mesodermal except in the iris, where the lesion arises from the dilator and sphincter muscles, which are neuroectodermal. Smooth-muscle tumors may also arise at sites where smooth muscle is not normally found.

In a reported case, a leiomyoma arose from the anterior surface of the iris near its root.[19] The author felt that it had no connection with the dilator or sphincter muscles or with the pigment epithelium. He concluded that the tumor originated from the stromal cells of the embryonic uvea, possibly misplaced cells that would ordinarily have formed part of the ciliary muscle. Mesenchymomas, occurring at any site, may have abundant smooth muscle. Leiomyomas may therefore be neuroectodermal; or they may be mesodermal, arising at any site from embryonic rests or mesodermal cells destined to form smooth muscle.

Leiomyomas without doubt occur in the ciliary body and iris, but most published cases have not been well enough documented to be accepted unequivocally. Among the pathologic characteristics that must be present to justify the diagnosis are a) a structure of interlacing, closely packed bundles of elongated, spindle-shaped cells; b) long oval nuclei that tend toward a palisade arrangement; c) granular eosinophilic cytoplasm of the cells; and d) myoglial fibrils. However, one investigator has suggested that such fibrils are present in neurinomas and therefore not pathognomonic of a myogenic tumor.[3] His belief that the very similar myogenic and neurogenic tumors can be differentiated only with the thionine inclusion stain supports the view that demonstration of myoglia is insufficient to confirm the diagnosis. The diagnosis can usually be confirmed by electron microscopy, as described in the section Electron Microscopy of Tumors of the Eye and Ocular Adnexa, by Ramon L. Font, in Chapter 12.

Demonstration of the myoglial fibrils (Fig. 9–1D, see p. 29), the most important criterion, is unfortunately lacking in most reported cases. The myoglial fibrils can be identified with the Mallory phosphotungstic acid hematoxylin stain, the Masson trichrome stain, or the gold impregnation stain. All these stains show longitudinal striations made up of fine, discrete fibrils along the body of the cell which tend to coalesce or fuse, forming larger and coarser fibrils at the cell terminal.

In contrast to the other so-called spindle-cell tumors, the myoma cells in leiomyomas are truly spindle shaped. On the other hand, cells of the uveal spindle-cell melanomas are seldom if ever distinctly spindle-shaped. They terminate in, or send off laterally, several ill-defined processes which join with neighboring cells and in this way form a more definite syncytium.[19]

A leiomyoma that is malignant, particularly after repeated attempts at excision, is less differentiated than when in the benign state. A tumor that does not fulfill the criteria for leiomyoma may nevertheless be a poorly differentiated leiomyoma or leiomyosarcoma. In one case the orbital leiomyoma presumably originated in Mueller's muscle; the first specimen was typical of this type of tumor, but this appearance was less marked with each of several recurrences and it finally resembled a sarcoma.[16]

LEIOMYOMA OF THE IRIS

(See also Ch. 2, 7 and 9)

In a study of 145 primary tumors of the iris, 21 were grouped as leiomyomas, 4 of them malignant. There were no deaths among the 21 cases.[1] These authors concluded that the tumors are invasive but not metastasizing.

Since the tumors have a common neuroecto-dermal ancestry, their histologic features may overlap, making clear-cut classifications difficult. For this reason, one author questioned the validity of most if not all published cases of leiomyoma of the iris.[3]

Although such tumors may be well localized and even somewhat pedunculated, they are more often rather diffuse and flat with a predilection for the pupillary half of the iris. They not infrequently infiltrate the iris stroma and tend to spread along the iris surface, even into the angle. A 28-year-old woman had always been aware of a discoloration and nodules partially encircling the pupillary margin of the left iris. Examination revealed glaucoma with cupping of the disc. An increase in size of the lesion led to enucleation (Fig. 9–2, see p. 30). Such tumors are cohesive with no evidence of disseminated tumor cells or implantation growths. The 30 to 50 age group is generally affected.

Some ectropion uveae over the tumor area is a common feature. A 46-year-old woman who had had regular eye examinations noted an iris lesion which doubled in size in six months, leading to enucleation (Fig. 9–1, see p. 29). It was suggested that the ectropion uveae in this and similar cases might be due to some contractility retained by the modified smooth-muscle fibers.[8]

The tumor is usually lightly pigmented and as a rule benign, as shown by the morphologic characteristics of the cells, the absence of mitoses, and reported cases of long duration with slow growth. For instance, in one patient a considerable portion of the tumor was left when excision was attempted but there was no appreciable growth for 16 years.[19] Another patient followed for 20 years showed no tumor growth.[6]

A reported case of pigmented leiomyoma of the iris had some characteristics of a neurofibroma.[7] This finding was attributed to the nature of the iris smooth muscle where both the sphincter and dilator muscles originate in the neuroectoderm. The sphincter seems to be fully differentiated into muscle cells, is nonpigmented, and could presumably give rise to a pure leiomyoma. But since the dilator muscle shows only partial differentiation, a leiomyoma rising from this layer could be expected to show both neural and muscular characteristics as well as pigmentation.

The cytologic picture in one case indicated transition from pigment epithelium to smooth muscle.[14] A leiomyoma of the iris containing a variety of tissues including nerve fibers was considered to be a mixed tumor arising from multipotential cells of the optic vesicle.[17] A 13-year-old boy with invasive leiomyosarcoma of the iris had no recurrence 11 years after enucleation of the eye, necessitated because the lesion was incompletely removed during an iridectomy.[5]

A leiomyoma or a leiomyosarcoma cannot be differentiated clinically from a melanoma. Even histologically there may be transitional cells between melanocytes and smooth muscle. The criteria for treatment are therefore the same. (See Melanoma of the Iris, in Ch. 7.)

Fluorescein angiography has been suggested as a valuable means of establishing the limits of an iris leiomyoma when excision is planned.[15]

It seems clear that we are not dealing with two absolute groups of iris tumors—myogenic and neurogenic—but rather with a blending of the two. The smooth muscle in the iris is believed to originate in cells of the primitive neural plate. Specifically, it arises from the outer layer of the optic vesicle, which is pigment epithelium in the retinal and ciliary portion of the eye and undergoes a transition to smooth muscle in the iris. In view of a neurogenic origin for smooth-muscle cells, tumors arising from this layer may show a muscle pattern, on the one hand, and a neuroepithelial pattern, on the other, with all gradations between.

The neurofibromatous appearance of a case of leiomyoma of the iris has been attributed to partial differentiation of a dilator anlage.[7] Besides the muscle-forming foci there were pigment-containing epithelial areas, and it was believed that such a matrix could combine anlagen of muscular and neural elements. The cells in some of our tissue cultures of iris melanomas seem to lie midway between smooth muscle and neuroepithelium.

If iris neurinomas have been confused with leiomyomas, we must assume a schwannian type of cell, yet the neuroepithelium from which the tumors arose comes from the optic vesicle. We do not believe that Schwann cells originate from such neuroepithelium. By far the larger proportion of Schwann cells are formed from the neural crest. They are also said to migrate directly from the spinal cord of the central nervous system or to stem from the mesoderm. So far as is known, Schwann cells cannot be formed directly from the tissue of the neural plate.

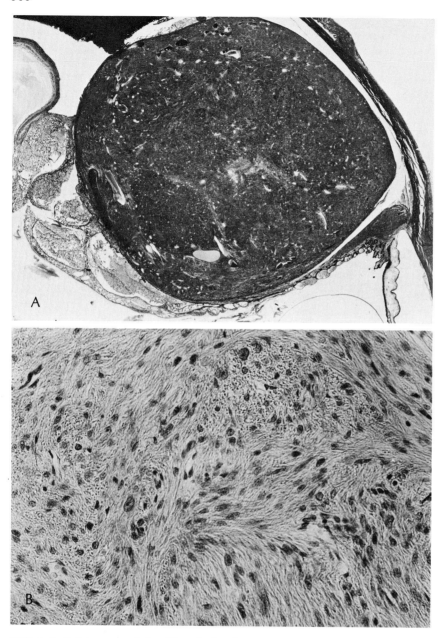

FIG. 9–3. Leiomyoma of the ciliary body. **A.**
Gross appearance. **B.** Interlacing bands of tissue.
Myoglial fibrils are demonstrated by the Masson
trichrome stain. (Courtesy of F. C. Blodi.[2])

LEIOMYOMA OF THE CILIARY BODY

Since the ciliary body has abundant smooth muscle, leiomyomas might be expected more frequently there than in the iris, but the opposite is true. A 1968 report from the Armed Forces Institute of Pathology showed only seven acceptable cases of leiomyoma of the ciliary body in their files. Electron microscopy confirmed the diagnosis based on findings by light microscopy.[12] A lesion of this type was removed by cyclectomy.[11]

Several cases of early myoma of the ciliary muscle have been found incidentally in enucleated eyes. The first case was reported in 1928 by Fuchs.[9] Others were diagnosed on the basis of the morphologic features and the staining reaction[13,18] or the typical appearance of a smooth-muscle tumor.[4] However, myoglia was not demonstrated in any of these cases.

A reported case of leiomyoma of the ciliary body that seems to fulfill the diagnostic criteria[2] appears in Figure 9–3. A 40-year-old woman complained of pain and impaired vision of six months' duration. Clinical examination showed a serous detachment of the retina and a black mass apparently in the ciliary body, seen at the periphery of the fundus, which interfered with transillumination. The clinical diagnosis was melanoma of the ciliary body and the eye was enucleated. Masson's trichrome stain revealed the characteristic purplish smooth-muscle tissue and the presence of myoglial fibrils.

It is probably impossible clinically to diagnose a leiomyoma of the ciliary body. In the early stages its slow growth causes no symptoms. The pigment epithelium, which remains unchanged or may even proliferate, covers the tumor and gives it the dark color seen clinically. It is therefore almost invariably assumed to be a malignant melanoma, and the eye is enucleated.

LEIOMYOMA OF THE ORBIT

Cases of leiomyoma said to arise from Müller's smooth muscle in the lids and orbit can be accepted only with reservations. In one instance this diagnosis was considered "highly suggestive" although the possibility of late metastasis from a uterine tumor could not be excluded.[16] This author believed that some tumors of the eyelids and orbit described as sarcomas were probably leiomyosarcomas.

LEIOMYOMA OF BLOOD VESSEL MEDIA

In one reported case a leiomyoma of the orbit in a 9-year-old girl was thought to have originated from vascular smooth muscle.[10]

REFERENCES

1. Ashton N, Wybar K: Primary tumours of the iris. Proc 2nd Congr European Soc Ophthalmol. Vienna 1964, pp 97–113
2. Blodi FC: Leiomyoma of the ciliary body. Am J Ophthalmol 33: 939–942, 1950
3. Böke W: Zur Kenntnis der gutartigen Iristumoren. Graefes Arch Klin Ophthalmol 157:368–379, 1956
4. Bossalino G: Di una non comune osservazione di leiomioma maligno del corpo ciliare e dell'iride. Boll Ocul 13:332–348, 1934
5. Dugmore WN: 11-year follow up of a case of iris leiomyosarcoma. Br J Ophthalmol 56:366–367, 1972
6. Ellett EC: (a) Leiomyoma and (b) hematoma of the iris. Arch Ophthalmol 21:497–504, 1939
7. Fleming N: A case of pigmented leiomyoma of the iris. Br J Ophthalmol 32:885–892, 1948
8. Frost AD: Leiomyoma of the iris. Am J Ophthalmol 20:347–353, 1937
9. Fuchs E: Ueber den Ciliarmuskel. Graefes Arch Klin Ophthalmol 120:733–742, 1928
10. Henderson JW, Harrison EG, Jr: Vascular leiomyoma of the orbit: report of a case. Trans Am Acad Ophthalmol Otolaryngol 74:970–974, 1970
11. Lowe RF, Greer CH: Leiomyoma of the ciliary body. Br J Ophthalmol 54:383–387, 1970
12. Meyer SL, Fine BS, Font RL, Zimmerman LE: Leiomyoma of the ciliary body; electron microscopic verification. Am J Ophthalmol 66:1061–1068, 1968
13. Pieck CFM: A so-called myoma of the ciliary body. Ophthalmologica 99:471–475, 1940
14. Salim I: De neurogene facetten van iris tumors. Amsterdam, NV Drukkerij Dico, 1956
15. Sevel D, Tobias MB: The value of fluorescein iridography with leiomyoma of the iris. Am J Ophthalmol 74:475–478, 1972
16. Terry TL: Sarcoma of eyelid. Arch Ophthalmol 12:689–692, 1934
17. Van Heuven GJ: Leiomyoblastoma iridis. Ophthalmologica 103:308–313, 1942
18. Velhagen K: Ein Fall von Leiomyom des Corpus ciliare. Klin Monatsbl Augenheilkd 91:456–461, 1933
19. Verhoeff FH: A case of mesoblastic leiomyoma of the iris. Arch Ophthalmol 52:132–139, 1923

10

RHABDOMYOSARCOMA, RHABDOMYOMA, BENIGN AND MALIGNANT GRANULAR-CELL MYOBLASTOMA

The term *rhabdomyosarcoma* was formerly used principally for tumors arising at sites of striated muscle, with cross striations demonstrable in the cells. Many tumors now recognized as rhabdomyosarcomas were then diagnosed as sarcomas merely with a prefix such as spindle-cell, round-cell, or anaplastic; others were incorrectly diagnosed as neuroblastomas, malignant lymphomas, or neurosarcomas.

It is now known that the morphologic and cytologic characteristics of these tumors vary widely, so that the diagnosis does not depend entirely on demonstrating cross striations which, in fact, are often not seen by light microscopy although they can be demonstrated by electron microscopy. Only in recent years has the high incidence of rhabdomyosarcoma been appreciated. It has been called the third most common malignant tumor in children, coming after leukemia and neuroblastoma. An alveolar rhabdomyosarcoma described in a 9-year-old boy seemed to have originated in an extraocular muscle, extended through the orbit, invaded the eyeball, and metastasized throughout the body.[39] A case of congenital embryonal orbital rhabdomyosarcoma was found at birth; metastasis, detected soon afterward, had probably occurred *in utero*.[14]

To ensure proper identification of longitudinal myofibrils, and particularly of cross striations, the tissue should be well fixed immediately upon removal. Sections no thicker than 5 microns should be subjected to differential stains, particularly the Masson trichrome stain. This stains the cytoplasm deep red, and there is little if any blue-staining material in the stroma.

Tumors with rhabdomyoblastic elements were formerly thought to occur only at sites where striated muscle is normally found, but it is now known that many other sites may be involved including the urinary bladder, uterus, prostate, biliary duct, meninges, and brain.

A rhabdomyosarcoma of the iris in a 4-year-old girl was characterized by cross striations and myofilaments in the cytoplasm of most cells. Although the histologic examination seemed to indicate malignancy there was no recurrence or metastasis in a four-year follow-up.[44] The majority of these protean tumors were believed to arise in embryonic tissue, with the potential for aberrant differentiation of muscle fibers, and only rarely to involve the adult skeletal muscle[43] or to arise from undifferentiated foci of mesenchymal cells, in which case they should be classified under embryonal sarcoma which may differentiate along various lines.[2] The consensus is that rhabdomyosarcoma appears at sites over the entire body. Despite marked pleomorphism (Fig. 10–1), the diagnosis does not, as previously stated, depend exclusively upon finding cross striations; in a series of 55 cases of orbital rhabdomyosarcoma,[30] they were demonstrable in all tumors of the "differentiated" type, 60% of the embryonal type, and 33% of the alveolar type. For some years more and more tumors have been classified as rhabdomyosarcomas, and the criteria have been elaborated.[32,36]

Rhabdomyosarcomas will be divided into three groups: pleomorphic, embryonal, and alveolar, although their cytologic characteristics in some instances overlap.

PLEOMORPHIC TYPE

The pleomorphic type (Fig. 10–2) is basically a spindle-cell tumor containing little collagen.[15,37] The cytology ranges from broad, elongated, ribbonlike or straplike cells with multiple nuclei arranged in tandem, to large syncytiumlike masses with multiple nuclei, brightly colored eosinophilic cytoplasm and vacuolated spider cells. The vacuoles contain glycogen. The cells with abundant cytoplasm may have longitudinal striations (myofibrils) and, less often, cross striations. Tissue cultures have revealed the rhabdomyoblastic nature of

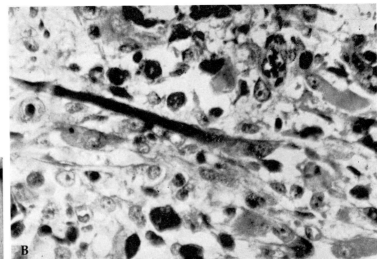

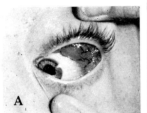

FIG. 10–1. Rhabdomyosarcoma of the orbit. **A.** Clinical appearance. **B.** Tumor cells from section at the time of exenteration. The patient was free of disease ten years later. (F. P. Calhoun, Jr. and A. B. Reese.[4])

FIG. 10–2. Rhabdomyosarcoma of the orbit with fatal outcome. **A.** Clinical appearance. **B.** Tumor cells from section taken at the time of recurrence after exenteration. Drawing in inset shows a cell with cross striations. (F. P. Calhoun, Jr. and A. B. Reese.[4])

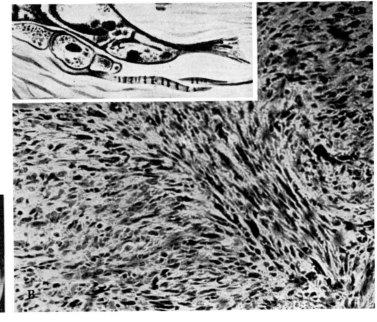

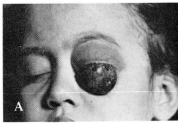

the tumor.[26] In the aforementioned series of 55 cases,[30] none of the patients, from birth to 25 years of age, was considered to belong to the pleomorphic group. However, some cases classified as "differentiated" might be of this type.

EMBRYONAL TYPE

This type is characterized by long, slim, tapering spindle-cells with bipolar processes[36] (Fig. 10–3). The cytoplasm is relatively abundant and eosinophilic. The cell is often enlarged around the nucleus, resembling a tadpole in shape if the nucleus is near one end. Some cells are very small, giving the tumor a myxomatous appearance; other numerous small round cells have little cytoplasm and lack distinguishing features. Longitudinal as well as cross striations may be found. These tumors occur usually in children 7 to 9 years of age, although a fatal case in a 57-year-old woman has been reported.[24]

Embryonal tumors accounted for 73% of the previously cited orbital rhabdomyosarcomas;[30] the 10% classified as "differentiated" (Fig. 10–4) had a good prognosis. Virtually all cells in this differentiated type have a ribbon of abundant, brightly colored eosinophilic myoplasm. The large, round, oval, or rectangular nuclei are often multiple and in tandem arrangement.

The so-called botryoid rhabdomyosarcoma belongs in this category as a morphologic variant. When originating just beneath the mucous membrane it has a grapelike multilobulated or polypoid pattern of growth.

FIG. 10–3. Embryonal rhabdomyosarcoma of the orbit. **A.** Syncytial arrangement and small spaces filled with faintly stained proteinaceous fluid. **B.** Undifferentiated area resembles embryonic mesenchyme. **C.** Hyperchromatic nuclei and ribbons of eosinophilic cytoplasm with faint cross striations. **D.** Many cells with cross striations. (Courtesy of J. F. Porterfield and L. E. Zimmerman.[30])

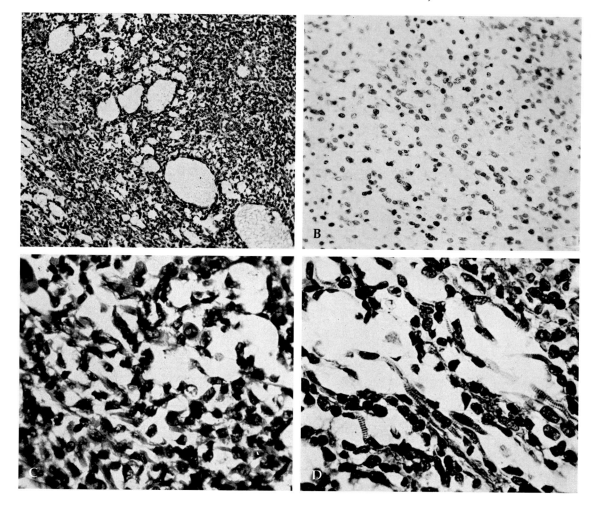

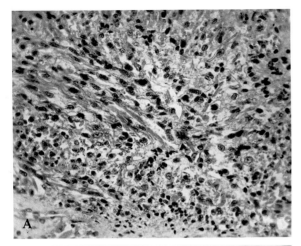

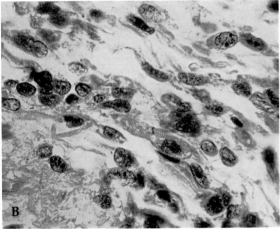

FIG. 10–4. Differentiated rhabdomyosarcoma of the orbit. **A.** Most cells have a ribbon of eosinophilic cytoplasm. **B.** Cytoplasmic striations and large, somewhat rectangular, centrally located nuclei are seen. (Courtesy of J. F. Porterfield and L. E. Zimmerman.[30])

ALVEOLAR TYPE

The alveolar pattern (Fig. 10–5) resembles that of epithelial tumors.[32] One or more layers of cells are usually closely applied to the connective tissue trabeculae separating the alveoli. The center of each alveolus is virtually empty except for varying numbers of free cells including some multinucleated giant cells with both longitudinal and cross striations. This tumor may be noted from birth to 20 years of age. Among the same 55 orbital rhabdomyosarcomas in one series,[30] 9 belonged in this group.

RELATIVE INCIDENCE OF THE THREE TYPES

Embryonal rhabdomyosarcoma, the type usually encountered in ophthalmology, is the most common malignant orbital tumor in young children. In a report on 12 cases of orbital rhabdomyosarcoma at various sites, 13 were classified as embryonal, of which 5 were in the orbit;[15] none of the other types in this series occurred there. Among 44 of our cases involving the orbit, 32 were embryonal, 4 alveolar, and 8 pleomorphic.

The orbital lesion becomes manifest as a very rapidly enlarging mass which first appears as a proptosis with a mass palpable through the lids or as a fleshy tumor under the conjunctiva. It usually grows markedly even within a few weeks. The embryonal type seems to have a predilection for the superior nasal quadrant[3,13] and the alveolar type for the lower part of the orbit.[30]

Rhabdomyosarcoma or granular-cell myoblastoma arising from the nasopharynx, paranasal sinuses, and central nervous system may involve the orbit secondarily, sometimes with ocular signs detected before the primary disease itself. The disease may be manifested as an optic neuritis,[10] a superior orbital fissure syndrome,[34] or a chiasmal syndrome.[38,42]

The expanding tumor may produce papilledema[4] or optic atrophy and enlargement of the optic foramen, in which case x rays may suggest an optic nerve tumor.[19]

In some series more males than females were affected,[3,15] but in others there was no sex-related difference.[13,29] Among our 44 cases, 26 patients were male and 18 female.

In one reported case a 14-year-old boy developed progressive ptosis and visual loss from an orbital tumor which proved to be a rhabdomyosarcoma. After some delay and various treatment methods an exenteration was performed. He died of generalized metastasis 20 months after the onset of symptoms. When his brother, two years younger, showed similar symptoms the orbit was exenterated within two months and six months later he had radiotherapy. He also died of the disease 20 months after the onset of symptoms.[17]

A unique case of rhabdomyosarcoma of the orbit was described in a 9-year-old girl.[21] She had undergone nephrectomy for rhabdomyosarcoma of the kidney at age 14 months. At age 21 she showed no evidence of recur-

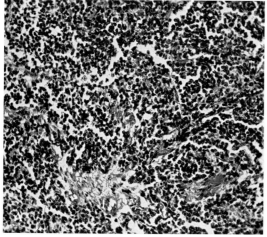

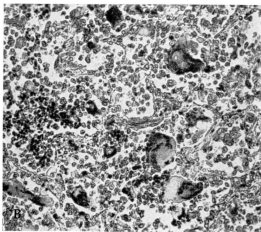

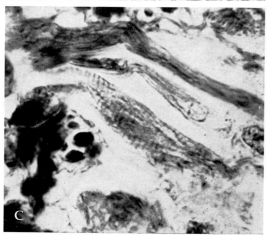

FIG.10–5. Alveolar rhabdomyosarcoma of the orbit. **A.** Cell pattern of the primary orbital tumor. **B.** Giant cells in metastatic lesion to lung. **C.** High magnification reveals longitudinal and cross striations in metastatic lung lesion. (Courtesy of J. F. Porterfield and L. E. Zimmerman.[30])

rence or metastasis from either of the two neoplasms, which were considered to be entirely independent.

The primary tumor, often with prominent striations, may give rise to extremely anaplastic metastases difficult to recognize as rhabdomyosarcoma.[4,19,27]

TREATMENT

If this tumor is diagnosed early in the orbit, exenteration may effect a cure. There is less chance of cure if it occurs elsewhere because the diagnosis may be delayed and the involved tissues may not be as readily expendable as in the orbit. The importance of early diagnosis and adequate surgery therefore cannot be overemphasized.

Successful results have been reported with radiotherapy, either alone,[23] with chemotherapy,[33] or as an adjunct to excision.[15] (See section Radiotherapy of Ocular and Orbital Tumors, by Patricia Tretter, in Chapter 12.) A report on the results of primary radiotherapy in 31 cases of orbital rhabdomyosarcoma[33] revealed that the supervoltage beam, unlike the orthovoltage beam, spares the skin and bone. It also permits better control of the depth dose and delivers a lower dose to uninvolved surrounding structures. A 5000–6000 r dose was given at the rate of 1000 r weekly over a five- to six-week period. Of the 31 children, 21 or 68% survived with a minimum follow-up of two years. Local tumor control was achieved in 28 patients (90%). When radiation is given in the amount and manner necessary in these cases there is always some keratinization of the cornea which results in constant desquamation of keratin and thus a punctate keratitis.

A young child with embryonal rhabdomyosarcoma of the orbit was treated with x ray for 25 days and developed numerous complications that led to enucleation.[22] The glass ball placed in the socket extruded; the socket healed and the lids fused. The patient was well and active 13 years later. In one series, however, none of the patients whose primary treatment was radiation was alive 3 years later.[30]

There have been reports of the successful use of actinomycin D alone and in combination with x ray.[12,28,40]

PROGNOSIS

When figures were available on survival after discovery of the tumor, the average interval was 1 year and 5 months. Among 20 fatalities in one of our series, 10 patients died within the first year, 8 lived 1 to 2 years, 1 lived 2½ years, and 1 lived 4 years. In another report[4] 2 of 5 patients were living with no signs of disease 20 and 21 years after exenteration. The other 3 had died. Two patients in the files of the Armed Forces Institute of Pathology were living 10 and 14 years after operation for rhabdomyosarcoma.

Ten of 13 patients with embryonal rhabdomyosarcoma in one group died within 15 months after the diagnosis. Five of them had orbital tumors, including 2 of the 3 survivors; the follow-up period was 12 years in one case and almost 3 years in the other.[15] Three of 12 patients with embryonal rhabdomyosarcoma of the orbit in another report[13] had immediate exenteration; 2 of the 3 were living without evidence of the disease 15 and 16 years later. Cross striations were evident in 2 of the 3 survivors but difficult to detect in the third. None of the tumors without striations responded to treatment.

The fact that all the fatalities occurred within 3 years in the aforementioned 55 cases[30] suggested a "cure" if the patient showed no sign of recurrence or metastasis within that interval. The prognosis was best for the differentiated tumor (half the patients living and well 5 or more years postoperatively), and next best for the embryonal type (almost one-fourth living and well at least 5 years). The prognosis was poorest for the alveolar type (only one patient survived more than 2 years).

Although the possibility of a cure for patients living 3 years was borne out in our series of 62 cases of orbital rhabdomyosarcoma,[20] one patient had a recurrence 6 years after surgery. Of the remainder, 30 were alive and well 1 month to 25 years after onset of the disease, with an average survival of 7 years; 25 died 6 months to 7 years after onset, with an average of 2.5 years. Six patients were living with the disease at the time of the report.

RHABDOMYOMA

A rhabdomyoma may arise from the extraocular muscles and from the lid and brow muscles. Other related lesions reported in the literature fall into three categories: a) Lesions containing adult muscle tissue but with so many signs of inflammation that their neoplastic nature might be doubted; these are probably instances of chronic granuloma. b) Lesions containing large amounts of fibrous, angiomatous, or nerve tissue in addition to adult muscle tissue; these are thought to be probably mixed tumors or neurofibromas. c) Benign lesions composed of adult striated muscle fibers.

GRANULAR-CELL TUMOR (GRANULAR-CELL MYOBLASTOMA, ALVEOLAR SOFT-PART SARCOMA)

The term *granular-cell tumor* has supplanted *granular-cell myoblastoma* because of increasing skepticism about the tumor's origin from muscle. Various concepts have their adherents: *e.g.,* the tumor is of myoblastic origin (Fig. 10–6), it belongs to the group of histiocytomas, or it belongs to the Schwann cell family. That it is benign and can be cured by complete excision is generally agreed.

In the past the terms *alveolar soft-part sarcoma* and *malignant granular-cell myoblastoma* were used interchangeably, but *alveolar soft-part sarcoma* is now usually reserved for a highly malignant tumor with a typical (alveolar) microscopic picture. Some observers have suggested that it arises from the paraganglia, but most pathologists assign it to an "unknown" category.

The appearance of striated muscle tumors at sites normally void of striated muscle is explained on the ground that they may arise from embryonic rests of primitive myoblasts. In what seem to be transitional examples, the cytologic characteristics approach those of rhabdomyomas; there are few granules and the cytoplasm tends to form ribbonlike syncytial extensions which have at times been described as cross and longitudinal striations. Despite these transitional forms indicating the relationship to rhabdomyoma and rhabdomyosarcoma, some authors have suggested placing them in a separate category,[18,37] but others do not think they are sharply demarcated.[5]

The relatively large amount of cytoplasm in these tumor cells with a granular appearance may lead to confusion with embryonic fat cells. The benign lesions are sometimes incorrectly diagnosed as xanthomas, but the absence of fat in the cell protoplasm and its definite granular character should establish the diagnosis.

Cultures of granular-cell myoblastoma more closely resemble those of various forms of normal and neoplastic skeletal muscle than

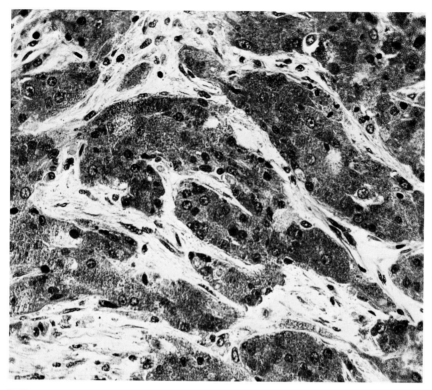

FIG. 10–6. Benign granular-cell myoblastoma of the orbit. Cords of tumor cells with abundant granular cytoplasm are interspersed with connective tissue stroma. (Courtesy of J. H. Dunnington.[11])

FIG. 10–7. Malignant granular-cell myoblastoma of the orbit. The mass, which progressed rapidly, was first excised and the diagnosis made. An exenteration for recurrence was carried out a few months later.

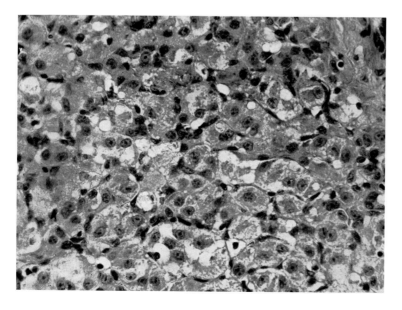

cultures of other tissue types from which they are sometimes said to originate.[26] This tumor is seen in both the benign and malignant stages. The benign types seems to occur frequently at sites of voluntary muscle, but the association of the malignant type with striated muscle is less certain. Among 30 such tumors in one report,[16] 12 were encapsulated and the others showed infiltrative tendencies. These authors felt that most of such tumors were benign but might recur if incompletely excised. There was no clinical evidence of malignant change in the 14 cases on which follow-up data were given. Increasing experience indicates that the malignant type of tumor not only recurs but metastasizes so that exenteration is indicated when the orbit is involved. Conversely, a definitely benign encapsulated tumor might be satisfactorily removed by local excision. There is no evidence that these tumors are radiosensitive.

Among designations for malignant tumors in this group are *malignant granular-cell myoblastoma,* which is preferred;[1,6,31] a less precise term, *alveolar soft-part sarcoma;* and the specific term *malignant nonchromaffin paraganglioma.*[35]

The tumors are composed of rather large polyhedral cells with abundant cytoplasm which stains faintly with eosin and contains many coarse granules varying greatly in number, size, density, and depth of eosino-philic staining (Fig. 10–7). The section in Figure 10–7 was from a mass in the left upper lid near the inner canthus in a 4½-year-old girl. The mass had grown appreciably since it was first noticed six weeks earlier. It continued to enlarge during the next 6 weeks and was excised; an exenteration was performed eight months after her first examination by an ophthalmologist.

In the malignant stage, cell groups in the typical organoid arrangement are separated by capillaries. The alveolar arrangement, shown particularly well by the reticulin stain, follows the same general pattern as that of an alveolar rhabdomyosarcoma. The tumor cells making up the alveolus, however, usually appear granular.

The benign granular-cell tumors can occur almost anywhere in the body. Among 162 cases of granular-cell myoblastoma in one series, 37.6% occurred in the tongue, 20.4% in the subcutaneous tissues, and smaller percentages at various other sites.[7]

Orbital granular-cell myoblastomas have been reported in the region of the lacrimal sac simulating dacryocystitis,[11,41] the iris and ciliary body,[9] the orbit,[11,25] and the eyelids[8] among other sites. In a case of chiasmal syndrome, neurosurgical exploration revealed the cause as a granular-cell myoblastoma of the neurohypophysis.[42] Two other such lesions have been reported.[38]

REFERENCES

1. ACKERMAN LV, PHELPS CR: Malignant granular cell myoblastoma of the gluteal region. Surgery 20:511–519, 1946
2. ASHTON N: Discussion in Blaxter PL, Smith JL, see reference 3
3. BLAXTER PL, SMITH JL: Rhabdomyosarcoma of the orbit. Trans Ophthalmol Soc UK 78:83–97, 1958
4. CALHOUN FP JR., REESE AB: Rhabdomyosarcoma of the orbit. Arch Ophthalmol 27:558–578, 1942
5. CAPPELL DF, MONTGOMERY GL: On rhabdomyoma and myoblastoma. J Pathol Bacteriol 44:517–548, 1937
6. CHRISTOPHERSON WM, FOOTE FW, STEWART FW: Alveolar soft-part sarcomas. Cancer 5:100–111, 1952
7. CRANE AR, TREMBLAY RF: Myoblastoma (granular cell myoblastoma or myoblastic myoma). Am J Pathol 21:357–375, 1945
8. CRISTINI G: Mioblastoma della palpebra (studio anatomoclinico). Rass Ital Ottal 15:207–223, 1946
9. CUNHA SL, LOBO FG: Granular-cell myoblastoma of the anterior uvea. Br J Ophthalmol 50:99–101, 1966
10. DABEZIES OH, NAUGLE TC, JR: Alveolar rhabdomyosarcoma of paranasal sinuses and orbit. Arch Ophthalmol 79:574–577, 1968
11. DUNNINGTON JH: Granular cell myoblastoma of the orbit. Arch Ophthalmol 40:14–22, 1948
12. FARBER S, TOCH R, SEARS E, PINKEL D: Advances in chemotherapy of cancer in man. Adv Cancer Res 4:1–71, 1956
13. FRAYER WC, ENTERLINE HT: Embryonal rhabdomyosarcoma of the orbit in children and young adults. Arch Ophthalmol 62:203–210, 1959
14. HIMMEL S, SIEGEL H: Congenital embryonal orbital rhabdomyosarcoma in a newborn. Arch Ophthalmol 77:662–665, 1967
15. HORN RC JR, ENTERLINE HT: Rhabdomyosarcoma: a clinicopathologic study and classification of 39 cases. Cancer 11:181–199, 1958
16. HORN RC, STOUT AP: Granular cell myoblastoma. Surg Gynecol Obstet 76:315–318, 1943
17. HOWARD GM, CASTEN VG: Rhabdomyosarcoma of the orbit in brothers. Arch Ophthalmol 70:319–322, 1963
18. HOWE CW, WARREN S: Myoblastoma. Surgery 16:319–347, 1944
19. JAIN NS, SETHI DV, MAHAJAN KC: Rhabdomyosarcoma of the orbit. Br J Ophthalmol 40:758–761, 1956

20. JONES IS, REESE AB, KROUT J: Orbital rhabdomyosarcoma: an analysis of sixty-two cases. Trans Am Ophthalmol Soc 63:224–232, 1965
21. KIRK RC, ZIMMERMAN LE: Rhabdomyosarcoma of the orbit. Arch Ophthalmol 81:559–564, 1969
22. LANDERS PH: X-ray treatment of embryonal rhabdomyosarcoma of orbit; case report of a 13-year survival without recurrence. Am J Ophthalmol 66:745–747, 1968
23. LEDERMAN M: Radiotherapy in the treatment of orbital tumours. Br J Ophthalmol 40:592–610, 1956
24. MASUDA Y, KUMAGAYA A, MORITA Y: Orbital rhabdomyosarcoma in a 57-year-old woman. Rinsho Ganka 22:1288, 1968
25. MORGAN LP, FRYER MP: Granular cell myoblastoma of the eye; case report. Plast Reconstr Surg 43:315–317, 1969
26. MURRAY MR: Cultural characteristics of three granular-cell myoblastomas. Cancer 3:857–865, 1951
27. OFFRET G: Les Tumeurs Primitives de l'Orbite. Paris, Masson et Cie, 1951, pp 391–405
28. PINKEL D: Actinomycin D in childhood cancer: preliminary report. Pediatrics 23:342–347, 1959
29. PINKEL D, PICKREN J: Rhabdomyosarcoma in children. JAMA 175:293–298, 1961
30. PORTERFIELD JF, ZIMMERMAN LE: Rhabdomyosarcoma of the orbit: a clinicopathologic study of 55 cases. Virchows Arch (Pathol Anat) 335:329–344, 1962
31. RAVICH A, STOUT AP, RAVICH RA: Malignant granular cell myoblastoma involving the urinary bladder. Ann Surg 121:361–372, 1945
32. RIOPELLE JL, THERIAULT JP: Sur une forme méconnue de sarcome des parties molles; le rhabdomyosarcome alveolaire. Ann Anat Pathol (Paris) 1:88–111, 1956
33. SAGERMAN RH, TRETTER P, ELLSWORTH RM: Orbital rhabdomyosarcoma in children. Trans Am Acad Ophthalmol Otolaryngol 78:602–605, 1974
34. SANANMAN ML, WEINTRAUB MI: Remitting ophthalmoplegia due to rhabdomyosarcoma. Arch Ophthalmol 86:459–461, 1971
35. SMETANA HF, SCOTT WF, JR: Malignant tumors of non-chromaffin paraganglia. Milit Surg 109:330–349, 1951
36. STOBBE GD, DARGEON HW: Embryonal rhabdomyosarcoma of the head and neck in children and adolescents. Cancer 3:826–836, 1950
37. STOUT AP: Tumors of soft tissues. In Atlas of Tumor Pathology, Fascicle 5, Section II, p 93, Armed Forces Institute of Pathology, published by the National Research Council, Washington DC 1953
38. SYMON L, GANS JC, BURSTON J: Granular cell myoblastoma of the neurohypophysis: report of two cases. J Neurosurg 35:82–89, 1971
39. TAKAYASU A, UCHIDA H, KIJIMA M, SONODA Y, HARADA K, FUKUYAMA M: Rhabdomyosarcoma in the eyeball and the orbit. Rinsho Ganka 22:616–626, 1968
40. TAN CTC, DARGEON HW, BURCHENAL JH: Effect of actinomycin D on cancer in childhood. Pediatrics 24:544–571, 1959
41. VON BAHR G: A case of myoblastic myoma of the lacrimal sac. Acta Ophthalmol (Kbh) 16:109–115, 1938
42. WALLER RR, RILEY FC, SUNDT TM JR: A rare cause of the chiasmal syndrome. Arch Ophthalmol 88:269–272, 1972
43. WILLIS RA: Pathology of Tumors. St Louis, CV Mosby, 1948, p 757
44. WOYKE S, CHWIROT R: Rhabdomyosarcoma of the iris; report of the first recorded case. Br J Ophthalmol 56:6–64, 1972

11

CONNECTIVE TISSUE AND OTHER MESENCHYMAL TUMORS

The numerous entities to be considered here fall under several headings: fibromatous and myxomatous tumors, histiocytic tumors, osseous and cartilaginous tumors, fibrous dysplasia of bone, lipomatosis, lipoma and liposarcoma, embryonal sarcoma, and mesenchymoma.

FIBROMATOUS AND MYXOMATOUS TUMORS

FIBROMA AND FIBROSARCOMA

These tumors stem from fibrocytes which, with the collagen they fabricate, constitute the connective tissue of the body. Complicating the problem, however, is the fact that any cell of mesenchymal origin is a facultative fibroblast.[95] A Schwann cell, reticulum cell, histiocyte, lipoblast, and rhabdomyoblast are all capable of acting as fibroblasts by producing reticulum and collagen.

This ability of various cells to function as fibroblasts and produce tumors simulating fibrosarcomas is of more than academic interest. The tumors formed by facultative fibroblasts do not necessarily behave biologically like fibrosarcomas but rather as if the tumor cells were masquerading as fibroblasts. The facultative fibrosarcomas are often composed of several different tumor types, thus giving rise to benign and malignant mixed mesenchymal tumors called mesenchymomas.

Further confusing the issue, the term *fibrosarcoma* is often applied to infiltrating as well as metastasizing tumors. Stout suggested reserving the term *fibrosarcoma* for truly malignant tumors capable of metastasis, using the term *fibromatosis* for infiltrating tumors, and the equivocal term *differentiated fibrosarcoma* for borderline tumors too cellular to be considered metastasizing or nonmetastasizing.

Pathologic classification of these fibrous tumors into infiltrating and metastasizing types helps the surgeon plan the scope of the operation. Among 246 cases of pure fibrous growths of mesenchymal tissues in children, 172 were classified as fibromatosis, 27 as differentiated fibrosarcomas, 25 as fibroids and keloids, 11 as pseudosarcomatous fasciitis, and 11 as undifferentiated fibrosarcomas.[95] The fact that known metastasis occurred in only 3 cases indicates that fibrous tumors in children may be infiltrating but are very seldom metastasizing.

Since these infiltrating fibrous tumors are radioresistant, cure must depend on total local excision. The extent of the excision is difficult to determine because they are not encapsulated but grow by insidious infiltration beyond their palpable limits.

Primary fibrosarcomas of the eye and orbit are extremely rare. Reviewers of reported cases concluded that all had been erroneously diagnosed or were insufficiently documented, and noted that the lesion often developed after radiotherapy for other neoplasms.[104] An epibulbar and ciliary body fibrosarcoma, interpreted as a malignant fibroxanthoma,[20] and a fibrosarcoma of the sclera[46] have been described. A 3-year-old girl with a primary orbital fibrosarcoma was treated by exenteration followed by irradiation; there was no evidence of recurrence six months later.[23] Electron microscopic studies revealed two fibrosarcomas secondarily involving the orbit which had been diagnosed by light microscopy studies as a malignant schwannoma and an amelanotic melanoma.[52]

Nonneoplastic lesions simulating a fibroma or a fibrous tumor, but not arising from the connective tissue, are relatively common, *e.g.,* neurofibroma or fibroma molluscum, both associated with von Recklinghausen's disease. Other epibulbar fibromas may represent congenital rests of mesodermal tissue (mesenchymoma) which developed into connective tissue rather than into various mesodermal derivatives. Some such tumors show only connective tissue in the sections studied, but sections at other levels may reveal fat, cartilage, bone, smooth muscle, angiomatous or myxomatous tissue. Furthermore, an epibulbar fibroma may represent a keloid tendency following inflammation,[68] trauma, filtering cicatrix, or an encapsulated foreign body.

In a review of 37 cases of fibrous tumors of the cornea, 27 were found to have followed inflammation, injury, or surgery.[89] The lesions were described as fibroma, keloid scar, or hypertrophic cicatrix. Some corneal tumors reported in the early literature as myxomatous might have been filtering cicatrices following a perforated ulcer, which may produce a rather large white tumorlike mass.

In most of the reports, the lesion originated in a staphyloma with marked fibrous hyperplasia; a true neoplasm in the nature of a fibroma apparently resulted in some instances. It is difficult to state definitely whether these patients had a keloid tendency or a true neoplasm.

True fibromas or fibrosarcomas are extremely rare in the orbit and lid, whereas fibrous tumors originating in the peripheral nerves or from neuroglia are not uncommon.

A myxoma, an extremely rare orbital tumor, contains mucin which stains red with mucicarmine. It arises from rests of muciform embryonic tissue—the parent substance of several varieties of the mesodermal group, especially fat, cartilage, bone, and connective tissue. The tumor is often associated with a lipoma. It is not well delimited and when completely removed may recur. It is found on the skin, in the periosteum, fascia, and connective tissue of nerves as well as in other areas such as the orbit, which contains loose connective tissue and fat. Any lesion characterized by edema and mucoid degeneration may simulate a myxoma. A biopsy specimen taken by chance from a myxomatous area of a mixed tumor of the lacrimal gland may lead to the erroneous diagnosis of myxoma. The same is true in cases of mesenchymoma.

Myxomas of the orbit tend to be diffuse and poorly demarcated; they infiltrate all orbital structures, grow slowly, and may cause marked exophthalmos. A number of verified cases have been reported. They frequently recur, in one case four years after the first excision,[41] but rarely cause death unless a myxosarcoma develops and invades vital structures.[97]

An admixture of liposarcomatous components is common. The tumor's ground substance is a mucopolysaccharide, as shown by the Alcian blue stain. The Sudan R stain reveals the frequent presence of a fat component.

Several cases of myxoma of the conjunctiva have been reported,[21,91] one of which[31] developed in a filtration scar of a trephine operation done six years earlier.

A myxoma, a liposarcoma, an infantile rhabdomyosarcoma, or a myxomatous portion of a mixed tumor is sometimes referred to as a myxosarcoma.

FIBROBLASTIC HYPERPLASIA (FIBROMATOSIS)

Fibromatosis, usually representing a reactive fibroblastic hyperplasia in children, may be seen in the lid or under the conjunctiva. It resembles and behaves like a tumor, and may recur repeatedly after excision. Although frequently mistaken for a fibrosarcoma, the clinical course is benign in spite of the recurrences. Stout called it juvenile fibromatosis and included in this group the different varieties of fibrous tissue proliferation that are difficult to distinguish from true neoplasms.[94] He reported 74 such lesions in children up to age 15, which were found in almost all body areas including the eyelids.

Juvenile fibromatoses may occur in the subepithelial soft parts at sites where scar tissue is known to have formed. Belonging in this group are keloids, desmoids, fibromatoses of the palmar and plantar fascia and of the sternomastoid muscle (congenital wryneck), radiation fibromatosis, and congenital progressive polyfibromatosis.

Similar growths found under the epithelium are not associated with known scars. The focus may have been unrecognized and unsuspected scar tissue lesions from a contusion.

Verhoeff's case reported in 1957 at a meeting of the Ophthalmic Pathology Club (later the Verhoeff Society) seems to belong to the group of fibromatoses. A 36-year-old woman had repeated gradual recurrences of growths excised from the inner surface of each upper lid, first noted at age one. He considered them to be fibromas or keloids. Each pedunculated tumor reached a large size then progressed no farther.

I have seen one case of juvenile fibromatosis of the cornea and limbus (Fig. 11–1). A fibroma of the cornea may be associated with congenital generalized fibromatosis,[1a] a rare juvenile disease that may also manifest itself in the orbit.[86]

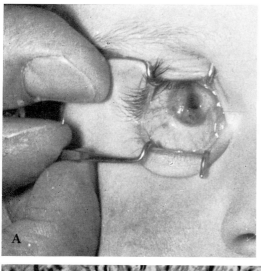
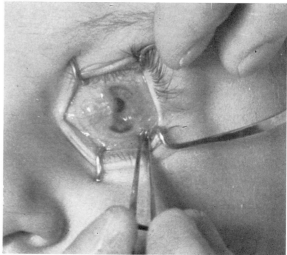
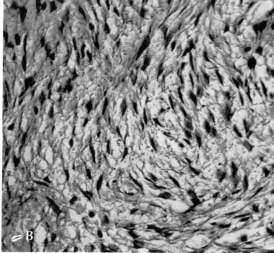
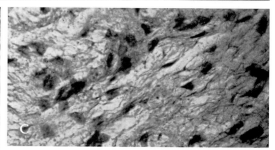

FIG. 11–1. Juvenile fibromatosis of the cornea and limbus. A 1-year-old female infant from birth had two slightly raised white spots, about 2 mm in diameter on each cornea 1 mm from the limbus, which gradually increased in size. The more advanced growths on the left cornea were removed but recurred two months later. The patient had a second and third excision, each followed by a recurrence. A. Clinical appearance when x-ray therapy was instituted. The growths regressed, and there were no recurrences after 15-month and 3-year follow-ups. B. Low-power magnification of a section from an excised lesion. C. High-power view of a part of the same section. A. P. Stout confirmed the diagnosis. (Courtesy of H. J. Wales, Christchurch, New Zealand.)

NODULAR FASCIITIS AND FIBROMATOSIS

First described in 1955,[54] nodular fasciitis is characterized by sudden onset, rapid growth, and an alarming histologic picture which, taken in combination, suggest a neoplasm. However, there is ample evidence that the lesion is benign. In ophthalmology, the lesion originates in the subcutaneous fascia and in Tenon's capsule.[30,98] Among the sites that may be involved are the lid, the orbit, and the limbus.

In a series of 77 cases of nodular fasciitis studied up to 1960, none involved the eye or its adnexa.[95] However, 10 such lesions involving the eyelid, eyebrow, eyeball, or periorbital tissue were reported 6 years later.[35]

Clinically, the disease appears as a rapidly growing nodular mass often with a histologic appearance leading to the suspicion of a sarcoma. The presenting complaint is usually a recently enlarged mass that may be painful and tender.

This condition must be differentiated histopathologically from a number of benign and

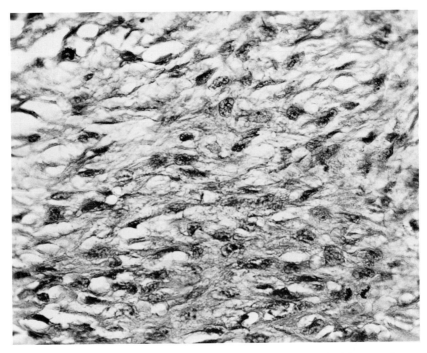

FIG. 11–2. Nodular fasciitis. Fibroblasts with plump vesicular nuclei, prominent nucleoli, and some mitotic activity may suggest sarcoma. (Font RL, Zimmerman LE: Arch Ophthalmol 75: 475–481, 1966; Copyright 1966–72, American Medical Association)

malignant fibrous connective tissue lesions including fibroma, fibrosarcoma, fibromatosis, fibrous xanthoma, myxoma, neurofibroma, and neurilemoma. It is generally considered to be a nodular reactive proliferation of fibroblasts and vascular tissue arising apparently from a fascial layer. The reason for this reactive hyperplasia is unknown. The fibroblasts, from plump to spindle-shaped, are sometimes arranged in parallel bundles and fascicles in a loose myxomatous ground substance. The presence of fibroblasts with plump vesicular nuclei, prominent nucleoli, and mitotic activity suggests sarcoma, and therefore the condition is at times referred to as subcutaneous pseudosarcoma (Fig. 11–2). Other histologic features are multiple cystlike spaces, abundant reticulum and collagen fibers, infiltration of lymphocytes and mononuclear cells, and areas of fat necrosis with foreign-body giant cells.

Simple excision is effective, and the prognosis is excellent. In an unusual case reported in a 6-month-old infant, a small tumor at the corneoscleral limbus clinically resembled a xanthogranuloma.[35] It enlarged slowly for two years and then rapidly. When the child was 3 years of age, an amber-colored elevated growth was excised. This had extended into the anterior chamber involving the base of the iris and adjacent ciliary body. Despite incomplete removal, there was no evidence of recurrence over a 13-year follow-up. Although the clinical appearance suggested xanthogranuloma, on microscopic examination the lesion proved to be nodular fasciitis.

In a 60-year-old woman with benign nodular fasciitis of Tenon's capsule, a well-defined, yellowish, disclike nodule 6 mm in diameter under the bulbar conjunctiva was successfully excised.[2] A case in a 14-year-old boy involved the upper part of the orbit.[58] A pseudotumor of the orbit may be a feature of familial multifocal fibrosclerosis, a possible variant of fasciitis.[16] Among the systemic manifestations are retroperitoneal fibrosis, mediastinal fibrosis, sclerosing cholangitis, Riedel's sclerosing thyroiditis, and Dupuytren's contracture. A case of inflammatory pseudotumor of the orbit associated with chronic fibrous mediastinitis was thought to be caused by an antiserotonin drug prescribed for migraine headache.[22]

OSSEOUS AND CARTILAGINOUS TUMORS

OSSIFICATION, OSTEOMA

Bone, a secondary manifestation in many neoplasms, sometimes is found in hemangiomas. Bone is also associated with teratoid or composite growths which contain pluripotential mesodermal rests with various combinations of connective tissue, bone, cartilage, muscle, and fat. Such bony tumefactions may occur at the limbus associated with teratoma, at the external canthus associated with dermolipoma, and in the nasal sinuses from an embryonic rest.

An osteoma originating in a sinus rest tends to recur in the anterior ethmoid cells and may extend slowly into the orbit, into the adjacent frontal sinus, or into both.[5] Among 740 tumors or tumorlike lesions of the orbit in one series, 38 were osteomas.[6] The often narrow base of such osteomas gives them a pedunculated configuration.

The tumor is benign and usually progresses very slowly if at all. In one case followed for five years, the tumor increased from 5 to 15 mm in diameter within two years and after four years caused a bulge in the nasal wall of the orbit.[67]

A small solitary nodule of essentially normal mature bone sometimes appears on the scleral surface in the upper outer quadrant or over the external rectus muscle. It is usually noted at birth on an otherwise normal eye. The lesion is viewed by some as a choristoma, by others as a progonoma, and by still others as a sequela of a congenital rest of primitive mesoderm and therefore related to the composite tumors. Several such cases have been reported,[55,76,101] in one of which there was a history of recurrent hemorrhage.[76]

Simple excision is adequate treatment. The anterior surgical route is preferred for orbital osteomas that are well circumscribed, lie far forward in the orbit, and show no signs of cranial extension. Osteomas in the frontal sinuses and maxillary sinuses often remain asymptomatic for long periods; surgery is indicated only if they grow. Sphenoid osteomas should be removed immediately, if possible, because the slow progressive growth may ultimately cause blindness. In a reported case of osteoma of the sphenoid body which was considered inoperable, the patient died from internal hydrocephalus.[64]

Surgical excision of osteomas located in the ethmoidal sinuses is usually successful and is often indicated because of their early encroachment on the orbit. However, if the tumors are asymptomatic and no rapid growth is evident, temporization is permissible. Ethmoidal tumors may be removed by an osteoplastic transtemporal approach as well as by the anterior orbital route.

Ethmoidoorbital osteomas vary in size and are usually mushroom-shaped with a constricted neck. The globular head extending into the orbit can thus be readily removed by using a direct approach through the lids, incising and reflecting the fibrous capsule, chiseling through the cortex of the neck of the tumor, and rocking the head with a rongeur until it breaks off.

In cases of frontal sinus mucocele, the overlying periosteum at times becomes detached and forms bone, so that on palpation the mucocele may be mistaken for an orbital osteoma.

Bone or cartilage is an infrequent congenital anomaly of the eye (Fig. 11-3). In a reported case, the presence of scleral bone with nerve fibers and striated muscle suggested a close relationship between these lesions and teratoid tumors.[84]

A number of rare, mysterious, and perhaps related bone lesions are found in young persons which affect the orbit and produce exophthalmos. There is no unanimity of opinion as to their nature, including whether they are actually neoplasms or granulomas. However, reports indicate that they are benign and can be cured by excision.

The term *aneurysmal bone cyst* has been suggested for a benign bone lesion resulting from some local circulatory disturbance which leads to increased venous pressure, producing a dilated and engorged vascular bed in the affected bone area.[51,59] The lesion had been confused with malignant giant-cell tumor, hemangioma, and osteogenic sarcoma.

Numerous cases have been reported[33,56,87] under various designations such as bone cyst, subperiosteal giant-cell tumor, benign bone aneurysm, hemangiomatous bone cyst, and infantile cortical hyperostosis. A case mentioned in the previous edition of this book as a giant-cell tumor of the orbital bones undoubtedly belongs in this group (Fig. 11–4).

Bone is sometimes found as a solitary epi-

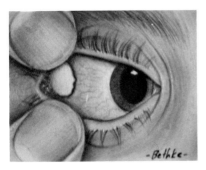

FIG. 11–3. Congenital ectopic bone. The white mass was noted at birth at the external canthus in an 18-month-old infant. The diagnosis was confirmed microscopically.

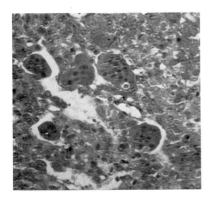

FIG. 11–4. Aneurysmal bone cyst. A 29-year-old woman with progressive proptosis over a three-year period showed erosion of the bony roof of the orbit on x-ray examination. (Courtesy of H. B. Owens.) The lesion, characterized by many large giant cells in a vascularized network of stromal tissue, was classified as a giant-cell tumor of the orbit in the previous edition of this text.

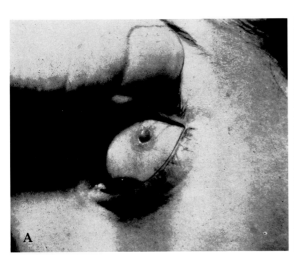

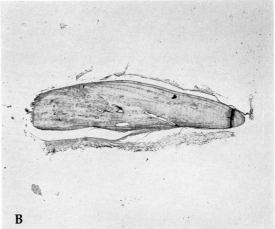

FIG. 11–5. Epibulbar osteoma. A. Pea-sized nodule in the upper temporal quadrant of the left eye about 8 mm from the limbus in a 9-year-old girl. Although noticed when she was very young, it had apparently grown only in the previous year or two. B. Gross specimen. (Courtesy of M. Boniuk and L. E. Zimmerman.[10])

bulbar nodule (Fig. 11–5) unaccompanied by any other eye abnormality. It is frequently located in the upper temporal quadrant about 5–10 mm from the limbus or over the lateral rectus muscle. It is usually noted at birth and remains essentially unchanged. Histologically, the mature compact bone is surrounded by fibrous connective tissue. Authors who reviewed 26 cases considered the lesions choristomas and called them episcleral osseous choristomas.[10] Others believe they develop from congenital rests of primitive mesoderm and are therefore related to teratoid or composite tumors.

Since cartilage or even bone is normally found in the sclera of many fish, amphibians, reptiles, and birds, such a constituent in the human sclera has been considered by some investigators to be atavistic. In a described case associated with a dermolipoma, the bone was located in the sclera and therefore closely related to the bony manifestations normally found in some lower vertebrates.[83]

Heterotopic ossification as a sequel to inflammation is seen in old atrophic globes. It may occur in organized fibrous tissue between the retina and the choroid, in a cyclitic membrane, in persistent hyperplastic vitreous, and in hemangiomas. In rare cases the bone formation is quite localized and large enough to appear as a localized osteoma (Fig. 11–6). An intraocular osteosarcoma originating in an ossified area of an old atrophic globe has been reported.[28] It has been pointed out[4] that just as bone, cartilage, and connective tissue derive from the primitive mesoderm, adult connective tissue can dedifferentiate into young, growing, primitive, undifferentiated connective tissue with the potential for producing bone.

OSTEOSARCOMA

Osteogenic sarcoma of the orbit, particularly when primary, is one of the rarest ocular tumors. It may develop secondary to fibrous dysplasia, to osteitis deformans, or to radiation therapy with the average interval between irradiation and the induced cancer 6.5 years.[37] The tumor is almost invariably fatal.

In one series, 3 of 430 cases of osteogenic sarcoma occurred in the head,[17] and in another 12 of 985 cases occurred in the skull.[14,15]

CHONDROMA, CHONDROSARCOMA, MESENCHYMAL CHONDROSARCOMA

Chondroma and chondrosarcoma constitute about 10% of all primary osseous tumors.[18] They are malignant in the sense that they infiltrate locally and may involve vital structures, resulting in a rather high mortality, but they do not metastasize. Histologically, the tumors also frequently manifest myxomatous, osseous, and fibrous elements. Chondromas usually arise from the bones adjacent to the orbit, extending to it secondarily, but in rare cases they are primary in the orbit[8,65,88] (Fig. 11–7). In one reported case bone and cartilage were embedded under the conjunctiva.[50]

Clinically, chondrosarcomas are manifested as a unilateral exophthalmos and nasal obstruction with massive and destructive local invasion into the floor of the cranium, the adjacent sinuses, and the nasal cavities (Fig. 11–8). Besides the conventional chondrosarcomas[48] there are three other main types: postradiation,[37] myxoid,[26] and the extraskeletal mesenchymal type which tends to occur in the orbit.[44] The tumors are very cellular with undifferentiated mesenchymal tissue containing islands of relatively well-differentiated cartilage. In one reported orbital case,[106] a 9-year-old boy had had an enucleation three years earlier supposedly for a retinoblastoma. However, histopathologic examination revealed a teratoid medulloepithelioma containing rhabdomyosarcomatous elements.

Mesenchymal chondrosarcoma has been described in the orbit.[12,75,79,99] This tumor is composed of islands of undifferentiated, small, round- to spindle-shaped cells together with well-differentiated hyalin cartilage which may undergo calcification and bone formation, with all the transitional stages between. Areas with numerous anastomosing capillaries may make the lesion resemble a hemangiopericytoma.[75] Recurrences or distal metastases are common.

The tumor involves soft tissue, bone, or both. In a series of 30 cases, 17 arose in soft tissue.[79]

PAGET'S DISEASE

Paget's disease is characterized by an uncontrolled proliferation of osteoblasts, osteoclasts, and fibroblasts; tumors may arise from

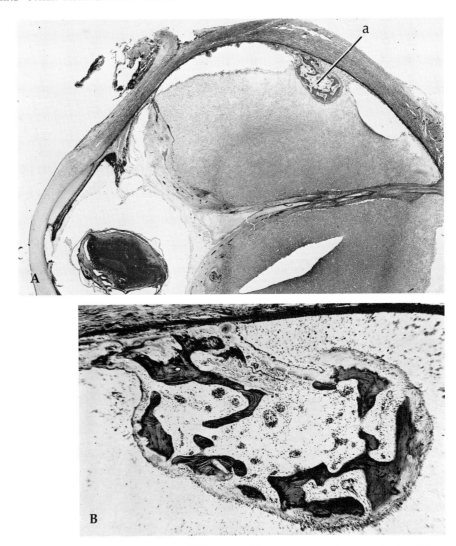

FIG. 11–6. Heterotopic ossification. **A.** An old degenerated globe resulting from exogenous inflammation, with a localized area of ossification at *a*. **B.** Higher magnification of the site *a*.

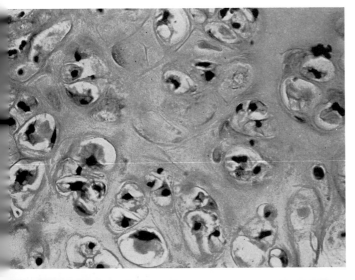

FIG. 11–7. Chondroma of the orbit. The multiple tumors in the orbit of a 12-year-old boy with a proptosed right eye were all connected with bone except one lying in the muscle cone. The optic nerve showed atrophy. The eye was enucleated and the tumors were excised. (Courtesy of F. C. Blodi.)

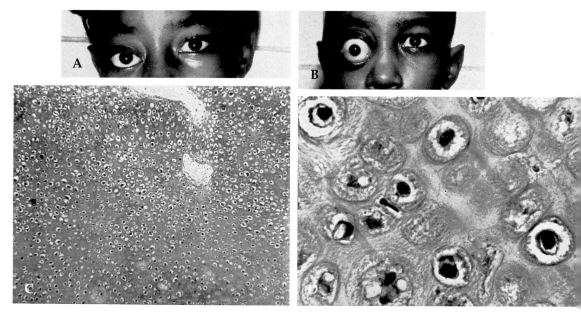

FIG. 11–8. Progressive chrondrosarcoma of the orbit. A. Proptosis of the right eye of three weeks' duration in a 9-year-old black girl. X rays of the skull and orbit revealed a densely calcified tumor arising from the lateral portion of the greater wing of the right sphenoid, involving the cranium as well as the orbit. B. Appearance three months later. C. The highly cellular neoplastic cartilage has occasional vascular spaces. D. Under high power, the rather large hyperchromic nuclei show cellular vacuolization and degeneration. (Courtesy of M. G. Holland, J. H. Allen, and H. Ichinose.[48])

each of these cellular elements.[57] The ophthalmologist is concerned with those arising in the facial or skull bones, of which several cases have been reported.[9] These sites are not usual for such tumors unless associated with Paget's disease, so that their presence is often the first indication of the disease. The tumor most often associated with Paget's disease is osteogenic sarcoma;[38,69] about one-third of patients with this type of sarcoma develop Paget's disease.[71]

HISTIOCYTIC TUMORS

Histiocytoses are characterized by proliferation of the so-called foam cells of the reticuloendothelial system which may be related to faulty fat metabolism or storage. The causation and pathogenesis are unknown but an infectious agent has been suspected. Xanthogranuloma and the histiocytosis X group of diseases are of main interest in this discussion.

XANTHOGRANULOMA

Xanthogranuloma seems preferable to the former term juvenile xanthogranuloma since the condition affects adults as well as children.[90a] Dermatologists have recognized this disease for over 50 years, but its importance in ophthalmology was long overlooked. A localized or diffuse vascular tumor of the iris or spontaneous hyphema with glaucoma was often the first manifestation appreciated by ophthalmologists[39,53a] (Fig. 11–9). Inflammation together with desquamated cells in the anterior chamber led to a diagnosis of uveitis with secondary glaucoma. Although the ocular lesion is usually unilateral, it may be bilateral.[13] Infants under one year of age are affected in the large majority of cases. The histologic picture of a lesion involving the iris and ciliary body appears in Figure 11–10.

Several cases involving the uveal tract have been presented at Verhoeff Society meetings. The first case affecting the iris[7] appeared in the pediatric literature in 1949, but the first report on an intraocular lesion[60] did not appear in the ophthalmic literature until 1956. Numerous reports followed. In one series of 20 cases the only ocular manifestations mentioned were in the uvea.[80] A comprehensive review added many detailed cases including 13 eyelid lesions, 7 epibulbar lesions, and 5 instances of intraorbital disease.[105]

It has only recently been recognized that xanthogranuloma occurs in the orbit as a diffuse or localized tumefaction simulating a rapidly growing tumor. The first such case was characterized by skin lesions and destruction of the orbital bones.[92] In describing three orbital cases, one with skin and bone lesions, the author stressed involvement of the intraocular muscles as an important complication.[81] Among other cases involving the orbit[12a,40,62] were 9 in infants.[34] A benign fibrous xanthoma of the conjunctiva[102] and flesh-colored lesions at the limbus involving the cornea and sclera[43] have been reported. Characteristic skin lesions may be found in the lid[22a], the epibulbar area,[64a] the axillae, the face, and other body areas[1] in patients with ocular findings.[3a]

Histologically, this infiltrative histiocytic lesion shows eosinophils and other inflammatory cells as well as Touton giant cells (Fig. 11–11).

Xanthogranuloma has been clinically confused with hemangioma of the iris[19,77] and uveitis with secondary glaucoma. It has been misdiagnosed both clinically and histologically in some cases as amelanotic malignant melanoma.[29,90,105]

In the event of a single bone lesion, a curettage not only establishes the diagnosis but also leads to prompt healing. In the event of multiple lesions, the affected sites may be treated by radiation after the diagnosis is established by biopsy. However, the lesions sometimes heal spontaneously without benefit of either curettage or radiation. The prognosis is good unless the patient develops either Hand-Schüller-Christian or Letterer-Siwe disease.

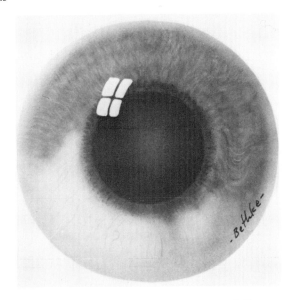

FIG. 11–9. Fibroxanthoma of the iris. A dull gray, slightly elevated, vascular lesion of the iris in an 11-month-old female infant produced intermittent hyphema.

FIG. 11–10. Xanthogranuloma of the iris and ciliary body. These structures are diffusely infiltrated by histiocytes, many of which have been shed into the anterior chamber. The lesion may be mistaken for a tumor such as melanoma, hemangioma, or an endogenous inflammation with or without glaucoma. (Courtesy of L. E. Zimmerman.[105])

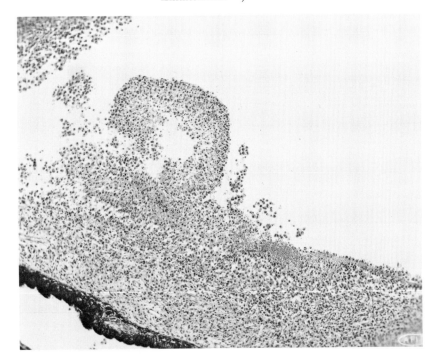

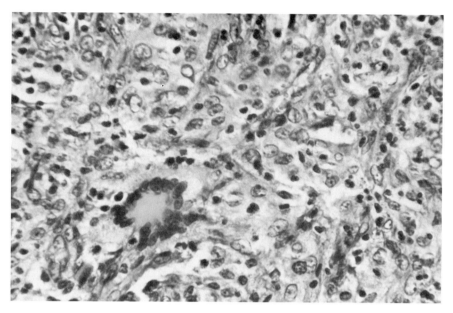

FIG. 11–11. Fibroxanthogranuloma of the orbit in a 4-month-old infant. Histologic picture shows a Touton giant cell. (Courtesy of T. E. Sanders.[81])

FIG. 11–12. Eosinophilic granuloma of the bony orbit. **A.** X-ray reveals a huge bony cavity of the left orbit in a 2-year-old boy with exophthalmos and a hard mass over the lateral half of the orbit. A lateral canthotomy was performed. Microscopic examination of the thick necrotic material in the cavity was unsatisfactory. **B.** Characteristic foam cells of eosinophilic granuloma of bone were found in biopsy material from the deep wall of the cavity.

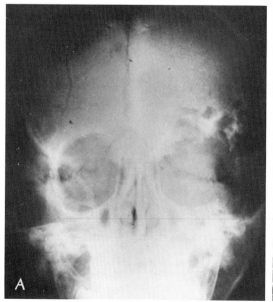

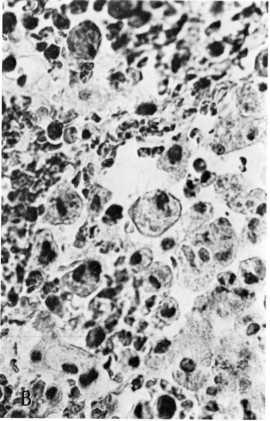

X-ray or steroid therapy may be indicated when the course is progressive.[40] The orbital bones may escape involvement.[100a]

HISTIOCYTOSIS X DISEASES

A relationship among eosinophilic granuloma, Hand-Schüller-Christian disease, and Letterer-Siwe disease—the so-called histiocytosis X group—has long been known. In all these conditions the primary tissue response is a proliferative reaction of histiocytes, leading to the conclusion that they are different stages of the same basic process. Essentially skeletal lesions are all characterized by cystic areas in bone which are filled with granulation tissue and contain numerous large phagocytic histiocytes, occasional multinuclear giant cells, and accumulations of eosinophils. Eosinophilic granuloma is the mildest and most localized; the other two, particularly Letterer-Siwe disease, are widespread and malignant types.

The three conditions were believed to be possibly associated with xanthogranuloma (nevoxanthoendothelioma) in one patient who first had an eosinophilic granuloma, then developed disseminated skin lesions and the Hand-Schüller-Christian triad: exophthalmos, bony skull defects, and diabetes insipidus.[96] However, another investigator, after comparing the ocular and orbital lesions of xanthogranuloma with those seen in Hand-Schüller-Christian disease, Letterer-Siwe disease, and eosinophilic granuloma of bone, concluded that xanthogranuloma is not related to the histiocytosis X group.[105]

Eosinophilic Granuloma

The clinical features include a rapidly developing, painful swelling over the skull, a rib, or a long bone. Multiple lesions are often found on x-ray examination (Fig. 11–12). These lesions occur primarily in children (the youngest patient found in the literature was 2 years old) and young adults, but cases have been recorded in a 34-year-old,[66] a 50-year-old,[100] and in a 53-year-old, associated with hypercholesteremia.[42]

When the orbital bones are involved, the granulation tissue may spread promptly to the orbit producing an exophthalmos.[63a,65a] This rapid development frequently leads

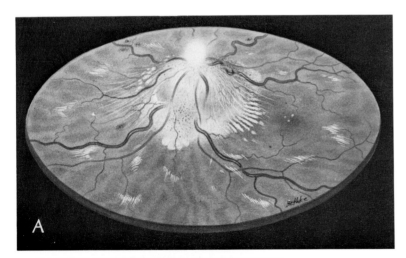

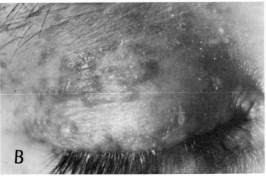

FIG. 11–14. Fibroxanthoma (Hand-Schüller-Christian disease). This disease of both optic nerves led to blindness in a 15-year-old boy who had multiple bone lesions, a diffuse yellow papular skin eruption over the body, and diabetes insipidus. **A.** Appearance of the left disc (identical with that of the fellow eye). **B.** Papules on the skin of the right upper lid. (Courtesy of J. H. Dunnington.)

to the suspicion of a malignant tumor. X rays show a localized lesion that begins in the bone and tends to erode and expand. These findings help to differentiate the lesion from bone cyst, myeloma, and metastatic tumor.

Hand-Schüller-Christian Disease

This disease has a more insidious onset and a more chronic course than eosinophilic granuloma. It occurs in children and youths, produces exophthalmos and skin lesions (Fig. 11–13, see p. 30), and in some instances is accompanied by diabetes insipidus (Fig. 11–14). X rays show bony defects in the skull.

Letterer-Siwe Disease

This is the most severe manifestation of histiocytosis X, sometimes referred to as aleukemic reticulosis or nonlipid histiocytosis. It usually affects children under age 2 and follows a rapid and fatal course. It is characterized by marked proliferation of the reticuloendothelial cells—particularly those of the skin, lymph nodes, and spleen.

These three diseases have been treated by various means. Although the effectiveness of corticosteroid therapy in adults is difficult to assess, prednisone has been found to reverse the skeletal and visceral manifestations of active disease in children.[3] Radiation, curettage of the bone lesion, and excision have also been recommended in different cases.

FIBROUS DYSPLASIA OF BONE

Fibrous dysplasia, a protean disease, may affect any part of the skeletal system, including the orbital bones.[39a,103] The causation is unknown but it is generally believed to be a congenital or developmental aberration with a familial tendency which may be triggered by trauma. It tends to develop in children, rarely in adults.

Three main clinical categories can be identified:

1. Monostotic—commonly involving the skull, maxilla, or ribs.[32]
2. Polyostotic—in which multiple sites are often associated with skin pigmentation[53] and the long bones, the ilium, and the craniofacial bones are largely affected.[32]
3. Albright's syndrome—in which the classical triad is polyostotic fibrous dysplasia,

skin pigmentation, and endocrine disorders, especially sexual precocity in female subjects, hyperparathyroidism, and hyperthyroidism.[53]

The disease has been variously designated, e.g., osteodystrophia fibrosa, juvenile Paget's disease, leontiasis ossea, osteogenesis imperfecta tarda, osteitis fibrosa disseminata, von Recklinghausen's disease of bone, fibrocystic disease, osteitis deformans juvenilis, osteitis fibrosa cystica, and osteopetrosis.

Diffuse thickening of the bone with encroachment on the paranasal sinuses, orbit, and foramina of the skull can produce various symptoms including visual loss, proptosis, diplopia, hearing loss, anosmia, nasal obstruction, and epiphora.[63] The disease may become more or less static, or it may progress.

The monostotic type of disease in some instances causes a decrease in orbital volume, and atresia of the optic foramen. An ophthalmologist is usually consulted because of the resulting exophthalmos with or without visual loss.

Optic nerve atrophy or papilledema may develop from atresia of the optic foramen. The affected bones thicken by acquiring fibrous tissue that may contain foci of calcified bone, hyalin, cartilage, cysts, and giant cells.[49] X rays reveal thickened and trabeculated bone, with some dense and some porous areas. While x rays are considered helpful in the diagnosis, an erroneous diagnosis in 25 of 90 reviewed cases emphasizes the diagnostic importance of adequate biopsy.[45] The lesions most commonly confused with fibrous dysplasia are hyperparathyroidism, Paget's disease, histiocytosis X, nonossifying fibroma, unicameral bone cyst, and aneurysmal bone cyst.

The maxilla has been considered to be the bone most commonly involved in the monostotic type.[32,74] The lesion is painless, slow-growing, and noninvasive. It becomes less aggressive in adulthood or stops growing completely. The first and principal symptom may be unilateral exophthalmos with or without cranial involvement. Visual impairment, due to atrophy of the optic nerve caused by atresia of the optic foramen, and hearing loss were the most common neurologic symptoms in 50 analyzed cases of fibrous dysplasia.[82] The visual impairment was bilateral in 38 of these patients; other authors reported a bilateral case.[11]

Reviewers of 91 cases of the polyostotic

variety concluded that such bone lesions are not usually associated with either skin pigmentation or precocious puberty.[59]

In a study of 148 patients from 4 months to 70 years of age,[72] the disease was traced to infancy in 7 cases, to childhood in 131, and to adolescence in 10. A report on the skeletal features of 37 patients with polyostotic fibrous dysplasia revealed that about 85% had had one fracture and more than 40% had had at least three.[45] The only significant abnormal laboratory finding was an elevated alkaline phosphatase level in one-third of them. The maxilla, the frontal bone, or the base of the skull was involved in all patients with craniofacial lesions.

Osteosarcoma is an occasional complication. About one-third of 28 patients in one series had previously received radiotherapy,[85] and 4 similar cases were described in another report,[103] indicating that this modality is contraindicated in fibrous dysplasia.

A well-localized lesion may be treated by surgical excision or curettage or both, with grafting if indicated. When the orbital volume is reduced, orbital decompression may be effective, or unroofing of the optic foramen when atresia is present. Bilateral unroofing of the foramen was necessary in one case[11] because of optic nerve changes.

Miscellaneous bone diseases simulating orbital tumors are discussed in Chapter 17.

LIPOMA AND LIPOSARCOMA

LIPOMA

The pathology laboratory sometimes receives specimens of orbital fat as the only tangible evidence of an unsuccessful exploration in cases of suspected orbital tumor. In such instances the normal orbital fat may be pushed forward by an expanding lesion that is located posteriorly and undetected by the surgeon. The report is often "lipoma" but the surgeon, if questioned, may admit that he did not encounter an actual tumor but removed some tissue at the site of the suspected pathologic process. Some specimens reported as orbital lipomas therefore represent normal fat.

True lipomas occur in the orbit, though very rarely, as localized, more or less encapsulated accumulations of adult fat. Two such lesions located in the posterior part of the orbit were discovered only when the eye was enucleated for another condition.[36]

LIPOSARCOMA

Liposarcoma does not arise characteristically from normal sites of adipose tissue such as the orbit, but rather from large connective tissue spaces where some areas have retained their potential for lipogenesis. The usual primary sites are the retroperitoneal, perirenal, thigh, and gluteal regions.[27, 93] These tumors vary so widely in cytologic characteristics and behavior that they must be viewed as a related group rather than a single entity. They have a close histologic relationship to myxosarcoma, chondrosarcoma, and mesenchymoma; fat may be a conspicuous element in any mesenchymal tumor.

Liposarcoma is frequently confused histologically with rhabdomyosarcoma because the glycogen-carrying rhabdomyoblasts resemble lipoblasts. Also to be considered in the differential diagnosis are fat necrosis, fibrous xanthoma, histiocytoma, xanthogranuloma, fasciitis, and necrotic areas of other types of tumors.

Any malignant soft-tissue tumor that forms fat as an integral part of its makeup has been classified as liposarcoma by authors who designated five types: well-differentiated myxoid, poorly differentiated myxoid, "lipomalike," myxoid mixed, and nonmyxoid.[24]

Of 13 so-called liposarcomas coded at the Armed Forces Institute of Pathology, only 3 were considered acceptable; 1 from Bogota, Colombia, 1 from the Mayo Clinic, and 1 from Algeria.[25] The remaining cases, coded decades earlier, include 7 now considered rhabdomyosarcomas and the other 3 probably reactive lesions such as fat necrosis, xanthogranuloma, histiocytoma, or fasciitis. One case called liposarcoma of the myxoid type[73] strongly suggested an embryonal rhabdomyosarcoma.

The Bogota patient, whom I saw in consultation through the courtesy of Dr. Rodriguez-Gonzales, was a 19-year-old girl with a two-week history of exophthalmos of the left eye. A biopsy was done, followed by exenteration of the orbit. The orbital bone at the apex and posterior ethmoid cells were found to be invaded by tumor tissue which had also invaded the sclera. The patient died of generalized metastasis. The oil-red-O stain revealed abundant intracellular fat.[78]

Liposarcomas are not known to develop in children under age 10. The reported cases appear to be localized or diffuse lipomatoses which mature to lipoma and become less and less aggressive with time.

EMBRYONAL SARCOMA

A completely undifferentiated embryonal sarcoma of the orbit may occur in infants. Some lesions are so anaplastic that the stem cell cannot be identified. One reported case was called merely an undifferentiated orbital sarcoma[61] and three appeared to be rhabdo-

myosarcomas.[47] No definite cross striations were found by light microscopy in 40% of the 55 cases of embryonal orbital rhabdomyosarcoma in one review.[70] Electron microscopy is helpful in identifying these sarcomas. (See special section, Electron Microscopy of Tumors of the Eye and Ocular Adnexa, by Ramon L. Font, in Chapter 12.)

REFERENCES

1. ALBERT DM, SMITH RS: Fibrous xanthomas of the conjunctiva. Arch Ophthalmol 80:474–479, 1968
1a. ANTINE BE, BROWN FM, ARISCO MJ: Fibroma of the cornea; report of a case associated with congenital generalized fibromatosis. Arch Ophthalmol 91:278–280, 1974
2. ANTON M: Nodular fasciitis. Cesk Oftalmol 23: 450–451, 1967
3. AVIOLI LV, LASERSOHN JT, LOPRESTI JM: Histiocytosis X (Schüller-Christian disease) a clinicopathological survey, review of ten patients and the results of prednisone therapy. Medicine (Baltimore) 42:19–47, 1963
3a. AZOURY FJ, REED RJ: Histiocytosis: Report of an unusual case. New Eng J Med 274:928–930, 1966
4. BALLANTYNE AJ: Two cases of epibulbar osteoma. Ophthalmologica 99:87–95, 1940
5. BELLIZZI AM: Tumores ósseos da órbit. Rev Bras Oftalmol 16:367–422, 1957
6. BENEDICT WL: Surgical treatment of tumors and cysts of the orbit. Am J Ophthalmol 32:763–773, 1949
7. BLANK H, EGLICK PG, BEERMAN H: Nevoxanthoendothelioma with ocular involvement. Pediatrics 4:349–354, 1949
8. BLODI FC: Personal communication
9. BLODI FC: Unusual orbital neoplasms. Am J Ophthalmol 68:407–412, 1969
10. BONIUK M, ZIMMERMAN LE: Epibulbar osteoma (episcleral osseous choristoma). Am J Ophthalmol 53:290–296, 1962
11. CALDERON M, BRADY HR: Fibrous dysplasia of bone with bilateral optic foramina involvement. Am J Ophthalmol 68:513–515, 1969
12. CARDENAS-RAMIREZ L, ALBORES-SAAVEDRA J, DE BUEN S: Mesenchymal chondrosarcoma of the orbit; report of the first case in orbital location. Arch Ophthalmol 86:410–413, 1971
12a. CODLING BW, SONI KC, BARRY DR, MARTIN-WALKER W: Histiocytosis presenting as swelling of orbit and eyelid. Br J Ophthalmol 56:517–530, 1972
13. COGAN DG, KUWABARA T, PARKE D: Epibulbar nevoxanthoendothelioma. Arch Ophthalmol 59: 717–721, 1958
14. COLEY BL: Neoplasms of Bone and Related Conditions, 2nd ed. New York, Harper & Row, 1960
15. COLEY BL, STEWART FW: Bone sarcoma in polyostotic fibrous dysplasia. Ann Surg 121:872–881, 1945
16. COMINGS DE, SKUBI KB, VAN EYES J, MOTULSKY AG: Familial multifocal fibrosclerosis: findings suggesting that retroperitoneal fibrosis, mediastinal fibrosis, sclerosing cholangitis, Reidel's thyroiditis, and pseudotumor of the orbit may be

different manifestations of a single disease. Ann Intern Med 66:884–892, 1967
17. COVENTRY MD, DAHLIN DC: Osteogenic sarcoma, a critical analysis of 430 cases. J Bone Joint Surg 39:741–757, 1957
18. DAHLIN DC, HENDERSON ED: Mesenchymal chondrosarcoma: further observations on a new entity. Cancer 15:410–417, 1962
19. DAILY RK: Hemangioma of the ciliary body: report of a case. Am J Ophthalmol 14:653–654, 1931
20. DELGADO-PARTIDA P, RODRIGUEZ-TRUJILLO F: Fibrosarcoma (malignant fibroxanthoma) involving conjunctiva and ciliary body. Am J Ophthalmol 74:479–485, 1972
21. DOUGHMAN DJ, WENK RE: Epibulbar myxoma. Am J Ophthalmol 69:483–485, 1970
22. DuPONT HL, VARCO RL, WINCHELL CP: Chronic fibrous mediastinitis simulating pulmonic stenosis, associated with inflammatory pseudotumor of the orbit. Am J Med 44:447–452, 1968
22a. EDWARDS WC, REED RE: Chronic disseminated histiocytosis X with involvement of the eyelid. Survey Ophthalmol 13:335–344, 1969
23. EIFRIG DE, FOOS RY: Fibrosarcoma of the orbit. Am J Ophthalmol 67:244–248, 1969
24. ENTERLINE HT, CULBERSON JD, ROCHLIN DB, BRADY LW: Liposarcoma: a clinical and pathological study of 53 cases. Cancer 13:932–950, 1960
25. ENZINGER FM: Personal communication 1971
26. ENZINGER FM, SHIRAKI M: Extraskeletal myxoid chondrosarcoma; an analysis of 34 cases. Hum Pathol 3:421–435, 1972
27. ENZINGER FM, WINSLOW DJ: Liposarcoma—a study of 103 cases. Virchows Arch (Pathol Anat) 335:367–388, 1962
28. EWING J: Personal communication
29. FERRY AP: Lesions mistaken for malignant melanoma of the iris. Arch Ophthalmol 74:9–18, 1965
30. FERRY AP, SHERMAN SE: Nodular fasciitis of the conjunctiva apparently originating in the fascia bulbi (Tenon's capsule). Am J Ophthalmol 78: 514–517, 1974
31. FFOOKS OO: Myxoma of the conjunctiva. Br J Ophthalmol 46:374–377, 1962
32. FIRAT D, STUTZMAN L: Fibrous dysplasia of the bone; review of twenty-four cases. Am J Med 44:421–429, 1968
33. FITE JD, SCHWARTZ JF, CALHOUN FP JR: Aneurysmal bone cyst of the orbit (a clinico-pathologic case report). Trans Am Acad Ophthalmol Otolaryngol 72:614–618, 1968
34. FLEISCHMAJER R, HYMAN AB: Juvenile giant cell

granuloma (nevoxanthogranuloma). In Fleischmajer R (ed): The Dyslipidoses. Springfield, Charles C Thomas, 1960, pp 329–372

35. Font RL, Zimmerman LE: Nodular fasciitis of the eye and adnexa; a report of 10 cases. Arch Ophthalmol 75:475–481, 1966

36. Forrest AW: Intraorbital tumors. Arch Ophthalmol 41:198–232, 1949

37. Forrest AW: Tumors following radiation about the eye. Trans Am Acad Ophthalmol Otolaryngol 65:694–715, 1961

38. Freydinger JE, Duhig JT, McDonald LW: Sarcoma complicating Paget's disease of bone; a study of seven cases with report of one long survival after surgery. Arch Pathol 75:496–500, 1963

39. Gass JDM: Management of juvenile xanthogranuloma of the iris. Arch Ophthalmol 71:344–347, 1964

39a. Gass JDM: Orbital and ocular involvement in fibrous dysplasia. South Med J 58:324–329, 1965

40. Gaynes PM, Cohen GS: Juvenile xanthogranuloma of the orbit. Am J Ophthalmol 63:755–757, 1967

41. Gifford SR: Multiple myxoma of the orbit. Arch Ophthalmol 5:445–448, 1931

42. Gornig H: Hypercholesterolaemia and eosinophil granuloma of the orbit. Klin Monatsbl Augenheilkd 152:517–524, 1968

43. Grayson J, Pieroni D: Solitary xanthoma of the limbus. Br J Ophthalmol 54:562–564, 1970

44. Guccion JG, Font RL, Enzinger FM, Zimmerman LE: Extraskeletal mesenchymal chondrosarcoma. Arch Pathol 95:336–340, 1973

45. Harris W, Dudley HR Jr, Barry RJ: The natural history of fibrous dysplasia; an orthopaedic, pathological, and roentgenographic study. J Bone Joint Surg 44:207–233, 1949

46. Heydenreich A: Fibrosarcoma of the sclera. Ophthalmologica 148:416–424, 1964

47. Himmel S, Siegel H: Congenital embryonal orbital rhabdomyosarcoma in a newborn. Arch Ophthalmol 77:662–665, 1967

48. Holland MG, Allen JH, Ichinose H: Chondrosarcoma of the orbit. Trans Am Acad Ophthalmol Otolaryngol 65:898–905, 1961

49. Hutter RVP, Foote FW Jr, Frazell EL, Francis KC: Giant cell tumors complicating Paget's disease of bone. Cancer 16:1044–1056, 1963

50. Jaensch PA: Subconjunctival chondroma in congenital coloboma of the superior lid associated with malformation of the lacrimal canaliculus. Klin Monatsbl Augenheilkd 117:615–620, 1950

51. Jaffe HL: Fibrous dysplasia of bone. Bull NY Acad Med 22: 588–604, 1946

52. Jakobiec FA, Tannenbaum MD: The ultrastructure of orbital fibrosarcoma. Am J Ophthalmol 77:899–917, 1974

53. Johnson RP, Mohnac AM: Polyostotic fibrous dysplasia. J Oral Surg 25:521–532, 1967

53a. Junemann G: Differential diagnosis and therapy of naevo-xanthoendothelioma of the iris. Ber Dtsch Ophthalmol Ges 69:136–139, 1968

54. Konwaler BE, Keasbey L, Kaplan L: Subcutaneous pseudosarcomatous fibromatosis (fasciitis). Am J Clin Pathol 25:241–252, 1955

55. Kreibig W, Nehm O: Über die episklerale Knochenlamelle. Klin Monatsbl Augenheilkd 155:707–712, 1969

56. Kubicz S, Sobieszczanska-Radoszewska L: A case of aneurysmal cyst of the ethmoid and frontal bone in an 8-year-old boy. Otolaryngol Pol 16:665–669, 1962 (Polish)

57. Lauchlan SC, Walsh MJ: Reticulum cell sarcoma complicating Paget's disease. Can Med Assoc J 88:891–892, 1963

58. Levitt JM, deVeer JA, Oguzhan MC: Orbital nodular fasciitis. Arch Ophthalmol 81:235–237, 1969

59. Lichtenstein L, Jaffe HL: Fibrous dysplasia of bone. Arch Pathol 33:777–816, 1942

60. Maumenee AE: Ocular lesions of nevoxanthoendothelioma (infantile xanthoma disseminatum). Trans Am Acad Ophthalmol Otolaryngol 60:401–405, 1956

61. Mendelblatt FI, Renpenning HJ: Congenital undifferentiated orbital sarcoma. Arch Ophthalmol 71:459–462, 1964

62. Mohan H, Sen DK, Chatterjee PK: Localized xanthomatosis of orbit. Am J Ophthalmol 69:1080–1082, 1970

63. Moore RT: Fibrous dysplasia of the orbit. Survey Ophthalmol 13:321–334, 1969

63a. Moreau PG, Putelat R, Courvoisier P: Orbital eosinophilic granuloma. J Med Lyon 45:505–515, 1964

64. Newell FW: Nevoxanthoendothelioma with ocular involvement: a report of two cases. Arch Ophthalmol 58:321–327, 1957

64a. Nordentoft B, Andersen SR: Juvenile xanthogranuloma of the cornea and conjunctiva. Acta Ophthalmol (Kbh) 45:720–726, 1967

65. Offret G: Les Tumeurs Primitives de l'Orbite. Paris, Masson et Cie, 1951, pp 297–303

65a. Okisaka S, Yazawa K: A case report of eosinophilic granuloma of the orbit. Folia Ophthalmol Jap 19:620–626, 1968

66. Otoni S, Ehrlich JC: Solitary granulomas of bone simulating primary neoplasm. Am J Pathol 16:479–490, 1940

67. Pfeiffer RL: Roentgenology of exophthalmos with notes on the roentgen ray in ophthalmology. Part III. Am J Ophthalmol 26:928–942, 1943

68. Picö G: Fibrotic hypertrophy of the plica semilunaris. Arch Ophthalmol 51:549–552, 1954

69. Porretta CA, Dahlin DC, Janes JM: Sarcoma in Paget's disease of bone. J Bone Joint Surg 39A:1314–1329, 1957

70. Porterfield JF, Zimmerman LE: Rhabdomyosarcoma of orbit; a clinicopathologic study of 55 cases. Virchows Arch (Pathol Anat) 335:329–344, 1962

71. Price CHG: The incidence of osteogenic sarcoma in southwest England and its relationship to Paget's disease of bone. J Bone Joint Surg 44B:366–375, 1962

72. Pritchard JE: Fibrous dysplasia of the bones. Am J Med Sci 222:313–332, 1951

73. Quéré AM, Camain R, Baylet R: Liposarcome orbitaire. Ann Ocul 196:994–1003, 1963

74. Ramsey HE, Strong EW, Frazell EL: Fibrous dysplasia of the craniofacial bones. Am J Surg 116:542–547, 1968

75. Reeh MJ: Hemangiopericytoma with cartilaginous differentiation involving the orbit. Arch Ophthalmol 75:82–83, 1966

76. Roch LM, Milauskas AT: Epibulbar osteomas. Arch Ophthalmol 79:578–579, 1968

77. RODIN FH: Angioma of the iris: first case to be reported with histologic examination. Arch Ophthalmol 2:679–690, 1929

78. RODRIGUEZ-GONZALES A: Personal communication

79. SALVADOR AH, BEABOUT JW, DAHLIN DC: Mesenchymal chondrosarcoma—observations on 30 new cases. Cancer 28:605–615, 1971

80. SANDERS TE: Intraocular juvenile xanthogranuloma (nevoxanthogranuloma); a survey of 20 cases. Trans Am Ophthalmol Soc 58:59–74, 1960

81. SANDERS TE: Infantile xanthogranuloma of the orbit; a report of three cases. Am J Ophthalmol 61:1299–1306, 1966

82. SASSIN JF, ROSENBERG RN: Neurological complications of fibrous dysplasia of the skull. Arch Neurol 18:363–369, 1968

83. SCHIECK F: Eine Bislang unbekannte Missbildung des Auges. Ber Dtsch Ophthalmol Ges, 1910, p. 11

84. SCHREIBER L: Zur Pathologie der Bindehaut. Graefes Arch Klin Ophthalmol 84:420–432, 1913

85. SCHWARTZ DT, ALPERT M: The malignant transformation of fibrous dysplasia. Am J Med Sci 247:1–20, 1964

86. SHNITKA TK, ASP DM, HORNER RH Congenital generalized fibromatosis. Cancer 11:627–639, 1958

87. SIEDENBIEDEL H: Brauner Tumor der Orbita: Gutartiger Riesenzellentumor. Klin Monatsbl Augenheilkd 122:86–90, 1953

88. SIMOES DE SÁ A: Two rare cases of exophthalmos (one a chondroma of the orbit). Arch Port Oftal 10:107–114, 1958

89. SMITH HC: Keloid of the cornea. Trans Am Ophthalmol Soc 38:519–538, 1940

90. SMITH JLS, INGRAM RM: Juvenile oculo-dermal xanthogranuloma. Br J Ophthalmol 52:696–703, 1968

90a. SMITH ME, SANDERS TE, BRESNICK GH: Juvenile xanthogranuloma of the ciliary body in an adult. Arch Ophthalmol 81:813–814, 1969

91. STAFFORD WR: Conjunctival myxoma. Arch Ophthalmol 85:443–444, 1971

92. STAPLE TW, MCALISTER WH, SANDERS TE, MILLER JE: Juvenile xanthogranuloma of the orbit; report of a case with bony destruction. Am J Roentgenol 91:629–632, 1964

93. STOUT AP: Liposarcoma—the malignant tumor of lipoblasts. Ann Surg 119:86–107, 1944

94. STOUT AP: Fibrosarcoma; the malignant tumors of fibroblasts. Cancer 1:30–63, 1948

95. STOUT AP: Fibrous tumors of the soft tissues. Minn Med 43:455–459, 1960

96. STRAATSMA BR: Eosinophilic granuloma of bone. Trans Am Acad Ophthalmol Otolaryngol 62:771–776, 1958

97. TJANIDIS T, GEORGIADES G, KONSTAS K: Evolution de certaines tumeurs peu fréquentes de l'orbite. Ophthalmologica (Additamentum) 151:986–999, 1966

98. TOLLS RE, MOHR S, SPENCER WH: Benign nodular fasciitis originating in Tenon's capsule. Arch Ophthalmol 75:482–483, 1966

99. TRZCINSKA-DABROWSKA Z, WITWICKI T, ZIELINSKA K: Primary "mesenchymal" chondrosarcoma of the orbit (chondrosarcoma mesenchymale primitivum orbitae) treated by biological resection. Ophthalmologica 157:24–35, 1969

100. VERSIANI L, FIGUERIO JM, JUNQUEIRA MA: Hand-Schüller-Christian syndrome and "eosinophilic or solitary granuloma of bone." Am J Med Sci 207:161–166, 1944

100a. VOGEL MH, MILLER H: Fibrous xanthoma (xanthofibroma) of the orbit. Klin Monatsbl Augenheilkd 155:552–555, 1969

101. WIESINGER H, GUERRY DuPONT. Zwei Fälle von epibulbären Osteomen. Klin Monatsbl Augenheilkd 141:281–284, 1962

102. WOOD JW, ELLIOTT JH, LAWRENCE GA: Conjunctival fibrous xanthoma. Arch Ophthalmol 84:306–311, 1970

103. YANNAPOULOS K, BOM AF, GRIFFITHS CO, CRIKELAIR GF: Osteosarcoma arising in fibrous dysplasia of the facial bones; case report and review of the literature. Am J Surg 107:556–564, 1964

104. YANOFF M, SCHEIE GH: Fibrosarcoma of orbit. Cancer 19:1711–1716, 1966

105. ZIMMERMAN LE: Ocular lesions of juvenile xanthogranuloma: nevoxanthoendothelioma. Trans Am Acad Ophthalmol Otolaryngol 69:412–439, 1965

106. ZIMMERMAN LE: Verhoeff's "terato-neuroma": a critical reappraisal in light of new observations and current concepts of embryonic tumors. Am J Ophthalmol 72:1039–1057, 1971

12

RECENT ADVANCES IN THE DIAGNOSIS AND MANAGEMENT OF OCULAR AND ORBITAL TUMORS

D. Jackson Coleman

ULTRASONIC EVALUATION OF OCULAR AND ORBITAL TUMORS

Diagnostic ultrasonography has become essential to the evaluation of ocular and orbital tumors. It is obviously useful in the orbit and in eyes with opaque media where no other visual or diagnostic technique can give information concerning the tissues behind the opacity. Even more importantly, ultrasound can add a new dimension to the characterization and identification of visualized and suspected tumor tissue.

Three display modes are currently used in ophthalmic ultrasonography: A-mode (a one-dimensional, amplitude versus time display), B-scan mode (a two-dimensional cross section of the tissue with echo amplitude modulating the brightness of the pattern), and M-mode (similar to A-mode but with modulation of the echo and real time character of the display to show motion of the tissues).[10] Of these, B-scan is the most easily interpreted by the clinician, since this two-dimensional display corresponds to the histologic cross section of the eye, and familiar anatomic landmarks may be recognized. The A- and B-display modes, used alone, or preferably together, provide the basis for most ultrasonic diagnostic techniques. The M-mode is used primarily as an adjunct to show vascular or respiratory movements of tissues.[2] Both M- and A-modes can display vascular or respiratory characteristics of a tumor, but these pulsatile changes are most graphically displayed on M-mode.

Ophthalmic ultrasound currently uses frequencies of 5 to 25 MHz to provide echoes from the physical interfaces between tissues and cells having sufficient acoustic discontinuities to reflect sound. Thus, with certain

exceptions, most anatomic planes can be seen. With the higher examining frequencies, resolution of both corneal surfaces, iris, lens, and zonules can be obtained. The greater sensitivity of 5 and 10 MHz is required to outline the orbital walls, optic nerve, and other orbital contents, but these frequencies have less resolution than the higher frequencies.

The amplitude or height of returned echoes can be shown best on A-mode, or as gray scale on the B-scan, to indicate specific differences in tissue reflectivity, which serves as an acoustic signature to identify tissue types. This reflective *signature*, combined with the *topographic cross section* of the tissue, provides the basis for ultrasonic diagnosis (Fig. 12–1). If the A-mode is not used in conjunction with the B-mode, adequate gray scale must be present to indicate the relative tissue reflectivity. In addition to good gray scale, color can be introduced to accentuate two-dimensional patterns and facilitate recognition of echo amplitude variations within tissues.[1,8] Isometric,[9] three-dimensional displays and computer analysis are also being utilized to aid in recognition of tissue patterns.

OCULAR SCANNING TECHNIQUES

Tumors are evaluated in a systematic method much like that used for radiographic tomography. As serial two-dimensional acoustic sections are obtained, the size and shape of any mass lesion present and its position relative to other ocular structures is readily appreciated, as in histologic sectioning. Likewise, any additional anatomic abnormalities such as secondary retinal detachment, vitreous hemorrhage, or impingement of a mass on adjacent tissues can be shown.

Accurate biometric determinations of tumor dimensions and volume can be made by sectioning through the crest or apex of a tumor. Since reliable realignment of a scan at a later examination date is difficult, ultrasonic slices should be taken through the maximum height of the tumor aligned parallel to the sclera. These measurements are helpful in documenting tumor growth or indicating the size and/or strength of cobalt plaques required for radiation treatment.

ULTRASONIC EVALUATION OF OCULAR TUMORS

This résumé will attempt to include our most significant findings and those of some of the other researchers—too numerous to mention here—who have provided a foundation for current diagnostic techniques in tumor evaluation.

ANTERIOR OCULAR TUMORS

Tumors of the anterior segment (iris and ciliary body) can be seen with ultrasound, but in this region are often too small to allow acoustic differentiation. If more than 1 mm thick, however, they can usually be quite readily detected.

In our experience, ultrasound has been most useful in differentiating solid from cystic lesions of the iris and ciliary body (Fig. 12–2). Large anterior tumors such as melanomas show characteristic transmission properties on A-mode similar to like tumors at the posterior pole.

CHOROIDAL TUMORS

The overwhelming majority of choroidal tumors are of four types: malignant melanoma, metastatic carcinoma, hemangioma, and subretinal hemorrhage. Differentiation of neoplastic lesions (hemangioma and subretinal hemorrhage) is of prime concern. Differentiation of metastatic disease from malignant melanoma is also desirable as a guide to proper treatment.

Ultrasound can aid in the differentiation of posterior pole tumors which appear similar visually.[6,7,12] More importantly, a lesion whose presence or location is obscured by opaque media may be characterized ultrasonically.

Since malignant melanoma is the most common intraocular tumor, its pattern of

FIG. 12–1. A. Schematic cross section of the eye with a tumor at the posterior pole. The structures in the path of the ultrasonic beam generate the A-scan echoes. B. B-scan ultrasonogram of an eye demonstrating the histologic cross section character of this type of display. The anterior chamber, lens, vitreous, and a tumor at the posterior pole may be identified. C. A-scan corresponding to the path noted in the schematic. Echoes are produced by tissue surfaces while relatively homogeneous tissue areas like the vitreous appear flat or anechoic.

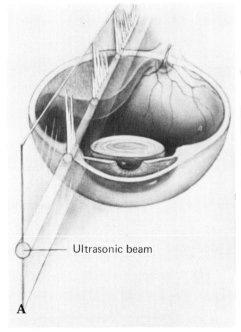

Ultrasonic beam

A

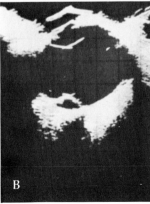

B

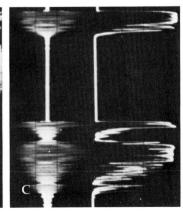

C

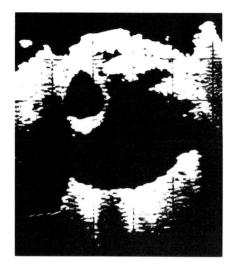 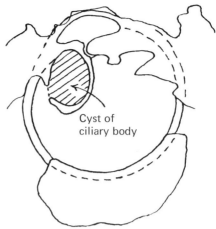

Cyst of
ciliary body

FIG. 12–2. B-scan ultrasonogram of a ciliary body cyst. The anechoic interior of the cyst produces little attenuation of the sound beam, and no shadowing of posterior structures is noted.

acoustic differentiation will be used as an index for comparison with that of other choroidal masses.

Malignant melanomas, which appear on B-scan as solid masses protruding into the vitreous from the interior ocular wall, range in size from 1mm in elevation to a mass filling most of the globe (Fig. 12–3). They are generally convex and smooth, due to restraint by Bruch's membrane. If a mass breaks through Bruch's membrane, however, it may have a polypoid or "collar-button" shape (Fig. 12–4): this is only rarely seen with metastatic lesions and has not, in our experience, been noted with hemangiomas. Malignant melanomas are found anywhere within the globe, but are most easily localized and studied acoustically when situated at the posterior pole.

Distortion of other ocular tissues caused by the melanoma can be observed acoustically, but except for choroidal replacement such changes do not significantly aid in diagnosis.

Chronologic increase in size of tumors can be a salient diagnostic point, indicating neoplastic activity. Metastatic carcinoma increases more rapidly than malignant melanoma, and mixed or epithelioid melanomas grow more rapidly than the spindle-cell types. Regression in size, either spontaneous or due to radiation, can be documented by A-mode or B-scan measurements.

Malignant melanomas have characteristic acoustic signatures. A- and B-scans of a solid tumor demonstrating the absorption pattern of a malignant melanoma appear in Figure 12–5. The A-mode echoes are closely spaced and of low amplitude after the initial high spike and acute fall-off slope. This acute angle may be due to the very homogeneous nature of melanomas. Ossoinig's special amplifier with calibration for quantitative characterization of this amplitude and slope provides a useful and reliable means of identifying tissues.

Vascular components of malignant melanomas may be observed either as a source of "spontaneous movements" on A-scan[12] or as pulsations on M-scan. Such pulsations do not commonly appear in hemangiomas.

An even more important phenomenon, observable in both A- and B-modes, is the internal acoustic texture of a mass. A textured internal appearance is produced by inhomogeneities which provide reflecting interfaces in the path of the sound beam. Homogeneous tissues, such as the lens, produce few internal reflections and appear acoustically hollow or "sonolucent." Among tumors, very homogeneous solid types, such as certain malignant melanomas, also show hollow areas. After the echo complex from the leading edge of the tumor, the echo amplitude drops so low that on the B-scan the posterior portion of the tumor appears sonolucent, or as an "acoustic quiet zone." This phenomenon may be seen more clearly at the higher examining frequencies of 15 or 20 MHz than at 5 and 10 MHz. If tumor tissue has replaced an area of

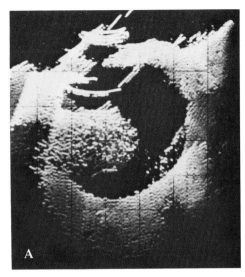

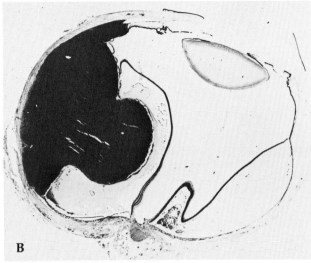

FIG. 12–3. A. B-scan of a large malignant melanoma occupying the temporal aspect of the globe. **B.** Histologic section of the same eye following enucleation, demonstrating the similarity in ultrasonic and pathologic appearance.

FIG. 12–4. A. Diascleral B-scan ultrasonogram of a malignant melanoma demonstrating the collar-button shape produced when the tumor breaks through Bruch's membrane. **B.** Histologic section of the same eye following enucleation.

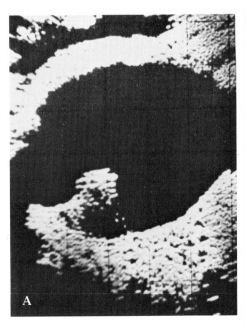

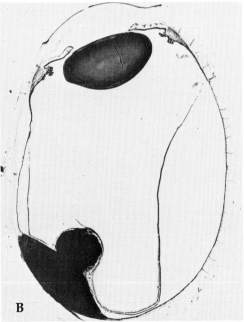

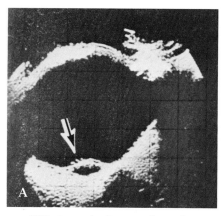
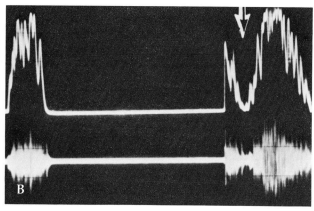

FIG. 12–5. A. B-scan of a melanoma (*arrow*) at the posterior pole. Homogeneity of the tumor produces the anechoic area noted in the posterior of the tumor which appears as "choroidal excavation" when tumor replaces the normal choroid. **B.** A-scan through the tumor demonstrating the sharp fall-slope (*arrow*) characteristic of a malignant melanoma.

FIG. 12–6. B-scan **(A)** and A-scan **(B)** of a malignant melanoma at the posterior pole, taken at 10 MHz (*top*), 15 MHz (*center*), and 20 MHz (*bottom*). Increased accentuation of both choroidal excavation and acoustic quiet zones is noted at the higher examining frequencies.

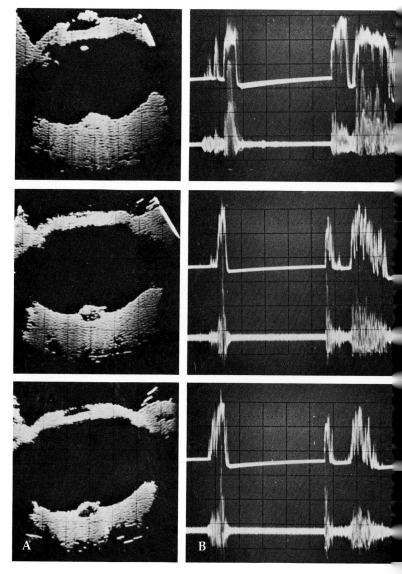

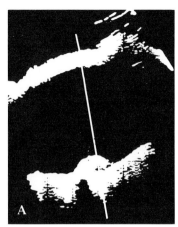
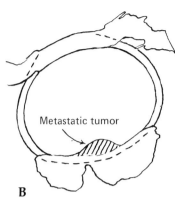
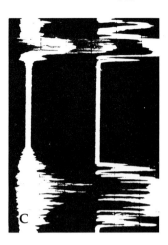

FIG. 12–7. A. B-scan ultrasonogram of a metastatic tumor adjacent to the optic nerve head. Line indicates path of A-scan. The mass appears solid at 10 MHz with no choroidal excavation. **B.** Schematic of B-scan. **C.** A-scan through the tumor showing densely spaced, moderate amplitude echoes throughout the mass.

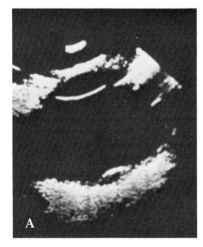
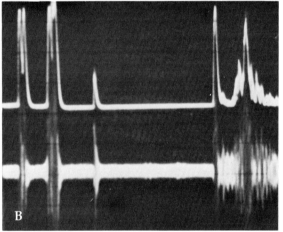

FIG. 12–8. A. B-scan ultrasonogram of a hemangioma at the posterior pole. The mass appears hollow at 15 MHz and shows no choroidal excavation. **B.** A-scan through the tumor showing the more widely spaced, moderate amplitude echoes representative of hemangiomas.

normal choroid, the quiet zone replaces the choroidal echoes, producing a B-scan pattern we have termed *choroidal excavation*[5] (Fig. 12–6). Choroidal excavation is useful in differentiating a solid tumor from hemorrhage overlying a normal choroid. It has been seen in approximately 45% of all malignant melanomas and in most melanomas posterior to the equator, but not in metastatic or non-neoplastic lesions.

Metastatic carcinomas are often similar to malignant melanomas in acoustic morphologic terms. They are usually convex, vary in size, and frequently cause nonrhegmatogenous retinal detachments. Metastatic carcinomas are most commonly located at or near

the posterior pole (Fig. 12–7). Certain acoustic patterns may aid in differentiation. The attenuation pattern through a metastatic lesion usually shows higher amplitude internal spikes than a malignant melanoma, and more closely spaced echoes than a hemangioma. In general, metastatic carcinomas are homogeneous tissues that absorb sound relatively well, but are usually less homogeneous than malignant melanomas. Echoes from within metastatic carcinoma are of higher sustained amplitude and do not usually show the acute fall-off slope on A-mode or the sonolucent area on B-mode in posterior portions of malignant melanomas. On B-scan, this sustained amplitude gives a solid appearance to metastatic tumors at all examining frequencies.

Hemangiomas morphologically may resemble both metastatic carcinoma and malignant melanoma, but they are usually only 0.5 mm to 2 mm in height and convex shape at the posterior pole (Fig. 12–8). The acoustic signatures of hemangiomas are usually a series of relatively widely spaced constant-amplitude echoes following the initial boundary spike, a reflection of their more grossly porous nature. On B-scan, smaller hemangiomas usually appear solid, but the larger ones have a quiet zone even at 5 and 10 MHz. Characteristic examples of absorption patterns through malignant melanoma and hemangioma are shown in Figure 12–9.

A subretinal hemorrhage (Fig. 12–10) has very low amplitude echoes from the subretinal space and should show no replacement of the choroidal echoes (choroidal excavation) by the tumor on B-scan.

Reliability of Ultrasonic Evaluation

While more than one examination may be required to arrive at a final ultrasonic diagnosis, most of the studies at various centers indicate a 95%–97% reliability for differentiating neoplasms from nonneoplastic changes. A report of 96% reliability,[12] identical with our findings, indicates that the technique is at least as effective as others in the detection and diagnosis of choroidal tumors, if not superior to them.

RETINOBLASTOMA

Retinoblastoma causes a change in both the retina and vitreous that is relatively diffuse, often making the acoustic pattern difficult to differentiate from vitreous hemorrhage. When the velocity of sound was compared in samples of retinoblastoma and organized blood, the two proved quite similar, especially when blood and vitreous were mixed.[14] Ultrasound does show several characteristics, however, that are indicative of retinoblastoma.[15]

There are two characteristic retinoblastoma patterns on B-scan: solid and cystic. These tumors vary from large lesions filling the vitreous compartment to small satellite or seed lesions along the retina. Calcium deposits produce high-amplitude spikes within the tumor which also cause shadowing in the orbit that may help in differentiation. The diagnosis of retinoblastoma is less reliable than of choroidal tumors; one author quoted approximately 80%, and we have found it to be 76%.[3]

ORBITAL TUMORS

SCANNING TECHNIQUES

As in ocular diagnosis, serial and kinetic B-scans in conjunction with A-mode monitoring are used in the evaluation of orbital tumors. Unlike ocular evaluation, where variations from the normal acoustic pattern clearly indicate pathology, changes in the orbital pattern may be more subtle, requiring comparative scans of the fellow eye to indicate abnormality.

CLASSIFICATION OF ORBITAL TUMORS

Orbital tumors can be identified as variations from the normal orbital fat pattern. Abnormal B-scan patterns are characterized by the morphology of the anterior surface of the tumor (the posterior outline usually being related to visualization of the orbital wall) and the acoustic transmission properties of the tumor.[12]

The first systematic classification of orbital tumors, based on their specific B-scan pattern, was provided in 1969.[13] Our method of characterizing such tumors (Fig. 12–11) is based on this original proposal. Tumors that transmit sound well are classified either as cystic (if they have a rounded anterior border) or as angiomatous (if they have an irregular anterior border). Tumors that transmit sound poorly are classified either as solid (if they have a rounded anterior border) or as infiltrative (if they have an irregular anterior border). These acoustic classes correspond well, although not perfectly, with certain tumor groups.

NEUROGENIC TUMORS

Neurogenic tumors such as meningiomas or gliomas characteristically show a "solid" rounded outline in the region of the optic

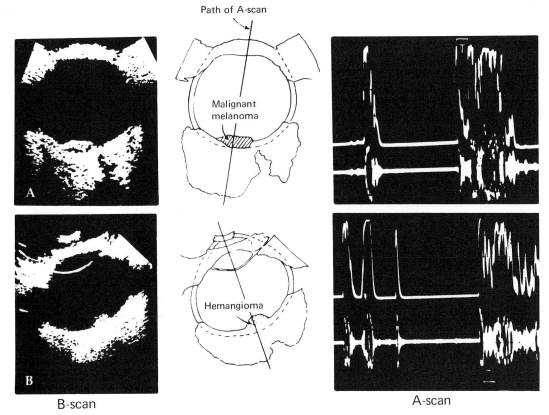

FIG. 12–9. A. A- and B-scans of a malignant melanoma with accompanying schematic diagram. B. A- and B-scans of a posterior pole hemangioma for comparison of sound attenuation pattern.

FIG. 12–10. A. B-scan ultrasonogram of a subretinal hemorrhage adjacent to the optic nerve head. B. A-scan exhibiting a sharp retinal echo (*arrow*) which drops sharply to base line and scattered low- to moderate-amplitude echoes preceding the high scleral echo.

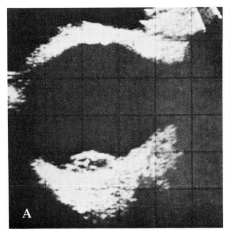

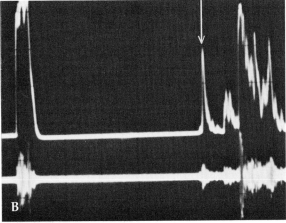

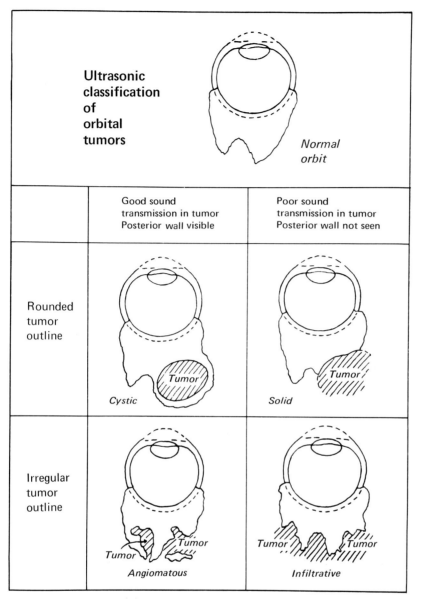

FIG. 12–11. Schematic diagram categorizing orbital tumors according to the ultrasonic characteristics of boundary properties and sound transmission.

nerve, blunting its anterior portion or widening its orbital course, or both. Separation of the sheath from the nerve due to tumor or inflammation is often indicated by a "doubled" echo outline. Neurofibromas of the orbit can cause irregularities in the fat pattern adjacent to or surrounding the nerve. Both types of neurogenic tumors conduct sound poorly. The use of kinetic scanning, *i.e.*, having the patient move his eye from side to side during sector scanning, can often differentiate neurogenic from other orbital tumors or from other abnormalities of the optic nerve. Occasionally, inflammatory swelling of the nerve, or congestive change secondary to an intracranial lesion, may resemble a sheath meningioma.

MUCOCELES, DERMOIDS, AND CAVERNOUS HEMANGIOMAS (CYSTIC TUMORS)

Cystic lesions of the orbit, such as mucoceles, and cavernous hemangiomas produce a characteristically rounded lesion which transmits sound well, as evidenced by good visualization of the retrotumor structures such as the orbital apex. These tumors, like the neurogenic tumors, are well outlined acoustically. The cystic or sonolucent space is the easiest to characterize acoustically and thus presents no significant ambiguity to ultrasonic evaluation. Echoes from within the lesion can be seen when organized cellular debris or vessels are present.

LYMPHANGIOMAS, ANGIOMAS (ANGIOMATOUS TUMORS)

Tumors that exhibit good sound transmission but are irregular in outline can be classified as angiomatous. These characteristically are lymphangiomas or diffuse hemangiomas that may be sectioned in such a way that fingers or extensions of the tumor throughout the orbital fat pattern appear as isolated orbital cysts. These tumors, like the two previous groups, are diagnosed ultrasonically with a high degree of confidence.

LYMPHOMAS, METASTATIC CARCINOMAS, PSEUDOTUMORS (INFILTRATIVE TUMORS)

The fourth category of tumors, demonstrating an irregular anterior outline and poor sound transmission, is more difficult to differentiate. Only the anterior border of the tumor is seen for contour analysis and absorption of sound within the tumor makes A-scan characterization less precise. Lymphomas, lymphosarcomas, metastatic carcinomas, and pseudotumors all may have a very similar morphologic appearance.

Diagnosis can be aided by the position of the pseudotumor as well as the presence of an associated inflammatory change, which often produces a characteristic sonolucent space in the perineural space or in the potential space of Tenon.

A-mode patterns provide another, more detailed method of portraying the sound trans-

mission properties of orbital tumors. Solid lesions such as lymphoma or lymphosarcoma tend to show relatively high attenuation compared with cavernous hemangioma or edematous normal tissue.

Measurement of A-scan amplitude reflectivity characteristics of orbital tumors has been calibrated against tissue models to aid in orbital tumor differentiation.[12] This author noted a reflectivity of less than 0.5% for serous cysts and sclerosing pseudotumor, 5% to 8% for lymphoma, granuloma or mucocele, 40% to 60% for glioma or abscess, 60% to 95% for normal tissue.

ORBITAL INFLAMMATION ((GRAVES'S DISEASE AND PSEUDOTUMORS)

Inflammatory changes of the orbit produce definite and reproducible changes in the B-scan pattern of the orbital fat and muscles. Graves's disease has a characteristic myositis pattern, and optic neuritis can be documented by an equally characteristic nerve pattern. The extraocular muscles appear as sonolucent areas adjacent to the orbital wall, which is itself accentuated. In addition to its relatively anechoic appearance, the muscle also appears thickened.

Among the inflammatory changes revealed are the appearance of abnormal sonolucent areas in Tenon's space (tenonitis or episcleritis), in the optic nerve sheath (optic neuritis), surrounding the optic nerve (vascular congestion), or in the rectus muscles (the eye changes of Graves's disease).

Pseudotumor also appears as a sonolucent area, but does not transmit sound as well as inflamed muscle. The orbital wall is seldom seen in pseudotumor, unlike the case in myositis. A careful search for other signs of inflammation may be the only way of acoustically distinguishing pseudotumor from a true lymphomatous lesion.

RELIABILITY OF ORBITAL DIAGNOSIS

The detection of orbital tumors with ultrasound has been reported as well over 90% reliable.[4] In our experience, diagnostic reliability is slightly less for orbital tumors in terms of differentiation of neoplastic from benign lesions. This is primarily due to the fact that lymphomas and granulomatous pseudotumors are too similar morphologically and histologically to allow good acoustic differentiation. However, delineation of tumors in the orbit, as to location and extent, is of great help in preoperative evaluation as well as in distinction of tumors from the most common cause of exophthalmos, Graves's disease.

The noninvasive character of ultrasound and its unique ability to outline otherwise nonevaluable tissue changes in both the globe and the orbit make it an essential test for the complete evaluation of all ophthalmic tumors.

Robert M. Ellsworth

DIATHERMY, LIGHT COAGULATION, AND CRYOTHERAPY IN THE MANAGEMENT OF INTRAOCULAR TUMORS

In the 1940s and 1950s malignant tumors of the eye and orbit were treated by enucleation or exenteration. Despite this, the mortality was high, over 50% in patients with malignant melanoma, for example. In the 1960s and 1970s radiation and chemotherapy, singly or in combination, came into increasing use. Recent improvements have enhanced the effectiveness of these treatments in controlling and even curing malignant tumors.

Light coagulation by xenon arc or lasers and cryotherapy are often effective and produce no extraocular side effects. In the case of retinoblastoma these techniques may be especially valuable. It now seems that all patients with familial retinoblastoma and all with bilateral disease have a germinal mutation believed to be on the long arm of chromosome 13. At least 20% of sporadic, unilateral retinoblastomas also have a similar mutation. The germinal change seems to predispose affected persons not only to retinoblastoma but also to other primary neoplasms later in life and to radiation-induced tumors at dosage levels that rarely bother those with a normal genetic constitution. Light coagulation, diathermy, and cryotherapy avoid the mutagenic effects of radiation. Early diagnosis is vital; most cases are too far advanced when detected to respond to locally acting agents.

The use of diathermy, light coagulation, and cryotherapy will be confined in this section to the three most common diseases: angiomatosis retinae, malignant melanoma of the uvea, and retinoblastoma. The principles involved may easily apply to other intraocular tumors.

ANGIOMATOSIS RETINAE

This disease, rightfully called the most benign from a purely ocular point of view, may plague an entire family line, visiting on its members central nervous system complications in early and mid adulthood. The most important consideration is therefore a total evaluation of the patient's ocular and central nervous system status. Because about 20% of patients with retinal angiomas have a family history of these tumors, and about 25% will develop lesions of the central nervous system, the physical status of the immediate family should also be evaluated.

Retinal angiomas under 2 dd in size are easily treated, but those over 6 dd are very difficult to control by any method without causing complications. As they grow, yellow exudate increases around them and an oval, yellow patch of about 3 × 5 dd may appear in the macula, even though the actual angioma is in the far periphery. The yellow, exudative macular lesion evolves over a period of months or years into a sharply demarcated, elevated, cystic lesion, often of about 2 dd, with an irregularly pigmented surface. It roughly resembles a toxocara granuloma; its presence should lead to a careful search of the retina for a peripheral angioma. A clear retinal cyst often forms adjacent to the angioma in time, progressing with increasing exudation to a total retinal detachment.

In the cyst and detachment stages, the angioma itself may be inconspicuous and its true nature be unsuspected. Angiomas in the fellow eye are also often missed. About 50%

of patients with a retinal angioma will develop a lesion in the fellow eye, and 50% develop new tumors in the same eye after treatment. Early angiomas may be detectable only by fluorescein angiography. They grow very slowly over many months. It is reasonable to wait until they reach about 1/10 dd in size and can be seen with the ophthalmoscope before starting treatment. Of the three modalities, light coagulation perhaps gives the best results. The appearance of a small, crooked, centripetal vessel turning back from the equator toward the disc is an early sign of an angioma. The search for a tiny red angioma against the red fundus background is exhausting for both patient and ophthalmologist; it may take 15–20 minutes even in a cooperative subject. Angiography is helpful but photographing the entire retina is also fatiguing for the patient.

DIATHERMY

Successful treatment of a 2/3 dd angioma with surface diathermy using a 2-mm probe was described in 1939 in a patient who had refused enucleation.[47] A patient with a 1-dd angioma treated by diathermy, with a 1.5-mm pin, was followed for 11 years.[43] The surrounding area was scarred in two months with obliteration of the retinal vessels. The yellow exudate disappeared within two years. This case appeared in a review of 47 eyes in 38 patients who had been treated with diathermy, with success in 33 eyes (70%). The treated angiomas were generally 1/2 to 3 1/2 dd with 1/2 to 3 diopters elevation. The technique was generally surface followed by penetrating diathermy, and minimal amperage was suggested. Multiple angiomas were treated over several sessions. Since complications included vitreous hemorrhage in 17 of 47 cases, perforating diathermy over the feeder vessels was considered to be undesirable. Thirteen eyes had exudative retinal detachments after treatment, 5 of them permanent.

LIGHT COAGULATION

Treatment of angiomas by light coagulation has been called the most rewarding field among intraocular tumors by an author who reported results on 59 eyes in 32 patients.[34, 35] Fourteen of the eyes were already blind, but 41 of the remaining 45 were cured. He considered light coagulation undoubtedly superior to diathermy because heat intensity can be more carefully controlled and the angiomas can be destroyed in stages. He noted, too, that angiomas near the disc and near the fovea can be treated with less destruction of adjacent retina and nerve.

Lesions of 1/2 dd were treated in one or two sittings with the beam diameter adjusted to the size of the tumor and one to three coagulations applied. Tumors of 1/2 to 2 dd were treated with three to six normal intensity coagulations (sufficient to produce a grayish spot in normal adjacent retina in one second). One to two months later the remnants were retreated with a smaller beam, repeated at two-month intervals until the entire mass was destroyed.

Lesions over 2 dd were treated with five to ten perhaps slightly more intense coagulations to the center of the angioma, again repeated at one- to two-month intervals. If the tumor became covered with exudate, white gliosis or a retinal detachment, further treatment was difficult and supplemental diathermy required. Lesions near the disc or macula were treated with minimal effective intensity.

Complications included hemorrhage, yellow retinal exudation, and retinal detachment. While small hemorrhages occurred regularly, only two patients had large vitreous hemorrhages. Exudative retinal detachment is usually noted 12–24 hours after treatment, and reattachment occurs spontaneously over several weeks. Treatment in stages minimizes this complication.

CRYOTHERAPY

It was originally believed that cryotherapy had no place in the treatment of angiomas because freezing has little or no effect upon blood vessels.[39] However, successful use of the method has been reported.[16] A 2-dd angioma was treated by the "triple freeze-thaw" method using a transscleral Amoils cryophobe at −70°C. A slow thaw was allowed between each freeze to the tumor and the surrounding retina.

Cryotherapy would seem to be useful only in treating small angiomas. Because small peripheral lesions are best seen with the indirect ophthalmoscope, it is probably preferable in such cases to use xenon-arc or argon coagulation.

PERSONAL TECHNIQUE

Light coagulation appears to be the easiest, safest, and most precise treatment for small angiomas. The technique involves treatment of the tumor alone, taking care to avoid the large afferent and efferent vessels which might bleed if treated directly. However, the occurrence of hemorrhage is less of a problem than the presence of white gliosis on the tumor surface. The surface is covered by normal intensity burns usually with a 3° spot. The 1.5° spot may not generate enough heat, and the 3° spot can be placed with greater precision than the 4.5° beam. If there is some doubt about intensity settings on the machine, a trial burn in adjacent nonvital retina is useful. At the time of exposure, there is little visible effect on the tumor, and a temptation to treat more heavily must be resisted. Red angiomas blanch a bit, and gray lesions may show a pink flush, but the effect is minimal.

With subsequent treatments there may be some pigment proliferation over the area and much more heat generated. The end point here is a sudden contraction of pigment granules which should make the operator quickly end the burn. Slightly longer exposure may produce an explosion, possibly leading to a major choroidal and vitreous hemorrhage. The retina immediately around the angioma is lightly treated in the hope of limiting exudative detachment, taking care to step through the feeder vessels with a 1.5° or 3° spot and not treat them heavily. Small hemorrhages frequently appear on the surface of the tumor during treatment and are almost always seen over the next three or four days as the tumor undergoes hemorrhagic necrosis. After treatment, exudate may increase or may appear around the tumor for the first time.

An unexplained complication, most frequent with angiomas on the temporal side, is the fresh appearance of yellow exudate in the macula following light coagulation. Eventual clearing of the exudate is rare. Macular function is compromised in 90% of the cases in which yellow exudate appears around the fovea. With larger lesions and heavier treatment, retinal detachment is common. It is usually transient as there are no breaks; reattachment occurs spontaneously in several days if the detachment is slight, and over several months if extensive.

Angiomas up to 1 dd can be destroyed in a single treatment, but larger tumors require several sessions at intervals of one to two months. Open feeder vessels provide evidence of a patent capillary bed, and further treatment is required. Again, light coagulation is directly applied to the tumor mass itself with normal intensity over pink areas and less intensity in pigmented areas. When the angioma has been destroyed, the feeder vessels shrink to normal size in a few months, and the surrounding exudates disappear over 4 to 12 months.

Angiomas over 4 dd in size, those with gray-white gliosis on the surface, and those with extensive retinal cyst formation or retinal detachment are difficult to control with light coagulation alone. Since it is associated with few complications, larger lesions may be treated in three or four sessions to see if they respond. If they shrink, the treatment is continued. A light coagulation scar around the lesion may minimize detachment or exudation if later diathermy is needed.

If light coagulation produces no real effect, supplemental diathermy is indicated. The Mira unit with 2-, 3-, or 4-mm perforating pins is preferred. The lesion is carefully marked on the scleral surface, and under constant visualization with the indirect ophthalmoscope, the shorter electrode (2 mm) is passed into the angioma. Starting with moderate intensity, a 2- to 10-second burn is produced. If there is no effect, the intensity is gradually increased to the maximum setting on the machine. If no shrinkage is seen, a 3-mm pin is next introduced with gradually increasing intensities followed by the 4-mm pin. The longer pin may perforate the tumor into the vitreous followed by a spiral of blood, but coagulation usually stops the bleeding. While rather intensive coagulation may be necessary to destroy large angiomas, it is safer to err on the side of light treatment. Diathermy coagulation can always be repeated, but the severe complications of hemorrhage and detachment cannot always be reversed.

In the treatment of large angiomas, macular function is almost always compromised. The objectives of treatment are cosmetic preservation of the globe and salvage of the peripheral field.

MALIGNANT MELANOMA

In spite of enucleation, and the fact that even tumor cells in the bloodstream do not certainly mean metastasis,[37,41] the five-year mortality rate for malignant melanoma of the choroid is nearly 50%. In some instances, as when the patient's only serviceable eye harbors a melanoma, treatment short of enucleation is advisable.

DIATHERMY

Diathermy was first used to treat malignant melanoma of the choroid in 1935. The 13-year mortality in this series was 12%.[48] A follow-up on 18 of these same patients 6 years later revealed no metastases even in the 2 who had died.[33] One woman who refused enucleation at age 25 was treated by diathermy and showed no recurrence after 8 years.[22]

A relatively short follow-up was reported on four cases treated by diathermy using the following technique:[21] Under direct ophthalmoscopic visualization, heavy dead-white confluent coagulations are made around the edge of the tumor and 2 mm beyond it. The sclera over the tumor is then treated with considerably increased intensity until the burn causes visible coagulation on the inner surface of the melanoma and destroys the overlying retina. Repeated applications to the same spot are usually necessary to achieve adequate burning. Following diathermy, the scleral surface is shrunken flat and severely burned; the inner surface is white.

Transscleral diathermy is used in patients with malignant melanomas up to 8–10 dd with an elevation of 2 mm or less, in any location away from the macula and optic nerve. An alarming amount of exudative detachment is often seen after treatment. Because of fragility of the burned retina, bed rest is advised for a week and limited activity for several weeks. Tumor elevation persists for many months or even a year, but the final result is an almost flat, pigmented, atrophic scar.

In view of the severe local reaction, melanomas near the macula and optic nerve cannot be treated by diathermy without major or total loss of retinal function. The sizes of the tumors in the aforementioned four cases were 5 dd with 2 mm elevation, 2 × 3 dd slightly elevated, 6 dd slightly elevated, and 7 dd with 1 mm elevation. The authors used perforating diathermy, pointing out sharp differences in

transscleral diathermy for retinal detachment and for malignant melanoma.[21] They indicated that intense coagulation of the entire melanoma destroys all the cells, preventing growth of the tumor into the orbit as sometimes occurs after a detachment procedure in an eye with unrecognized melanoma.

LIGHT COAGULATION

Malignant melanoma of the choroid was first treated by light coagulation in 1952, with encouraging results in 61 cases treated by 1961.[19] During this period the technique was being developed and the success rate is difficult to interpret, since many eyes were enucleated at different intervals after light coagulation to assess the treatment results histologically.

Pathologic evaluation of four eyes with malignant melanomas of the choroid treated with light coagulation 2, 6, 8, and 17 days, respectively, before preplanned enucleation has been reported.[20] The surgeons, interested in the histologic aspect of the burns, found a mixture of viable and nonviable cells in all cases but did not attempt to destroy the tumors completely, as was done by other operators. They concluded that flat tumors could be more easily destroyed than highly elevated ones, that necrosis was not influenced by pigmentation of the tumor, and that overlying retinal detachment did not influence treatment results as long as the subretinal fluid was clear.

The histologic findings in eyes in which an attempt was made to destroy the tumor have also been reported.[45]

An eye with a malignant melanoma unsuccessfully treated by serial light coagulation, diathermy, repeated light coagulation, and radon seeds in a plastic shell[19] showed many complications due to treatment. When ultimately studied microscopically, viable tumor cells were found. In another report,[32] the authors noted that none of the four choroidal melanomas was completely destroyed despite intensive treatment, leading to the conclusion that photocoagulation alone is not suitable treatment for melanoma.

The histologic characteristics of malignant melanomas after photocoagulation have been described by several investigators.[24,27,45]

The following indications for treatment by light coagulation have been suggested:[44]

1. The diagnosis must be made with all available methods (fluorescein, ^{32}P uptake, etc.). If in doubt, observation is continued until unequivocal growth can be determined.

2. Informed consent by patient
3. Tumors less than 5 diopters
4. Tumors less than 6 dd
5. No retinal detachment
6. Localization of tumor amenable to complete surrounding by light coagulation (not near disc or posterior pole)
7. Clear media
8. Widely dilated pupil
9. Location away from major retinal vessels, as their obliteration may lead to neovascularization and retinitis proliferans.

These qualifications represent the ideal situation and in each case some factors must be compromised.

This author[44] suggests a technique somewhat different from that for other intraocular tumors. At the first session a double ring of heavy coagulations is made around the mass, avoiding large retinal vessels. At the next session a month later, the ring is reinforced over the pigmented scar and the entire tumor surface is covered by gentle coagulations, producing a visible whitish discoloration. During the third session another month later, the mass itself is treated more intensely. In a heavily pigmented tumor, explosion may occur. If a choroidal hemorrhage is produced, the bleeding site should be swiftly coagulated to prevent a major vitreous hemorrhage. A month later, at the fourth session, the tumor mass is treated by heavy coagulations with small explosions until bare sclera is seen. The final session of coagulation is advisable to judge the possible activity of a tumor rest. When the area is covered by high-intensity coagulations, an explosion or bleeding suggests viable tumor remnants. Mere contraction of pigment, baring white sclera, indicates that the tumor has been destroyed.

A 10-year follow-up of 54 patients treated by this method[44] showed survival of 34 (63%). Only 8 of the 20 deaths were due to metastases; the rest were due to other or unknown causes. Of the 34 survivors, 25 were considered to have been cured.

The successfully treated tumors were from 4 to 10 dd and from 2 to 9 diopters. The patients had two to eight treatment sessions, with an average of six. Tumors in the unsuccessful cases were slightly larger with more mass and up to 14 diopters. Location over the short ciliary vessels at the posterior pole may be a factor in failure.

Complications in this series included rare hemorrhage during treatment, injury to the iris sphincter in six cases, and retinal detachment in one case. Recurrences were usually manifested within two years but have been seen as late as eight years after light coagulation; those near the disc are especially likely to show late recurrence.

CRYOTHERAPY

Cryotherapy is ineffectual in the treatment of intraocular malignant melanoma.[28-30]

COBALT-60 PLAQUE

Local treatment can also be carried out by application of the ^{60}Co plaques, which appear to be the treatment of choice for malignant melanomas of the choroid.[18,31,40] (See section Radiotherapy of Ocular and Orbital Tumors, by Patricia Tretter in this chapter.)

PERSONAL EXPERIENCE

Six malignant melanomas have been light-coagulated using the previously described method; there was one death. During routine ophthalmologic examination of a 40-year-old woman, a highly elevated, 8 dd, mushroom-shaped tumor was found in the lower nasal quadrant. It was destroyed in 20 treatment sessions over two years. She has had no recurrence for 10 years. Pigment dispersion into the vitreous had no unfortunate sequelae. This case provides evidence that persistent and intense light coagulations can destroy melanomas up to or slightly over 6 dd even if highly elevated.

Malignant melanomas may grow very slowly or not at all for many years, then undergo some transformation marked by rapid growth. They are usually diagnosed during this phase because of tumor or subretinal fluid encroachment on the macula. A rapidly growing tumor may not be burned from the top down as fast as it grows from the bottom up. In this event supplemental diathermy or a ^{60}Co plaque may be used. Slowly growing melanomas are more amenable to light coagulation but are usually asymptomatic and therefore undetected when small.

During the past ten years, increasing reliance has been placed on ^{60}Co plaques rather than light coagulation. If late complications should occur, diathermy and light coagulation would again be the method of choice for smaller lesions.

Since many melanomas are paramacular, there is reason to believe that foveal function is more likely spared by ^{60}Co plaques than by diathermy or light coagulation, which destroys the fovea. A melanoma over 6 dd should be treated only by ^{60}Co plaques.

RETINOBLASTOMA

Among the six modalities commonly used for the treatment of retinoblastoma, external beam supervoltage radiation and systemic chemotherapy treat the entire retina. The others—diathermy, light coagulation, cryotherapy, and ^{60}Co applicators—treat only the affected area of the retina. There is strong evidence that children with hereditary retinoblastoma and anyone with bilateral retinoblastoma have a genetic mutation affecting every cell in the body. As mentioned earlier, these children may develop other primary tumors, as well as retinoblastoma, and seem more likely to have radiation-induced tumors than do normal individuals receiving the same dosages.

The use of diathermy, light coagulation, and cryotherapy circumvents the danger of producing osteogenic sarcomas. The second eye in a bilateral case might harbor one or several small tumors amenable to these measures, and they may also be effective for new tumors in a hereditary case suspected and followed from birth. A tumor of only 2 or 3 dd may arise in the macula producing early strabismus. With increasing awareness of the dangers of external beam radiation in recent years, we have leaned more toward light coagulation or cryotherapy for small lesions, especially at the periphery.

New retinoblastomas rarely develop after the age of 2; if they do arise they are likely to be at the periphery, especially below where undifferentiated retinal cells may still be present.[26] Diathermy, light coagulation, or cryotherapy in these areas will not produce an objectionable field defect. On the other hand, small tumors near the macula are better treated by external beam radiation if foveal function is to be preserved. This also applies to lesions near the optic nerve where light coagulation or diathermy may produce large field defects.

DIATHERMY

Results in the earliest cases of retinoblastoma treated by diathermy were disappointing[46,47] but have been encouraging with the newer techniques.[17,22,36] Surface diathermy is preferred, and only small tumors are amenable to treatment. The procedure may be combined with irradiation and chemotherapy.

LIGHT COAGULATION

The first series of retinoblastoma treated by light coagulation[35] showed success in 14 out of 18 cases. Eight other patients were successfully treated by a combination of light coagulation, radiation, and chemotherapy. Seven patients previously treated by radiation were subsequently cured by light coagulation.

Light coagulation can destroy a retinoblastoma that is relatively small.[32] The suggestion that this procedure may destroy the lamina vitrea, thereby permitting tumor extension into the choroid,[25] has not been substantiated.

Small retinoblastomas depend on the retinal circulation alone for nutrition during a considerable period of their growth, and can be destroyed by light coagulation if the retinal circulation is completely interrupted. The technique consists of surrounding them by two or three rows of coagulations carried down along the proximal vessels if necessary to occlude them. The light-colored tumors are usually highly resistant to direct coagulation. One tumor personally treated had an explosion, but this is extremely rare. Treatments are repeated at intervals of three to four weeks until there is a complete avascular scar around the lesion. Complications include rare hemorrhage and exudative detachment at the time of treatment or several days later. The latter is usually seen with large tumors heavily treated; since such retinas have no holes, they usually reattach spontaneously over the next few weeks or months.

CRYOTHERAPY

Cold of $-40°C$ applied to the scleral surface produces a temperature of 0 to $-20°C$.[28-30] It destroys the nuclear and ganglion cell layers and the layer of rods and cones, but does not obliterate the larger blood vessels. Numerous case reports of retinoblastoma treated by cryotherapy have appeared.[23,29,38]

In one suggested technique[42] using the Amoils carbon dioxide apparatus,[16] the author correctly stressed the necessity of firmly indenting the sclera to blanch the choroid and allow freezing through the tumor. The temperature range was $-60°$ to $-70°C$, and the tip of the ice ball was seen coming through the tumor. With strong indentation, the tumor is frozen, allowed to thaw partially, and then refrozen. The ice ball is maintained for about one minute. The tumor is treated at monthly intervals until the scleral scar is completely flat. It was felt that partial thawing might prevent the choroidal and scleral congestion that could make refreezing more difficult.

PERSONAL TECHNIQUE

Personal experience is based on the light coagulation of 125 cases and cryotherapy of 41 cases of retinoblastoma. No patients have been treated by diathermy.

Light coagulation has proved the most valuable adjunct. The great majority of children are given an initial course of supervoltage radiation, using the 22.5 mev betatron, the dose ranging from 3500 to 4500 rads in three to four weeks. They are examined under anesthesia eight weeks after completion of radiation. Because the lens must be avoided, the anterior annulus of the retina between the equator and the ora serrata may not receive a full homogeneous dose. This factor, and the greater likelihood of new tumors arising from the less differentiated retinal cells at the periphery, point up the importance of directing attention to the anterior retina. Small tumors in this area that remain pink and opaque are suspect and treated with light coagulation. Use of this technique in the anterior retina carries little threat of hemorrhage or other complications and does not produce a significant field defect. In many such cases light coagulation may not be strictly necessary but it is relatively harmless and may obviate a second course of radiation.

Light coagulation is indicated for recurrent retinoblastoma following radiation either at the original site or elsewhere in the retina. Tumors of up to 6 dd can be successfully controlled if they are well separated from the optic nerve and from the major retinal vessels. A heavy double or triple row of coagulations surrounds the tumor and is carried proximally along the vessels in areas where there is little risk of producing a field defect. The tumor is treated at intervals of three to four weeks until all its vessels are destroyed. Initially, the retinal blood vessels may go into spasm and appear to be destroyed only to reopen minutes or hours after treatment. Light coagulation is continued until the pigmented scar around the tumor shows no retinal blood vessels. The choroidal circulation can also be obliterated by intense, repeated coagulations, but this is unnecessary in the treatment of retinoblastoma. In one to six months the tumor rest in the scar resorbs completely. Retrogression, or an increase in elevation, suggests extension into the choroid; light coagulation will no longer be effective and a ^{60}Co plaque should be used.

The immediate complications are retinal detachment and hemorrhages. The latter often occur on the tumor surface but are rarely a major problem. The blood vessels nourishing a retinoblastoma can usually be treated directly without great danger of hemorrhage. With large tumors and extensive light coagulation, a limited retinal detachment is occasionally observed, but it usually resolves over the next several weeks or months without having interfered with function. At times yellow fatty exudates appear following light coagulation, especially if the nutrient vessels are large. Because of possible damage to the lamina vitrea, light coagulation should not be used as a "last ditch" measure in an only eye.[25] If the tumor is not over 6 dd choroidal extension is probably not an important factor. In the past few years light coagulation has been our primary form of treatment for one or two small tumors in an involved eye, despite a positive family history and the expectation that more tumors may develop. Close supervision of these children is mandatory; they are often examined at one- to two-month intervals under anesthesia. In general, tumors behind the equator should not be treated by light coagulation because of the production of field defects, the danger of hemorrhage, and the fact that such lesions are more easily treated by radiation. There is generally less damage to retinal structures in an eye successfully treated by radiation than in an eye successfully treated by diathermy, light coagulation, cryotherapy, or ^{60}Co applicators, but the risk of radiation-induced tumors, principally osteogenic sarcomas, is ever-present.

Cryotherapy is approximately as effective as light coagulation for retinoblastomas but not for other types of tumors. Destruction is achieved by intracellular crystal formation, dehydration, and interruption of the tumor's internal capillary circulation rather than by interrupting the retinal circulation. A retinoblastoma treated by light coagulation which has a vessel-free annulus and the rest unabsorbed is an excellent choice for cryotherapy. Any tumor treated by either light coagulation or cryotherapy should disappear entirely with no visible rest. Conversely, after radiation treatment elevated opaque rests may persist throughout the patient's life without apparent danger.

Recurrent tumors behind the equator are treated with light coagulation and those anterior to the equator with cryotherapy because of easier visualization with the indirect ophthalmoscope. With a Searcy pick, however, and an indirect ophthalmoscope, light coagulation can be applied up to the ora serrata and indeed several millimeters onto the pars plana with a little practice.

My preference is for light coagulation first, followed by cryotherapy if the rest within the light coagulation scar has not disappeared completely within a reasonable time.

SUMMARY

Briefly, small retinal angiomas are best treated by light coagulation and larger lesions by combined light coagulation and diathermy.

Malignant melanomas are best treated by ^{60}Co applicators, but small flat lesions can be handled by diathermy and when slightly larger by light coagulation. It cannot be overemphasized that only repeated and very intense coagulation completely destroys the tumor cells.

Small retinoblastomas can be destroyed by diathermy, light coagulation, or cryotherapy. Unfortunately, most tumors are so large when first seen as to require external beam radiation. Light coagulation and cryotherapy are both valuable adjuncts and have specific indications in treatment. Small retinoblastomas, especially those in the anterior portion of the retina, are best treated by primary light coagulation or cryotherapy in an attempt to avoid the carcinogenic effects of radiation on bone and on other orbital structures.

Ramon L. Font

ELECTRON MICROSCOPY OF TUMORS OF THE EYE AND OCULAR ADNEXA

For many years routine histologic techniques have been applied to conventional light microscopy for the study of normal and pathologic processes. In the past two decades, electron microscopy has become an increasingly popular means of broadening our understanding of numerous problems encountered in ophthalmic as well as general pathology.

The anatomist and the researcher ideally prefer optimal methods of fixation of tissues processed for electron microscopy. While these methods produce excellent results with good cytologic preservation of the cellular organelles and extracellular components, electron microscopy should not be excluded merely because the tissue has been fixed in formalin and routinely embedded in paraffin for light microscopy. In such cases, valuable information toward the solution of various problems can still be obtained. For example, when conventional methods for light microscopy fail to establish an unequivocal histopathologic diagnosis, electron microscopy may lead to a more definitive diagnosis. Several examples involving differential diagnoses follow:

1. Spindle-cell tumors, *e.g.*, leiomyoma vs neurofibroma vs spindle-cell amelanotic malignant melanoma; fibrosarcoma vs spindle-cell squamous carcinoma vs fibrous histiocytoma.
2. Poorly differentiated neoplasms, *e.g.*, epithelial tumors vs reticulum-cell sarcoma; rhabdomyosarcoma vs amelanotic malignant melanoma. Certain orbital tumors with alveolar pattern, *e.g.*, alveolar rhabdomyosarcoma vs alveolar soft-part sarcoma vs nonchromaffin paraganglioma.

3. Certain melanotic tumors, *e.g.*, tumors of the retinal pigment epithelium vs those arising from uveal melanocytes; melanoma cells vs melanophages; lipid-filled macrophages vs lipid-containing melanoma cells.
4. Certain intraocular tumors showing highly characteristic specialized structures, *e.g.*, retinoblastoma with photoreceptor differentiation.
5. Certain metastatic lesions, *e.g.*, carcinoid tumors that may demonstrate the presence of neurosecretory granules.

In the examples selected for this presentation, electron microscopy has proved of great value in solving a very specific diagnostic or research problem. Details of the technique of processing the tissue for electron microscopy have been previously reported from our laboratory.[52,71]

Figure 12–12 illustrates a problem in the cytologic interpretation of large cells with abundant acidophilic cytoplasm (circle, inset) that were contained within an embryonal medulloepithelioma (Fig. 12–13). The cells in question (Fig. 12–12, circle) were suspected of being ganglion cells, mainly because of their shape and large size; however, by electron microscopy they were found to be rhabdomyoblasts. The rhabdomyoblasts were characterized by their cytoplasmic content of interlacing bundles of thick (myosin) and thin (actin) myofilaments with formation of I bands and Z lines (Fig. 12–14). Numerous glycogen particles were distributed along the myofilaments.

This case plus three additional examples of embryonal intraocular medulloepitheliomas with rhabdomyosarcomatous differentiation

351

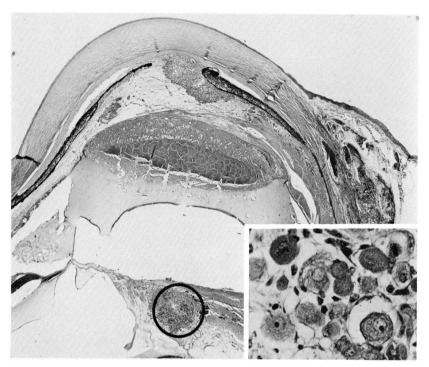

FIG. 12–12. A malignant neoplasm filling the posterior chamber and pupillary region has infiltrated through the ciliary body (on the right) and extended to the episclera subconjunctivally. (Hematoxylin and eosin, × 12, AFIP Neg. 70-7855.) *Inset:* High magnification of the area in circle shows large ganglioform cells (actually rhabdomyoblasts) among the smaller undifferentiated cells. (Hematoxylin and eosin, × 305, AFIP Neg. 69-9903)

FIG. 12–13. Higher magnification of the intraocular tumor in Figure 12–12 reveals a malignant medulloepithelioma containing a few neuroepithelial rosettes, masses of poorly differentiated medullary epithelium, and an abundance of spindle-shaped cells. Arrow points to a round myoblast (below the rosette). (Hematoxylin and eosin, × 210, AFIP Neg. 71-6850) (From Zimmerman LE, et al. Cancer 30:817–835, 1972)

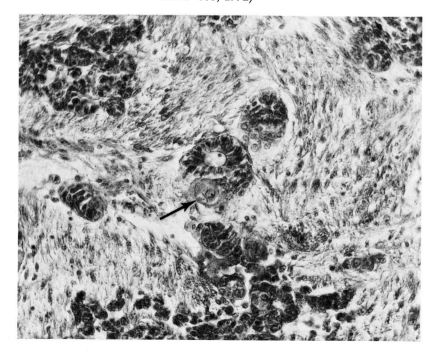

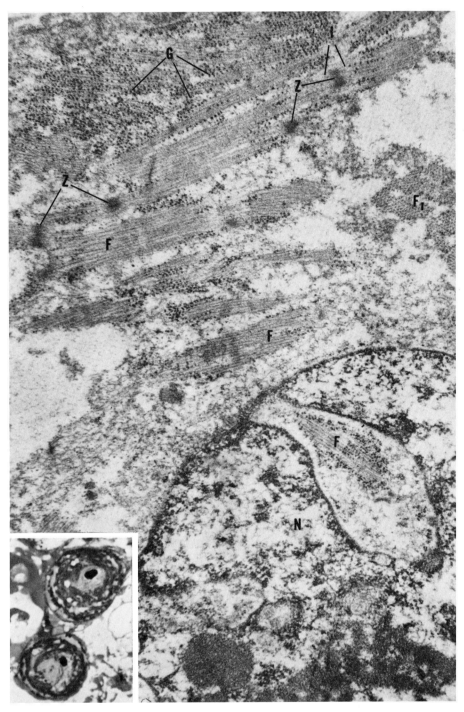

FIG. 12–14. Rhabdomyoblast showing numerous
bundles of cytoplasmic myofilaments cut
longitudinally (*F*) and transversely (*F₁*).
Numerous glycogen particles (*G*) are oriented
along the myofilaments. I bands (*I*) and Z lines
(*Z*) are readily recognizable. Myofilaments can be
seen in a portion of the cytoplasm that is
entrapped in an indentation of the nucleus (*N*).
(× 34,000, AFIP Neg. 60-9143-2.) Inset shows
the large round cells (Fig. 12–12, circle and
inset) present within the medulloepithelioma of
the ciliary body. (Epon-embedded, 1.5 micron
section, toluidine blue, × 750, AFIP Neg.
69-9830) (From Zimmerman et al.): Cancer 30:
817–835, 1972)

have been reported.[70] One of these authors proposed a classification of intraocular medulloepithelioma[69] and emphasized the marked polymorphism of these tumors of the ciliary epithelium.[68] A cytologic classification of orbital rhabdomyosarcomas has also been proposed, based on electron microscopic observations.[57]

Certain poorly differentiated neoplasms may exhibit an alveolar pattern (Fig. 12–15), creating diagnostic confusion with other apparently similar tumors (e.g., alveolar rhabdomyosarcoma vs alveolar soft-part sarcoma vs nonchromaffin paraganglioma).

A distinctive and highly characteristic finding in favor of alveolar soft-part sarcoma, not seen in other tumors with an alveolar pattern, is the presence of PAS-positive, diastase-resistant crystalline inclusions. The crystals vary in size, shape (retangular, rhomboidal, rodlike, spiked) (Fig. 12–16, right inset), and distribution from tumor to tumor and even in various areas of the same tumor. Crystals were found in 9 out of 13 tumors in one study.[61] The authors concluded that the crystals were composed of protein-carbohydrate complex.

Earlier histochemical studies of the granules in the cytoplasm of these tumors suggested a neural origin.[53] Our own electron microscopic studies are similar to those reported by others.[54,61] The crystals in some areas were incompletely formed (Figs. 12–16 and 12–17) and demonstrated longitudinal striations with a periodicity of 80 to 100 A (Fig. 12–16, left lower inset). In addition, the almost total lack of myofilaments and/or sarcomere formation in alveolar soft-part sarcomas distinguishes them from the more common embryonal and alveolar forms of rhabdomyosarcoma. Electron microscopy, however, has failed to produce any clues about their histogenesis. Isolated case reports of alveolar soft-part sarcomas of the orbit[49,50] have further emphasized the diagnostic significance of these crystalline inclusions. Judging from the published photomicrographs alone, one case reported as malignant nonchromaffin paraganglioma of the orbit[58] is probably another example of an alveolar soft-part sarcoma.

Another important practical application of electron microscopy is the study and classification of intraocular melanotic lesions. We have reported findings in a case of pigmented adenoma of the retinal pigment epithelium of the vacuolated type,[56] and a similar tumor of the ciliary pigment epithelium has been described by others.[62]

Figure 12–18 is from a moderately pigmented tumor of the iris that proved to be a low-grade spindle-cell melanoma. By electron microscopy the spindle-shaped melanoma cells (Fig. 12–18, circle) demonstrate the presence of immature and mature melanosomes (Fig. 12–19) in their cytoplasm. Figure 12–20 by contrast shows the presence of melanin-laden macrophages or melanophages (Fig. 12–18, square) containing myriad melanosomes within phagocytic vacuoles, many of which are clearly enclosed by a single membrane (Fig. 12–20, inset).

Figure 12–21 shows another type of melanin-filled macrophage containing melanosomal complexes that indicate origin of the melanosomes from the pigment epithelium in contrast to the pigment granules derived from uveal melanocytes as demonstrated in the macrophage in Figure 12–20. By light microscopy the origin of pigment-containing cells in the trabecular meshwork spaces can be difficult to determine with certainty (Fig. 12–22, inset). Electron microscopy clearly differentiates between melanophages and melanoma cells (Figs. 12–20 and 12–21).

Certain uveal melanomas contain lipid-laden cells (balloon cells) (Fig. 12–23, inset). There are two main possibilities concerning the origin of these cells: a) lipid-laden macrophages and b) a peculiar lipoidal degeneration of melanocytic cells. Figures 12–23 and 12–24 demonstrate that they contain numerous intracytoplasmic, round to oval, single membrane-bound vacuoles. The convolutions of the nuclear membrane, the prominent nucleoli, and the presence of immature and mature melanosomes between the cytoplasmic vacuoles are strong evidence in favor of a lipoidal degeneration of melanoma cells and against their being lipid-laden macrophages. The cytoplasmic vacuoles in these figures appear empty because the lipid had been dissolved owing to storage of the wet tissue in 60% alcohol. The lipid can be vividly demonstrated, however, on frozen sections stained with oil red 0 (Fig. 12–25A) as well as under polarized light showing a striking birefringence of the intracytoplasmic material (Fig. 12–25B). The latter finding probably represents an in vitro crystallization of the lipoidal material in the tumor cells.

Balloon cells have been described in nevi of the skin, the choroid, and the conjunctiva; they have also been noted in primary and

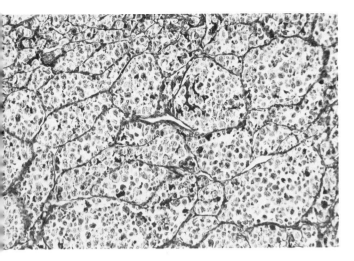

FIG. 12–15. Orbital tumor with a prominent alveolar pattern delineated by thin fibrous septa. The round or polygonal cells contain abundant cytoplasm with many PAS-positive granules as well as scattered crystalline inclusions. (PAS, × 80, AFIP Neg. 69-1298)

FIG. 12–16. Electron micrograph of alveolar soft-part sarcoma showing several rectangular or rhomboidal crystals (*C*) and abundant rough-surfaced endoplasmic reticulum (*ER*). Nucleus (*N*). (× 30,000, AFIP Neg. 74-10013-1) Inset at right reveals numerous intracytoplasmic crystalline inclusions within tumor cells. (Toluidine blue, × 485, AFIP Neg. 74-9100.) Inset at left shows one of the crystals with a periodicity of 80 Å. (× 63,000)

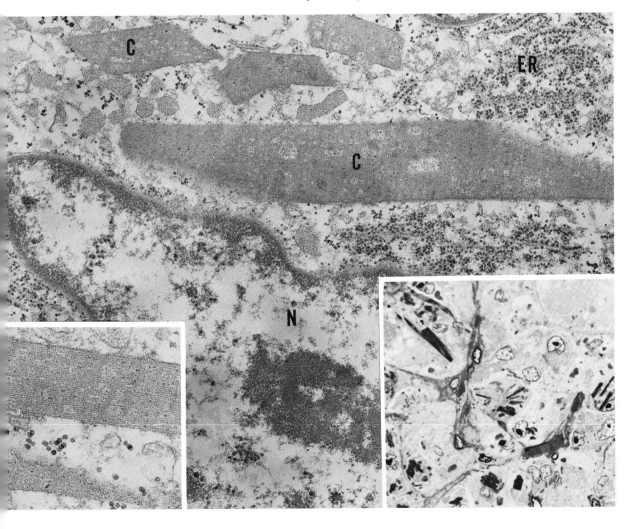

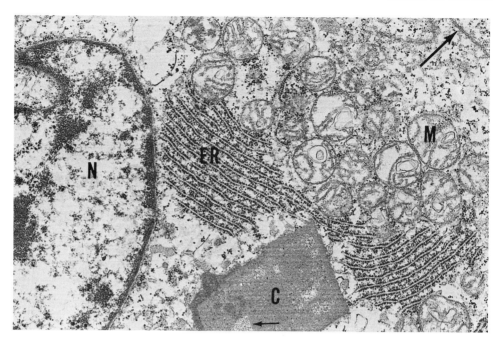

FIG. 12–17. Another tumor cell showing a rectangular, incompletely formed crystal. A small square defect (*small arrow*) contains dense osmophilic granules. There are numerous lamellae of rough-surfaced endoplasmic reticulum (*ER*). Some mitochondria (*M*) demonstrate irregular or concentrically arranged cristae. Plasmalemma (*large arrow*); nucleus (*N*); crystalloid (*C*). (× 18,000, AFIP Neg. 10013-2)

FIG. 12–18. Spindle-cell melanoma of the iris (low-grade malignancy). The tumor cells have formed a placoid, cohesive mass extending along the anterior surface of the iris. The circle encloses spindle-shaped melanoma cells (Fig. 12–19). Scattered melanophages are present within the square (Fig. 12–20). (Paraphenylenediamine, × 140, AFIP Neg. 74-9102)

FIG. 12–20. Pigment-laden macrophage (melanophage) located within square in Figure 12–18, containing numerous phagocytic vacuoles or phagosomes predominantly filled with immature melanosomes. The nucleus (*N*) is eccentric (× 18,000, AFIP Neg. 10013-4). Inset shows several melanosomes in phagocytic vacuoles each surrounded by a single membrane (*arrow*). (× 36,000)

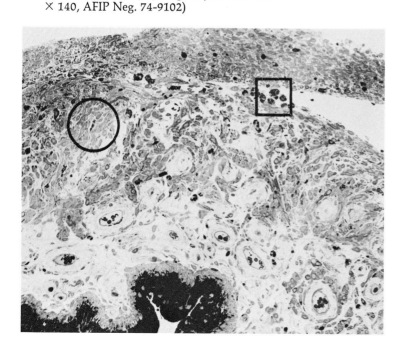

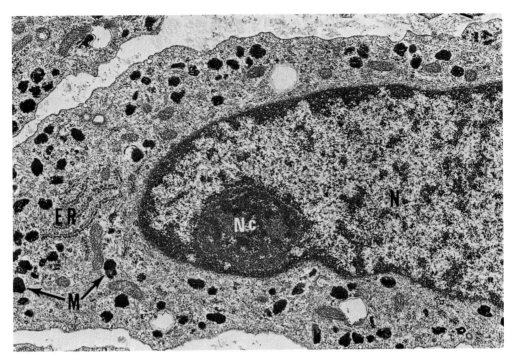

FIG. 12–19. Spindle B-type melanoma cell (Fig. 12–18, circle) has a moderate number of melanosomes (*M*) and rather scanty endoplasmic reticulum (*ER*). The plasmalemma shows minimal interdigitations with adjacent cells. Nucleus (*N*); nucleolus (*Nc*). (× 14,400, AFIP Neg. 10013-3)

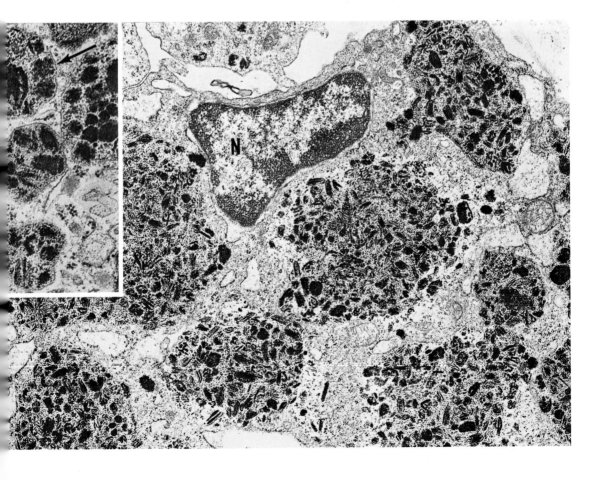

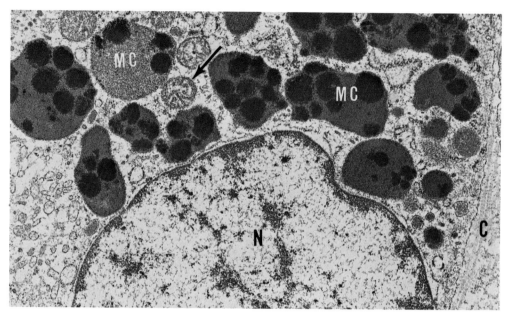

FIG. 12–21. Another pigment-laden macrophage (melanophage) filled with melanosomal complexes (*MC*). The pigment granules here indicate their origin from pigment epithelium (compare with uveal melanin granules in macrophage of Fig. 12–20). Arrow points to mitochondria. Nucleus (*N*); collagen (*C*). (× 18,000, AFIP Neg. 10013-5)

FIG. 12–22. Pigment-containing cells in the trabecular meshwork spaces (*inset*) are melanoma cells and not macrophages, a distinction not readily made by light microscopy. Immature melanosomes (*M*) are seen in the nonfilamentous cytoplasm (epithelial cell type). Lipid vacuoles (*L*); trabecular spaces (*Tr*); nucleus (*N*). (× 16,500; inset, paraphenylenediamine, × 750, AFIP Neg. 10013-6) (Courtesy of M. Yanoff and B. S. Fine.[67])

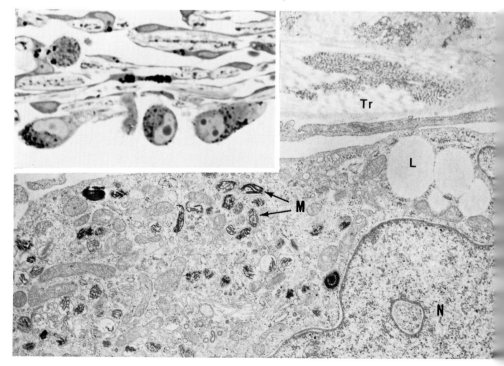

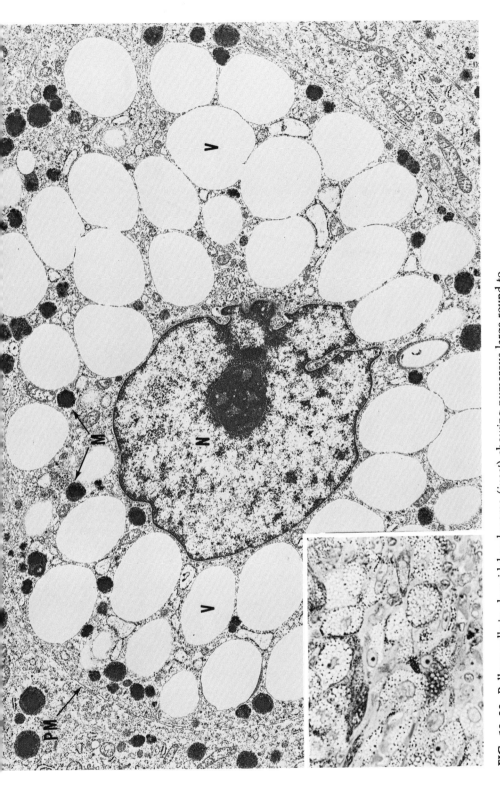

FIG. 12–23. Balloon cells in choroidal melanoma (*inset*) showing numerous large round to oval empty vacuoles (*V*). The lipid has been mainly dissolved out since the specimen was stored in 60% alcohol. The indentations of the nuclear membrane, the prominent nucleolus, and the presence of melanosomes (*M*) are strong evidence indicating lipoidal degeneration of a melanoma cell rather than lipid engorgement by a macrophage. Plasma membrane (*PM*); nucleus (*N*). (× 10,800, AFIP Neg. 10013-7); inset, paraphenylenediamine, × 440, AFIP Neg. 72–12985)

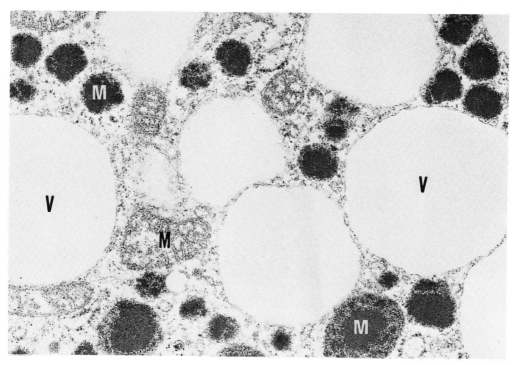

FIG. 12–24. High-power field of adjacent balloon cell showing single membrane-bound vacuoles (*V*) and melanosomes (white *M*) in different stages of development. Mitochondria (*M*). (× 30,000, AFIP Neg. 10013-8)

FIG. 12–25. A. Lightly pigmented malignant melanoma of ciliary body containing numerous balloon cells. Frozen section reveals abundant lipoidal material in the cell cytoplasm. (Oil red O, × 290, AFIP Neg. 74-9104.) **B.** The same field reveals numerous birefringent crystals within the cytoplasm of the tumor cells. This finding probably represents an *in vitro* crystallization of the intracytoplasmic lipoidal material. (Polarized light, × 290, AFIP Neg. 74-9105)

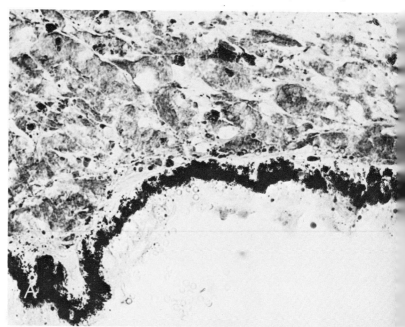

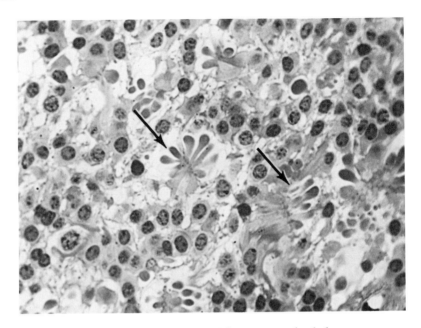

FIG. 12–26. Light micrograph of photoreceptor elements in retinoblastoma (1.5 microns, Epon-embedded section). The flowerlike clusters (fleurettes) of the photoreceptor cell processes (*arrows*) are clearly evident. (Paraphenylenediamine, × 575, AFIP Neg. 68-9466) (Courtesy of M. O. M. Ts'o et al.[66])

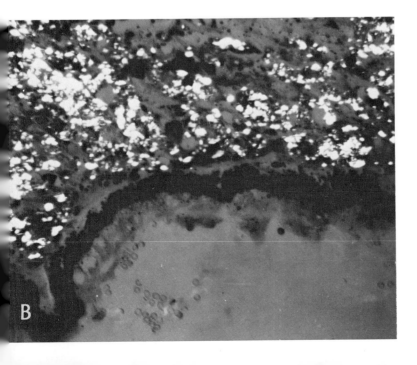

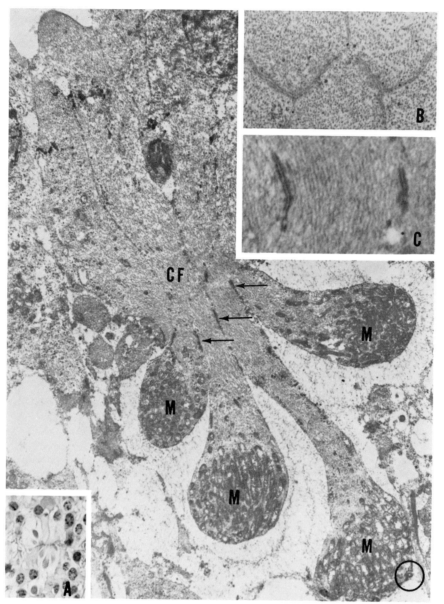

FIG. 12–27. Photoreceptor cell elements (fleurettes) in retinoblastoma. Tumor cells with long conducting fibers (*CF*) are joined together by dense cell attachments (*arrows*). The cell processes extend beyond the plane of cell attachments for a variable distance. Longitudinally oriented mitochondria (*M*) in large numbers are packed in the outer bulbous end of the cytoplasmic processes. A cilium (cut in cross section [*circle*]) is seen at one of the cell processes. (× 5382 before 15% reduction.) Inset A shows a similar fleurette by light microscopy. (× 400 before 15% reduction.) Inset B shows a portion of the hexagonal pattern observed in a tangential section of the cell attachments. (× 6739 before 15% reduction.) A cross section of similar cell attachments (terminal bars) appears in inset C. (× 16,100 before 15% reduction, AFIP Neg. 69-4552-8.) (Courtesy of M. O. M. Ts'o et al.[66])

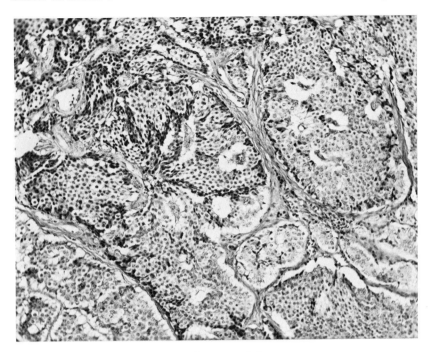

FIG. 12–28. A metastatic carcinoid tumor of the orbit composed of irregular lobules separated by thin septa of fibrous connective tissue. The cells in the periphery of each lobule have a darker eosinophilic cytoplasm that interdigitates with the more centrally located clear cells. (Hematoxylin and eosin, × 115, AFIP Neg. 72-12549)

FIG. 12–29. Higher magnification of the tumor shown in Figure 12–28 reveals dark and light cells. Distinct granules are more clearly seen in the cytoplasm of the light cells, but are present in the dark cells which also contain fine vacuoles. (Toluidine blue, × 1600, AFIP Neg. 74-9515)

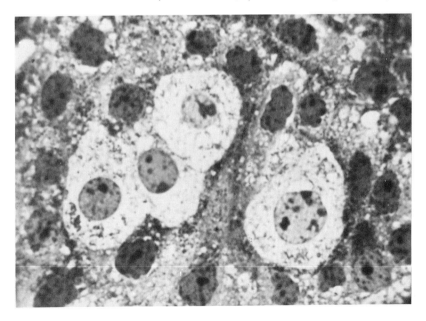

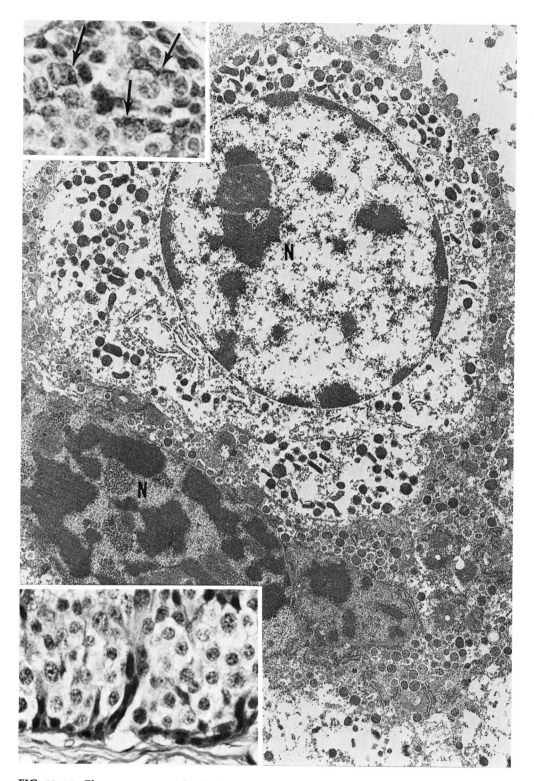

FIG. 12–30. Electron micrograph of a light cell (above) surrounded by a dark cell (below). Both cells contain numerous neurosecretory granules that vary in shape, density, and distribution. Nucleus (*N*). ($\times$ 14,000, AFIP Neg. 10013-9) The inset below reveals both dark and light cells at the periphery of one of the tumor lobules. (Hematoxylin and eosin, $\times$ 440, AFIP Neg. 74-9513) The inset above demonstrates a positive argentaffin reaction (black cytoplasmic granules indicated by *arrows*). (Fontana reaction, $\times$ 575, AFIP Neg. 74-9511)

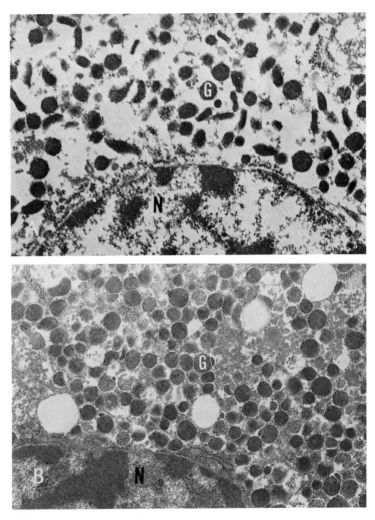

FIG. 12–31. A. Light cell containing more electron-dense spherical or elongated (rod-shaped) granules (G). The cytoplasm is more translucent and the granules widely dispersed throughout. Nucleus (N). (× 21,000, AFIP Neg. 10013-11) **B.** Dark cell disclosing more closely packed, less electron-dense spherical granules (G) and scattered cytoplasmic vacuoles which are also present in Figure 12–29. N indicates nucleus. (× 21,000, AFIP Neg. 10013-10)

metastatic malignant melanomas of the skin. A 10% incidence in 200 cases of choroidal melanomas has been reported.[59] Electron microscopic studies of balloon-cell nevus of the skin and conjunctiva and of metastatic balloon-cell melanoma have raised some doubt as to whether an early arrest in melanogenesis occurs.

Electron microscopy has also established the nature of a peculiar orange pigment that is sometimes observed clinically on the surface of a choroidal melanoma.[55]

The origin of retinoblastomas has long been a controversial subject. In studies using principally paraffin-embedded tissues, it has been clearly established that they are neuronal neoplasms.[63-66] The areas exhibiting photoreceptor differentiation are usually small and often undetectable prior to microscopic examination of the eye. Fleurettes (Fig. 12–26) were first described within these areas by the same authors, who demonstrated the ultrastructural features characteristic of inner and outer photoreceptor segments of the human retina (Fig. 12–27). They concluded that the fleurette is more differentiated than the Flexner-Wintersteiner rosette and therefore phylogenetically more closely related to the mature adult retina.

Certain metastatic tumors of the eye and orbit may reveal characteristic histochemical and electron microscopic findings permitting a more precise diagnosis. For example, Figure 12–28 represents a metastatic tumor of the orbit in an otherwise healthy, middle-aged patient. The three main histopathologic diagnoses considered were primary carcinoma of the lacrimal gland, metastatic carcinoma, and metastatic carcinoid tumor. Sections 1–2 microns thick clearly revealed the presence of light and dark cells, both containing intracytoplasmic granules (Fig. 12–29). The darker cells were predominantly confined to the periphery of the tumor lobules (Fig. 12–30,

lower inset). Special stains demonstrated the presence of a positive argentaffin reaction (Fig. 12–30, upper inset). Electron microscopy of the paraffin-embedded tissue revealed two cell types, both containing myriad neurosecretory granules of variable shape and density (Fig. 12–30). The granules in the light cells were less numerous, more electron-dense and varied from round to elongated to rod-shaped structures (Fig. 12–31A), while the granules in the dark cells were more densely packed, less electron-dense, and varied from spheroidal to oval in shape (Fig. 12-31B). In addition, the darker cells contained distinct intracytoplasmic small vacuoles that were not observed in the light cells.

Electron microscopic studies of the neurosecretory granules of carcinoid tumors have been described.[51,60]

Other practical applications of electron microscopy are a) establishing the differences between nevocytic and melanocytic malignant melanomas (arising from a freckle of Hutchinson), b) determining the histiogenesis of certain tumors, such as granular-cell myoblastoma, and c) detecting viral particles, although no viral particles have yet been found in any neoplasm of the human eye and ocular adnexa.

J. Donald M. Gass

STEREOFUNDUS PHOTOGRAPHY AND FLUORESCEIN ANGIOGRAPHY IN THE DIAGNOSIS OF INTRAOCULAR TUMORS

In some patients a primary intraocular neoplasm can be accurately diagnosed with the aid of ophthalmoscopy, biomicroscopy and transillumination, whereas in others special techniques of examination may be required. While such techniques including fluorescein angiography may assist in the clinical diagnosis, they are subject to pitfalls in interpretation, and the information that they provide should be used only to supplement the physician's own ophthalmoscopic and biomicroscopic observations, which in the last analysis are the most important findings in determining the correct diagnosis.

STEREOFUNDUS PHOTOGRAPHY AND STEREOANGIOGRAPHY

Following the intravenous injection of fluorescein into the antecubital vein the physician can obtain useful information by direct observation of the fundus with the ophthalmoscope and biomicroscope equipped with appropriate blue filters.[76] This technique, however, has several major disadvantages, including the following: a) the physician must be partly dark-adapted; b) the early events occur rapidly and there is inadequate time for study of the sequential events; c) the distinction between abnormal fluorescence due to alterations in the pigment epithelium and that due to escape of dye from the choroidal and retinal vessels is difficult; d) there is no permanent record for comparison with future studies; and e) the technique requires much practice before the clinician acquires skill in the interpretation of his observations.

The availability of stereofundus photography and fluorescein angiography provides the physician with the following advantages: a) greater accuracy in diagnosis is possible by deliberate study of stereo color photographs of the tumor for anatomic details that are often overlooked during the course of patient examination, and by study of stereoangiograms that provide additional anatomic as well as physiologic information concerning the tumor and the structures surrounding it; b) the photographs may be used to obtain rapid consultation by mail; c) the photographs are part of the patient's permanent record and are invaluable in detecting future anatomic and physiologic changes in the tumor; d) copies of the photographs of unusual or suspicious lesions can be provided to the patient for his own personal record or to other physicians responsible for the patient's care; e) diagnostic skills are improved by detailed correlation of the photographic and the histopathologic findings of tumors following enucleation of the eye; and f) the availability of photographs is invaluable in the instruction of other physicians in the diagnosis, natural course, and treatment of intraocular tumors.

Equipment and Technique

Various fundal cameras are available. The techniques of stereophotography and fluorescein angiography of the fundus have been published elsewhere.[72,76-81]

Safety Precautions

The intravenous injection of sodium fluorescein has proven to be a safe clinical procedure. A rare patient, however, may manifest an allergic reaction. Epinephrine and cortisone for injection and an emergency respiratory apparatus should be available. Skin testing with fluorescein is not done unless there is some reason to suspect a possible reaction to the injection.

GENERAL PRINCIPLES OF INTERPRETATION OF FLUORESCEIN ANGIOGRAPHY

The reader should consult previous publications[73-75] for a review of the normal ocular anatomy and physiology as it relates to fluorescein angiography, as well as principles of interpretation of fluorescein angiography in eyes containing intraocular tumors. Fluorescein angiography is primarily of value in demonstrating some of the gross anatomic and physiologic features of a tumor, as well as in detecting and defining some of the alterations in the tissues surrounding the tumor. Because of variations in growth patterns produced by a particular tumor, and because of the similarity of anatomic and physiologic alterations that can be produced by different tumors, angiography alone cannot provide a definitive clinical diagnosis. The information, however, when coupled with careful clinical observations and a knowledge of the histopathologic features and growth patterns of tumors, can be important in arriving at a correct diagnosis.

FINDINGS

Malignant Melanoma of the Choroid

Malignant melanoma of the choroid shows great variation in its growth pattern and degree of pigmentation. The angiographic picture produced by each tumor is a reflection of these variations. Very early in its growth, a melanoma produces alterations in the pigment epithelium including loss of pigmentation, cellular destruction, reactive proliferation, and fibrous metaplasia. Because of early changes in the pigment epithelium, melanomas typically show some evidence of fluorescence during the early phases of angiographic examination (Fig. 12–32).

Associated with damage to the pigment epithelium, varying degrees of exudation occur in the area separating the tumor from the overlying retina. Fluorescein escapes from the blood vessels of the tumor and choroid and typically leaks from multiple areas, often pinpoint in size, staining the exudate and cellular debris on the surface of the tumor. The area and intensity of fluorescence increase during the course of the study. Patches of orange-red or rust-colored granular pigment often seen ophthalmoscopically on the surface of choroidal melanomas or within the outer retinal layers appear angiographically hypofluorescent or nonfluorescent on a background of irregular fluorescence. While these pigment patches frequently overlie choroidal melanoma, they may also occur over other choroidal tumors, including nevi, serous detachment of the pigment epithelium, and choroidal hemangiomas.

As a melanoma enlarges, the vascular network within the tumor becomes more prominent and may become visible ophthalmoscopically and angiographically (Fig. 12–32A and B). This is seen best in relatively hypopigmented melanomas and in highly elevated tumors that have broken through Bruch's membrane. In highly pigmented tumors these vessels may not be visible ophthalmoscopically, and their demonstration with angiography may be helpful in differentiating the tumor from a large mass of darkly colored blood (Fig. 12–32A and B). The presence of these vessels within the tumor mass is not pathognomonic for melanomas. They may be observed in hemangiomas, disciform scars, and occasionally in tumors metastatic to the choroid. As melanomas increase in size, they often destroy the overlying pigment epithelium and also invade and erode the outer retinal layers. If the surface of the tumor contains considerable pigment, and if the tumor is in direct contact with overlying retinal tissue without any intervening exudation, the melanoma may appear quite hypofluorescent throughout the angiographic study. Almost invariably, however, there is some degree of exudative detachment at the margin of the tumor, and fluorescein will stain this exudate during the later stages of the study. In some instances, particularly in very slowly growing melanomas, cystoid degeneration and edema of the overlying retina may occur. In such cases the dye leaking from the tumor vessels and retinal vessels pools within these cystoid spaces, producing the characteristic

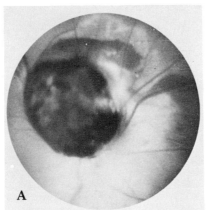 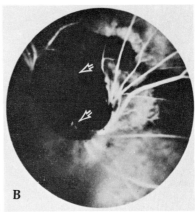

FIG. 12–32. A. A small highly pigmented juxtapapillary choroidal melanoma extended through the retina into the vitreous cavity. Subretinal blood was present at its base. The tumor was misinterpreted as a hematoma. **B.** Angiography revealed evidence of blood vessels (*arrows*) within the dome of the tumor. This finding should have alerted the physician that this black lesion was a malignant melanoma and not a hematoma. (From Gass JDM: Differential Diagnosis of Intraocular Tumors: a Stereoscopic Presentation. St. Louis, CV Mosby, 1974, p 95)

multiloculated angiographic picture of cystoid retinal degeneration and edema.

Extensive cystoid degeneration of the entire retina overlying a melanoma is rare and is much more likely to occur over a long-standing hemangioma of the choroid. If the melanoma completely destroys the overlying retina and its bare surface extends into the vitreous cavity, fluorescein dye escaping from the surface of the tumor will diffuse into the vitreous body, and angiographically that portion of the tumor may appear as a relatively hypofluorescent mass outlined by a haze of intravitreal fluorescence (Fig. 12–32A and B).

Tumors That May Simulate Malignant Melanoma of the Choroid

Choroidal Melanocytic Hamartomas (Nevi or Benign Melanomas). While most nevi are blue-black in color, some may be only partly pigmented or may be completely amelanotic. Choroidal nevi may be confined to the outer layers of the choroid and may be unassociated with alterations in the overlying choriocapillaris, pigment epithelium, or retina. In such instances the tumor often produces a hypofluorescent filling defect in the normal pattern of background fluorescence. Many nevi are associated with deposition of eosinophilic material beneath the overlying pigment epithelium in either a discrete (drusen) or irregular pattern. These deposits appear hyperfluorescent angiographically because of thinning of the pigment epithelium and because of dye staining of the subpigment epithelial material. Nevi may be the underlying cause of serous detachment of the overlying retina (Fig. 12–33A and B). Angiography will

identify the site where the serous exudate is passing from the choroid into the subretinal space (Fig. 12–33B).

Breaks in Bruch's membrane and ingrowth of new capillaries from the choriocapillaris beneath the pigment epithelium are more advanced degenerative changes caused by choroidal nevi (Fig. 12–33C). They may occasionally be the underlying cause of hemorrhagic disciform detachment of the pigment epithelium and retina. Angiography is helpful in demonstrating the fine network of subpigment epithelial neovascularization overlying nevi (Fig. 12–33D). In some instances this network has a cartwheel pattern. In others its pattern is more irregular but it is distinctly different from the sinusoidal pattern of the choriocapillaris or the network of large vascular trunks seen within the substance of a choroidal tumor.

While choroidal melanocytic hamartomas or nevi are typically small and relatively flat, some may be 4 to 5 disc diameters in size, or larger, and they may be elevated. Such lesions are more likely to be associated with degenerative changes in the overlying pigment epithelium and, because of their size, may be mistaken for malignant melanoma.

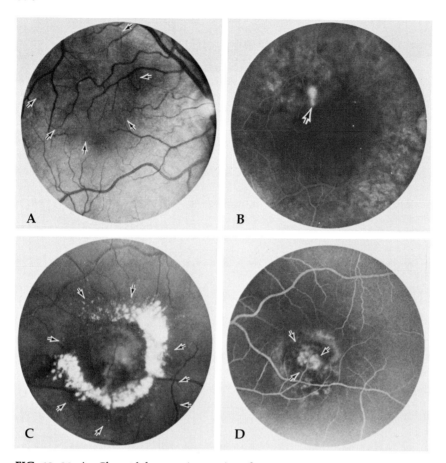

FIG. 12–33. A. Choroidal nevus (*arrows*) with a secondary serous detachment of the retina extending inferiorly into the foveal area. **B.** Angiography demonstrated abnormalities in the pigment epithelium and a focal area of dye leakage (*arrow*). Note the dye streaming superiorly into the subretinal exudate from the site of the leak. The detachment resolved spontaneously and the patient's visual acuity returned to normal. A three-year follow-up has revealed no change in the tumor size. **C.** This 70-year-old white woman had a two-year history of loss of central vision in the left eye. She had an exudative detachment of the macula and a choroidal neovascular membrane caused by an underlying pigmented choroidal nevus (*arrows*). Note the extensive circinate pattern of subretinal and outer retinal exudate derived from the neovascular membrane. **D.** Angiography showed early staining in the region of the choroidal neovascular membrane (*arrows*).

Discrete zones of hypopigmentation of the pigment epithelium secondary to previous long-standing localized serous retinal detachment often surround the inferior margins of these larger nevi. These zones may be most evident as hyperfluorescent areas during the early phases of angiography. The clinical or angiographic demonstration of extensive drusen deposition or choroidal neovascularization overlying a pigmented choroidal tumor, or the demonstration of circumscribed zones of pigment epithelial depigmentation adjacent to the tumor, is evidence that the tumor has been present for many months or years and that it is probably benign.

Melanocytomas of the Optic Nerve Head. These highly pigmented melanocytic hamartomas are closely related to choroidal nevi and are derived from similar melanocytes found normally in the region of the lamina cribrosa in more darkly pigmented individuals (Fig. 12–34A). They vary widely in size. The small lesions appear relatively

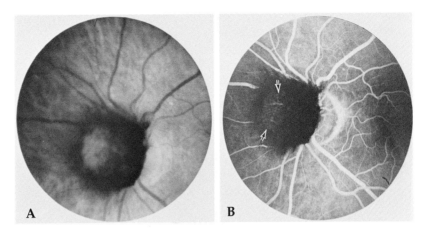

FIG. 12–34. A. This highly elevated black melanocytoma arose from the nasal half of the optic nerve head in a 69-year-old white female. B. Note the fine capillary network (*arrows*) within the tumor.

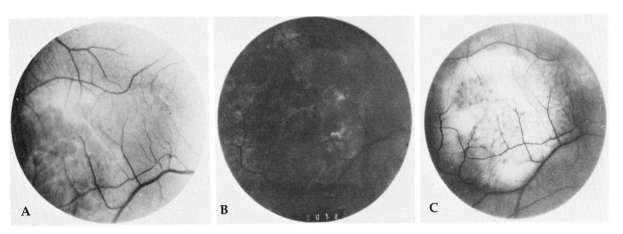

FIG. 12–35. A. Cavernous hemangioma of the choroid. B. Prearterial phase angiogram showing large vascular channels within the tumor. C. One-hour angiogram showing multiloculated pattern of fluorescein pooled within the cystoid spaces of the retina overlying the tumor.

hypofluorescent throughout the course of fluorescein angiography. The capillaries within the larger tumors may be visible angiographically, and they are permeable to fluorescein (Fig. 12–34B).

Localized Cavernous Hemangiomas of the Choroid. These vascular hamartomas are typically 3 to 6 disc diameters in size, are slightly or moderately elevated, and have a characteristic orange-red color (Fig. 12–35A). An irregular or mottled pattern of yellowish exudative material and metaplastic pigment epithelium as well as extensive cystic degeneration of the retina is usually evident on the tumor surface biomicroscopically.

The characteristic, although not pathognomonic, angiographic findings in choroidal hemangioma are a) a coarse vascular pattern of fluorescence corresponding to the location of the tumor in the prearterial and arterial phase of angiography, b) widespread and irregular areas of fluorescence secondary to diffusion of dye from the surface of the tumor during the course of angiography, and c) a diffuse multiloculated pattern of fluorescein accumulation in the outer retina characteristic of polycystic degeneration and edema during the later stages of angiography (Fig. 12–35B and C). The subretinal exudate surrounding the tumor shows a diffuse pattern of less intense fluorescence. A circular zone of hypofluorescence is often present near the tumor margin during the early and middle phases of angiography.

Metastatic Carcinoma to the Choroid. The growth patterns, the secondary ocular changes, and the angiographic changes caused by metastatic carcinoma can simulate in every way those caused by a malignant melanoma of the choroid. In the absence of evidence of a primary extraocular tumor, it is presently impossible by either clinical, fluorescein angiographic, or radioactive phosphorus uptake studies, or other special ocular tests to differentiate a metastatic tumor from an amelanotic melanoma of the choroid.

Serous Detachment of the Pigment Epithelium. These typically sharply circumscribed yellow or orange, round or kidney-shaped mounds with a smooth surface and a solid appearance may simulate a solid choroidal tumor. The angiographic picture is pathognomonic. During the early stages the dye diffuses across the entire breadth of Bruch's membrane underlying the pigment epithelial detachment and stains the subpigment epithelial fluid. This produces an area of hyperfluorescence that corresponds precisely with the area of pigment epithelial detachment and persists for an hour or longer after dye injection.

Hemorrhagic Detachment of the Pigment Epithelium and Retina. These lesions are typically sharply circumscribed, oval or round, black tumefactions (Fig. 12–36A). Within several days or weeks a red halo of subretinal blood appears at the margin of the lesion. Fluorescein angiography reveals a nonfluorescent area corresponding to the lesion, which remains nonfluorescent throughout the course of angiographic examination (Fig. 12–36B). This is helpful in distinguishing this lesion from a heavily pigmented melanoma of the choroid, which invariably is associated with some evidence of fluorescence due to destruction of the pigment epithelium and exudation. Focal areas of the underlying choroidal disease not obscured by the hemorrhagic detachment may cause some degree of abnormal fluorescence at its margin. Examination of the posterior pole of the opposite eye usually reveals evidence of the underlying degenerative choroidal disease.

Hypertrophy of the Pigment Epithelium. These flat, discoid, sharply outlined, greenish-black lesions may be mistaken for a choroidal melanoma, particularly when they are 5 disc diameters in size or larger. There may be fenestrated areas of depigmentation within the lesion, and a narrow band of depigmentation near its margin. The pigmented portion of the lesion remains nonfluorescent or hypofluorescent throughout the course of angiography. Its nonpigmented portion fluoresces because of staining of the underlying choroid and sclera.

Combined Pigment Epithelial and Retinal Hamartomas. These peculiar tumors, which are composed of pigment epithelial cells, glial cells, and blood vessels, occur most frequently in the juxtapapillary malignant melanoma or a melanocytoma. Usually they are only slightly or moderately elevated, and they have a mottled, dark or light charcoal gray appearance depending on the amount of pigment epithelium within the lesion. They often replace the normal architecture of the retina and optic nerve head and may be associated with changes at the vitreoretinal interface. When these lesions occur around the optic nerve head or posterior pole, spontaneous contraction or shrinkage of the surface of the lesion may cause loss of central vision because of traction and distortion of the macula. This generally occurs either in late childhood or in early adulthood. The abnormal capillaries within these tumors are readily visualized angiographically and they are permeable to fluorescein.

Retinoblastoma. There are no angiographic features that will readily differentiate a relatively small retinoblastoma from a benign astrocytic hamartoma of the retina. Angiography may be of some value in differentiating a large exophytic retinoblastoma from other causes of massive exudative detachment of the retina such as retinal telangiectasis.

The reader should consult the references at the end of the chapter for additional information concerning the angiographic features of intraocular tumors.

Patricia Tretter

RADIOTHERAPY OF OCULAR AND ORBITAL TUMORS

RETINOBLASTOMA

Since the first treatment of retinoblastoma with x ray early in the century[83] and an important paper about 25 years later,[86] various authors have published their results and modes of therapy. The first patients treated at the Eye Tumor Clinic of the Columbia-Presbyterian Medical Center were given doses ranging from 7000 to 17,000 roentgens over an extended period of time.[85] As the results of high doses of x rays to the eye became apparent and the relative radiosensitivity of this tumor was appreciated, the dose was reduced to 6000 roentgens in the early 1950s. It was lowered still further in the mid-1950s to the present range of 3500–4000 rads* given three times weekly over a three- to four-week period.

With the advent of supervoltage equipment and the development of the philosophy of treatment now being used at this center, the present treatment policy has evolved. In cases of bilateral retinoblastoma the eye containing advanced disease is generally enucleated, since the tumors are usually so massive with or without such extensive retinal detachment that the likelihood of cure with useful vision is remote.

The eye with less advanced tumor is treated with radiotherapy. Patients with groups I, II, and III tumors receive 3500 rads in three weeks with treatment given three

days weekly. (See page 118 for retinoblastoma groups.) Those with tumors in groups IV and V receive 4500 rads in four weeks on a three-day-a-week schedule. These dosages are infrequently modified. It is essential to use a sharp beam such as that obtained from a betatron or linear accelerator, and the field routinely used is 3 × 4 cm rectangular or 3 × 4 cm D-shaped, placed temporally with the anterior edge of the beam at the bony canthus. With lesions more anteriorly placed the beam may be moved forward 1–2 mm, and with very advanced tumors it may even be necessary to deliver about one-fourth of the treatment through a 3-cm circular anterior field.

The beam is usually passed through the eye posterior to the lens, but if a small portion of the posterior pole of the lens is included at the edge of the beam, a cataract probably will not develop. When employing a betatron or linear accelerator, there is only a slight divergence of the beam, and since the opposite eye has been enucleated, it is not necessary to angle the beam posteriorly during treatment.

If a patient presents with small tumors bilaterally, these can be treated through bilateral portals, angled slightly posteriorly depending on the divergence of the beam, to a tumor dose of 3500 rads in three weeks. The use of a black pointer enhances the reproducibility of such a setup.

Less frequently, a child is seen with advanced bilateral disease in which both eyes are almost equally affected. Treatment may be given through bilateral portals to a tumor

---

* For over two decades rad has been the radiation unit in common use.

dose of 4500 rads in four weeks. If indicated, the eye responding less well, whose future is equivocal, is enucleated several months later.

Unilateral retinoblastoma, if discovered early, can be treated effectively with radiotherapy in an attempt to preserve vision in both eyes. The modes of treatment for unilateral disease can be varied according to the availability of equipment and skill of the radiotherapist. The important consideration is to deliver as little radiation as possible to the uninvolved eye. Although Griem's method of using 10 mev through a single anterior field with a central shield to protect the cornea and lens is acceptable, a simpler approach is to use a temporal beam angled approximately 5° posteriorly, again employing a linear accelerator.

Orbital recurrence of retinoblastoma carries a very poor prognosis and often heralds the onset of widely disseminated metastases. Once a mass is noted in the orbit it should be biopsied, and the tumor irradiated. Although with exenteration of the orbit in some early cases there is reasonable hope that the retinoblastoma will not recur locally, the disease can usually be controlled by delivering a dose of 5000 rads in five weeks (or 4500 rads in four weeks) through a single anterior field covering the bony walls of the orbit or with appropriate wedged fields.

For tumor discovered in the optic nerve after enucleation, it is necessary to treat the orbit and the remaining portion of the optic nerve to include the area of the optic chiasm in a similar fashion, by delivering a tumor dose of 4500 rads in four weeks or 5000 rads in five weeks.

Radioactive applicators can be employed successfully in the treatment of solitary retinoblastomas involving one eye. Cobalt discs have been used extensively in England.[82,87] The discs are available in circular, semicircular, and horseshoe shapes and in general are used for lesions no larger than 10 mm in diameter. Our policy is to use a cobalt disc for those patients who have received a full course of radiotherapy and then develop a solitary recurrence in an area where the disc can be safely applied. Discs are not the treatment of choice for a solitary lesion because the eye often harbors multiple tumors. The usual tumor dose for retinoblastoma with the application of a cobalt disc is 4000 rads given over a seven-day period.

To achieve the most reproducible and accurate treatment, it is recommended that one person knowing the tumor location prepare the treatment setups each day. Our patients receiving external beam treatment are never anesthetized and rarely sedated for their treatment. They are securely mummied, fastened to the treatment table, their heads held in position with the chin slightly elevated by a Flexicast, and a colorful mobile is suspended directly over the head. Most children tolerate this procedure very well, and after the excitement of the preliminary setup, they become docile and cooperative. Very little eye movement, if any, is observed during treatment.

Since techniques for treating the eye with anterior fields using an electron beam require the patient's full cooperation, they are probably unsuitable for children who are heavily sedated or anesthetized.

Once the disease has metastasized, radiotherapy still provides palliation for enlarging lymph nodes, soft-tissue masses, or painful bone involvement. A tumor dose of about 2000 rads is usually adequate for effective palliation. For central nervous system involvement, a dose of 3000–4000 rads may be necessary for adequate control.

RHABDOMYOSARCOMA OF THE ORBIT

Radiotherapy for rhabdomyosarcoma of the orbit has become an aggressive approach only during the past few years. The disease was previously considered to result fatally soon after primary surgical or radiation treatment. In a series of 62 cases of orbital rhabdomyosarcoma reported in 1965,[84] about half appeared to be cured by orbital exenteration, in a few instances combined with radiation or radiation and chemotherapy. In the early 1960s adoption of the present tumor dose of 5000–6000 rads delivered in five to six weeks led to much better control of local disease in the orbit, most patients having no further evidence of the tumor.

When biopsied or locally excised, the rhabdomyosarcoma appears to be encapsulated, but this appearance is misleading. The orbital contents should be considered involved, and the entire orbit treated.

During the general work-up for patients with metastatic disease, polytomes or laminograms of the involved orbit and surrounding paranasal sinuses are essential to detect possible bone destruction and sinus invasion.

Both can be present despite a very short known history of the tumor.

If all of the tumor site is encompassed in the treatment fields, local control can be achieved in a high percentage of patients. A tumor dose of 5000–6000 rads is necessary. Paired wedged fields are effectively utilized, delivering 5000 rads in five weeks through a single anterior field, with the last 1000 rads given through a lateral field to achieve the desired dose to the posterior portion of the orbit. Supervoltage equipment is used, preferably cobalt for the first five weeks and, if available, a sharper-edged beam for the posterior orbital supplement. Since irradiation of the eye cannot be avoided, treatment should be given with the lids open if at all possible, so that the cornea will receive the smallest possible dose (skin-sparing effect). Bolus is placed over the skin scar to prevent recurrence at the biopsy site.

The rate of regression during and following treatment varies greatly. Some tumors respond almost immediately to the first few hundred rads, and others show little response during the entire treatment course, although steady gradual improvement may be noted within the next three months. In the absence of orbital pain which might indicate persistence of tumor, it is reasonable to wait for the full radiotherapeutic effect before considering surgery.

Metastases due to lymphatic spread usually occur in the cervical region. A few patients have been salvaged with surgery or radiotherapy or both, at times combined with chemotherapy. The recommended tumor dose to the involved side of the neck is 5000–6000 rads given in five to six weeks.

The disease may also metastasize to the lungs and bone marrow. Metastatic lung lesions, especially if solitary, should be pursued vigorously with radiotherapy and chemotherapy. In incurable widespread metastatic disease, radiotherapy has a valuable palliative effect.

Recurrent orbital disease as well as metastases becomes apparent during the first year after the completion of radiotherapy without chemotherapy. Recurrent disease in the orbit should be treated by exenteration. Further radiotherapy to this region is reserved for necessary palliation.

At present all patients in our tumor clinic are treated with adjuvant chemotherapy upon completion of radiotherapy. The complications attributable to irradiation range from a small stationary cataract, which does not interfere significantly with vision, to perforation of the globe. Other manifestations include some degree of photophobia which may be transient, conjunctival neovascularization, xerophthalmia, telangiectases involving the retina, retinal hemorrhage, keratitis, and corneal ulceration. In the young child, orbital growth may be impaired and there may be some enophthalmos. Eyelashes and brows are epilated at least temporarily but usually show sparse to reasonable regrowth a few months after the completion of radiotherapy. A few complications have been severe enough to lead to enucleation. Most patients do quite well after the long-term effects of irradiation have stabilized; a few require partial lid closure in an attempt to heal corneal ulcerations.

To date 31 children have been followed for at least two years. Of these, 68% have survived with a local control rate of 90%. Five of seven patients with bone destruction, with or without paranasal sinus involvement, have survived.

LYMPHOMA

Lymphomas of the orbit, conjunctiva and uvea, when localized, respond well to radiotherapy but not when the tumor is a manifestation of systemic disease. In any event the radiation dose should be sufficient to control the lymphoma locally and effect a cure in patients with no evidence of the disease elsewhere.

Since lymphomas can be controlled with a moderate dose of radiation, it is essential that the lens and cornea be protected from the primary beam. When using orthovoltage, an external lead eye shield to protect the eye or an external lead shield 1.5 cm in diameter to protect the cornea and lens is used, depending on the nature of the involvement. The internal lead shield consists of molded lead 1/32 to 1/16 inch thick and covered with smooth paraffin to prevent corneal and conjunctival irritation. It is lubricated with a small amount of steroid ointment before insertion under the lids and over the globe, to which a suitable topical anesthetic agent has just been applied. If the disease is confined to the conjunctiva but approaches the limbus, it may be necessary to deliver a few hundred rads to the unprotected eye to encompass the entire involved area.

In patients with conjunctival involvement

which appears to be limited to the fornices, all the conjunctival surface should be treated, since the exact extent of disease is not always apparent. This is usually accomplished by employing orthovoltage with a 5 cm circular field anteriorly, delivering a tumor dose of 3000 rads in three weeks. If orthovoltage is not available, ^{60}Co or a suitable electron beam may be used with appropriate corneal and lens shielding.

When retroorbital disease causes proptosis or when there is both conjunctival and orbital involvement, it is necessary to treat a volume of tissue from the lids anteriorly to include the apex of the orbit posteriorly. A similar dose of 3000 rads is given in three weeks with anterior and lateral fields; the temporal field is so placed and angled posteriorly that the radiation beam does not pass through the lens of either eye. Using orthovoltage, the orbital dose is inhomogeneous with a small "hot spot" developing anterolaterally, but it is tolerated very well in this dose range. With supervoltage equipment a simple anterior and angled lateral field or paired wedged fields are sufficient.

After orthovoltage treatment the patient develops moderately severe erythema, particularly in the anterior field, with swelling of the lids which comes and goes for several months. The use of ^{60}Co causes no erythema or appreciable lid swelling in this dose range.

In the case of reticulum-cell sarcoma the disease is likely to be generalized. The treatment scheme is similar to that used for other lymphosarcomas, but at least 3500 rads should be given in three-and-a-half weeks or 4000 rads in four weeks for local control.

The diagnosis of malignant lymphoma of the conjunctiva or orbit may be difficult for the pathologist. If there is any question about the diagnosis and the clinical picture is compatible with that of a malignant lymphoma, it is wiser to assume this diagnosis and treat accordingly.

Lymphomas may also involve the caruncle, lids and brows, ciliary body, choroid, and iris; the radiotherapeutic approach for the control of these lesions should be tailored to the presenting problem.

Hodgkin's disease occurring in the orbit or the extraocular structure should be treated—bearing in mind the areas that require shielding and the clinical picture—with dosages of 3000–3500 rads given in three to three-and-a-half weeks.

Orbital infiltration is sometimes seen in lymphatic leukemia, particularly in acute lymphatic leukemia of children. The proptosis caused by the infiltration can usually be lessened with irradiation by delivering about 600 rads, but it is seldom necessary since multiple-drug chemotherapy used in the general treatment seems to control this manifestation. Occasionally, subconjunctival leukemic infiltrates are found in older patients with chronic lymphatic leukemia. Palliation probably requires a dose as high as 2000–3000 rads.

BASAL-CELL EPITHELIOMAS

Small basal-cell epitheliomas of the eyelid tend to progress insidiously over a long period of time. They may be treated successfully with surgery or radiotherapy. The majority of patients present early with relatively small tumors, but others delay until the orbit is filled with tumor causing fixation of the globe or ulceration of the lids. Occasionally, a large tumor mass involves the entire lid or extends onto the nose or cheek.

In all of these instances radiotherapy is of value. The smaller lesions can be well controlled in a high percentage of cases by treatment with superficial x ray (120–140 kv, 1–3 mm A1 HVL) after suitable preparation. An appropriate lead cutout is prepared to allow treatment of at least 5 mm of normal tissue around small lesions or 1 cm of normal tissue around larger lesions or those with indistinct margins. It should be molded to fit securely the anatomy of the brow, cheek, nose and handle on the internal lead eye shield, so that it will not slip out of position during treatment even though it is taped well to the patient's skin.

Since the x-ray beams are now well collimated, a face mask is not necessary to prevent scattered rays from reaching normal structures. After instillation of a drop of a topical anesthetic, an appropriate waxed lead internal eye shield (the largest that will fit comfortably) is placed over the globe and under the lids. It can be held in place by taping to the patient's face two lengths of string extending from the handle, one superiorly and one inferiorly. The cutout is then applied and the treatment cone adjusted into place. The head should be immobilized with sandbags and the patient carefully monitored during treatment so that any movement away from the beam during treatment can be corrected. The dose for small lesions can be given rapidly; a skin dose of 4500 rads in 19 days, 3 to 5 days weekly. With larger lesions the thicker filter should be used. Lesions over 2.5 to 3 cm in diameter require orthovoltage.

When the lesion is extensive, infiltrates the orbit, and fixes the globe, treatment with ^{60}Co using wedge filters is better tolerated and more effective, and the dose more homogeneous; 5000–5500 rads given at the rate of 200 rads daily should be adequate. Bolus must be used over any area where the skin itself is involved to ensure the skin-sparing effect of ^{60}Co.

The occasional massive lesions involving the orbit should be thoroughly evaluated by polytomography or laminography to determine possible bone invasion or destruction, in which case surgery is preferable to radiotherapy. Patients whose general condition contraindicates extensive local surgery should have radiotherapy.

Lesions arising at the inner canthus are particularly amenable to radiotherapy. Surgery in this area is usually not feasible. However, stenosis of the lacrimal duct often occurs after irradiation.

Except for the occasional locally aggressive or metastasizing basal-cell epithelioma, the cure rate for this lesion is high.

Lesions treated surgically which recur are amenable to radiotherapy, as are those in which the tumor was incompletely excised. In the latter instance, postoperative radiotherapy may be given after the wound had healed or delayed until the first sign of recurrence.

There are few complications following proper irradiation of small lesions. If the eye is adequately protected, a cataract should not develop. Corneal abrasions that may occur from trauma caused by the internal eye shield usually heal promptly without sequelae. If the treated area includes the lid margin, the lashes will be permanently epilated and the skin will probably develop an atrophic appearance to some degree, possibly with telangiectasis.

HEMANGIOMAS

The use of radiotherapy for the treatment of hemangiomas of infants which normally regress spontaneously is controversial. We favor treating only those tumors that interfere with vision and thereby cause amblyopia ex anopsia.

Hemangiomas of one or both lids, with or without the orbital involvement, may be localized or represent only part of a mass covering much of the head. In such instances we treat the area affecting the lids, the orbit, or both, with small doses in the hope of promoting the normal expected sclerosis of the vessels and thereby hastening the regressive process. We prefer to treat these tumors even before other sclerosing methods are used, in order to obtain a better cosmetic result.

Most lid lesions will begin to respond to a skin dose as low as 150–300 rads delivered with superficial x ray with a half-value layer of 1–3 mm Al. For orbital involvement, it is necessary to employ a harder, more penetrating beam such as that produced by orthovoltage equipment (200–300 kv). Using an appropriate lead cutout, the lid lesions are treated in an area including as little normal skin as possible. A lead eye shield affords protection. The patient is observed in three to four weeks when the decision regarding further treatment must be made. A total dose of 600–800 rads delivered over two to four months should not be exceeded. With this dose there should be no future bone hypoplasia, and if the eye is protected adequately during treatment, no cataract is expected to develop.

The use of radon seeds or any form of interstitial irradiation has largely been abandoned because of persistent radioactivity in the case of radon seeds and the inability to protect the eye treated with radon seeds or other types of interstitial radiation.

There is little or no place for radiotherapy in the treatment of hemangiomas in adults.

Stephen L. Trokel

SPECIAL RADIODIAGNOSTIC STUDIES OF THE ORBIT INCLUDING COMPUTERIZED TOMOGRAPHY (EMI SCANNER)

The importance of an adequate plain film examination of the orbit is stressed in Chapter 17. At least five views—Caldwell, Waters, optic canal, base, and lateral—have been found necessary to demonstrate the orbital structures. The Caldwell view should be modified so that the petrous pyramids are located at the level of the orbital floor to allow an *en face* view of the orbital cavity. Stereoscopic views help to detect changes in the orbital walls and contents that indicate the presence of a mass lesion.

In recent years radiographic techniques have been expanded, and sophisticated procedures have been developed to study intracranial disease. These techniques have all been applied in the study of patients with exophthalmos and ocular disease with increasing success.

SPECIAL RADIOGRAPHIC TECHNIQUES

TOMOGRAMS

Tomography makes anatomic details in a given plane more visible by blurring unwanted portions of the radiographic image that exist on either side of the plane of interest. It thereby supplements the plain film study and makes apparent structural changes that may be obscured or barely viewable in the plain films.

A patient with exophthalmos shows minimal clouding of the right ethmoid sinus on the Caldwell view (Fig. 12–37A). A tomo-graphic section through the midorbit (Fig. 12–37B) reveals extensive destruction of the orbit's medial wall and floor and the nasal septum and turbinates due to a rhabdomyosarcoma. Normal structures overlying the area of destruction obscured these changes on the plain films.

A number of different tomographic methods are commercially available, but linear and hypocycloidal tomography is most widely used to study the orbit. The names of the tomographic methods refer to the blurring pattern used to eliminate the image outside the plane of interest. Hypocycloidal tomography, the most efficient blurring pattern, is capable of resolving structural planes 1 mm thick and is preferred for analysis of the complex orbital structures.

An important clinical factor in the management of patients with orbital tumors is whether the tumor is restricted to the orbit or involves an adjacent sinus or the cranial fossa. This can be determined with certainty after tomographic analysis. When the orbital walls are intact, any mass lesion must be restricted to the orbital cavity.

PHLEBOGRAPHY

The orbital veins have a characteristic course through the orbit and may be displaced by an orbital tumor. Orbital varices may cause exophthalmos which is intermittent, varying with position or with venous pressure. Characteristically, the Valsalva maneuver will induce the exophthalmos and indicate the need

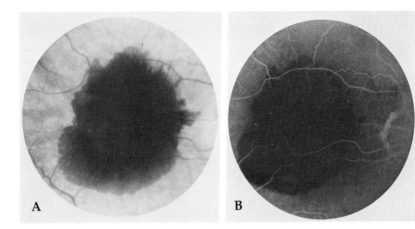

FIG. 12–36. **A.** A black submacular tumor secondary to hemorrhagic detachment of the pigment epithelium and retina in an elderly patient who had small drusen in the macula of the opposite eye. The margins of the tumor were dark reddish in color. **B.** The lesion was nonfluorescent throughout the course of angiography.

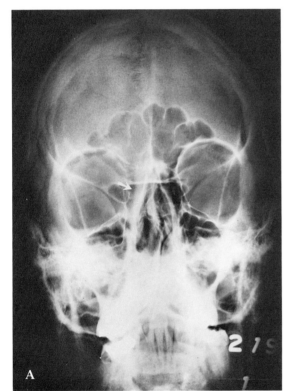

FIG. 12–37. **A.** Caldwell view of a 28-year-old woman with right exophthalmos of several weeks' duration showing clouding of the right ethmoid sinus (*arrow*). **B.** Tomographic section through midorbit reveals extensive destruction of medial wall (*black arrow*), floor (*curved arrow*), nasal septum and turbinates (*open arrow*). Biopsy showed this to be due to a rhabdomyosarcoma.

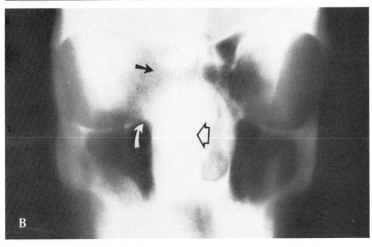

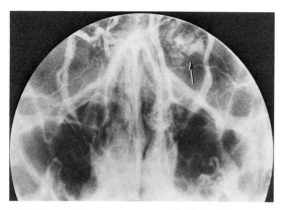

FIG. 12–38. Venous varices in the left orbit (*arrow*) of a 26-year-old woman. Exophthalmos of 6 mm could be induced with a Valsalva maneuver.

FIG. 12–39. Downward displacement of the superior ophthalmic vein (*arrow*) by orbital tumor arising within the roof of orbit.

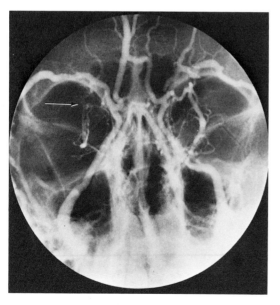

for phlebography. Figure 12–38 pictures a tangle of abnormal veins in the orbit of a 26-year-old woman in whom 6 mm of exophthalmos was induced with a Valsalva maneuver.

The orbital veins may be displaced by an orbital tumor, but in our experience not by a tumor restricted to the muscle cone. Figure 12–39 shows the downward displacement of the superior ophthalmic vein by a dermoid mass arising within the orbital roof.

A number of orbital inflammatory conditions which cause exophthalmos and accompanying neuroophthalmologic signs may show characteristic changes in the veins. A 42-year-old woman developed exophthalmos with a partial third-nerve palsy over a ten-day period. A phlebogram revealed partly obstructed orbital veins with evidence of thrombi and recanalization (Fig. 12–40). We have found these changes only in orbits where an inflammatory disease is present.

ARTERIOGRAPHY

The intracranial blood vessels are located in the cranial vault so that small displacements are readily apparent. This allows the accurate detection of small masses by the shift of known anatomic locations. The ophthalmic artery has a tortuous course in the orbit, and only large tumor masses will cause an identifiable displacement. Arteriography has therefore proved less sensitive in detecting orbital masses than intracranial masses. With improvements in radiographic technology, we are better able to visualize the smaller blood vessels within the orbit and hence to demonstrate neovascularization, tumor stain, and displacement of the smaller branches of the ophthalmic artery. Injection of 10 ml of iodinated contrast material into the internal carotid may be repeated at 10-minute intervals to produce different views of the orbit's arterial anatomy. The standard anteroposterior and lateral views may be followed by Caldwell (orbital), Waters, and base view.

MAGNIFICATION

One of the technical advances facilitating the visualization of small blood vessels is the availability of fine focal spot x-ray tubes. The image can be magnified by moving the film away from the patient or moving the patient closer to the source of the x rays. The resulting image is enlarged or magnified. Air ab-

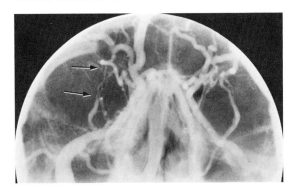

FIG. 12–40. Partly obstructed orbital veins with thrombi and recanalization (*arrows*)—changes found only in patients with orbital inflammatory disease.

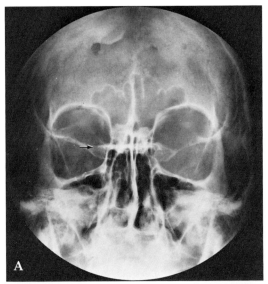

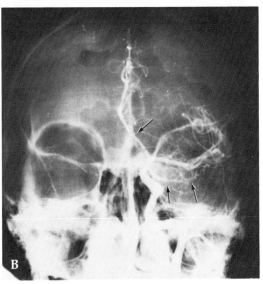

sorption of soft secondary radiation increases contrast and visibility of detail in the image. Fine focal spot equipment is essential for sharpness of the primary image and absence of a penumbra. This technique permits visualization of orbital blood vessels as small as 0.15 mm.

SUBTRACTION

Subtraction is a photographic process that makes details of the contrast-filled blood vessels more visible by eliminating (or subtracting) the bone background. The initial radiograph in an angiographic series is taken without contrast in the blood vessels. This radiograph is printed in a reversal of tone to produce a "subtraction mask." The subtraction mask is superimposed on the x rays that contain contrast material, and a print is made of the combination. The subtraction process makes the bone structure less visible, and details of the vascular anatomy are enhanced.

OCULAR TUMORS

The foregoing technical advances permit visualization of smaller vessels. Ziedses des Plantes[93] has reported visualization of hemangioma, malignant melanoma, and metastatic tumor in the choroid. Whether differential diagnosis of these choroidal tumors is aided by angiography is yet to be demonstrated.

ORBITAL TUMORS

Tumors That Involve an Adjacent Cranial Fossa

Figure 12–41 is from the radiographic study of a 53-year-old woman with no light percep-

FIG. 12–41. A. Plain film of a 53-year-old woman with an exophthalmic blind left eye of eight years' duration and a recent right visual field loss. The large left orbit shows thickening of the planum sphenoidale (*arrow*). **B.** Arteriogram showing displacement of intracranial vessels (*curved arrow*) by an intracranial extension of the tumor mass. Extensive displacement of the ophthalmic artery (*thin arrows*) is caused by the intraorbital portion of the tumor. A large meningioma was present involving the planum sphenoidale with intracranial and orbital components.

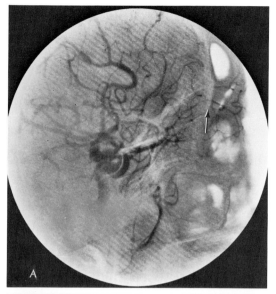

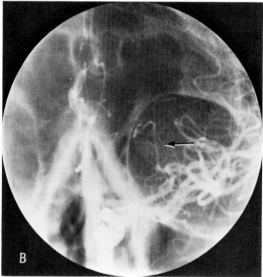

tion in the left eye and a recent progressive visual field loss in the right eye.

The plain film view (Fig. 12–41A) shows an enlarged left orbit and a thickened planum sphenoidale. Angiographic studies in Figure 12–41B show characteristic radiographic findings associated with a meningioma that involves the intracranial space and has a large orbital component made dramatically apparent by the marked displacement of the ophthalmic artery. Similarly, the intracranial component of the tumor displaces the anterior cerebral artery. The full extent of the tumor can be appreciated in the capillary phase when the tumor becomes visible as it fills with contrast. The visibility of the tumor vascularity forms the so-called tumor stain.

Tumors Restricted to the Orbit

Tumors in the orbital apex, large muscle-cone tumors, and vascular tumors that are restricted to the orbit can be detected by arteriographic study. Tumors in the muscle cone that are smaller—hemangiomas, lymphangiomas, or neurogenic tumors—usually do not cause enough vascular displacement to be detected by arteriography even with use of magnification and subtraction. A 42-year-old man with progressive exophthalmos showed upward displacement of the ophthalmic artery (Fig. 12–42A, B). This proved to be due to a lipoblastic meningioma arising from the orbital floor.

NONNEOPLASTIC CAUSES OF EXOPHTHALMOS

VASCULAR DISORDERS

Arteriography offers the only means of demonstrating caroticocavernous fistulas and arteriovenous malformations. Associated clinical findings that suggest the presence of these conditions are tortuous dilatation of the episcleral vessels extending to the corneoscleral limbus, dilated retinal veins, bruit, and glaucoma. Episcleral venous dilatation is the most common finding and indicates the need for carotid arteriography.

The arteriogram of a 42-year-old woman with progressive exophthalmos and vascular engorgement revealed that a caroticocavernous fistula was responsible for these symptoms (Fig. 12–43).

FIG. 12–42. A. The ophthalmic artery is displaced upward (*arrow*) by a tumor whose bulk is in the lower part of the orbit. A mass must be large to cause this degree of visible displacement. B. In the Caldwell projection, the stretched ophthalmic artery is displaced superomedially.

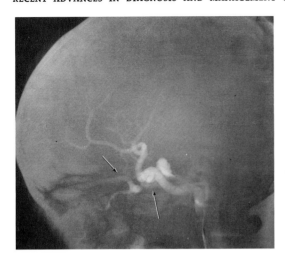

FIG. 12–43. Carotid arteriogram of patient with typical dilated episcleral veins extending to the limbus, indicating increased arterial pressure within the orbital veins. The cavernous sinus (*straight arrow*) and superior ophthalmic vein (*curved arrow*) are filled directly from the carotid artery in the arterial phase. A caroticocavernous fistula, as in this case, and less commonly local or distant arteriovenous malformations are detected by this means.

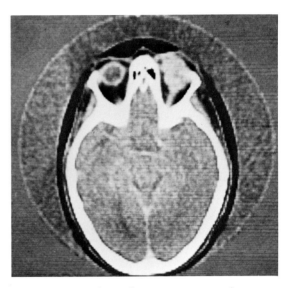

FIG. 12–44. Technetium-99m pertechnetate orbital scintigram in patient with ophthalmic Graves's disease. Thick arrow indicates normal right orbit (black represents low radioactivity). Thin arrows indicate inflamed medial rectus and inferior rectus muscles within left orbit (white represents high radioactivity). Isotope uptake by the swollen individual extraocular muscles can be shown because of the improved resolution obtained by this scanning method. (Courtesy of A. S. Grove, Jr.)

FIG. 12–45. High resolution computerized tomogram. Tomographic section through the upper third of the orbit of a 62-year-old woman with proptosis of the right globe. A mass was palpable through the right upper lid. The large mass surrounding the upper portion of the globe extending into the upper lid proved to be a lymphosarcoma. It was treated with radiotherapy after biopsy. (Courtesy of S. K. Hilal.)

ORBITAL INFLAMMATION AND PSEUDOTUMOR

Inflammatory conditions that cause exophthalmos usually show a normal arteriogram. A mild hypervascularity that may be present is nonspecific and represents a subjective evaluation on the part of the angiographer.

The extraocular muscles may become extremely swollen in myositis or exophthalmos associated with Graves's disease. In the more severe forms the swollen muscles displace the smaller muscular branches of the ophthalmic artery. This occurrence should not be confused with a tumor mass.

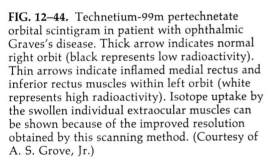

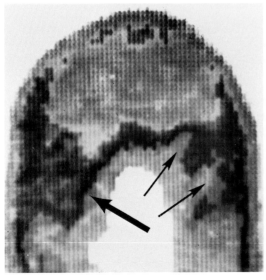

RADIOISOTOPE SCANNING

Because of the high percentage of unilateral exophthalmos caused by thyroid disease and inflammation, screening laboratory procedures that detect neoplasms with low morbidity may be of great importance. Measurement of radiation from absorbed radioisotopes has been helpful in the detection and localization of intracranial neoplasms. Similarly, orbital tumors producing exophthalmos may be distinguished from thyrotropic exophthalmos and orbital granuloma. The technique has been improved with the use of multiple radionuclides and scanning devices permitting increased resolution that is sufficient to demonstrate the focal concentration of technetium by the swollen muscles in thyroid disease (Fig. 12–44).

COMPUTERIZED TOMOGRAPHY (EMI SCANNING)

A new and different radiographic technique[88,91,92] will undoubtedly prove important in the investigation of the orbit and adjacent areas. The skull and orbit are scanned in layers by a fine collimated x-ray beam. The transmission of the x-ray photons is measured in a layer with detector crystals by rotating the source of the x rays and the detector in a fixed spatial plane. A picture of the internal structures of the scanned tissues is constructed by a computer (Fig. 12–45).

This instrument, developed by the EMI Company in England, is known as the EMI Scanner. Heretofore, x rays have been useful in distinguishing structures only if there were large differences in radiographic density. Analysis of soft tissues was extremely limited. With computer methods, x-ray studies can differentiate tissues of similar radiographic density, making possible the pictorial representation of soft-tissue structures. The computer introduces a tremendous flexibility in the range of densities that may be visualized; it can be set to print from air to bone density with a range centered on water density.

In studies of the orbit [89,90] the presence of orbital fat provides a ready-made bed of lower radiographic absorption which facilitates demonstration of orbital tumors.

The method does not require contrast material or injections. Considerably less radiation is involved than with conventional tomographic and angiographic methods.

REFERENCES

ULTRASONIC EVALUATION OF OCULAR AND ORBITAL TUMORS

1. BAUM G: Quantitized ultrasonography. Ultrasonics 10:14–15, 1972
2. COLEMAN DJ: Measurement of choroidal pulsations with M-scan ultrasound. Am J Ophthalmol 71:363–365, 1971
3. COLEMAN DJ: Reliability of ocular and orbital diagnosis with B-scan ultrasound. 1. Ocular diagnosis. Am J Ophthalmol 73:501–516, 1972
4. COLEMAN DJ: Reliability of ocular and orbital diagnosis with B-scan ultrasound. 2. Orbital diagnosis. Am J Ophthalmol 74:704–718, 1972
5. COLEMAN DJ: Reliability of ocular tumor diagnosis with ultrasound. Trans Am Acad Ophthalmol Otolaryngol 77:677–683, 1973
6. COLEMAN DJ, ABRAMSON DH: Correlation of ultrasonic characteristics and tissue morphology of malignant melanoma. In Massin M, Poujol J (eds): Diagnostic Ultrasonics in Ophthalmologica; Proc. SIDUO IV, 1971. Centre National D'Ophtalmologie des Quinze-Vingts, Paris, 1973, pp 215–218
7. COLEMAN DJ, ABRAMSON DH, JACK RL, FRANZEN LA: Ultrasonic diagnosis of tumors of the choroid. Arch Ophthalmol 91:344–354, 1974
8. COLEMAN DJ, KATZ L: Color-coding of B-scan ultrasonograms. Arch Ophthalmol 91:429–431, 1974

9. COLEMAN DJ, KATZ L, LIZZI F: Isometric three-dimensional viewing of ultrasonograms. Arch Ophthalmol 93:1362–1365, 1975
10. COLEMAN DJ, KONIG WF, KATZ L: A hand-operated ultrasound scan system for ophthalmic evaluation. Am J Ophthalmol 68:256–263, 1969
11. OSSOINIG K: Clinical echo-ophthalmology. Current Concepts of Ophthalmology 3:101–130, 1972
12. OSSOINIG K: Quantitative echography—the basis of tissue differentiation. J Clin Ultrasound 2:33–46, 1974
13. PURNELL E: Ultrasonic interpretation of orbital disease. In Gitter K et al (eds): Ophthalmic Ultrasound. St. Louis, CV Mosby, 1969, pp 249–255
14. STERNS GK, COLEMAN DJ, ELLSWORTH RM: The ultrasonographic characteristics of retinoblastoma. Am J Ophthalmol 78:606–611, 1974
15. TILL P, OSSOINIG K: Zur Echographie des Retinoblastoma. Dtsch Ophthalmol Ges 69:203–208, 1968

DIATHERMY, LIGHT COAGULATION, AND CRYOTHERAPY IN THE MANAGEMENT OF INTRAOCULAR TUMORS

16. AMOILS SP, SMITH TR: Cryotherapy of angiomatosis retinae. Arch Ophthalmol 81:689–691, 1969
17. ASAYAMA R, AKUTOGAWA T, UTSUGI F: Experience

with diathermy coagulation of retinoblastoma. Folia Ophthalmol (Jap) 17:1182–1187, 1966

18. BEDFORD MA, BEDOTTO C, MACFAUL PA: Radiation retinopathy after application of a cobalt plaque; report of three cases. Br J Ophthalmol 54:505–509, 1970

19. BONIUK M, GIRARD LJ: Malignant melanoma of the choroid treated with photocoagulation, transscleral diathermy and implanted radon seeds. Am J Ophthalmol 59:212–216, 1965

20. CURTIN VT, NORTON EWD: Pathological changes in malignant melanomas after photocoagulation. Arch Ophthalmol 70:150–157, 1963

21. DAVIDORF FH, NEWMAN G, HAVENER W, MAKLEY TA JR: Conservative management of malignant melanoma. Arch Ophthalmol 83:273–280, 1970

22. DUNPHY E: Management of intraocular malignancy. Am J Ophthalmol 44:313–322, 1957

23. HALE PN, CHRISTENSEN RE: Cryotherapy of retinoblastoma. Trans Pac Coast Otoophthalmol Soc 49:197–211, 1968

24. HEPLER RS, ALLEN RA, STRAATSMA BR: Photocoagulation of choroidal melanoma. Arch Ophthalmol 79:177–181, 1968

25. HOWARD GM: Ocular effects of radiation and photoagulation. Arch Ophthalmol 76:7–10, 1966

26. KITCHIN FD, SALMONSEN P: Personal communication

27. LUND O: Changes in choroidal tumors after light coagulation (and diathermy coagulation). Arch Ophthalmol 75:458–465, 1966

28. LINCOFF H: Report on the freezing of intraocular tumors. Mod Probl Ophthalmol 7:348–358, 1968

29. LINCOFF H, KREISSIG I: The management of intraocular tumors. Contemporary Ophthalmology Honoring Sir Stewart Duke-Elder. Baltimore, Williams & Wilkins, 1972, pp 382–388

30. LINCOFF H, MCLEON J, LONG R: The cryosurgical treatment of intraocular tumors. Am J Ophthalmol 63:389–399, 1967

31. LONG RS, GALIN MA, ROTMAN M: Conservative treatment of intraocular malignant melanoma. Trans Amer Acad Ophthalmol Otolaryngol 75:84–93, 1971

32. MAKLEY TA JR, HAVENER WH, NEWBERG J: Light coagulation of intraocular tumors. Am J Ophthalmol 60:1082–1089, 1965

33. MELCHERS M: Diathermy treatment of intraocular tumors. Schotanuson Jens. Utrecht, Netherlands, 1953

34. MEYER-SCHWICKERATH G: Further progress in the field of light coagulation. Trans Ophthalmol Soc UK 77:421–440, 1957

35. MEYER-SCHWICKERATH G: The preservation of vision by treatment of intraocular tumors with light coagulation. Arch Ophthalmol 66:458–466, 1961

36. PERERA CA: Treatment of retinoblastoma by diathermic coagulation. Am J Ophthalmol 34:1275–1278, 1951

37. REESE AB: Tumors of the Eye, 2nd ed. New York Harper & Row 1963, pp. 237, 241

38. RUBIN ML: Treatment of retinoblastoma with cryopexy. Mod Probl Ophthalmol 7:359–361, 1968

39. SHEA M: Cryotherapy in retinal detachment surgery: Int Ophthalmol Clin 7:429–443, 1967

40. STALLARD HB: Radiotherapy for malignant melnoma of the choroid. Br J Ophthalmol 50:147–155, 1966

41. STANFORD GB, REESE AB: Malignant cells in the blood of eye patients. Trans Am Acad Ophthalmol Otolaryngol 75:102–109, 1971

42. TOLENTINO FI, TABLANTE RT: Cryotherapy of retinoblastoma. Arch Ophthalmol 87:52–55, 1972

43. VAIL D.: Angiomatosis retinae; eleven years after diathermy coagulation. Trans Am Ophthalmol Soc 55:217–238, 1957

44. VOGEL MH: Treatment of malignant choroidal melanomas with photocoagulation. Am J Ophthalmol 74:1–11, 1972

45. VOGEL MH: Histopathologic observations of photocoagulated malignant melanomas of the choroid. Am J Ophthalmol 74:466–474, 1972

46. WEVE H: Uber augenerkronkungen in fruhester jeigend. Ned Tijdschr Geneeskd, 1932, p 5328.

47. WEVE H: On diathermy in ophthalmic practice. Trans Ophthalmol Soc UK 59:43–80, 1939

48. WEVE H: Derde geval van melanosarcoma genezen door diathermische behandeling. Ned Tijdschr Geneeskd, 1948, p 3472

ELECTRON MICROSCOPY OF TUMORS OF THE EYE AND OCULAR ADNEXA

49. ABRAHAMS IW, FENTON RH, VIDONE R: Alveolar soft part sarcoma of the orbit. Arch Ophthalmol 79:185–188, 1968

50. ALTAMIRANO-DIMAS M, ALBORES-SAAVEDRA J: Alveolar soft part sarcoma of the orbit. Arch Ophthalmol 75:496–499, 1966

51. BENSCH KG, GORDON GB, MILLER LR: Electron microscopic and biochemical studies on the bronchial carcinoid tumor. Cancer 18:592–602, 1965

52. FINE BS, TS'O MOM, FONT RL, ZIMMERMAN LE: Electron microscopy of pathologic ocular tissue. Int Ophthalmol Clin. 11:57–86, 1971

53. FISHER ER: Histochemical observations of an alveolar soft part sarcoma with reference to histogenesis. Am J Pathol 32:721–731, 1956

54. FISHER ER, REIDBORD H: Electron microscopic evidence suggesting the myogenous derivation of the so-called alveolar soft part sarcoma. Cancer 27:150–159, 1971

55. FONT RL, ZIMMERMAN LE, ARMALY MF: The nature of the orange pigment over a choroidal melanoma. Arch Ophthalmol 91:359–362, 1974

56. FONT RL, ZIMMERMAN LE, FINE BS: Adenoma of the retinal pigment epithelium, histochemical and electron microscopic observations. Am J Ophthalmol 73:544–554, 1972

57. KROLL AJ: Fine structural classification of orbital rhabdomyosarcoma. Invest Ophthalmol 6:531–543, 1967

58. NIRANKARI MS, GREER CH, CHADDAH MR: Malignant nonchromaffin paraganglioma of the orbit. Br J Ophthalmol 47:357–363, 1963

59. RILEY FC: Balloon cell melanoma of the choroid. Arch Ophthalmol 92:131–133, 1974

60. ROSAI J, RODRIGUEZ HA: Application of electron microscopy to the differential diagnosis of tumors. Am J Clin Pathol 50:555–562, 1968

61. SHIPKEY FH, LIEBERMAN PH, FOOTE FW JR, STEWART FW: Ultrastructure of alveolar soft part sarcoma. Cancer 17:821–830, 1964

62. STREETEN BW, McGRAW JL: Tumor of the ciliary pigment epithelium. Am J Ophthalmol 74:420–429, 1972

63. Ts'o MOM, Fine BS, Zimmerman LE: The Flexner-Wintersteiner rosettes in retinoblastoma. Arch Pathol 88:664–671, 1969

64. Ts'o MOM, Fine BS, Zimmerman LE, Vogel MH: Photoreceptor elements in retinoblastoma; a preliminary report. Arch Ophthalmol 82:57–59, 1969

65. Ts'o MOM, Zimmerman LE, Fine BS: The nature of retinoblastoma. I. Photoreceptor differentiation: a clinical and histpathologic study. Am J Ophthalmol 69:339–349, 1970

66. Ts'o MOM, Fine BS, Zimmerman LE: The nature of retinoblastoma. II. Photoreceptor differentiation: an electron microscopic study. Am J Ophthalmol 69:350–359, 1970

67. Yanoff M, Fine BS: Ocular Pathology; a Text and Atlas. Hagerstown, Harper & Row, 1975, p 674

68. Zimmerman LE: The remarkable polymorphism of tumors of the ciliary epithelium. Trans 1970 Congr Austral Coll Ophthalmol 2:114–125, 1970

69. Zimmerman LE: Verhoeff's "teratoneuroma." Am J Ophthalmol 72:1039–1057, 1971

70. Zimmerman LE, Font RL, Andersen SR: Rhabdomyosarcomatous differentiation in malignant intraocular medulloepitheliomas. Cancer 30:817–835, 1972

71. Zimmerman LE, Font RL, Ts'o MOM, Fine BS: Application of electron microscopy to histopathologic diagnosis. Trans Am Acad Ophthalmol Otolaryngol 76:101–107, 1972

STEREOFUNDUS PHOTOGRAPHY AND FLUORESCEIN ANGIOGRAPHY IN THE DIAGNOSIS OF INTRAOCULAR TUMORS

72. Allen L, Kirkendall M, Snyder WB, Frazier O: Instant positive photographs and stereoangiograms of ocular fundus fluorescence. Arch Ophthalmol 75:192–198, 1966

73. Gass JDM: A Stereoscopic Atlas of Macular Diseases. St Louis, CV Mosby, 1970, pp 1–12

74. Gass JDM: Fluorescein angiography: an aid in the differential diagnosis of intraocular tumors. Int Ophthalmol Clin 12(1):85–120, 1972

75. Gass JDM: Differential Diagnosis of Intraocular Tumors: a Stereoscopic Presentation. St Louis CV Mosby, 1974, p 95

76. Gass JDM, Sever RD, Sparks D, Goren J: A combined technique of fluorescein funduscopy and angiography of the eye. Arch Ophthalmol 78:455–461, 1967

77. Haining WM, Lancaster RC: Advanced technique for fluorescein angiography. Arch Ophthalmol 79:10–15, 1968

78. Novotny HR, Alvis DL: A method of photographing fluorescence in circulating blood in the human retina. Circulation 24:82–86, 1961

79. Rosen ES: Fluorescence Photography of the Eye. London, Appleton-Century-Crofts, 1969, pp 2–5

80. Schikano S, Shimizu K: Atlas of Fluorescence Fundus Angiography. Tokyo, Igaku Shoin, Ltd, 1968, pp 2–24

81. Wessing A: Fluorescein Angiography of the Retina (translated by von Noorden GK). St Louis, CV Mosby, 1969, pp 9–30

RADIOTHERAPY OF OCULAR AND ORBITAL TUMORS

82. Bedford MA, Bedotto C, MacFaul PA: Radiation retinopathy after application of a cobalt plaque; report of three cases. Br J Ophthalmol 54:505–509, 1970

83. Hilgartner HL: Report of a case of double glioma treated by x-rays. Texas Med J 18:322, 1903

84. Jones IS, Reese AB, Krout J: Orbital rhabdomyosarcoma: an analysis of 62 cases. Trans Am Ophthalmol Soc 63:223–255, 1965

85. Martin HE, Reese AB: Treatment of retinal gliomas by the fractionated or divided dose principle of roentgen radiation; a preliminary report. Arch Ophthalmol 16:733–761, 1936

86. Moore RF, Scott RS: Clinical and pathological report of bilateral glioma retinae. Proc R Soc Med (Sect Ophthalmol) 22:39–50, 1929

87. Stallard HB: Retinoblastoma treated by radon seeds and radioactive disks. Ann R Coll Surg Engl 16:349–366, 1955

SPECIAL RADIODIAGNOSTIC STUDIES OF THE ORBIT INCLUDING COMPUTERIZED TOMOGRAPHY (EMI SCANNER)

88. Ambrose J: Computerized transverse axial scanning (tomography). Part 2. Clinical application. Br J Radiol 46:1023–1047, 1973

89. Baker HL Jr, Kearns TP, Campbell JK, Henderson JW: Computerized transaxial tomography in neuro-ophthalmology. Trans Am Ophthalmol Soc 72:49–64, 1974

90. Hanafee WN: Symposium on modern examination methods in orbital disease. Selection of contrast studies of the orbit. Trans Am Acad Ophthalmol Otolaryngol 78:599–601, 1974

91. Hounsfield GN: Computerized transverse axial scanning (tomography). Part 1. Description of system. Br J Radiol 46:1016–1022, 1973

92. Perry BJ, Bridges C: Computerized transverse aixal scanning (tomography). Part 3. Radiation dose considerations. Br J Radiol 46:1048–1051, 1973

93. Ziedses des Plantes BG: Subtraction angiography of the orbit. In Bleeker GM, Garston JB, Kronenberg B, Lyle TK (eds): Orbital disorders, Vol 14, Modern Problems in Ophthalmology. Basel, Karger, 1975, pp 74–82

13

TUMORS OF THE HEMATOPOIETIC SYSTEM

Normally, lymphoid tissue around the eye is found subconjunctivally and in the lacrimal gland. Lymphomatous diseases are thus most likely to occur there but are also encountered elsewhere in the eye or the adnexa, including the uveal tract and the deep orbital structures.

A tumor under the conjunctiva presents a unique clinical picture. The single or multiple elevated tumor mass is uniformly salmon-colored, with no gross blood vessels, a perfectly smooth overlying conjunctiva, and a sharply demarcated border.

The lesion assumes the contour of the affected site. At the limbus its contour is usually followed for varying distances. Over the bulbar conjunctiva, the lesion is usually round or oval. When the fornices are involved, the lesion is horizontal and conforms more or less to the fornix. In the area of the lacrimal gland, it appears as a deep mass which is smooth, soft, and tends to favor the conjunctival side. In contrast, mixed tumors of the lacrimal gland tend to appear on the skin side. Amyloidosis of the conjunctiva may bear some resemblance to a lymphoma.

In the past, malignant lymphomas have been overdiagnosed.[68] The present trend is toward interpreting some lesions formerly considered in this group as reactive hyperplasias or as belonging to an indeterminate group somewhere between neoplasms and hyperplasia. The final decision in equivocal cases may rest on the presence of related lesions elsewhere in the body.

The tumor may be primary in any ocular structure or become manifest during the course of an already generalized lymphomatous disease. Lymphomatous diseases may occur at any age, but more commonly affect the 30 to 40-year age group. The eye lesions are so insidious that the patient usually seeks medical advice not because of symptoms but because of an unexplained mass under the conjunctiva or skin or because of exophthalmos.

A primary tumor at sites where there is normally no lymphoid tissue is usually of the reticulum-cell type. Metastatic lesions are found at any site.

A lymphomatous disease may cause unilateral exophthalmos with no overt evidence of the lesion and no palpable mass (Fig. 13–1, see p. 31). In rare instances a primary tumor in the nasopharynx and nasal cavity spreads secondarily to the orbit.

Some malignant lymphomas progress rapidly and terminate fatally in a short time. In one of our cases the primary lesion was located in the area of the lacrimal sac giving rise to an acute inflammatory process (Fig. 13-2). Many reports of sarcoma of the lacrimal sac seem to be instances of malignant lymphoma.

It is rare for a lymphomatous tumor to be primary in the eye. When the tumors are multiple, the primary and secondary sites cannot be distinguished. Reports have described a primary malignant lymphoma in the mediastinum and also in the choroid; a tumor primary in the choroid with secondary involvement of the orbit; an iris lesion thought to be secondary to a primary malignant lymphoma of the ovary; a generalized lymphomatous process with bilateral intraorbital involvement and, in one case, the kidney as well.[67]

Reactive proliferation of lymphoid tissue may clinically resemble a neoplasm such as a diffuse or flat uveal melanoma, an orbital tumor, or a leukemic infiltration. The spectrum of lymphoid lesions poses a problem for the pathologist; at one extreme is the clearly malignant lesion and at the other are the inflammatory nonneoplastic pseudotumors, with all the perplexing gradations lying between the two.[55]

One published case was originally diagnosed as choroidal lymphosarcoma or possibly reactive lymphoid hyperplasia of the uveal tract simulating malignant lymphoma.[15] The patient was alive and well six years after enucleation. True intraocular malignant lymphomas, which are rare, have been reported.[13, 32]

The clinical picture when the uvea is involved is often interpreted as uveitis; a lymphoma is suspected only if there are tumor areas elsewhere. Some degree of uveal infiltration, even though subclinical, seems to be a feature of all cases of lymphatic leukemia.

Leukemic involvement of the uvea, especially the iris, may be an early manifestation of the disease. A bilateral case in the iris in a child of 2 has been reported.[36] Infiltration in the uvea may be nodular and diffuse with or without a hypopyon. The reticuloses and histiocytoses must be considered in the differential diagnosis.

Brief histories of four cases in which the intraocular structures participated in a lymphomatous process follow:

Case 1 (Fig. 13–3, see p. 31): A radical mastectomy was performed on a 50-year-old woman with the histologic diagnosis of carcinoma. Two years later her left eye became irritated and painful. A tumor was found in the iris. The eye was enucleated under the assumption of a metastatic carcinoma. Histologic examination revealed a malignant lymphoma of the iris, considered to be a lymphocytic-cell type with follicles.[44]

Case 2 (Fig. 13–4, see p. 32): A 47-year-old man complained of blurred vision, pain, and redness in the right eye of two weeks' duration. Five weeks before the eye symptoms appeared he had noted a lump in the right submandibular region. At examination, the lower two-thirds of the anterior chamber of the right eye contained cream-colored material resembling a hypopyon. The patient could distinguish only hand movements, and light projection was poor nasally and above. The cornea was somewhat steamy, and the intraocular pressure was 35 mm Hg. A large, nontender, smooth, firm mass was visible and palpable at the angle of the right mandible.

The clinical impression was that a partially necrotic tumor of the iris had produced an inflammation with a purulent discharge. The eye lesion, as well as the enlarged node, was believed to be due to metastatic cancer. The primary site was unknown.

The pathology report revealed a malignant lymphoma (reticulum-cell type) of the iris, ciliary body, and anterior choroid. Necrotic areas in the tumor had given rise to a marked exudation of polymorphonuclear leukocytes.

An aspiration biopsy taken from the submandibular node showed reticulum-cell lymphoma. The patient died seven months later. No blood changes were evident, and there was no x-ray evidence of mediastinal tumor. An autopsy report was not available.

Case 3: A 64-year-old woman complained of photophobia and pain in one eye. The examina-

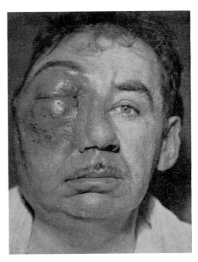

FIG. 13–2. Malignant lymphoma (reticulum-cell type). The tumor, arising in the region of the lacrimal sac, was already considered inflammatory when the photograph was taken on admission of this patient who died 40 days later. In addition to orbital involvement, the autopsy findings included lymphomatous invasion of the lymph nodes, face, neck, heart, lungs, kidneys, liver, spleen, pancreas, stomach, and large and small intestines.

tion revealed a tumor occupying the circumference of the iris, with hemorrhage over its surface. Repeated severe hemorrhages finally necessitated enucleation of the eye. Histologic examination showed a malignant lymphoma (reticulum-cell type) of the iris which involved part of the ciliary body and anterior choroid. No signs of a neoplasm were detected elsewhere in the body. Soon after enucleation the same type of lesion appeared in the remaining eye, which was treated by radiotherapy. The patient died of tumor involvement of the abdomen six months later.

Case 4: A 58-year-old man had iritis with posterior synechiae. Within six weeks his vision was reduced from 20/40 to no light perception. A cloudy vitreous prevented a view of the fundus. He had been treated for malignant lymphoma at multiple sites over the body. The affected eye was enucleated. Examination revealed a large, globular, partially necrotic malignant lymphoma (reticulum-cell type) of the choroid.

HODGKIN'S DISEASE

Hodgkin's is a protean disease whose characteristics seem to place it somewhere between a chronic granuloma and a malignant lymphoma. That little is known about its nature and etiology is apparent from the confused nomenclature, which includes lymphadenoma, malignant lymphoma, malignant granuloma, lymphogranuloma, and lymphogranulomatosis.

Although it is a disorder of the entire reticuloendothelial system, the lymphatic elements are affected predominantly. The neck nodes are usually involved first, and successive exacerbations and remissions often associated with fever characterize the progress of the disease. If the patient lives long enough, generalized involvement of the deeper nodes, the viscera, and bones is inevitable.

Lymphomatus diseases are now divided into non-Hodgkin's lymphoma and Hodgkin's disease. The older classification of Hodgkin's disease according to granuloma, paragranuloma, and sarcoma has been replaced by a classification that takes into consideration the neoplastic character of the disease. The cytologic examination invariably shows anaplastic malignant cells, known as Reed-Sternberg cells. These are binucleate histiocytes, or reticulum cells, characteristic of Hodgkin's disease. They are necessary for the diagnosis of the condition even if atypical malignant mononuclear reticulum cells are present.[42,54]

Hodgkin's disease is now typed on cytologic grounds into four categories:

1. *Lymphocyte predominance*, in which lymphocytes are numerous and Reed-Sternberg and atypical cells less prominent
2. *Mixed cellularity*, in which lymphocytes, plasma cells, and eosinophils coexist with neoplastic reticulum cells
3. *Nodular sclerosing*, in which the tumor cells are divided into compartments by bands of collagenous tissue
4. *Lymphocyte depletion*, in which atypical reticulum cells and Reed-Sternberg cells overrun the basic tissue of the lesion at the expense of lymphocytes

As a rule, types 1 and 3 offer the best prognosis.

The viral causation of the disease has not been established, but it is a true lymphoma which, if left untreated, inevitably spreads along contiguous lymph nodes, seeds parenchymal organs, and may even involve the skin, brain, eye, and ocular adnexa.

OCULAR MANIFESTATIONS

Ocular manifestations of Hodgkin's disease are usually seen in the orbit, in the lids, and in the region of the lacrimal gland. The adjacent sinuses may also be involved. The ocular and orbital structures are less likely to be affected in Hodgkin's disease than in lymphoma and lymphatic leukemias. However, case reports have described corneal infiltration (varying forms of keratitis), fundal changes, subconjunctival and limbal manifestations, uveitis, and episcleritis. In one instance, the disease manifested itself as a bilateral granuloma of the conjunctiva.[21]

I have seen two instances of Horner's syndrome caused by Hodgkin's disease. Lymph nodes of the neck were involved in one case and the cervical spinal cord (from tumor in the vertebrae) in the other. Two other patients showed papilledema and retinal hemorrhages. The changes in one were due to invasion of the optic nerve from an intracranial lesion, and in the other to invasion of the sphenoidal region. Still another patient had papilledema and optic atrophy due to involvement of the apex of the orbit or the middle cranial fossa or both.

Brief résumés of three other patients with orbital involvement follow:

Case 1: A 40-year-old woman noticed a swelling of the left eyelid and double vision. X rays showed some cloudiness of the ethmoids and antrum on the left side. Operation on both sinuses resulted in no improvement. Later the left eye became proptosed and displaced downward: the patient experienced a considerable degree of pain over the left side of the head.

A mass could be palpated in the upper outer quadrant of the orbit. Orbital tissue removed for microscopic study showed a chronic granulomatous reaction in the lacrimal gland. Two years later the cervical lymph nodes on the left side became enlarged, and x-ray treatment was given. One year later the patient developed an intestinal obstruction. A mass of enlarged mesenteric lymph nodes was found at operation. Nodes elsewhere over the body were enlarged, particularly in the axillary region. The patient died of Hodgkin's disease one year later. No autopsy was performed. In this case the disease was first evident in the lacrimal gland and later was found in the orbit.

Case 2: A 56-year-old woman presented with exophthalmos due to an orbital mass palpable through the lower lid. The orbital and sinus involvement progressed, accompanied by some enlargement of regional lymph nodes and two attacks diagnosed as pneumonitis. Hodgkin's disease primary in the orbit, which was diagnosed histologically, resulted fatally.

Case 3 (Fig. 13–5, see p. 32): A 45-year-old man was treated for Hodgkin's disease. The diagnosis was established by repeated histologic examinations. The lacrimal gland became involved during the course of the disease.

MALIGNANT LYMPHOMA

To understand tumors of the reticuloendothelial system, particularly lymphomas, it is essential to appreciate the pluripotential nature of the primitive cells making up this system. Only then is it possible to grasp the numerous cellular combinations and transformations that characterize these tumors. The functions of these cells and their derivatives include phagocytosis, antibody production, formation and destruction of blood cells.

It is in order to discuss the relationship of lymphoma to Sjögren's syndrome. There is ample evidence relating Sjögren's syndrome to immune activity of the serum.[19] The rheumatoid factor is found in the great majority of patients with this syndrome; antithyroglobulin antibodies are present in one-third, and hyperglobulinemia in about half; antibodies capable of reacting with various tissue antigens are prevalent. The association of Sjögren's syndrome with reticulum-cell sarcoma has been reported in several patients,[53, 62] also two cases of Waldenström's macroglobulinemia, five cases with widespread lymphoid abnormalities suggesting lymphoma, and another case of reticulum-cell sarcoma.[63]

Rappaport[50] classifies lymphomatous tumors according to cell type, architectural arrangement, and extent:

1. *Cell type*
   This category, based on cell maturity, includes
   a. Undifferentiated lymphoma
   b. Histiocytic lymphoma (formerly called reticulum-cell sarcoma)
   c. Mixed lymphohistiocytic lymphoma
   d. Poorly differentiated lymphocytic lymphoma
   e. Well-differentiated lymphocytic lymphoma
2. *Architectural arrangement*
   a. Follicular
   b. Nodular
   c. Diffuse
3. *Extent*
   a. Amount of lymph node involvement
   b. Site—bone marrow, above or below diaphragm, *etc.*

Follicular lymphoma is less common than the diffuse type, and offers a much better prognosis.

Lymphoma follicles do not have the cellular composition of normal germinal centers. They are viewed as abortive attempts of neoplastic lymphocytes to form follicles. The lymphoma may progress from the follicular form into one of the diffuse forms (lymphocytic, reticulum-cell, or Hodgkin's type), but the variations, once determined, are limited to degree of differentiation and not to a shift in the type.[50]

The basic relationship of all variants of the group of malignant lymphomas cannot be overemphasized. They must be viewed as a single entity adopting one or more histologic patterns.

The clinical and histologic pictures are characteristically in a state of flux. Microscopic examination in the early stages may suggest a chronic lymphogranuloma, whereas later the same lesion appears to be a type of malignant lymphoma. A giant-follicle lymphoma may develop into a lymphocytic-cell type or a reticulum-cell type, but the reverse is never true. Repeated biopsies and bone marrow studies are therefore necessary in such cases, particularly in the event of multiple areas.

A histologic diagnosis of benign lymphoma can be made only when germinal centers are present, and a diagnosis of lymphosarcoma only when lymphoblasts infiltrate the tissues.[45] According to this author the remaining tumors, representing the large majority, can be diagnosed as benign or malignant only after a prolonged follow-up. He based these conclusions on a study of 26 cases of lymphocytic tumors of the conjunctiva followed for more than five years. Of the 18 cases diagnosed as benign, 2 showed metastasis; of 8 diagnosed as malignant, 4 did not disseminate.

Certain clinical and histologic features of malignant lymphomas suggest an infectious cause. Lesions with histologic characteristics of an inflammatory granuloma may later develop into a malignant lymphoma. In this category are the interesting cases of Burkitt's tumor reported in recent years.

Burkitt's tumor or lymphoma, an undifferentiated lymphosarcoma, arises characteristically in extralymph-nodal areas, particularly the maxilla and the orbit in children and youths, 2 to 16 years of age. Proptosis is common when the maxillary bones are involved. Unlike the common childhood lymphomas, it is usually aleukemic. The tumor was first described as endemic in Central Africa and New Guinea where malaria is common.[6] The reticuloendothelial system was believed to become vulnerable to some preinfectious agents; i.e., a favorable environmental condition fostered an appropriate vector, probably the Epstein-Barr (EB) virus.

Several equivocal cases probably belong in the Burkitt-type lymphoma.[18,39,41,49] Sixty-five cases occurring outside of Africa were reviewed in one series[7] and 20 in another.[12] Several patients in these series had ocular involvement.

The case of a 22-month-old Caucasian girl with intraocular involvement was reported.[22] Analysis of 60 cases of proptosis in Ugandan children suggested an orbital tumor as the cause;[64] nearly half were thought to be due to Burkitt's lymphoma. A 12-year-old African boy with this tumor had massive intraocular involvement; the blood picture was aleukemic, and the blood smear for malaria was positive.[38]

It had been suggested that Burkitt's lymphoma might be associated with immunosuppressive antimalarial drugs inasmuch as the first case was reported four years after pyrimethamine was introduced in tropical Africa, and lymphomas have developed in other groups receiving immunosuppressive drugs, e.g., patients undergoing a kidney transplant or those with collagen disease.[56] However, this disease was seen long before such drugs were administered in affected areas. The records at Mengo Hospital in Uganda show cases dating from 1905.[17]

The possible etiologic importance of an interaction between the EB virus and malaria has been suggested.[8] When the 82 cases accepted by the Papua New Guinea Tumor Registry from 1960 to February 1973 were reviewed,[2] the most acceptable hypothesis seemed to be that Burkitt's lymphoma is due to the effect of an oncogenic virus, probably the EB virus, on an immune system altered by chronic malaria infection.

RETICULUM-CELL SARCOMA OF THE RETINA AND UVEA

Reticulum-cell sarcoma may manifest itself initially as either a unilateral or bilateral uveitis or a chorioretinitis associated with retinal hemorrhage, or both. The conditions are often of unknown cause.[13,16,65] The tumor may be primary in the eye or secondary to generalized malignant lymphoma or to reticulum-cell sarcoma of the central nervous system. In five of eight patients seen at one center after 1968,[40] the eye symptoms were the first indication of reticulum-cell sarcoma. Three such lesions affecting the uvea alone were mentioned in the previous edition of this book.

The tumor is manifested in middle age, resembling inflammation of the fundus. Five of six patients in one series were treated for uveitis for five months to five years before the diagnosis was made.[65]

An unsuspected reticulum-cell sarcoma of the choroid of each eye in the guise of a uveitis was treated by systemic corticosteroids.[47] Death resulted from a fungal infection contracted as a complication of therapy. The correct diagnosis was made from pathologic examination of the eyes after autopsy. There was no other evidence of neoplasm.

Six cases of reticulum-cell lymphosarcoma of the brain were described, all showing a transition from a granulomatous process to sarcoma.[66] In seven patients with uveitis associated with reticulum-cell sarcoma of the brain,[46] the eye symptoms antedated the neurologic symptoms by three months to eight years. Primary reticulum-cell sarcomas arising in the meninges of either the optic nerve or the base of the brain may present ophthalmologic problems.[34]

The fundus shows a characteristic perivascular pattern of tumor areas with hemorrhagic necrosis, a fluffy outline, and in some instances a grayish-green color. In the typical cytologic picture, the reticulum cells are arranged around blood vessels and intimately surrounded by reticulum fibers.

LYMPHATIC LEUKEMIA

Acute or chronic lymphatic leukemia is one of the manifestations of malignant lymphoma. The only distinguishing characteristic is an appreciable number of malignant lymphocytes in the circulating blood. The Gomori stain may be helpful in demonstrating the leukocytic alkaline phosphatase.

Leukemic manifestations may be apparent at the outset, appear concomitantly with localized tumor masses, be transitory, be noted only in the terminal phase of the disease, or fail to appear at all. The incidence of leukemia in cases of malignant lymphoma has been reported as 2.3%,[58] 6.6%,[60] and 10%.[27]

Some degree of orbital infiltration is commonly encountered in acute or chronic lymphatic leukemia and probably accounts for exophthalmos (in about 2% of the cases), conjunctival and orbital hemorrhages, and inflammatory processes. Fundal changes that may occur include retinal hemorrhages and a pale milky appearance of the entire fundus. Vascular occlusion is often found. According to one report,[1] 50% of patients with leukemia and allied conditions show ocular involvement, particularly those with acute leukemia. Eye manifestations—such as proptosis, which may be very marked (Fig. 13–6), visual decrease from uveitis, retinal vascular changes, vitreous infiltration, optic nerve and intracranial infiltration, and secondary glaucoma—may lead to the correct diagnosis.

A case has been described in which glaucoma was the presenting sign of chronic lymphatic leukemia, probably due to leukemic infiltration of limbal tissues.[29] Sudden loss of vision in a case of unsuspected leukemia was due to infiltration by the choroidal tumor,[5] suggesting the advisability of a blood count before enucleation in patients with a rapidly growing choroidal tumor. Leukemia patients may have ocular disorders threatening vision despite complete hematologic and bone marrow remission;[48] in such cases early radiotherapy may prevent visual loss.

MYCOSIS FUNGOIDES

Mycosis fungoides, a dermatosis of undetermined origin, has an inflammatory nature in the early stage, becoming neoplastic in later stages. It is classified as a type of malignant lymphoma. The lid and conjunctiva are the ocular structures most likely to be affected, but intraocular lesions have been reported.[23,26,28]

PLASMA-CELL TUMORS

The two types of plasma-cell tumors, both encountered in ophthalmology, are plasma-cell myeloma and benign plasmoma, which seems to develop in the wake of chronic inflammation.

PLASMA-CELL MYELOMA

Plasma-cell myeloma usually arises from the bone marrow but occasionally from extra-osseous tissues. X rays may show typical osteolytic bone lesions. The urine occasionally contains Bence Jones proteins, but in over 90% of cases the most important typical finding is a spike in the gamma globulin area on paper protein electrophoresis of the serum or urine or both. The blood sedimentation rate is often high. Aspirated bone marrow usually reveals an increased number of normal and immature plasma cells. The process may be fatal in a few months or the patient may survive for years. The average survival time is reported to be about two years.[11] Even though the tumor appears at one site, other evidence of the disease is invariably found if carefully sought.

In a histologic study of the eyes of 15 autopsied patients with multiple myeloma, 12 were found to have intraocular lesions.[57]

One author divided orbital myelomas into those primary in the orbit and those involving it secondarily, citing 13 cases in which primary or extraosseous myeloma of the orbit initiated the disease.[11]

Secondary myeloma of the orbit may develop from a primary focus in the cranial bones, paranasal sinuses, nose, nasopharynx, or mucous membrane of the upper respiratory pathways. The cranial bones are said to be involved eventually in over 70% of patients with myeloma.[3]

FIG. 13–6. Exophthalmos due to acute leukemia (undifferentiated cell type). A 4-year-old boy had had increasing lassitude, pallor, and ankle pain for three months. Exophthalmos, apparent almost from the onset of the other symptoms, progressed steadily. The lymph nodes, liver, and spleen were enlarged.

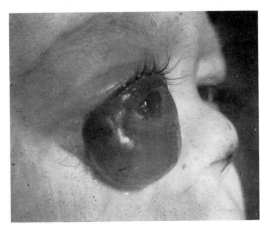

BENIGN PLASMOMA

Because benign infiltrations of lymphocytes, plasma cells, and reticulum cells are localized in certain body areas, presumably in response to chronic inflammation, lesions are formed that must be differentiated from malignant lymphomas. Such tumors occur in the orbit and the conjunctiva as well as in the rectum, the skin, the salivary glands, and the oral cavity. They can be distinguished from malignant lymphoma because they are composed solely of differentiated adult cells with or without lymph follicles.

Plasmoma (plasma-cell granuloma, reactive lymphocytic hyperplasia) can be distinguished from lymphoma because the plasma cells are broken up into small groups by the proliferating capillaries and fibroblasts of the granuloma. If Russell bodies are found, the lesion is almost certainly a granuloma. A plasma-cell myeloma has very few vessels; and the plasma cells, which may be poorly differentiated, collect in large masses.

Plasmomas and benign lymphomas may involve the conjunctiva, lacrimal gland and sac, lids, caruncle, and orbit. A plasmocytoma of the conjunctiva may later develop into amyloidosis.[30]

A type of benign lymphoma consisting of a cluster of lymphoid follicles under the skin is sometimes referred to as Spiegler-Fendt disease. It belongs to the general group of reactive lymphocytic hyperplasias, and is preferably called lymphoma cutis. It is encountered in ophthalmology in the skin of the lids, in the conjunctiva, and probably in the orbit.

MYELOGENOUS LEUKEMIA

Although orbital or subconjunctival infiltration is common in acute or chronic lymphatic leukemia, both are rare in myelogenous leukemia.[10] In one reported case the first manifestations were a disturbance of vision with fundal changes followed by exophthalmos.[43] The fundus is frequently involved in this type of leukemia, showing marked dilatation and tortuosity of the retinal veins, with white fluffy material along their margins, white deposits surrounded by thin rims of blood, called Roth spots, and hemorrhage. The entire fundus is sometimes pale and often faintly green—a valuable diagnostic finding. Two-thirds of the patients in one series[43]

had some blurring of vision with accompanying fundal changes.

Myelogenous leukemia may be manifested first in the conjunctiva. A 52-year-old woman showed subconjunctival nodular infiltration of the right then left eye which progressed steadily (Fig. 13–7). A thorough medical examination did not reveal the disease early in its course.

A 21-year-old woman with fever, malaise, and increasing fatigue for two or three months was treated for severe anemia. The blood count and bone marrow aspiration revealed no suggestion of leukemia. Within six weeks she developed subconjunctival masses in each eye (Fig. 13–8) and was referred to me. The white blood count rose precipitously, and myelogenous leukemia was established.

Orbital infiltration certainly occurs in myelogenous leukemia, but to my knowledge it has not been established by biopsy or histologic study of autopsied tissue in the reported cases.

A sudden hemorrhage in the orbit may lead to extreme exophthalmos in the course of myelogenous leukemia.

Inasmuch as leukemia, particularly acute lymphatic leukemia, is a common malignant tumor in children, the possibility of leukemic

FIG. 13–7. Nodular infiltrations under the conjunctiva as the first manifestation of myelogenous leukemia. A 52-year-old woman had noted swelling and redness of both eyes for three months. Subconjunctival infiltration in the lower nasal quadrant of the right eye was followed by similar involvement of the left eye. The condition progressed in both eyes and, when she consulted me, was as shown here. A thorough medical examination did not reveal the cause. The white blood count was 14,000 with 54% polymorphonuclear leukocytes, 26% lymphocytes, and 19% eosinophils. Early in the disease, brawny scleritis and scleromalacia perforans were considered in the diagnosis. The clinical picture was similar to that seen in leukemia. The patient developed myelogenous leukemia and died six years after the drawings were made.

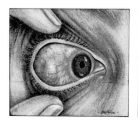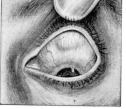

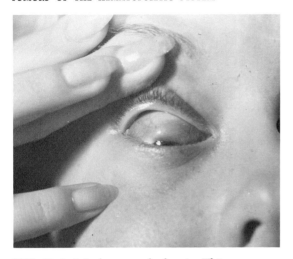

FIG. 13–8. Myelogenous leukemia. This 21-year-old woman had a salmon-colored subconjunctival mass surrounding the upper half of the cornea of each eye. The diagnosis was confirmed by bone marrow tests. The disease resulted fatally within four weeks.

infiltration of the orbit as the cause of proptosis in this age group should be considered. Exophthalmos or fundal changes may be the first sign of the disease. In some cases a routine blood count does not reveal the presence of leukemia. In this aleukemic phase, bone marrow studies should establish the diagnosis. Hematopoiesis, especially in the uvea, was found in the eyes of 14% of stillborn infants or infants who died shortly after birth.[52] This blood-forming faculty was noted primarily in the choroid. Occasionally the cells assumed tumorlike proportions, but the foci tended to be small to medium in size. The high incidence found in this group suggests that the uvea may be one of the physiologic sites of hematopoiesis during fetal life. Uveal infiltration and the resulting fundal changes seen by ophthalmoscope in leukemia patients may be due to activation or resumption of the uvea's blood-forming properties (Fig. 13–9) rather than to simple infiltration. Since ectopic hematopoietic sites elsewhere become reactivated in the course of myelogenous leukemia, it seems logical that the uvea might be involved.[52]

CHLOROMA

This tumor, which may spread secondarily to the orbit from adjacent bones, is regarded as a localized form of myelogenous leukemia. Their relationship is comparable to that of malignant lymphoma and lymphatic leukemia. A chloroma has a predilection for the

FIG. 13–9. Hematopoiesis in the choroid. Section of an eye of a premature male (birthweight 1021 g) who survived only 67 days. A large focus of hematopoiesis is manifested as a dense accumulation of immature cells which produce a tumorlike thickening of the choroid. (A. B. Reese and F. C. Blodi.[52])

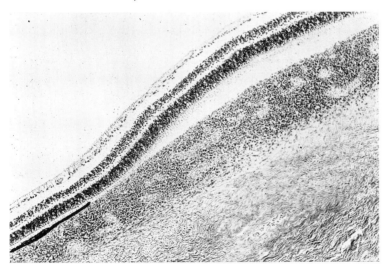

meninges, the periosteum, and mucous membranes. In two reported cases[31] exophthalmos produced by the orbital extension was the first sign of the disease.

The tumor's characteristic green color is considered to be due to a pigment related chemically to the porphyrins.[31] At autopsy the pigment is found not only in the tumor tissue but also distributed uniformly in connective tissue, in endothelial linings, and over mucosal surfaces. It is probably carried in the blood plasma and represents an intermediate product in the breakdown of hemoglobin to bilirubin.

TREATMENT

Surgery is usually employed for the eye manifestations of lymphomatous tumors only to establish the diagnosis. Simple excision may suffice for a localized lesion under the conjunctiva or skin. If a lesion is deep in the orbit, producing progressive exophthalmos and showing signs of jeopardizing vision by pressure on the optic nerve, a Krönlein operation may be indicated.

Irradiation results in a dramatic regression of lymphomatous tumors. In fact, these tumors are so radiosensitive that it is unwise to attempt local excision if they are large. When any lymphomatous lesion is surgically excised, postoperative irradiation is advisable even if it was apparently completely removed. (See Radiotherapy of Ocular and Orbital Tumors by Patricia Tretter, in Chapter 12.)

It must be emphasized that although a given tumor regresses completely there may be systemic manifestations of the disease. Since the patients may develop nodal or extranodal lesions anywhere over the body, or a lymphatic leukemia, they should have periodic medical check-ups including a differential blood count and bone marrow study.

Of 33 cases of primary lymphoma of the orbit in one series, 30 were treated initially by radiotherapy and 3 by surgery alone.[25] There were 5 local recurrences, all successfully retreated. Nine patients developed generalized disease, which in two resulted fatally. Patients with reticulum-cell or mixed-cell-type tumors were more susceptible to generalized disease.

A series of 100 cases of orbital lymphoma seen at the Institute of Ophthalmology, New York,[20,37] was increased to 140 nine years later.[61] These authors concluded that it is often difficult to tell whether a lesion is basically malignant or benign, because of certain pathologic problems:

1. There is no completely certain histologic basis for predicting the clinical course.
2. There is no reliable evidence as to whether the disease is monocentric or multicentric.
3. There is no reliable means of distinguishing between primary and secondary tumors by biopsy.
4. The nature of the so-called pseudotumor is obscure, whereas the lymphoma is eventually fatal.

The following simplified histologic classification has been suggested by these authors:

1. Benign lymphoid hyperplasia (6%)
2. Lymphosarcoma
   a. Giant follicular (2%)
   b. Lymphocytic cell (58%)
   c. Reticulum cell (34%)
3. Hodgkin's disease

Chemotherapy

In the treatment of plasma-cell myeloma a combination of agents leading to approximately 40% of active remissions includes the use of corticosteroids in small doses and an alkylating agent such as melphalan (Alkeran, PAM) or cyclophosphamide (Cytoxan), the hemogram permitting. Daunorubicin has proved effective in the treatment of acute myelogenous leukemia, and L-asparaginase following vincristine (Oncovin) and prednisone induction in the treatment of acute lymphatic leukemia.[35]

PROGNOSIS

The generally accepted policy is to refer to five-year survivals rather than cures because the disease is chronic and unpredictable.

In each cytologic group, a follicular pattern is of prognostic significance. Patients whose tumors have a follicular element have a higher survival rate than those with diffuse tumors of the same cell type.[33,50] The rate appears to be highest in patients with well-differentiated lymphocytic tumors and lowest in those with reticulum-cell tumors.

The survival rate is low in patients with reticulum-cell lymphoma, Hodgkin's disease, or acute leukemia.

An overall five-year survival of 26% was reported in a series of 308 radiation-treated patients.[14] The disease was first noted only in the head and neck region in 40 of the 81 survivors. The somewhat better prognosis in malignant lymphoma of the head and neck than in the generalized form of this disease is borne out by another report of 52% survival in 50 patients.[9] At the initial examination 46% of them presented only the primary tumor; 61% of this group survived at least five years. The other 54% of the patients had one or more enlarged cervical nodes in addition to the primary mass when first examined; 44% of them survived at least five years. In 40% of the cases the disease became generalized; only one patient in this group survived five years.

Patients with lymphosarcoma treated by radiotherapy or surgery were found to

survive much longer than those left untreated.[58, 59] In the treated group 28.8% survived five years and 14.8% were free of symptoms. In the untreated group only 3.2% survived more than five years, and none was free of disease. According to all available reports, the prognosis is much better for patients treated while the disease is still localized than for those with multiple manifestations. The chances for survival are poor if the neoplasm develops before age 20, and best in the age group over 40. Cases associated with leukemia inevitably result fatally.

Four of 19 patients with primary malignant lymphoma of the orbit treated at the Mayo Clinic were alive and well 11, 9, 6, and 5 years after therapy.[4] In another report,[24] among 7 patients with orbital malignant lymphoma, follow-up was available in 4, all of whom died in two to nine months.

REFERENCES

1. ALLEN RA, STRAATSMA BR: Ocular involvement in leukemia and allied disorders. Arch Ophthalmol 66:490–508, 1961
2. BARNES P: Letters to the Editor (aetiological significance of pyrimethamine in Burkitt's lymphoma). Lancet 1:68, 1974
3. BAYRD ED, HECK FJ: Multiple myeloma. JAMA 133:147–157, 1947
4. BENEDICT WL, MARTENE TG: Malignant lymphocytic tumors of the orbit. Surg Clin North Am 26:871–875, 1946
5. BLODI FC: Unusual tumors in and around the eye. Trans Pac Coast Otoophthalmol Soc 50:195–224, 1969
6. BURKITT D: A sarcoma involving the jaws in African children. Br J Surg 46:218–222, 1958
7. BURKITT D: Burkitt's lymphoma outside the known endemic areas of Africa and New Guinea. Int J Cancer 2:562–565, 1967
8. BURKITT DP: Etiology of Burkitt's lymphoma—an alternative hypothesis to a vectored virus. J Nat Cancer Inst 42:19–28, 1969
9. CATLIN D: Lymphosarcoma of the head and neck. Am J Roentgenol 59:354–358, 1948
10. CHATTERJEE BM, SEN NN: Acute myeloid leukemia with leukemic deposit in the orbit. Br J Ophthalmol 44:440–442, 1960
11. CLARKE E: Plasma cell myeloma of the orbit. Br J Ophthalmol 37:543–554, 1953
12. COHEN MH, BENNETT JM, BERARD CW, ZIEGLER JL, VOGEL CL, SHEAGREN JN, CARBONE PP: Burkitt's tumor in the United States. Cancer 23:1259–1272, 1969
13. COOPER EL, RIKER JL: Malignant lymphoma of the uveal tract. Am J Ophthalmol 34:1153–1158, 1961
14. CRAVER LF: Malignant Lymphomas and Leukemias. New York, American Cancer Society, 1952
15. CROOKES GP, MULLANEY J: Lymphoid hyperplasia of the uveal tract simulating malignant lymphoma. Am J Ophthalmol 63:962–967, 1967

16. CURREY TA, DEUTSCH AR: Reticulum cell sarcoma of the uvea. South Med J 58:919–922, 1965
17. DAVIES JNP: Antimalarial drugs and Burkitt's lymphoma. Lancet 1:67–68, 1974
18. DORFMAN RF: Childhood lymphosarcoma in St Louis, Missouri, clinically and histologically resembling Burkitt's tumor. Cancer 18:418–430, 1965
19. EDITORIAL: Sjögren's syndrome. JAMA 202:902, 1967
20. ELLSWORTH RM (ed): Lymphoma of the orbit. Symposium on Surgery of the Orbit and Adnexa. Trans New Orleans Acad Ophthalmol. St Louis, CV Mosby, 1974, pp 48–52
21. FAULBORN J: Malignant lymphogranulomatosis of the conjunctiva. Klin Monatsbl Augenheilkd 156:409–416, 1970
22. FEMAN FS, NIWAYAMA G, HEPLER RS, FOOS RY: "Burkitt tumor" with intraocular involvement. Survey Ophthalmol 14:106–111, 1969
23. FOERSTER HC: Mycosis fungoides with intraocular involvement. Trans Am Acad Ophthalmol Otolaryngol 64:308–313, 1960
24. FORREST AW: Intraorbital tumors. Arch Ophthalmol 41:198–232, 1949
25. FOSTER SC, WILSON CS, TRETTER PK: Radiotherapy of primary lymphoma of the orbit. Am J Roentgenol Radium Ther Nucl Med 111:343–349, 1971
26. FRANCESCHETTI A: Micosi fungoide con manifestazioni oculari (un caso con retinopatia disorcia). Ann Ottalmol Clin Ocul 76:413–420, 1950
27. GALL EA, MALLORY TB: Malignant lymphoma; a clinico-pathologic survey of 618 cases. Am J Pathol 18:381–429, 1942
28. GARTNER J: Mycosis fungoides mit Beteiligung der Aderhaut. Klin Monatsbl Augenheilkd 131:61–69, 1957
29. GLASER B, SMITH JL: Leukaemic glaucoma. Br J Ophthalmol 50:92–94, 1966

30. GLASS R, SCHEIE HG, YANOFF M: Conjunctival amyloidosis arising from a plasmacytoma. Ann Ophthalmol 3:823–825, 1971

31. GOODMAN EG, IVERSON L: Chloroma: clinical study of two cases. Am J Med Sci 211:205, 1946

32. HARTSHORNE I: Lymphosarcoma of the orbit probably arising in choroid. Am J Ophthalmol 5:604, 1922

33. HELWIG CA: Malignant lymphoma: analysis of 202 cases. Am J Clin Pathol 16:546, 1946

34. HOGAN MJ, SPENCER WH, HOYT WF: Primary reticuloendothelial sarcomas of the orbital and cranial meninges: ophthalmologic aspects. Am J Ophthalmol 61:1146–1158, 1966

35. HYMAN, GA: Personal communication

36. JOHNSTON SS, WARE CF: Iris involvement in leukaemia. Br J Ophthalmol 37:320–324, 1973

37. JONES W, ELLSWORTH RM: Cited in Ellsworth RM, ref 20

38. KARP LA, ZIMMERMAN LE, PAYNE T: Intraocular involvement in Burkitt's lymphoma. Arch Ophthalmol 85:295–298, 1971

39. KLEIN G, CLIFFORD P, KLEIN E, STJERNSWARD J: Search for tumor-specific immune reactions in Burkitt lymphoma patients by the membrane immunofluorescence reaction. Proc Natl Acad Sci USA 55:1628–1635, 1966

40. KLINGELE TG, HOGAN MJ: Ocular reticulum cell sarcoma. Am J Ophthalmol 79:39–47, 1975

41. LEVY JA, HENLE G: Indirect immunofluorescence tests with sera from African children and cultured Burkitt lymphoma cells. J Bacteriol 92:275–276, 1966

42. LUKES RJ, BUTLER JJ, HICKS EB: Natural history of Hodgkin's disease as related to its pathologic picture. Cancer 19:317–344, 1966

43. MANCHESTER PT, GIDDINGS GA: The eye signs of leukemia. J Med Assoc Ga 46:198–199, 1957

44. MCGAVIC JS: Lymphomatoid diseases involving the eye and its adnexa. Arch Ophthalmol 30:179–193, 1943

45. MORGAN G: Lymphocytic tumors of the conjunctiva. J Clin Pathol 24:585–595, 1971

46. NEAULT RW, VAN SCOY RE, OKAZAKI H, ET AL: Uveitis associated with isolated reticulum cell sarcoma of the brain. Am J Ophthalmol 73:431–436, 1972

47. NEVINS RC JR, FREY WW, ELLIOTT JH: Primary, solitary, intraocular reticulum cell sarcoma (microgliomatosis). A clinicopathologic case report. Trans Am Acad Ophthalmol Otolaryngol 72:867–876, 1968

48. NEWMAN NM, SMITH ME, GAY AJ: An unusual case of leukemia involving the eye: a clinico-pathological study. Survey Ophthalmol 16:316–321, 1972

49. O'CONOR GT, RAPPAPORT H, SMITH EB: Childhood lymphoma resembling "Burkitt tumor" in the United States. Cancer 18:411–417, 1965

50. RAPPAPORT H: Tumors of the hematopoietic system. In Atlas of Tumor Pathology, Fascicle 8, Section III, pp 98–206, Armed Forces Institute of Pathology, published by the National Research Council, Washington DC, 1966

51. REESE AB, GUY L: Exophthalmos in leukaemia. Am J Ophthalmol 16:718–720, 1933

52. REESE AB, BLODI FC: Hematopoiesis in and around the eye. Am J Ophthalmol 38:214–221, 1954

53. ROTHMAN S, BLOCK M, HAUSER FV: Sjögren's syndrome associated with lymphoblastoma and hypersplenism. Arch Dermatol Syphilol 63:642–643, 1951

54. RUBIN P: Updated Hodgkin's disease: A. Introduction. JAMA 222:1292–1306, 1972

55. RYAN SJ, ZIMMERMAN LE, KING FM: Reactive lymphoid hyperplasia; an unusual form of intraocular pseudotumor. Trans Am Acad Ophthalmol Otolaryngol 76:652–671, 1972

56. SADOFF L: Aetiology of Burkitt's lymphoma. Lancet 2:1414, 1972

57. SANDERS TE, PODOS SM, ROSENBAUM LJ: Intraocular manifestations of multiple myeloma. Arch Ophthalmol 77:789–794, 1967

58. STOUT AP: Is lymphosarcoma curable? JAMA 118:968–970, 1942

59. STOUT AP: Results of treatment of lymphosarcoma. NY State J Med 47:158–164, 1947

60. SUGARBAKER ED, CRAVER LF: Lymphosarcoma. JAMA 115:17–23, 112–117, 1940

61. SULLIVAN TB: Lymphomatous involvement of the eye and adnexa. Thesis, Department of Ophthalmology, University of Iowa, 1972, p 4 (cited in ref 20)

62. TALAL N, BUNIM JJ: The development of malignant lymphoma in the course of Sjögren's syndrome. Am J Med 36:529–540, 1964

63. TALAL N, SOKOLOFF L, BARTH WF: Extrasalivary lymphoid abnormalities in Sjögren's syndrome (reticulum cell sarcoma, "pseudo-lymphoma," macroglobulinemia). Am J Med 43:50–65, 1967

64. TEMPLETON AC: Orbital tumours in African children. Br J Ophthalmol 55:254–261, 1971

65. VOGEL MH, FONT RL, ZIMMERMAN LE, LEVINE RA: Reticulum cell sarcoma of the retina and uvea; report of six cases and review of the literature. Am J Ophthalmol 66:205–215, 1968

66. WILKE G: Über primäre Reticuloendotheliosen des Gehirns. Dtsch Z Nervenheilkd 164:332, 1950

67. YANOFF M, SCHEIE HG: Malignant lymphoma of the orbit; difficulties in diagnosis. Survey Ophthalmol 12:134–140, 1967

68. ZIMMERMAN LE: Personal communication

14

TUMORS OF THE LACRIMAL GLAND

The incidence of benign and malignant epithelial tumors of the lacrimal gland is about the same. The benign group includes mixed tumors and adenomas. In the malignant group are mixed tumors, adenocarcinomas (adenocystic carcinoma or cylindroma), and squamous-cell carcinomas.

EPITHELIAL TUMORS

MIXED TUMORS

As mixed tumors are pleomorphic, there is considerable discussion about their nature. Despite the many descriptive terms designating mixed tumors in which one or more tissues predominate, and despite variations in their structure, they are basically the same type of lesion.

They contain both epithelial and mesenchymal elements, and some appear to have transitional tissue. In the transitional zones, the tumor cells seem to be neither epithelial nor myxomatous. In view of this unusual relationship of tissues, supposedly derived from separate germ layers, the confusion regarding histogenesis is understandable.

According to one of the earliest theories regarding mixed tumors, their parenchyma was derived from endothelium so they were for a long time called endotheliomas. Later, it was believed that ectodermal and mesodermal elements of the lacrimal gland remained as embryonic rests which gave rise to various types of tissue. Other theories advanced over the years include the following:

1. The parenchyma of the tumor is epithelium and the apparent mesenchymal element is not really mesodermal but represents ectodermal products that have undergone metaplasia.
2. The parenchyma of the tumor is epithelium which, through its so-called organizer action, induces abnormal differentiation of the undifferentiated mesoderm. The basis for this theory is that normal development depends upon a close interrelationship between all tissues involved. Functional inadequacy of one tissue during the developmental phase may cause structural changes in other related tissues. This organizer or provocative effect of epithelium acts on undifferentiated mesoderm and *vice versa*. Not only does one embryonic tissue affect another during development, but also even adult tissues appear to retain some of the organizer influence.

Mesenchymal mucus can be differentiated from epithelial mucus by a special staining technique; both types are found in mixed tumors of the parotid gland, emphasizing their truly mixed nature.

Embryologic, histologic, and topographic studies suggest that mixed tumors of the salivary glands are derived from misplaced elements of the notochord, a theory that would explain not only their complex structure but also their marked predilection for the parotid glands.

Most investigators believe that the precursor cells of mixed tumors represent an embryonic displacement or rest. During human development, some cells destined to form the lacrimal gland become isolated and remain dormant until such time as they are reactivated by an unknown stimulus and become neoplastic.

To adherents of the metaplasia hypothesis, these rests are merely epithelial cells. To adherents of the organizer theory, the epithelial cells represent the tumor matrix, with the mesenchymal elements secondary to the organizer effect of the epithelium on the undifferentiated mesoderm. The organizer concept seems tenable to me, and the fact that recurrent mixed tumors and metastatic foci are epithelial indicates the basically epithelial nature of the tumor.

Histologically, the tumors are composed of epithelium arranged in alveoli, cords, or islands (Figs. 14–1, 14–2, 14–3). Mucus is often present in a central lumen or outside of the epithelial foci. Cartilage and bone are

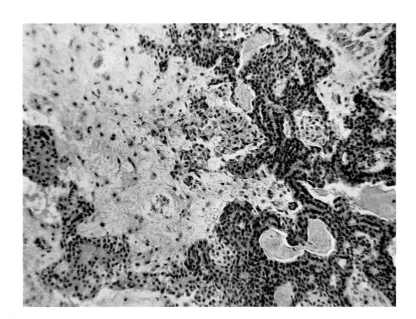

FIG. 14–1. Benign mixed tumor of the lacrimal gland. The basal layer of epithelium shows an orderly growth pattern, and the stroma is myxomatous.

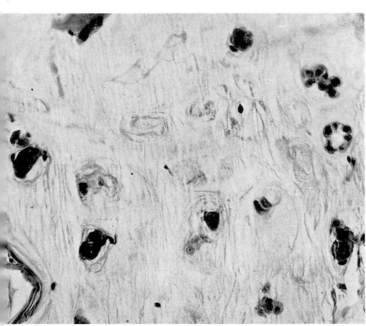

FIG. 14–2. Benign mixed tumor of the lacrimal gland. The stroma is myxomatous, with cartilage and only small islands of epithelial tissue.

FIG. 14–3. Benign mixed tumor of the lacrimal gland. The epithelium shows a benign cytology; the stroma is myxomatous.

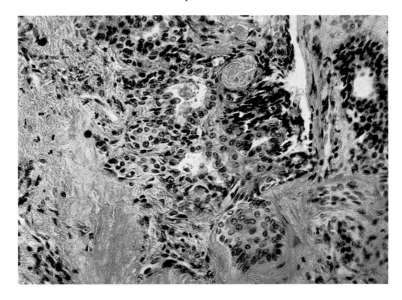

sometimes found in a myxomatous stroma between the epithelial elements, which are often two cells thick. The inner layer gives rise to the mucous element and the outer to the mesenchymal element. A tumor with a great amount of myxomatous tissue resembles a colloid carcinoma. The tumors are usually definitely encapsulated, but the capsule is often invaded by epithelial elements (Fig. 14–4).

It has been suggested that a myoepithelial cell component of a malignant mixed tumor of the lacrimal gland might represent atavistic remains of Harder's gland, seen normally in birds and some mammals.[34]

Histologically, tumors arising in the lacrimal gland and the salivary glands are analogous. They have the same structure and represent the majority of neoplastic lesions in these glands. In spite of the similarity, however, the clinical behavior and prognosis differ.

Mixed tumors in general may be benign or malignant. They occur most commonly in the salivary glands, particularly the parotid gland, but also may develop in the lips, gums, tongue, floor and roof of the mouth, pharynx and larynx, as well as the lacrimal gland. In fact, they can arise at any site in the head and neck where there are mucous or serous glands. Only about 10% develop from glandular elements of the mucous membrane in the nose and paranasal sinuses; the majority originate in the parotid, sublingual, and submaxillary salivary glands, with only a very small percentage originating in the lacrimal gland. A mixed tumor may arise from the lacrimal sac or spread to it from a primary site in the nose.

Benign Type

This tumor has a definite capsule, benign cytology, and is not capable of metastasis. However, when an initially benign tumor recurs it may be malignant and manifest seeding and bone invasion. The benign type of mixed tumor is by far the most common epithelial tumor of the lacrimal gland.

Two cases of benign mixed tumors of the palpebral portion of the lacrimal gland, one of which was diagnosed clinically as a sebaceous cyst and the other as a hematoma, have been reported.[30]

Malignant Type

This tumor has the same general pattern as the benign type but shows areas of frank carcinoma (Fig. 14–5), which may be present initially or represent recent increased growth.

ADENOID CYSTIC CARCINOMA

Adenoid cystic carcinoma (cylindroma), the most common type of carcinoma of the lacrimal gland (Fig. 14–6), has no relation to mixed tumor. It has a basal-cell type of growth with hyaloid stroma. The cells are small, stain darkly, and have relatively little cytoplasm. They grow in anastomosing cords between which are acellular areas varying considerably in size, which may be empty or contain mucus, hyalin, or mucohyaline material. Some of the tumors are solid with highly malignant cells and few or no areas showing the cystic glandular pattern (Fig. 14–7).

SQUAMOUS-CELL CARCINOMA

Such tumors in the lacrimal gland have the same structural characteristics as those occurring elsewhere in the body.

ADENOMA

There is no reason why a true adenoma should not occur in the lacrimal gland, but the so-called adenomas I have seen have been interpreted as aberrant or ectopic lacrimal glands.

MUCOEPIDERMOID CARCINOMA

The last edition of this book included one case described as a mucoepidermoid carcinoma of the lacrimal gland which I now believe was misinterpreted. At present there is no reason to suppose that the mucoepidermoid tumor seen in the salivary glands has a counterpart in the lacrimal gland.[4]

CONGENITAL LESIONS; CYSTS

ABERRANT OR ECTOPIC LACRIMAL GLAND

An ectopic lacrimal gland may appear practically anywhere in or around the eye and at times be clinically mistaken for a true neo-

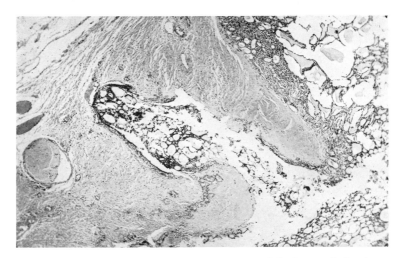

FIG. 14–4. Mixed tumor of the lacrimal gland invading its capsule. (Courtesy of A. W. Forrest.[16])

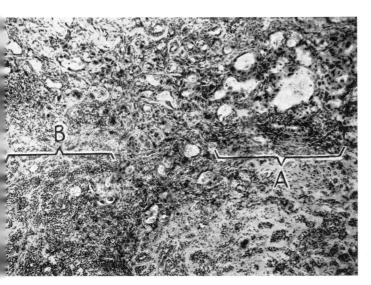

FIG. 14–5. Malignant mixed tumor of the lacrimal gland. Areas at *B* and *A* show marked epithelial activity including anaplasia and mitotic figures in an otherwise benign tumor. Multiple sections may be necessary to demonstrate such areas. (Courtesy of A. W. Forrest.)

FIG. 14–6. Adenoid cystic carcinoma of the lacrimal gland.

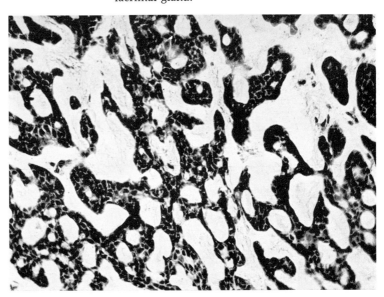

plasm. Many cases have been reported in the conjunctiva and lids, [1,9,21,26,39] and fewer involving the intraocular structures[8,10,11,23] (Fig. 14–8).

Ectopic lacrimal glands rarely occur in the conjunctiva. One author[24] found small glands of this type at the corneal limbus in 3 of 25 normal subjects. Because of their similarity to the gland of Manz, which is normal in the pig, he believes that they represent

glandular primordium and described a case in which the tissue started to grow, for unknown reasons, in a 20-year-old (Fig. 14-9).

Cases in the orbit are rare.[5,7,22] Reexamination of 35 cases coded at the Armed Forces Institute of Pathology as aberrant or ectopic lacrimal gland revealed 8 with orbital involvement.[22] All had accompanying chronic inflammation, which the authors postulated might be due to stasis of the glandular secre-

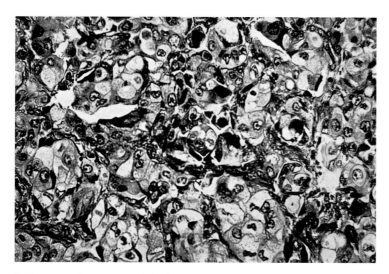

FIG. 14–7. Carcinoma of the lacrimal gland.

FIG. 14–8. Aberrant lacrimal gland in the iris and ciliary body. A. Clinical appearance of mass in the iris. B. Aberrant normal lacrimal gland tissue in the iris seen under high-power magnification. (Courtesy of G. M. Bruce.[8])

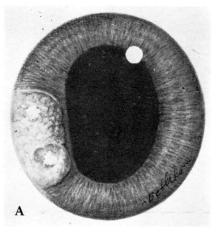
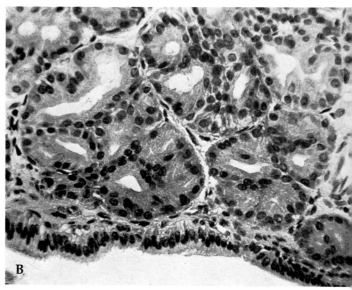

tion. Cyst formation in several cases added to the tumor volume. In the other 27 cases, 18 of the ectopic lacrimal glands were in the bulbar conjunctiva (10 involving the cornea), 6 in the outer canthus or upper lid, 2 in the lower lid, and 1 was intraocular. Two of the 35 cases were bilateral.

DERMOID TUMORS

Dermoid tumors occurring usually at the limbus may contain lacrimal gland tissue in conjunction with other elements such as muscle and nerve tissue, cartilage, bone, and dermoid appendages (see Ch. 15). In one reported case an aberrant lacrimal gland was associated with a dermoid tumor at the outer canthus.[6]

Cysts as well as neoplasms (adenocarcinomas) may arise from an ectopic lacrimal gland.[1,9,19,22]

CYSTS

Clear cysts, probably retention cysts, sometimes occur in the lacrimal gland. They are lined with epithelium resembling that seen in ducts of normal lacrimal glands. The origin and nature of these clear cysts are not known; they may be confused with a tumor.

SIGNS AND SYMPTOMS

The various expanding lesions in the lacrimal gland have no distinguishing features. In general, the tumors are slow-growing and

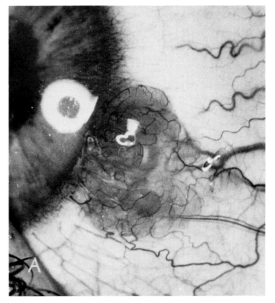

FIG. 14–9. Ectopic lacrimal gland tissue involving the conjunctiva. **A.** Tissue located at the corneal limbus. **B.** Photomicrograph showing well-differentiated glandular acini and branched excretory ducts. (Courtesy of S. V. Kessing.[24])

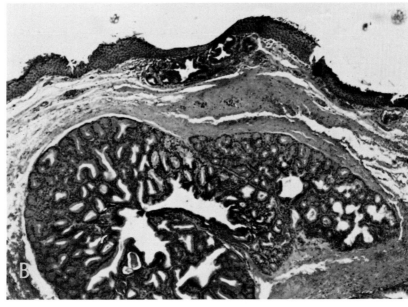

cause no symptoms. The patient may seek medical advice because of exophthalmos, but more often because of a fullness or lump in the outer upper lid. Acquired unilateral ptosis in an adult should arouse suspicion of a possible lacrimal gland lesion.

MIXED TUMORS

Mixed tumors of the lacrimal gland may have a particularly insidious onset. In one such case a palpable nodule in the upper quadrant of the orbit remained unchanged for 30 years, then steadily increased in size over a one-year period.[2] If untreated, such tumors may become huge (Fig. 14–10).

Mixed tumors usually affect the 40–50 age group, although I have seen a 70-year-old patient, and a case in a 13-year-old has been reported.[35]

The tumor has a strong tendency to invade the bone of the lacrimal fossa. Sometimes a smooth, firm osteoblastic process can be felt before it can be demonstrated by x rays. Bone invasion should be looked for in every case; it is of the utmost importance in the treatment and prognosis of the disease. X rays are, of course, helpful in detecting bone invasion, although it is not ruled out if the findings are negative. (See section Special Radiodiagnostic Studies of the Orbit, Including Computerized Tomography by Stephen L. Trokel, in Chapter 12.)

ADENOID CYSTIC CARCINOMA

Pain is a particularly prominent symptom of adenoid cystic carcinoma since the nerves are frequently involved. Exophthalmos appears later than in most expanding orbital lesions; it may be accompanied by papilledema and blurred vision when the lesion reaches the apex of the orbit and affects the optic nerve or deforms the globe.

DIFFERENTIAL DIAGNOSIS

All tumefactions arising in the lacrimal gland, or at least in the lacrimal fossa, are by no means neoplastic. Table 14–1 lists 115 expanding lesions, confirmed by microscopic sections, from consecutive cases seen at the Eye Institute prior to the last edition of this

FIG. 14–10. Growth of an untreated mixed tumor of the lacrimal gland. **A.** Seven years before the photograph was taken, the patient noted a pea-sized, hard nodule in the region of the right lacrimal gland. She refused surgery. **B.** Photograph taken ten years later. Rapid growth in the previous six years resulted in a large, heavy tumor that had to be supported with her hands. She again refused surgery, and died eight years later of nontumor-related disease. (Courtesy of F. B. Fralick.)

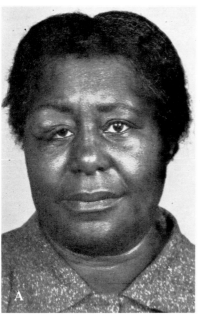
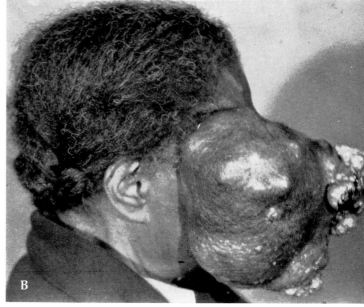

book. Clinically, the lesions were well demarcated, localized, firm masses palpable through the upper lid in the region of the lacrimal gland. They were closely associated with contiguous bone and it was sometimes difficult to demarcate the orbital margin and the lesions by palpation. Exophthalmos was not a prominent feature; ptosis and swelling or fullness of the upper lid were more often the presenting signs. To my knowledge, a correct clinical diagnosis can be made in these cases only by taking a biopsy.

A chronic dacryoadenitis or granuloma is the most common cause of an expanding lesion in the lacrimal gland fossa, a process similar to chronic granuloma of the orbit, often called a pseudotumor. The frequent occurrence of such a lesion confined to the region of the lacrimal gland is not generally appreciated. Dermoid cysts and other mass lesions in the area of the lacrimal gland fossa must be considered in the differential diagnosis. An amyloid tumor in the lacrimal gland has been reported.[32]

BENIGN LYMPHOEPITHELIAL LESION (BLL) (MIKULICZ'S DISEASE)

In the past Mikulicz's syndrome or disease has been loosely used for this type of adenopathy, but the term *benign lymphoepithelial lesion* (BLL) proposed for the lesion affecting the parotid gland[20] is now generally preferred.[27] Bilateral or unilateral enlargement of the lacrimal gland, with or without enlargement of one or more of the salivary glands, is often associated with Sjögren's syndrome—keratoconjunctivitis sicca, xerostomia, and rheumatoid arthritis.

The characteristic histologic picture shows a benign lymphoepithelial reaction involving particularly the glandular ducts.[13,27] According to one report, the histologic picture is characterized by replacement of acinar parenchyma by lymphoid tissue, and by intraductal proliferation of two cell elements—epithelial and myoepithelial—with formation of so-called epimyoepithelial islands,[29] which these authors considered the most dependable means of distinguishing true Mikulicz's disease from malignant lymphoma and other simulating processes. Four such cases were described, three of them unilateral, of which one also had orbital involvement producing proptosis.[28]

The close association of BLL with Sjögren's

syndrome has been demonstrated,[13] but it is also known to be associated at times with other systemic diseases such as leukemia, lymphoma, sarcoidosis, rheumatoid arthritis, macroglobulinemia, and collagen disease.

Sjögren[38] was prompted to consider the syndrome an autoimmune disease in view of the associated increase in gamma globulin. Hypergammaglobulinemia was found in patients with Sjögren's syndrome who had no rheumatoid arthropathy.[25]

Total fibrosis of the thyroid and both lacrimal glands was reported in a patient with Riedel's thyroiditis.[37]

As lacrimal gland disease may affect ectopic lacrimal glands outside the fossa, this possibility should be kept in mind for any tumor in the orbit.

TREATMENT AND PROGNOSIS

A review of the various expanding lesions of the lacrimal gland (Table 14–1) immediately suggests that treatment depends on the type of lesion. Approximately one-third of the expanding lesions in the lacrimal gland are nonneoplastic, and 38% of the neoplastic group are malignant lymphomas, presenting no sur-

TABLE 14–1. Incidence of Expanding Lesions of the Lacrimal Gland Based on 115 Consecutive Cases

Granuloma	31	(26%)
Nonspecific dacryoadenitis*	26	
Sarcoid	5	
Malignant Lymphoma	28	(25%)
Carcinoma†	27	(24%)
Mixed Tumor‡	25	(21%)
Dermoid Cyst§	2	(2%)
Adenoma¶	2	(2%)
Total	115	

* Some of these cases may represent Mikulicz's disease (see text).

† It seemed unnecessary for our purpose to break down the carcinoma group, e.g., adenoid cystic (cylindroma), mucoepidermoid, and those arising from mixed tumors. The adenoid cystic type was by far the most common.

‡ "Mixed tumor" refers to the so-called benign type; those with malignant cells were grouped with carcinomas.

§ Recent experience has shown a higher incidence of dermoid cysts in the lacrimal gland than is shown here. Such cysts cannot be differentiated clinically from the other lesions listed.

¶ Whether these are true adenomas instead of normal or ectopic lacrimal glands is a question.

gical problems after the diagnosis is established. Therefore only about half the lesions arising in the gland—50% of them benign cytologically and 50% malignant—require surgical removal.

In a study of 226 epithelial tumors of the lacrimal gland,[36,41] 58.6% were benign mixed tumors, 25% adenoid cystic carcinomas, 8.6% malignant mixed tumors, and 7.8% other carcinomas. The prognosis for benign mixed tumors was good, and for all malignant tumors very poor. Histopathologic examination may reveal a recurrent benign mixed tumor to be carcinomatous or sarcomatous, in which case the prognosis is poor.

The same histopathologic features were found in such tumors as had been reported in salivary gland tumors.[15] Of the 116 lacrimal gland tumors 33% were carcinomas, compared with 10% in the parotid glands. Lacrimal gland carcinomas can easily invade the adjacent bone of the lacrimal gland fossa, and the surgical approach is difficult. These factors, as well as the higher incidence of such tumors here than in the parotid gland, account for the poorer prognosis.

No local treatment is effective for chronic granuloma, which in any case usually has a regressive clinical course. However, local radiation may be beneficial if microscopy reveals extensive lymphocytic infiltration. Also, it must be kept in mind that granulomas are sometimes the forerunners of malignant lymphomas.

Exenteration is usually necessary for a patient with a carcinoma or a malignant mixed tumor; in most if not all instances the bony orbital wall of the lacrimal gland fossa and surrounding orbit should be resected even if no gross involvement can be seen, palpated, or demonstrated by x ray.

In the case of a benign mixed tumor, exposure at the time of operation should be adequate to permit inspection of contiguous bone and resection of any involved areas.

If a dermoid cyst or cholesteatoma is present, excision, or drainage with ablation, is indicated.

The diagnosis cannot be made short of a biopsy. Taking a biopsy from any encapsulated tumor with a malignant potential is to be discouraged as a general practice, since the tumor may grow and disseminate if the capsule is broken. However, it is absolutely necessary to determine the nature of an expanding lesion of the lacrimal gland before deciding on the ultimate treatment. Granuloma,

malignant lymphoma, epithelial tumor of the lacrimal gland, and dermoid cyst are all treated differently. Furthermore, the nature of the epithelial tumor determines the type of surgery: local excision with or without bone resection, or exenteration of the orbit with or without bone resection.

Attempts to use frozen sections of the biopsied tissue, with the idea of carrying out the indicated surgery immediately, have not proved satisfactory in my experience because the method does not permit a sufficiently accurate diagnosis.

For relatively small lesions confined to the area of the lacrimal gland, it is advisable to establish the diagnosis by an excisional biopsy. The histologic examination indicates whether further treatment is necessary. For lesions that are extensive, as revealed by palpation or by exophthalmos, biopsy tissue should be removed; again the histologic examination indicates whether further treatment is advisable. The biopsy must be taken with great care to avoid seeding tumor cells. The tissue wedge should extend deeply because normal lacrimal gland tissue is often displaced anteriorly by the lesion, with the risk of taking the biopsy from it rather than from the tumor itself. If there is a capsule it should be accurately and firmly resutured after biopsy. Extensive sectioning of lacrimal gland tumors is necessary to discover small areas of malignant change.[18]

Almost all tumors of the salivary glands have their counterparts in the lacrimal gland. The incidence of various types of salivary gland tumors in a series of 873 cases[14] appears in Table 14–2. All but acinar-cell adenocarcinoma, Warthin's tumor, and muco-

TABLE 14–2. Incidence of Salivary Gland Tumors*

Mixed tumor		63 %
Benign	56.5%	
Malignant	6.5%	
Mucoepidermoid		11 %
Adenocarcinoma		11 %
Adenoid cystic		
Acinar cell		
Miscellaneous		
Warthin's tumor (papillary cystadenoma		
lymphomatosum)		6 %
Squamous-cell carcinoma		4.5%
Unclassified (mostly malignant)		4.5%

* Based on Foote and Frazell's classification of 873 cases.[14]

epidermoid have been identified in the lacrimal gland. The incidence of epithelial tumors of the salivary glands and of the lacrimal gland is about the same except that the adenoid cystic (cylindroma) type of adenocarcinoma is more common in the lacrimal gland.

If all epithelial tumors of the salivary glands are grouped under the general heading of mixed tumors (as with tumors of the lacrimal gland in Table 14–1), it can be seen that approximately half are benign and half are malignant, comparable with the percentages for lacrimal gland tumors. Table 14–3 gives the incidence of epithelial tumors of the lacrimal gland based on our cases and on a comparable group reported in the literature.

In view of the similarities between salivary gland and lacrimal gland tumors, the difference in cure rate of the same type of lesion at the two sites is striking. The prognosis in cases of salivary gland tumors is good, but poor in cases of lacrimal gland tumors. No recurrence was reported in 96% of patients with mixed tumors of the salivary glands from 5 to 15 years postoperatively, and no recurrence in 25%–30% of patients with carcinoma of these glands followed 5 or more years.[14] In marked contrast, a review of our own and other cases revealed that only 50% of patients with mixed tumor of the lacrimal gland were living free of disease 5 or more years postoperatively. One patient with carcinoma had a recurrence in the bone 5 years after exenteration. He was treated by radical bone resection and was alive and well 9 years later.

Follow-up information was obtained on 10 of 25 patients with mixed tumors of the lacrimal gland from files of the Registry of Ophthalmic Pathology of the Armed Forces Institute of Pathology.[16] Recurrence in 9 of them had necessitated a second operation within 1 to 6 years after the first.

Statistics on 80 patients with epithelial tumors of the lacrimal gland, from the files of the same registry, appear in Table 14–4.[40]

Of 13 patients with mixed tumor of the lacrimal gland, all 5 who could be followed for 5 years or more had died; of the 8 followed for shorter periods, 2 had recurrences.[2]

There seems to be evidence that when a benign tumor recurs its power to grow and to infiltrate surrounding structures is considerably enhanced. After each incomplete excision the tumor becomes more locally destructive, more invasive, and more likely to metastasize, resulting in frank carcinoma that proves fatal.

The tumor has recurred as long as 22 years after surgery.[12] In one of our cases there was a recurrence 22 months after removal of a well-encapsulated tumor. An attempt at removal failed, because of the tumor's infiltrative and diffuse nature. The tumor receded after x-ray therapy, and had not recurred after 16 years.

Treatment of these patients seems inadequate for a number of reasons:

1. *Incorrect diagnosis.* When treatment is attempted the precise diagnosis is often not known.

2. *Failure to consider the tumor's characteristics when deciding on the surgical approach.* Epithelial tumors of the lacrimal gland (both mixed and carcinomatous) have five characteristics that bear on the choice of surgical procedure:

a. A tendency to invade or extend through the capsule, in which case the capsule should be removed with the tumor.

b. A tendency to seed, against which every precaution should be taken. The primary mixed tumors in the aforementioned large series of salivary gland tumors were al-

TABLE 14–3. Composite Group of Lacrimal Gland Tumors*

Benign mixed tumor		43%
Malignant mixed tumor		4%
Other carcinomas		53%
Adenoid cystic	38%	
Miscellaneous	15%	

* Based on our cases and those in the literature.

TABLE 14–4. Prognosis in Epithelial Tumors of the Lacrimal Gland*

Follow-up status	Total	Benign mixed	Malignant mixed	Carcinoma
Living and well	16	12	3	1
Living (with history of recurrence)	10	4	3	3
Dead from tumor	17	0	2	15
Indeterminate	37	23	5	9
Total	80	39	13	28

* From Zimmerman LE[40]

ways unilobular;[14] however, recurrent manifestations were always multilobular, with discrete nodules sometimes widely separated. This multilobular characteristic of recurrent tumors is attributed to seeding.

c. A tendency to invade bone, which should be resected where specifically indicated and routinely in firmly established cases of adenoid cystic carcinoma (Fig. 14–11).

d. A tendency of carcinomas, particularly the adenoid cystic type, to extend along nerves. The supraorbital nerve, which is usually included in exenteration, should be removed up to its exit from the orbit.

e. A tendency of benign and malignant mixed tumors to develop diffuse foci which may be missed during surgery. The need for thorough examination of exenterated specimens for residual tumor cells at the surgically cut surfaces has been emphasized.[17] Application of India ink to these surfaces facilitates microscopic differentiation from subsequent laboratory cut surfaces. If residual tumor tissue is identified, further surgery carried out immediately holds more hope for a cure than the alternate policy of watchful waiting for possible recurrence of the tumor.[18]

3. *Inadequate surgical exposure.* The direct approach through a skin incision parallel to the orbital margin over the area of the lacrimal gland gives an unsatisfactory exposure. In the fossa, lying back of an overhanging bony margin, an expanding lesion apparently exerts tension on the orbital septum, producing an exostosis of this overhanging margin which makes the fossa even more inaccessible. The Krönlein operation alone does not suffice, and the transcranial approach is not feasible because only a small portion of the involved area lies adjacent to the anterior cranial fossa. I prefer the Benedict approach through the upper lid with reflection of the periosteum, but even this does not give the necessary exposure.

A technique that has merit is as follows (Fig. 14–12):

The usual Krönlein incision is made, and a second incision extending from under the brow following the curve of the bony orbital margin and joining the original horizontal incision at a point beyond the external canthus. The skin and fascia are dissected back to expose the entire lateral wall of the orbit, particularly the upper outer portion over the

lacrimal gland. Dissection of the lid to expose the upper margin of the orbit must be kept in the plane of the levator muscle. The periosteum is incised along the outer orbital margin. With an elevator, the periosteum is reflected away from the bone along with the lesion in the lacrimal gland. The lateral wall of the orbit is resected with an oscillating Stryker saw according to the usual Krönlein technique. The lesion is then excised with its adjacent periosteum. The operation can be done without causing ptosis.

Figure 14–13 shows the overhanging bony margin of the fossa which must be rongeured to provide access to the gland.

An anteriorly localized orbital lesion which lies apposed to the periosteum can be satisfactorily excised by the following method,[3]

FIG. 14–11. Resected specimen of the lacrimal gland fossa after removal of a mixed tumor that had invaded bone. The invasion, determined by direct inspection, was not detected by palpation or x-ray examination. **A.** Inner surface of orbit: (*a*) bone invasion, (*b*) superior orbital margin, (*c*) nasal margin, (*d*) temporal margin. **B.** Oblique view of above specimen: (*a*) bone invasion, (*b*) superior orbital margin, (*c*) anterior cranial fossa, (*d*) nasal margin, (*e*) temporal margin.

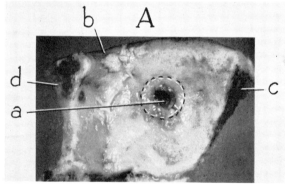

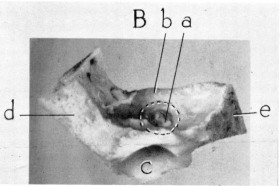

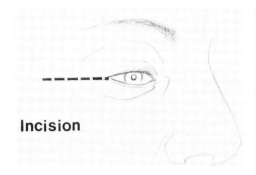

Incision

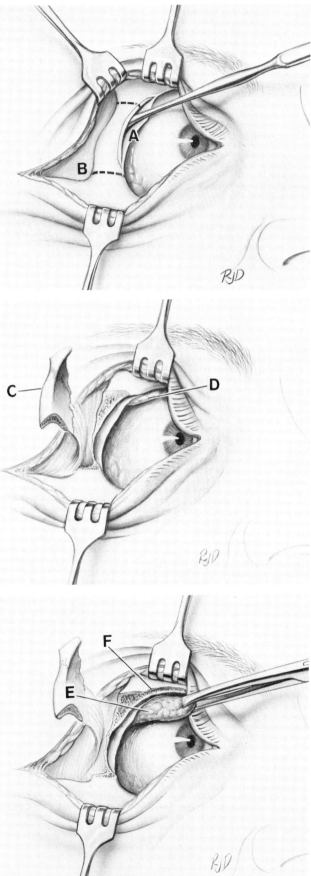

FIG. 14–12. Excision of a lacrimal gland tumor. *Step 1.* Top left, the longitudinal skin incision from the external canthus. The periosteum (*A*) is incised along the external orbital margin and reflected from the bone with a spatula. The dotted lines show where two horizontal incisions are to be made in the external wall of the bony orbit. The fascia of the temporalis muscle is shown at *B. Step 2.* After the two horizontal bone incisions have been made with the oscillating saw, the lateral wall of the bony orbit (*C*) is reflected, hinged to the temporalis muscle. The lacrimal gland is seen at *D.* The overhanging edge of the orbital margin is removed by rongeurs (see Fig. 14–13). The proximity of the foramen of the supraorbital nerve is indicated, as it might be inadvertently included in the area of rongeured bone. *Step 3.* The lacrimal gland is delivered by fixation forceps (*E*). The rongeured orbital margin is indicated at *F.*

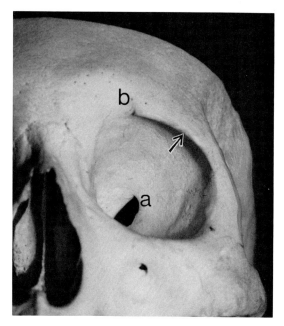

FIG. 14–13. Orbit showing lacrimal gland fossa. Arrow indicates the overhanging bony margin of the fossa which must be rongeured to make the lacrimal gland accessible. The superior orbital fissure is seen at *a* and the bony notch for the superior orbital nerve at *b*.

FIG. 14–14. Extent of bone resection for epithelial tumors of the lacrimal gland. *Step 1.* Bone resection is begun by two cuts through the lateral wall (*E*) with the oscillating saw, as in the Krönlein operation; (*A*) the optic foramen, (*B*) the superior orbital fissure, (*C*) the inferior orbital fissure, (*D*) the inferior orbital canal and foramen. *Step 2.* The bone flap is broken and removed. The remaining lateral wall is rongeured as far back as possible. *Step 3.* A cut by the oscillating saw parallel to the orbital rim continues the bone resection to the midpoint of the superior rim. If a full-thickness bone resection of the lacrimal gland fossa is indicated, a small exposure of the dura in the anterior cranial fossa is necessary (Fig. 14–11). *Step 4.* The plate of bone cortex of the lacrimal gland fossa is removed. The broken posterior edge is removed with rongeurs to the extent necessary. *Step 5.* Bone resection is continued below by outlining the adjacent inferolateral wall with two cuts of the Stryker saw. *Step 6.* Removal of the remaining bone to the end of the inferior orbital fissure completes the resection.

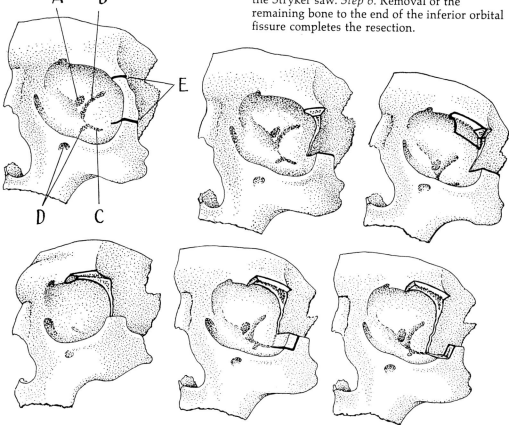

often suitable for tumors in the lacrimal fossa: The skin incision follows the curve of the bony orbital margin. The periosteum is exposed and incised in a similar manner. Both the tough periosteum and the lesion are resected from the bone, delivered anteriorly by blunt and sharp dissection, and then excised. The advantage of this method is that traction through the periosteum facilitates resection and delivery of deep tumors that would otherwise be difficult to remove.

When an excisional biopsy is done on a lesion confined essentially to the area of the lacrimal gland, the extra incision from under the brow to join the horizontal incision may not be necessary; more exposure may be obtained by dissecting the upper lid away from the area around the fossa. Also, it may not be necessary to resect the lateral wall of the orbit when the lesion is small. Traction on the tough periosteum which has been reflected with the lesion is a great help in dissecting and delivering the tumor.

Although removing the contents of the lacrimal gland fossa sometimes leads to keratitis sicca, this complication is rare, due no doubt to the adequate areas of supplemental lacrimal gland tissue.

When exenteration is indicated for carcinoma, the bony orbital wall in and around the lacrimal gland fossa is usually resected, as described previously, even though no gross involvement can be seen or demonstrated by x rays. When the orbital wall is resected, it must be remembered that the anterior cranial cavity is just posterior to the lacrimal gland fossa, so that the dura may be exposed. The frontal sinus is not usually encountered if the bone resection is confined to the outer third of the superior orbital wall. It is well to take x rays preoperatively, to establish the extent of the frontal sinus.

If the bone is involved beyond the region of the lacrimal gland fossa—a particularly likely complication in recurrent disease—a more extensive resection may be necessary.

The prognosis is not hopeless in cases of bone invasion by an epithelial tumor of the lacrimal gland if sufficient resection is carried out while the tumor is still in expendable bone. This type of invasion may be noted either primarily or with a recurrence, and still the patient can be cured by adequate surgery. Four of our patients with mixed tumors of the lacrimal gland invading bone were alive and well four to nine years after orbital exenteration and bone resection. Bone invasion was noted at the time of the original surgery in three patients and in one at the time of a recurrence. In two patients the original tumor seemed to arise in an ectopic lacrimal gland palpable either just above or just below the external canthus. When the tumor arose in an ectopic lacrimal gland, no mass was palpable in the region of the lacrimal gland either before or during surgery.[33]

Steps for resection of the bone are outlined in Figure 14–14.

An operative approach via a frontal flap, with removal of the entire orbital roof to the frontal sinus anteriorly and to the ethmoid sinuses medially, has been suggested.[31] At the posterolateral portion of the orbit beneath the anterior part of the temporalis muscle, the bone should be removed up to the orbital rim and back to the orbital fissure.

We have found that radiotherapy usually does not effect a cure of epithelial tumors of the lacrimal gland. However, it sometimes alleviates pain and results in a palliative regression in cases of extensive bone involvement, where no other form of treatment is availing.

REFERENCES

1. BECH K, JENSEN OA: Mixed tumor of the lower orbital region. Arch Ophthalmol 74:226–228, 1965
2. BENEDICT WL: Discussion in Sanders TE (ref 35)
3. BENEDICT WL: Surgical treatment of tumors and cysts of the orbit. Am J Ophthalmol 32:763–773, 1949
4. BÖCK J, FEYRTER F: Über die benignen epithelialen Geschwülste der menschlichen Orbita. III. Zur Frage des orbitalen Mukoepidermoidtumors. Doc Ophthalmol 15:351–370, 1961

5. BOUDET C, BERTEZÈNE M: Exophtalmie par adénome lacrymal en position ectopique (angiographie de l'orbite). Bull Soc Ophtalmol Fr 64:624–627, 1964
6. BRACCIOLINE MR: Aberrant lacrimal gland associated with dermoid of the outer canthus and other malformations. Minerva Oftalmol 9:116–119, 1967
7. BRAUN-VALLON S: Une curieuse anomalie du muscle droit externe. Bull Soc Fr Ophtalmol 4:212–215, 1955

8. BRUCE GM: Aberrant glandular tissue in the iris. Trans Am Acad Ophthalmol Otolaryngol 56:47–51, 1952

9. CHENG PH: Pleomorphic adenoma of lid. Chin Med J 83: 49–51, 1964

10. CHRISTENSEN L, ANDERSON ED: Aberrant intraocular adenomata and epithelization of the anterior chamber. Arch Ophthalmol 48:19–29, 1952

11. DALLACHY R: Ectopic lacrimal glandular tissue within the eyeball. Br J Ophthalmol 45:808–815, 1961

12. DiMARZIO Q: Tumori dell'orbita; cilindroma della ghiandola lacrimale. Riv Otoneurooftalmol 14:65, 1937

13. FONT RL, YANOFF M, ZIMMERMAN LE: Benign lymphoepithelial lesion of the lacrimal gland and its relationship to Sjögren's syndrome. Am J Clin Pathol 48:365–376, 1967

14. FOOTE FW, FRAZELL EL: Tumors of the major salivary glands. Cancer 6:1065–1138, 1953

15. FOOTE FW, FRAZELL EL: Tumors of the major salivary glands. In Atlas of Tumor Pathology. Armed Forces Institute of Pathology, Section IV, Fascicle II, Washington DC, 1954

16. FORREST AW: Intraorbital tumors. Arch Ophthalmol 41:198–232, 1949

17. FORREST AW: Epithelial lacrimal gland tumors. Trans Am Acad Ophthalmol Otolaryngol 58:848–866, 1954

18. FORREST AW: Pathologic criteria for effective management of epithelial lacrimal gland tumors. Am J Ophthalmol 71:178–192, 1971

19. FREYDINGER JE, DUHIG JT: Carcinoma of accessory lacrimal gland. Arch Pathol 77:643–645, 1964

20. GODWIN JT: Benign lymphoepithelial lesion of the parotid gland (adenolymphoma, chronic inflammation, lymphoepithelioma, lymphocytic tumor. Mikulicz disease); report of 11 cases. Cancer 5:1089–1103, 1952

21. GÖRDÜREN S: Aberrant lacrimal gland associated with other congenital abnormalities. Br J Ophthalmol 46:277–280, 1962

22. GREEN WR, ZIMMERMAN LE: Ectopic lacrimal gland tissue; report of eight cases with orbital involvement. Arch Ophthalmol 78:318–327, 1967

23. HUNTER WS: Aberrant intra-ocular lacrimal gland tissue. Br J Ophthalmol 44:619–625, 1960

24. KESSING SV: Ectopic lacrimal gland tissue at the corneal limbus (gland of Manz). Acta Ophthalmol (Kbh) 46:398–403, 1968

25. McLENACHAN J: New aspects of the aetiology of Sjögren's syndrome. Trans Ophthalmol Soc UK 76:413–426, 1956

26. METTIER SR JR: Aberrant lacrimal gland. Arch Ophthalmol 60:488–490, 1958

27. MEYER D, YANOFF M, HANNO H: Differential diagnosis in Mikulicz's syndrome, Mikulicz's disease, and similar disease entities. Am J Ophthalmol 71:516–524, 1971

28. MILAM DF JR: Mikulicz's disease of the lacrimal gland. Arch Ophthalmol 57:236–240, 1957

29. MORGAN WS, CASTLEMAN B: A clinicopathologic study of Mikulicz's disease. Am J Pathol 29:471–503, 1953

30. MURPHY MB, RODRIGUES MM: Benign mixed tumor of the (palpebral) lacrimal gland presenting as a nodular eyelid lesion. Am J Ophthalmol 77:108–111, 1974

31. NAFFZIGER HC: Discussion of Sanders TE (ref 35)

32. RADNÓT M, LAPIS K, FEHÉR J: Amyloid tumor in the lacrymal gland. Ann Ophthalmol 3:727–742, 1971

33. REESE AB, JONES IS: Bone resection in the excision of epithelial tumors of the lacrimal gland. Arch Ophthalmol 71:382–385, 1964

34. REIXACH-GRANES R, BECKER PF: Malignant mixed tumor of lacrimal gland; clinicosurgical and histopathologic study. Hospital 69:603–614, 1967

35. SANDERS TE: Mixed tumor of the lacrimal gland. Arch Ophthalmol 21:239–260, 1939

36. SANDERS TE, ACKERMAN LV, ZIMMERMAN LE: Epithelial tumors of the lacrimal gland; a comparison of the pathologic and clinical behavior with those of the salivary glands. Am J Surg 104:657–665, 1962

37. SCLARE G. LUXTON RW: Fibrosis of the thyroid and lacrimal glands. Br J Ophthalmol 51:173–177, 1967

38. SJÖGREN H: Some new investigations concerning the sicca-syndrome. Acta Ophthalmol (Kbh) 39:619–622, 1961

39. SOMMER G: Beitrag zur Ektopie der Tränendrüse. Klin Monatsbl Augenheilkd 130:415–417, 1958

40. ZIMMERMAN LE: Discussion of Spaeth EB: Tumors of the lacrimal gland. Trans Am Acad Ophthalmol Otolaryngol 63:739–751, 1959

41. ZIMMERMAN LE, SANDERS TE, ACKERMAN LV: Epithelial tumors of the lacrimal gland; prognostic and therapeutic significance of histologic types. In Tumors of the Eye and Adnexa. International Ophthalmology Clinics. Boston, Little, Brown & Co., 1962, pp 337–367

15

HAMARTOMAS, PROGONOMAS, CHORISTOMAS, MISCELLANEOUS TUMORS AND TUMEFACTIONS

Three terms have been adopted with increasing frequency in our oncology literature: *choristoma, hamartoma,* and *progonoma.* The custom of classifying tumors in these three general groups has its shortcomings because of considerable overlapping. For example, a choristoma may also be a hamartoma or a progonoma.

Choristoma refers to normal tissue at an abnormal site, *e.g.,* dermoid cyst, osteoma, chondroma, teratoid tumor, and aberrant lacrimal gland. *Hamartoma* refers to faulty embryonal development in size or pattern in an area for which it would otherwise be normal, *e.g.,* primary hyperplastic vitreous, angiomas, and fibrous masses at the disc stemming from remains of the hyaloid system and Bergmeister's papilla. *Progonoma* refers to a mass resulting from atavistic remains, it is not normal in the life history of the organism of a particular species but has occurred in an ancestral member; examples are nictitating membrane, remains of the subcutaneous pigment system seen in man as a blue nevus, nevus of Ota or Ito, mongolian spot, and skin nevus.

The following entities will be considered here: dermoid cyst, dermoid tumor, dermolipoma, mesenchymoma, teratoma and teratoid tumor, cysts of the iris and ciliary body, pilomatrixoma, and phakomatous choristoma.

DERMOID CYST

A dermoid cyst (epidermoid cyst, oil cyst, or cholesteatoma) arises from a congenital rest of primitive ectoderm at the site of closure of a fetal cleft. A dermoid tumor whose surface is covered with abnormal epidermis and its glandular appendages should be distinguished from a dermoid cyst whose epidermis is invaginated.

Microscopically, the cyst wall is composed of an inner epidermal layer and an outer connective tissue layer, corresponding to the dermis, in which sebaceous glands, hair follicles, fat, smooth muscle, and elastic fibers may be found. The epidermal layer varies in thickness: a single layer of cells or all layers found in the epidermis. The retained sebaceous material may give rise to a foreign-body inflammatory reaction in the cyst wall, manifested by macrophages and giant cells lining a portion of the wall and sometimes even replacing the epithelium.

Division of these cysts into dermoid and epidermoid types seems to be largely academic. The epidermoids are derived largely from ectodermal tissue, while dermoids also have derivatives of mesodermal tissue. Both are primarily epithelial lesions developing from aberrant inclusions and causing either an epidermoid cyst, when epidermoid tissue is included, or a dermoid cyst, when the deeper dermal layer is also involved. Inasmuch as there are transitional types as well, the differentiation is of little importance.

The simpler type, the epidermoid cyst, may have few or no skin appendages such as hair follicles and sebaceous glands, and it is sometimes confused with a sebaceous cyst. It often has merely an epithelial layer surrounding a solid mass of desquamated epithelial products arranged in homogeneous and at times concentric layers containing numerous cholesterol crystals. For this reason the lesion has sometimes been referred to as a cholesteatoma.

An epidermoid cyst of the iris and ciliary body arises from a congenital rest of primitive ectoderm at the closure site of a fetal cleft. I have reported such a cyst in a 2½-year-old girl who had had from birth a small tumor in the anterior chamber at 6 o'clock. Because the mass was increasing in size and might be a diktyoma, excision was advised. A corneoscleroiridectomy was performed, with a corneal transplant to cover the resulting defect.

Microscopic examination of the excised specimen confirmed the diagnosis of an epidermoid cyst of the iris and ciliary body, which contained flakes of keratin. In a two-year follow-up the eye was in good condition.

The Armed Forces Institute of Pathology had three similar cases.[29]

Dermoid cysts contain a brown oily fluid, often with cholesterol crystals, masses of yellowish debris, and at times hairs that may protrude from the cyst wall. The oily substance comes from the sebaceous glands; its brown color is due to the hemosiderin secondary to hemorrhage, probably the result of inflammation from the cyst's toxic contents.

A 23-year-old man had noted swelling and ptosis of the left eyelid for eight years, with recent exacerbation. A cystic tumor was removed. Sections showed the wall of a dermoid cyst surrounded by extensive areas of fat necrosis and a lipogranulomatous reaction.[29]

The cyst may be in the brow, the lids, or the orbit; it may extend from the orbit to the cranium, the sinuses, or the temporal fossa. Conversely, a dermoid cyst primarily of the cranium may also involve the orbit.

Dermoid cysts of the orbit tend to occur along the bone suture lines; the extent of these cysts is often much greater than is suggested by either the clinical appearance or the radiologic findings.[8] When the cranial cavity is involved, the lesion is in the province of the neurosurgeon.

Dermoid cysts are soft, vary greatly in size, and may be oval, round, or hourglass in shape. They are not usually associated with other congenital anomalies.

Even though the cyst is congenital, it sometimes does not become sufficiently large to be detected until about the third decade of life. Expansion may then result in pressure not only on the contiguous bone but also on the eyeball. The growth usually becomes stationary at some period.

A dermoid or an epidermoid cyst may arise in the diploë of the skull or orbital bones; as it grows, both the inner and outer bony tables are expanded, resulting in characteristic bone defects.

The frontal bone was involved in seven of nine patients with dermoids of the orbit described in one report.[20] The growth in six of the seven apparently arose in the diploë of the bone forming the orbital roof. In two there was a through-and-through defect so that pulsation of the dura was observed at operation. One patient had an hourglass lesion with portions in both the frontal fossa and the orbit. In two of the nine patients, the growth was on the lateral wall of the orbit or the greater wing of the sphenoid.

Although a mucocele or retention cyst of the frontal sinus must be considered in the differential diagnosis (Ch. 17), it can be readily recognized by its connection with the sinus, cloudiness of the sinus itself, and absence of dermoid characteristics. Other conditions that may suggest a dermoid are xanthogranuloma or eosinophilic granuloma of bone, invasion of bone by a malignant tumor, meningioma of the sphenoid ridge, meningocele, nodular fasciitis, and rhabdomyosarcoma.

When a dermoid cyst is incompletely excised, the remaining epithelium may become necrotic and act as a foreign body, appearing clinically as a recurrence.

TREATMENT

A dermoid cyst located superficially around the orbital margin and attached to the bone can be excised through a skin incision directly over the lesion. This method is suitable for small cysts often seen on the brow and confused with sebaceous cysts. A dermoid cyst of the iris and ciliary body may be treated by a corneal graft and iridectomy (Fig. 15–1). However, the Krönlein operation is indicated for a deep cyst arising from the diploë of bone. If the entire cyst cannot be removed, part of the remaining wall should be cauterized with carbolic acid and neutralized with alcohol. Following this, all or as much as possible of the eschar should be excised. In two of the nine aforementioned cases[20] the anterior cranial fossa was involved, calling for the service of a neurosurgeon. In six of these cases a direct approach through the margin of the orbit over the presenting mass was adequate. The bone was followed back to the lesion, which was incised and evacuated. The interior of the cyst wall was swabbed with carbolic acid, then neutralized with alcohol and irrigated with saline solution. The charred cyst wall was excised; the wound was closed tightly, and a pressure dressing applied.

DERMOID TUMOR

Dermoid tumors are congenital and occur primarily at the limbus (Fig. 15–2A). They are localized, elevated, white masses situated partly over the cornea and partly over the sclera. Hairs are usually noted over the keratinized surface (Fig. 15–2B), and in some in-

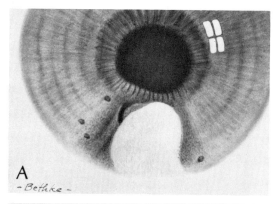

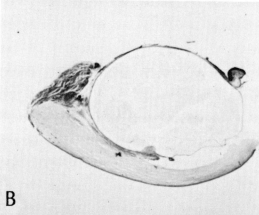

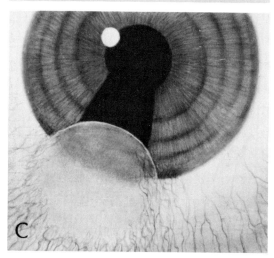

FIG. 15–1. Dermoid cyst of the iris and ciliary body. **A.** Preoperative appearance. **B.** Excised cyst with adjacent cornea, iris, and ciliary body. **C.** Corneal graft and iridectomy.

stances there is evidence of secretion from the glandular appendages of epidermis. In rare cases multiple or even bilateral tumors have been reported.[12] A limbal dermoid tumor with intraocular extension has been described.[24]

Histologic examination reveals dense, collagenous connective tissue covered by epidermis which is stratified and contains a granular layer with keratin on the surface. Hair follicles and sebaceous glands extend into the underlying tissue. Nerve bundles and sweat glands are occasionally noted.

The tissue derivatives in these tumors vary considerably. I have seen bone and lacrimal gland tissue in one case of limbal dermoid tumor, cartilage and lacrimal gland tissue in another (Fig. 15–3), and various mesodermal elements along with ectodermal elements forming abortive lacrimal gland tissue in still another. In some instances the sclera or cornea under the tumor may be thin or absent.

In one reported case, ectopic brain tissue was found in a limbal dermoid associated with a scleral staphyloma.[16] In another case a congenital dermoid tumor with surface hairs and containing bone was located over the lateral rectus muscle.[10]

The lesion may interfere with vision in several ways, *e.g.*, by producing astigmatism or extending to the pupillary area. The extension may be progressive after trauma or irritation, particularly at the time of puberty. Lipid infiltration of the cornea adjacent to the tumor site in some cases simulates an arcus senilis concentric to the tumor base, which tends to progress as long as the tumor is present. Over a period of years corneal opacification reduced the vision from 20/30 to 20/100 in one case and from 20/40 to 20/200 in another.[27]

Goldenhar's Syndrome

A limbal dermoid is sometimes associated with a preauricular tumor, with microphthalmos[12,21,23] and scleral ectasia. Goldenhar in 1952 first described the syndrome that bears his name: epibulbar dermoids, preauricular appendages, and pretragal fistulas present from birth. Vertebral anomalies were later recognized, and the condition was called oculoauriculovertebral dysplasia.[14] The syndrome has been attributed to faulty differentiation of the first and second branchial arches.[9]

In one series of 13 cases of Goldenhar's

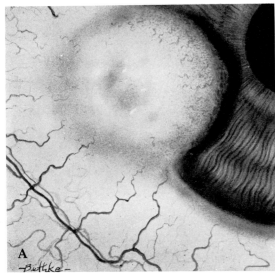

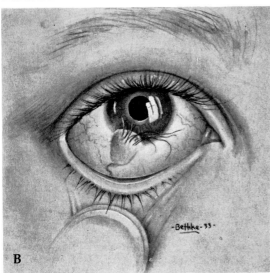

FIG. 15–2. Dermoid tumor of the limbus.
A. Lesion without hair. B. Lesion with hair.
(Courtesy of J. H. Dunnington.)

FIG. 15–3. Teratoid or mixed tumor of the
limbus. A round mass 8 mm in diameter
straddling the limbus had been present since
birth in an 8-year-old boy. The tumor showed
neovascularization, and some nutrient vessels
were coursing to the site. Opposite this site, a
yellowish opacity with a clear margin between
the corneal lesion and the tumor was interpreted
as a secondary degenerative arcus in the adjacent
cornea. A. Clinical appearance. B. Microscopic
section shows (a) normal-appearing lacrimal
gland tissue with cysts of the accompanying
ducts; (b) an area of cartilage; (c) epidermaliza-
tion of the conjunctiva; and (d) lymphocytic foci
commonly seen in congenital aberrations.
(Courtesy of the Armed Forces Institute of
Pathology.)

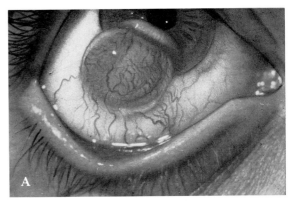

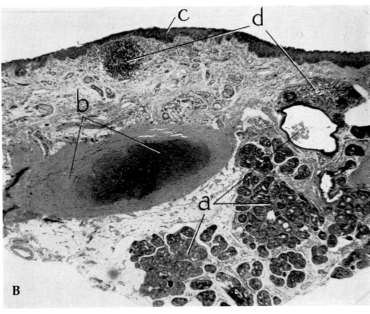

syndrome with ocular involvement,[3] preauricular appendages were found in all the patients, unilateral auricular involvement in 70%, hearing loss in 54%, and vertebral anomalies in 62% These authors also reviewed 114 cases from the literature. Of the total of 127 patients, 78% had epibulbar dermoids, 47% had lipodermoids, and 24% had colobomas of the upper lid. Other cases have been reported.[4,18] One unusual case was characterized by conductive deafness and facial hemiatrophy,[25] and another by hemifacial microsomia and decreased corneal sensation which led to intractable corneal ulceration.[26]

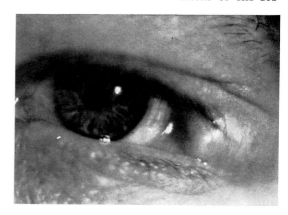

FIG. 15–4. Dermolipoma at the external canthus.

TREATMENT

Dermoid tumors should be excised by a superficial lamellar keratectomy with a lamellar graft over the site of the lesion to prevent scar formation on the cornea. Since the sclera or cornea may be thin or almost absent over the base of the dermoid, care must be taken to avoid perforating these structures during dissection.

DERMOLIPOMA

A dermolipoma is a congenital lesion occurring in and under the bulbar conjunctiva at the external canthus (Fig. 15–4). It is not usually noticeable with the eyes in the primary position but is apparent when the involved eye is adducted. It appears as a fatty herniation covered by a thick epidermal epithelium that may contain hairs and evidences of glandular appendages with their secretions. The tumor is harmless and does not tend to progress, although surgical excision may be required for cosmetic reasons. Excision should include the overlying epithelium consisting of thick keratinized epidermis with hairs and glands.

MESENCHYMOMA

The term *mesenchymoma* was proposed for benign and malignant tumors composed of two or more elements derived from the mesenchyme. Such tumors affect both children and adults.[19] Of 42 cases of malignant mesenchymoma, 2 involved the orbit. One of the 2 showed rhabdomyoma, leiomyosarcoma and undifferentiated tissue, and the other showed chondrosarcoma and undifferentiated tissue. A mesenchymoma of the orbit may also harbor vascular (hemangiopericytoma) and chondroblastic tissue.[22] In another case, a malignant mesenchymoma of the orbit was composed of rhabdomyosarcoma and liposarcoma.[28]

OTHER CONGENITAL TUMORS

Hamartomas and related tumors that represent congenital rests of pluripotential tissue are variously referred to as choristomas, mixed tumors, teratomas, teratoid tumors (Fig. 15–3), and mesotheliomas. Tissues derived from these mesodermal and ectodermal rests vary tremendously. These tumors may be seen at the limbus, on the cornea, at the internal canthus, in the eyelids, in the orbit, and at the base of the nose.

PHAKOMATOUS CHORISTOMA OF THE EYELID

A previously unrecognized benign tumor of the lower lid has been described.[30] The author named the lesion *phakomatous choristoma* because it obviously stems from a lenticular anlage, and reported three cases, all in infants. In another case[11] the tumor noted at birth enlarged within five months and was removed. It was attached to palpebral conjunctiva of the lower fornix and to fascia surrounding the lacrimal sac, extending along the inferomedial border of the orbital floor (Fig. 15–5).

PILOMATRIXOMA

A hard, localized benign tumor originating in hair structures (pilomatrixoma or benign calcifying epithelioma of Malherbe) occurs on the eyebrow, on the lids, and in the orbit.[1,7] It is now generally considered to be derived from a sebaceous gland anlage.

Among 35 cases coded at the Armed Forces Institute of Pathology as aberrant or ectopic lacrimal gland which were reexamined, the authors reported 2 cases associated with hamartomatous malformations in the posterior portion of the orbit.[15]

TERATOMA

Teratomas of the orbit, with or without exophthalmos, are usually noted at birth. Tumor sections show a great variety of tissue including fat, bone, cartilage, and many cysts lined with epithelium in different forms. The epithelium may be squamous with hair follicles, sebaceous and sweat glands; ciliated; or mucous with papillary structures similar to those in the intestinal tract.[17] A malignant ovarian teratoma was found to contain a well-formed optic cup, the inner wall of which showed almost normal development of a 14 mm embryonal retina.[5] In the most spectacular cases, the teratomas contain various fetal structures including hands and legs or abortive organs. An orbital teratoma simulating an orbital encephalocele was successfully excised without sacrifice of the eye.[13] Another orbital teratoma noted at birth was removed through a Krönlein exposure, leaving the globe and optic nerve in place.[2] A teratoma of the orbit half as large as the infant's head has been described.[6]

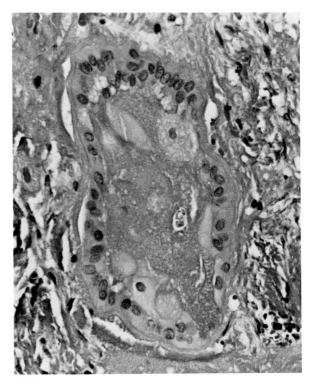

FIG. 15–5. Phakomatous choristoma of the eyelid. This lenticular anlage shows all the lens elements: a rudimentary hyalin capsule and subcapsular epithelium surrounding cortical lens matter. (Filipic M, Silva M: Arch Ophthalmol 88:172–175, 1972, copyright 1966–72, American Medical Association)

REFERENCES

1. ASHTON N: Benign calcified epithelioma of eyelid. Trans Ophthalmol Soc UK 71:301–307, 1951
2. BARBER JC, BARBER LF, GUERRY D III, GEERAETS WJ: Congenital orbital teratoma. Arch Ophthalmol 91:45–48, 1974
3. BAUM JL, FEINGOLD M: Ocular aspects of Goldenhar's syndrome. Am J Ophthalmol 75:250–257, 1973
4. BOWEN DI, COLLUM LMT, REES DO: Clinical aspects of oculo-auriculo-vertebral dysplasia. Br J Ophthalmol 55:145–154, 1971
5. BREININ GM: The eye in teratomas. Arch Ophthalmol 43:482–499, 1950

6. CASANOVAS R: Congenital teratoma of the orbit. Arch Ophthalmol 77:795–797, 1967
7. CHARLIN C: Pilomatrixoma cilio-palpebral (epitelioma benigno calcificado de Malherbe). Arc Soc Esp Oftalmol 33:753–764, 1973
8. CULLEN JF: Orbital diploic dermoids. Br J Ophthalmol 58:105–106, 1974
9. FEINGOLD M, GELLIS SS: Ocular abnormalities associated with the first and second arch syndromes. Survey Ophthalmol 14:30–42, 1969
10. FERRY AP, HEIN HF: Epibulbar osseous choristoma within an epibulbar dermoid. Am J Ophthalmol 70:764–766, 1970

11. FILIPIC M, SILVA M: Phakomatous choristoma of the eyelid; a tumor of lenticular anlage. Arch Ophthalmol 88:172–175, 1972

12. GARNER LL: Dermoid of the limbus involving the iris angle and lens. Arch Ophthalmol 46:69–72, 1951

13. GIRARD LJ, FOUNTAIN EM, MOORE CM, THOMAS JR: Teratoma of the orbit. Trans Am Acad Ophthalmol Otolaryngol 62:226–233, 1958

14. GORLIN RJ, JUE KL, JACOBSEN U, GOLDSCHMIDT E: Oculoauriculovertebral dysplasia. J Pediat 63:991–999, 1963

15. GREEN WR, ZIMMERMAN LE: Ectopic lacrimal gland tissue; report of eight cases with orbital involvement. Arch Ophthalmol 78:318–327, 1967

16. HUTCHISON DS, GREEN WR, ILIFF CE: Ectopic brain tissue in a limbal dermoid associated with a scleral staphyloma. Am J Ophthalmol 76:984–986, 1973

17. JENSEN OA: Teratoma of the orbit. Acta Ophthalmol (Kbh) 47:317–327 (Fasc 2), 1969

18. MORTADA A: Orbital dermo-lipoma with Goldenhar's syndrome and exophthalmos. Br J Ophthalmol 53:786–788, 1969

19. NASH A, STOUT AP: Malignant mesenchymomas in children. Cancer 14:524–533, 1961

20. PFEIFFER RL, NICHOLL RJ: Dermoids and epidermoids of the orbit. Trans Am Ophthalmol Soc 46:218–243, 1948

21. RAIFORD M, DIXON JM: Cystic dermoid tumor replacing the anterior segment of the eye with microphthalmos. Am J Ophthalmol 36:508–510, 1953

22. REEH MJ: Hemangiopericytoma with cartilaginous differentiation involving orbit. Arch Ophthalmol 75:82–83, 1966

23. SCHULTZ GR, WENDLER PF, WESELEY AC: Ocular dermoids and auricular appendages. Am J Ophthalmol 63:938–941, 1967

24. SCHULZE RR: Limbal dermoid tumor with intraocular extension. Arch Ophthalmol 75:803–805, 1966

25. SEN DK, MOHAN H, GUPTA DK: The syndrome of Goldenhar (oculoauricular dysplasia). Acta Ophthalmol (Kbh) 47:1044–1048, 1969

26. SUGAR HS: An unusual example of the oculo-auriculo-vertebral dysplasia syndrome of Goldenhar. J Pediat Ophthalmol 4:9–12, 1967

27. SWAN KC, EMMENS TH, CHRISTENSEN L: Experience with tumors of the limbus. Trans Am Acad Ophthalmol Otolaryngol 52:458–469, 1947–1948

28. VALVO A: Malignant mesodermal mixed tumor (mesenchymoma) of the orbit. Am J Ophthalmol 66:919–923, 1968

29. ZIMMERMAN LE: Personal communication

30. ZIMMERMAN LE: Phakomatous choristoma of the eyelid; a tumor of lenticular anlage. Am J Ophthalmol 71:169–177, 1971

16

METASTATIC TUMORS OF THE EYE AND ADNEXA

Malignant tumor cells enter the bloodstream not only through direct invasion of the wall of blood or lymph vessels but also by intravasation. This occurs when the extravascular pressure even momentarily exceeds the intravascular. It may occur from the usual increased tissue pressure of expanding cancer as well as from manipulation at the time of surgery, from the explosive effect of the laser and the photocoagulator, and especially through surgically opened vessels. Bone spicules, muscle, fat, and foreign matter may also arrive at ectopic sites through this route.

In a series of 213 adults and 46 children with generalized malignancy, the most common site of ocular metastases proved to be the uvea in adults and the orbit in children.[2]

In the uvea, metastasis from carcinoma is much more frequent than from sarcoma or malignant melanoma, reflecting the higher incidence of carcinoma.

METASTATIC TUMORS OF THE UVEA

Among 227 cases of ocular and orbital metastasis in one series,[18] the principal involvement was the eye in 196, the orbit in 28, the optic nerve in 3. The primary sites were breast 40%, lung 29%, kidney 4%, testicle 3%, prostate 1%, and pancreas, colon, stomach, thyroid and ileum less than 1%. In 41 of the cases (18%) the primary site was not discovered. Of the 217 patients who could be followed, 192 died, with a median survival time of 7.4 months after operation. Other rare primary locations are the ovary, the parotid gland, the liver, the uterus (chorioepithelioma),[32] and the face (squamous-cell carcinoma). Metastasis of a carcinoma of the male breast to the choroid has been described,[25] and metastasis from the cortex of the suprarenal gland to the choroid.[23]

In another report six out of seven tumors metastasizing to the uvea were primary in the breast, and one originated in the esophagus.[42]

For many years malignant melanoma has been considered the most common malignant tumor of the eye. Of late, however, doubts have been cast on the validity of the statistical process in reaching that conclusion. It has been pointed out that statistics on bilaterality may be misleading, because usually only one eye is removed, and possible involvement of its fellow may not be considered.[18] On the other hand, metastatic carcinoma results in enucleation only in the presence of intractable pain, although not a few eyes containing the tumor have been removed following an erroneous diagnosis of malignant melanoma. Ocular symptoms are often overlooked in a seriously ill patient; and if the eyes are examined at all the task is likely to be performed by a surgeon or an internist, seldom by an ophthalmologist. Moreover, when the eyes come to autopsy, permission is often given only for examination of the posterior pole. With these facts in mind, various investigators[2,10,18,26] have studied eyes of patients with metastatic carcinoma and concluded that this is the most common malignant tumor of the eye.

In a series of 305 reported cases of uveal melanoma in Denmark,[31] an additional malignancy was found in 19 cases, or 6.2%. A uveal tumor might be a melanoma or other neoplasm instead of a metastatic tumor, especially in patients with a history of previous malignant disease.[43] These authors described a patient with three primary malignancies, one of which was an intraocular tumor.

I believe it must be assumed that in most cancer patients some of the tumor cells enter the bloodstream but only rarely remain viable and grow at the implantation sites.[62] Different types of cancer cells vary widely in their ability to remain viable away from the primary site, and may even vary from time to time within certain inconstant factors of host resistance. Breast cancer cells, known to be very hardy, can survive and even propagate under circumstances unfavorable to other types of cancer cells. The high incidence of ocular metastases from primary breast cancer can probably be explained on this basis.

The numerous reports on metastases from the lungs and bronchi in recent years seem to reflect the increased incidence of this type of cancer. Metastasis to the iris and ciliary body from a primary carcinoma at either site is frequently confused clinically with iridocyclitis with and without secondary glaucoma. I have seen two patients in whom the iris was principally involved; the clinical picture simulated that of a hypopyon iritis with secondary glaucoma (Fig. 16–1, see p. 33; Fig. 16–2). In a case of mucoepidermoid carcinoma that metastasized to the ciliary body from a squamous-cell carcinoma of the lung, the diagnosis was made by examination of cells in the aqueous humor.[44] In three of four reported cases of primary cancer of the lung, the first manifestation was a metastatic tumor in the anterior ocular segment.[15] Bronchogenic cancer metastasizing to the uvea has been reported.[27,41,53,56] In one case metastasis to the anterior uvea caused iridocyclitis which was thought to be due to tuberculosis because of suspicious lung changes on the x rays.[65] At autopsy, tumor deposits were found in the iris, ciliary body, Schlemm's canal, angle of the anterior chamber, and posterior surface of the cornea, although the cornea was not involved.

A ring tumor of the angle may be metastatic (Fig. 16–3, see p. 33). Reports have appeared of ocular metastases from so-called bronchial adenomas.[21]

There have been many published cases of a primary malignant melanoma of the conjunctiva or the skin (Fig. 16–4) metastasizing to the uvea of one or both eyes[17,22] or to the ciliary body of the fellow eye; a similar tumor has also metastasized from the uvea to the uvea of the fellow eye. In one patient with two separate metastases from a malignant melanoma of the skin—to the ciliary body and to the choroid of the same eye—there were clinical manifestations of absolute glaucoma.[63] Primary sarcomas of the breast and of the ovary have metastasized to the uvea and a choriocarcinoma of the uterus to the choroid.[34] In one reported case an osteogenic sarcoma originating in the left fibula metastasized to the choroid.[60] Some of the cases of uveal metastasis that have been reported from a primary round-cell sarcoma in the mediastinum were probably malignant lymphomas.

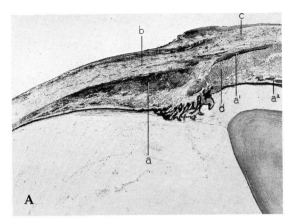

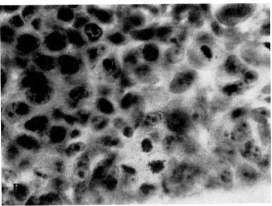

FIG. 16–2. Metastatic carcinoma of the iris and ciliary body. The clinical picture suggested iridocyclitis with hypopyon and secondary glaucoma. The eye manifestations were noted before the primary site in the lung was discovered. **A.** Section of the anterior portion of the globe shows (*a*) the ciliary body, partly necrotic and partly viable carcinoma associated with an inflammatory reaction. (*a¹*) Viable carcinoma extends along the posterior surface of the iris, (*a²*) invading and replacing the stroma of the iris and growing along the posterior surface of the pigment epithelium. Adjacent scleritis is seen at *b*, adjacent keratitis at *c*, and a hypopyon at *d*. **B.** Higher-power magnification reveals the structure of the tumor tissue, from *a¹* area, in which several mitotic figures can be distinguished.

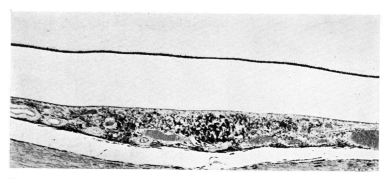

FIG. 16–4. Metastatic melanoma of the choroid. The primary site was in the skin of the shoulder. (Courtesy of W. Kreibig.[34a])

PREDILECTION FOR POSTERIOR POLE

The majority of neoplastic metastases occur in the posterior portion of the uvea. Most of the tumor emboli would naturally be carried through the 20-odd short posterior ciliary arteries rather than the two long posterior or the five or more anterior arteries. These tumor metastases appeared to have a predilection for the posterior portion of the choroid, specifically the temporal side near the macular region where the short posterior arteries are relatively large and numerous. The left eye was formerly considered to be more often involved, in accord with the higher incidence of left cerebral embolism, but in a report on 227 cases no left-sided preponderance was found.[18]

BILATERALITY

Various authors agree on a 20%–25% incidence of bilateral metastasis.[13,36] Both eyes are seldom involved simultaneously, although simultaneous involvement of the brain and eye is common.

INCIDENCE

Uveal metastases are rarely detected clinically. Subclinical cancerous emboli to the uvea are unquestionably common, especially in the late stages. Since the ophthalmic artery branches at almost a right angle from the internal carotid, cancer cells in the bloodstream tend to be swept past the ophthalmic artery and deposited in the brain and meninges.

The choroid is more frequently involved than the iris and ciliary body, no doubt because of the more abundant arterial distribution to the posterior uvea than to the anterior uvea. The ratio in one series[58] was 156 to 17. The ratio of iris involvement to pure ciliary body involvement is about 7 to 1. In an early review[36] of 229 cases of uveal metastasis, of which 21% were bilateral, involvement of the choroid was found in 156.

INTERVAL BETWEEN DIAGNOSIS OF PRIMARY TUMOR AND METASTASIS

A period of weeks to years may elapse between diagnosis of the primary tumor and discovery of the uveal metastasis—14 years in one patient whose primary site was in the thyroid gland[67] and 10 years in another whose primary site was in the rectum.[68] In many instances metastasis to the eye manifests itself before the primary site is known[18] (Figs. 16–1, 16–5, see pp. 33, 34; also Fig. 16–2).

DISSEMINATION FROM PRIMARY SITE

The fact that tumor cells are carried from the primary to the metastatic site by the bloodstream is difficult to explain without assuming lung involvement. In a series[36] of 59 autopsied cases with eye involvement, pulmonary metastasis was found in 83%. Such metastases cannot usually be demonstrated clinically. However, metastases occasionally appear in the eye with no evidence of lung involvement. This finding has been explained on the basis of Batson's theory that a neoplasm of the breast, lung, pelvis, shoulder, pelvic girdle or other sites may metastasize at any point along the vertebral system without involving the portal, pulmonary, or caval system. The reversed blood flow in veins, frequently occurring during coughing and straining, may be an important factor.

CLINICAL COURSE

The patients usually complain of defective vision, and examination reveals a more or less solid-appearing detachment of the retina, invariably in the posterior pole. The elevated area is pinkish white, fading off into the normal-appearing surrounding retina. The tumor surface is frequently mottled (Fig. 16–6, see p. 34). An occasional hemorrhage and some slight pigmentary changes may be seen over the involved area. Such lesions are often pale gray, pale yellow, or yellowish gray. Multiple tumor foci are in some instances noted throughout the fundus. In the early stages the lesion is characteristically rather flat, in keeping with the usual growth pattern of epithelium. In the later stages the retina generally becomes detached. Direct inspection of the lesion is then impossible, and the diagnosis becomes presumptive. In some cases the growth spreads flatly in all directions; it may simulate a papilledema when the disc becomes surrounded. After the tumor has ben detected in the choroid, other nodules may be noted in the iris, the ciliary body, or both.

Necrosis of the metastatic tumor may lead to inflammation (Fig. 16–7, see p. 34). This inflammatory feature can cause pigmentary changes over and around the lesion suggesting a melanoma. In cases where the anterior uvea is involved, a marked inflammation may result in secondary glaucoma. If the tumor affects the iris, the ciliary body, or both, even the sclera and cornea may participate when the inflammatory element is pronounced. Clinical diagnosis then becomes difficult, particularly in the presence of secondary glaucoma.

Cases of hepatoma with metastasis to the choroid have been reported.[64] The fundus appeared dark green from bile in the metastatic cells.

The possibility that a retinal detachment may be caused by a metastatic lesion in the choroid must be kept in mind. Patients do not always volunteer information about previous cancer surgery, particularly a mastectomy. It is therefore well to inquire about any such operations when taking the history of a patient with a detached retina. Choroidal metastasis in the early stages before retinal detachment has occurred may appear flat and solid. Transillumination is of no diagnostic value.

A neoplastic metastasis to the uvea, which may be confused with a primary malignant melanoma, has the following characteristics: a) The lesion is usually not sharply circumscribed and does not show a globular elevation; b) light is transmitted by retroillumination; c) the growth is rather rapid; d) pain may be an early feature and glaucoma may ensue; e) the retina over the tumor site is opaque and shows a tendency to early detachment; f) necrosis with secondary inflammation may occur; g) bilaterality is not uncommon; h) in most instances there is a history of primary carcinoma; i) the tumor rarely perforates the lamina vitrea and therefore does not fungate toward the vitreous cavity.

PATHOLOGY

The most characteristic pathologic feature is the tendency of cancerous tissue in the choroid to spread and produce a rather flat, diffuse lesion (Fig. 16–8). This is to be expected because of the nature of epithelium and is particularly evident when the cancer is primary in the breast. Uveal metastasis from a primary tumor in the stomach or thyroid gland either may grow in a rather localized elevated fashion (Fig. 16-5, see p. 34) or become diffuse.

TREATMENT AND PROGNOSIS

Radiation and endocrine therapy have been advised for choroidal metastases from a primary site in the breast.[39] Three of seven women with carcinoma metastatic to the choroid showed marked improvement with radiation therapy, three improved slightly, and one was not benefited.[47] Although the prognosis in tumor metastases to the eye may be hopeless from the standpoint of prolonged survival, attempts to improve the patients' vision with lenses and reduce pain by irradiation improve morale. These patients are often unaware of the grave prognosis and welcome any efforts to improve the eye condition, which usually concerns them more than the primary tumor. Such treatment is more than merely morale-building when the patient's only useful eye is affected, for adequate vision can sometimes be maintained for the remaining six months to two years of his life. If he develops painful glaucoma, enucleation may be indicated.

In one series the average life expectancy of patients with metastatic carcinoma to the choroid and iris was 8 months, and the

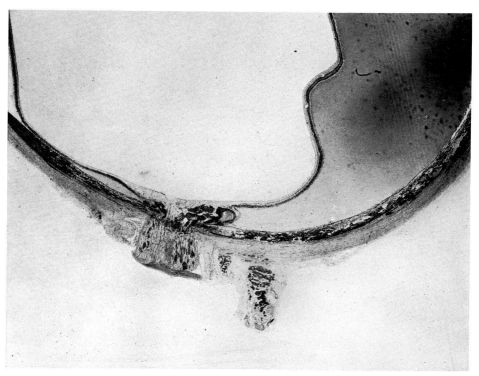

FIG. 16–8. Metastatic carcinoma of the choroid from a primary site in the breast. The tumor has grown diffusely throughout the choroid and extended into the optic nerve. The retina is detached.

FIG. 16–9. Metastatic carcinoma of the sclera from a primary site in the breast. The localized, elevated tumor nodule is in the upper nasal quadrant of the sclera.

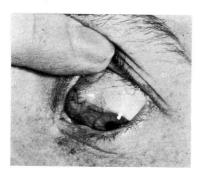

longest survival about 2 years.[66] In another report the average survival after the onset of ocular symptoms was 9.3 months and the longest survival 16 months.[47]

METASTATIC TUMORS OF THE RETINA AND IRIS

Carcinoma

A number of reports have appeared on metastatic carcinoma to the retina from various primary sites: the pancreas,[6] the esophagus and stomach,[59] the rectum,[33] the uterus,[16] and the breast.[20,37] A carcinoma of the breast has also metastasized to the iris.[11]

Malignant Melanoma

Malignant melanoma may metastasize to the retina.[38]

METASTATIC TUMORS OF THE OPTIC NERVE

Metastases of carcinoma to the optic nerve proper have been reported from primary tumors in the kidney, the lung, the breast[45,46] and the pancreas.[55] In one case of metastatic involvement of the intracranial segment of the optic nerves, the primary site was unknown but may possibly have been a mole removed from the skin of the back four years earlier.[69]

Metastatic meningeal carcinomatosis may occur in one or both optic nerves. In a bilateral case, the primary tumor proved at autopsy to be a small adenocarcinoma of the lung.[14]

Metastases to the retrobulbar and intraorbital portions of the nerve sheath have occurred from various primary sites, e.g., the ovaries and the stomach, also metastases to the intracerebral portion of the sheath from various primaries including the breast, the stomach, and the bronchi. In one instance carcinoma of the gastric wall was found at autopsy in a patient with bilateral papilledema.[61] The cells were identical morphologically with those in the perineural sheaths of the optic nerves. No other metastases were found, although similar cells were scattered in the meninges of the brain.

METASTATIC TUMORS OF THE EYELID

In a study of 13 cases of mammary carcinoma metastatic to the eyelid with a histiocytoid appearance, 7 presented diagnostic problems.[28] The authors suggested that once this peculiar appearance is appreciated, the tumor can usually be recognized. Metastasis of an adenocarcinoma to the eyelid has been reported[50] and of a thyroid carcinoma to the lids and orbit.[4]

Only 3 of a series of 214 malignant lid lesions were metastatic carcinomas; the primary site was not specified.[7] A review of the literature revealed 15 cases of metastatic tumor to the lids, and 15 other cases were added from the Mayo Clinic tumor registry over a 47-year period.[54] The most frequent primary sites were the breast (10 cases), the lung (5 cases), and cutaneous melanoma (5 cases), with smaller percentages for the stomach, colon, thyroid, parotid, and trachea.

METASTATIC TUMORS OF THE SCLERA AND CONJUNCTIVA

One of our patients had metastatic carcinoma of the sclera from a primary tumor in the breast (Fig. 16-9). A carcinoma of the colon in one case metastasized to the conjunctiva.[49]

METASTATIC TUMORS OF THE ORBIT

A neuroblastoma of the suprarenal medulla or the retroperitoneal ganglia commonly metastasizes to the orbit. In a report of two cases of Hutchison's syndrome in young children, the ocular symptoms were attributed to intraorbital neuroblastoma as part of a multilocular sympathetic neuroblastomatosis.[51]

Reports of Wilms's tumor metastatic to the orbit[3,5,24] indicate that it must be considered a primary locus, in addition to neuroblastoma. Wilms's tumor is no longer considered fatal even if metastasis has occurred; about 50% of such patients survive.

A rare, well-differentiated myxoid type of liposarcoma was diagnosed in the orbit of a 43-year-old man two years after discovery of the primary lesion in the thigh.[1] At autopsy, the thigh and orbital masses, lungs and lymph nodes had identical histologic characteristics.

Among numerous reports of metastatic carcinoma to the orbit, the most frequent primary site was the breast.[30] Among other primary sites reported were the uterus and cervix, the kidney (hypernephroma), the bronchi,[35] the thyroid gland, the prostate gland, the rectum,[52] the pancreas, the lung, and the stomach.[12] In one case,[8] a carcinoma of the breast metastasized to the extraocular muscles, from which orbital metastases probably often arise. Metastasis to the orbit from a bronchogenic carcinoma was found only at autopsy in one case.[19]

Exophthalmos is the usual response to an orbital metastasis, although enophthalmos may develop in instances of scirrhous carcinoma.[9,40,48] In three reported cases,[48] the first indication of a malignant scirrhous carcinoma of the breast was an unexplained enophthalmos and diplopia. This author felt that enophthalmos from metastatic scirrhous carcinoma to the orbit was characterized by absence of pain and inflammatory signs. Also, he stressed the value of sonograms in making the diagnosis. Usually, diplopia is the only symptom except for the enophthalmos, although a painful ophthalmoplegia was present in one case[57] and papilledema and choroidal striae in another.[29]

REFERENCES

1. ABDALLA MI, GHALY AF, HOSNI F: Liposarcoma with orbital metastases; case report. Br J Ophthalmol 50:426–428, 1966

2. ALBERT DM, RUBENSTEIN RA, SCHEIE HG: Tumor metastasis to the eye. Part I. Incidence in 213 adult patients with generalized malignancy. Am J Ophthalmol 63:723–726, 1967

3. ALGAN B, VITTE G, DEFINES M: Métastase orbitaire d'un nephroblastome. Bull Soc Ophtalmol Fr 5:323–324, 1955

4. APPALANARSAYYA K, SATYENDRAN OM: Metastases in the lid and orbit from thyroid carcinoma. Orient Arch Ophthalmol 2:183–184, 1964

5. APPLE DJ: Wilms' tumor metastatic to the orbit. Arch Ophthalmol 80:480–483, 1968

6. ARISAWA U: Metastatisches Aderhautkarzinom bei latentem Primärtumor. Klin Monatsbl Augenheilkd 52:695–701, 1914

7. AURORA AL, BLODI FC: Lesions of the eyelids: a clinicopathologic study. Survey Ophthalmol 15:94–104, 1970

8. BEDFORD PD, DANIEL PM: Discrete carcinomatous metastases in the extrinsic ocular muscles. Am J Ophthalmol 49:723–726, 1960

9. BIRÖ I: Mit Enophthalmus einhergehende Mammakrebsmetastase in der Orbita. Acta Ophthalmol (Kbh) 19:255–260, 1941

10. BLOCH RS, GARTNER S: The incidence of ocular metastatic carcinoma. Arch Ophthalmol 85:673–675, 1971

11. BONNET JL, DE MARIGNY G, MARTHOURET M: Metastasis in the iris of a cancer of the breast. Bull Soc Ophtalmol Fr 70:283–285, 1970

12. CHATTERJEE BM, DEB M: Metastatic carcinoma of the orbit. Am J Ophthalmol 59:103–105, 1965

13. CORDES FC: Bilateral metastatic carcinoma of the choroid with X-ray therapy to one eye. Am J Ophthalmol 27:1355–1370, 1944

14. CURTIN VT: Metastatic adenocarcinoma of the optic nerves. Presented at the Verhoeff Society, Washington, DC, April 1973

15. DUKE JR, KENNEDY JJ: Metastatic carcinoma of the iris and ciliary body. Arch Ophthalmol 60:1092–1103, 1958

16. DUKE JR, WALSH FB: Metastatic carcinoma to the retina. Am J Ophthalmol 47:44–48, 1959

17. FERRY AP: Primary malignant melanoma of the skin metastatic to the eye. Am J Ophthalmol 74:12–19, 1972

18. FERRY AP, FONT RL: Carcinoma metastatic to the eye and orbit: a clinicopathologic study of 227 cases. Arch Ophthalmol 92:276–286, 1974

19. FERRY AP, NAGHDI MR: Bronchogenic carcinoma metastatic to the orbit. Arch Ophthalmol 77:214–216, 1967

20. FLINDALL RJ, FLEMING KO: Metastatic tumour of the retina. Can J Ophthalmol 2:130–132, 1967

21. FONT RL, KAUFER G, WINSTANLEY RA: Metastasis of bronchial carcinoid tumor to the eye. Am J Ophthalmol 62:723–727, 1966

22. FONT RL, NAUMANN G, ZIMMERMAN LE: Primary malignant melanoma of the skin metastatic to the eye and orbit; report of ten cases and review of the literature. Am J Ophthalmol 63:738–754, 1967

23. FRANÇOIS J, BOELS W, RABAEY M: Cancers métastiques de la choroïde, dont un d'origine cor- tico-surrenalienne. Ann Ocul 185:497–514, 1952

24. GOULDING HB: Orbital metastases from Wilms' tumor. Trans Ophthalmol Soc UK 67:491–492, 1947

25. GREER CH: Choroidal carcinoma metastatic from the male breast. Br J Ophthalmol 38:312–315, 1954

26. GUTHERT H, JANISCH W, ROSSBACH K: Über die Häufigkeit der Augenmetastasen. Munch Med Wochenschr 107:939–941, 1965

27. HAFT AS, WORKEN B: Metastatic carcinoma of the choroid (bronchogenic) simulating primary tumor of the eye. Arch Ophthalmol 51:445–450, 1954

28. HOOD CI, FONT RL, ZIMMERMAN LE: Metastatic mammary carcinoma in the eyelid with histiocytoid appearance. Cancer 31:793–800, 1973

29. HOYT WF, BEESTON D: The Ocular Fundus in Neurologic Disease: A Diagnostic Manual and Stereo Atlas. St Louis, CV Mosby, 1966, p 40

30. HUDA N, VENABLE HP: Metastasis of carcinoma of the breast to both orbits. Am J Ophthalmol 64:779–780, 1967

31. JENSEN OA: Malignant melanomas of the uvea in Denmark; a clinical, histo-pathological and prognostic study. Acta Ophthalmol (Kbh) (Suppl) 75:1–220, 1963

32. KEATES RH, BILLIG SL: Metastatic uveal choriocarcinoma; report of a case with improvement after chemotherapy. Arch Ophthalmol 84:381–384, 1970

33. KENNEDY RJ, RUMMEL WD, MCCARTHY JL, HAZARD JB: Metastatic carcinoma of the retina. Arch Ophthalmol 60:12–17, 1958

34. KIENDLER W: Solitary choroidal metastasis as the sole clinical manifestation of a chorionepithelial tumor of the uterus. Klin Monatsbl Augenheilkd 154:850–854, 1969

34a. KREIBIG W: Zur Kenntnis intraokulärer Sarkommetastasen. Z Augenheilkd 87:265–284, 1935

35. KULVIN MM, SAWCHAK WG: Tumor of orbit metastatic from malignant bronchial adenoma. Am J Ophthalmol 49:833–838, 1960

36. LEMOINE AN, MCLEOD J: Bilateral metastatic carcinoma of the choroid. Arch Ophthalmol 16:804–821, 1936

37. LEVY RM, DEVENECIA G: Trypsin digest study of retinal metastasis and tumor cell emboli. Am J Ophthalmol 70:778–782, 1970

38. LIDDICOAT DA, WOLTER JR, WILKINSON WC: Retinal metastasis of malignant melanoblastoma. Am J Ophthalmol 58:172–177, 1959

39. MACMICHAEL IM: Management of choroidal metastases from breast carcinoma. Br J Ophthalmol 53:782–785, 1969

40. MANOR RS: Enophthalmos caused by metastatic breast carcinoma. Acta Ophthalmol (Kbh) 52:881–884, 1974

41. MAXWELL E: Metastatic tumors of the uveal tract. Am J Ophthalmol 37:867–873, 1954

42. MEUR G, SZYPER C, JOSSE P: A propos de sept cas de tumeurs métastatiques de l'uvée. Bull Soc Belge Ophtalmol 167:679–692, 1974

43. MORGAN SS, HEIDENRY R, BOWEN SF: Malignant melanoma of the iris and ciliary body occurring as a third primary malignancy. Am J Ophthalmol 76:26–29, 1973

44. MORGAN WE III, MALMGREN RA, ALBERT DM: Metastatic carcinoma of the ciliary body simulating uveitis; diagnosis by cytologic examination of aqueous humor. Arch Ophthalmol 83:54–58, 1970

45. NICHOLLS JVV: Metastatic carcinoma of the optic nerve. Trans Can Ophthalmol Soc 24:18–30, 1961

46. NORTON HJ: Adenocarcinoma metastatic to the distal nerve and optic disc. Am J Ophthalmol 47: 195–199, 1959

47. ORENSTEIN MM, ANDERSON DP, STEIN JJ: Choroid metastasis. Cancer 29:1101–1107, 1972

48. OSSOINIG K: Enophthalmos from metastatic orbital tumors. Dtsch Ophthalmol Ges 70:82–85, 1969

49. OSTRIKER PJ: Metastasis of adenocarcinoma of colon to conjunctival surface of lid. Arch Ophthalmol 57:279–281, 1957

50. PARKHILL EN: Adenocarcinoma metastatic to eyelid. Presented at the Verhoeff Society, Washington, DC, April 1965

51. PESCH KJ: On the pathogenesis of Hutchison's syndrome. Klin Monatsbl Augenheilkd 145:376–386, 1964

52. RICHARDS RD: Unilateral exophthalmos caused by metastatic carcinoma. Am J Ophthalmol 49: 1034–1037, 1960

53. RICKETTS MM, PRICE T, THOMAS M: Choroidal metastasis of bronchial adenoma. Am J Ophthalmol 39:33–36, 1955

54. RILEY FC: Metastatic tumors of the eyelids. Am J Ophthalmol 69:259–264, 1970

55. RING HG: Pancreatic carcinoma with metastasis to the optic nerve. Arch Ophthalmol 77:789–800, 1967

56. ROSENBLUTH J, LAVAL J, WEIL JV: Metastasis of bronchial adenoma of the eye. Arch Ophthalmol 62:47–50, 1960

57. SACKS JG, O'GRADY RB: Painful ophthalmoplegia and enophthalmos due to metastatic carcinoma: simulation of essential facial hemiatrophy. Trans Am Acad Ophthalmol Otolaryngol 75:351–354, 1971

58. SANDERS TE: Metastatic carcinoma of the iris. Am J Ophthalmol 21: 646–651, 1938

59. SMOLEROFF JW, AGATSTON SA: Metastatic carcinoma of the retina. Arch Ophthalmol 12:359–365, 1934

60. SPAULDING AG, WOODFIN MC JR: Osteogenic sarcoma metastatic to the choroid. Arch Ophthalmol 80:84–86, 1968

61. SPENCER WH: Papilledema (bilateral) secondary to metastatic meningeal carcinomatosis. Presented at the Verhoeff Society, Washington, DC, April 1967

62. STANFORD GB, REESE AB: Malignant cells in the blood of eye patients. Trans Am Acad Ophthalmol Otolaryngol 75:102–109, 1971

63. SZEPS J, PATTERSON TD: Metastatic malignant melanoma of ciliary body and choroid from a primary melanoma of skin. Can J Ophthalmol 4:394–399, 1969

64. TAAKE WH, ALLEN RA, STRAATSMA BR: Metastasis of a hepatoma to the choroid. Am J Ophthalmol 56:208–213, 1963

65. TALEGAONKAR SK: Anterior uveal tract metastasis as the presenting feature of bronchial carcinoma. Br J Ophthalmol 53:123–126, 1969

66. USHER CH: Cases of metastatic carcinoma of the choroid and iris. Br J Ophthalmol 7:10–54, 1923

67. VENCO L: Metastasi nella coroide di un tumore tiroideo. Ann Ottal 63:401–436, 1935

68. VON SALLMANN L: Gelatinous cancer of the choroid following carcinoma of the rectum. Arch Ophthalmol 25:89–92, 1941

69. WEIZENBLATT S: Metastatic disease of the optic nerve. Am J Ophthalmol 47:77–83, 1959

17

ORBITAL NEOPLASMS AND LESIONS SIMULATING THEM

Orbital lesions most commonly manifest themselves by exophthalmos. Whether a given lesion produces exophthalmos, and if so to what degree, depends on the size of the lesion, its character, its position in the orbit, and its effect on the extraocular muscles.

If the lesion is localized posterior to the equator of the globe and is sufficiently large, the eye is pushed forward. Even a relatively small lesion (5 to 8 mm in diameter), if located in the muscle funnel, may produce some degree of exophthalmos. Depending on the position of the lesion in the orbit, the globe's displacement may be in a medial, lateral, superior, or inferior direction. A lesion located more anteriorly may cause eccentric displacement of the globe, fullness of the overlying lid, ptosis, or dysfunction of the ocular muscles, instead of exophthalmos.

As the rectus muscles retract the globe, paralysis of one or more of them may cause the globe to protrude as much as 2 mm. When the paralysis occurs with an expanding lesion of the orbit, the degree of exophthalmos is greater than would otherwise be the case. In addition, a tumor that interferes with the extraocular muscles limits the motion of the globe; when the lesion is extensive and diffuse, the globe may become fixed.

Other secondary factors that may cause or contribute to proptosis include passive congestion from pressure of the tumor on veins, an inflammatory process in the orbit such as that produced by necrosis of an unrecognized intraocular melanoma, and, in rare instances, thrombosis of one of the larger veins.

An orbital mass may indent the sclera at the site where it is in contact with the globe, occasionally before the proptosis is apparent. The indentation, particularly if in the macular area, may lead to hyperopia or hyperopic astigmatism so irregular that lenses will not correct the refractive error. Cases of hyperopia of 8 diopters caused by an orbital osteoma, and of astigmatism of 13 diopters caused by a mucocele pressing the eyeball against the lower orbital margin, have been reported.[57]

PRESSURE FOLDS

The pressure of an expanding lesion of the orbit on the adjacent sclera may produce striae in the fundus seen with the ophthalmoscope (Fig. 17–1). On histologic section, actual folds may be observed in the retina proper as well as a wrinkling of the internal limiting layer (Fig. 17–2). The horizontal folds are seen over the region of scleral pressure. A well-localized orbital tumor may cause retinal striae radiating from the area of focal pressure. Such pressure lines may also appear when there is a generalized increase in orbital pressure in patients with endocrine ophthalmopathy. When the indentation is at the posterior pole, the lines may run concentric to the disc. Localization of retinal striae in one area of the fundus is a reliable sign of an expanding orbital lesion, and usually justifies proceeding with the Krönlein operation.

Biomicroscopy and fluorescein angiography have revealed the broader folds in the choroid and pigment epithelium (see section Stereofundus Photography and Fluorescein Angiography in the Diagnosis of Intraocular Tumors, by J. Donald M. Gass, in Chapter 12). When not visible by the ophthalmoscope, the folds may be seen by angiography.

Several observers have commented on the persistence of these retinal striae long after surgical relief of the scleral pressure—three years in one case,[99] and in another case four months when last seen.[47] Conversely, the striae may disappear immediately after the pressure is relieved. The important factor is probably how long the pressure was applied. Persistence of the folds has been attributed to permanent shrinkage of the sclera from prolonged indentation.[99]

The indented sclera may simulate a flat detachment of the retina.

An expanding lesion in the posterior part of the orbit may push some orbital fat forward, causing it to present anteriorly as a mass under the conjunctiva or back of the lid. This fat may be excised on the supposition that it is the primary lesion, whereas the causative lesion, such as a dermoid cyst or a tumor of the lacrimal gland, actually lurks posteriorly.

Glaucoma may develop when the orbital lesion disturbs the venous return through the vortex veins or when myopathy of the rectus muscles in thyroid disease compresses the globe.

An expanding lesion around the posterior pole of the eye may produce venous stasis in the retina or even occlude the central retinal vein or one of its branches. Moreover, pressure around the optic nerve can give rise to papilledema (Fig. 17–1) or optic atrophy.

The development of bilateral exophthalmos has been described following steroid therapy in four patients[87] and was previously reported in animals receiving steroids.[98] Exophthalmos was found in 6%–8% of patients with Cushing's syndrome who showed elevated endogenous steroid production.[75] In another case exophthalmos was the first manifestation.[67] An exophthalmos-producing factor was demonstrated in five cases of Cushing's syndrome.[85] Because of these interesting new developments, steroid therapy should be used cautiously in cases of Graves's disease and pseudotumor (granuloma) of the orbit, the two conditions for which it is frequently prescribed.

Exposure of the cornea may be a complication of marked exophthalmos. The earliest manifestations of corneal exposure are irritation of the eye and punctate areas over the lower third of the corneal epithelium, which stain with fluorescein. These may be the forerunners of corneal ulceration which, if not arrested, can lead to perforation and loss of the eye. Some corneal pathology including ulceration may be neurotrophic, secondary to involvement of the orbital nerves in various pathologic processes.

Sometimes an orbital mass cannot be palpated without obtaining good relaxation of the lid muscles by local or general anesthesia. It may be advantageous to palpate the fornices with a glass rod.

Although it is common practice to have the patient look up when palpating through the lower lid, and look down when palpating through the upper lid, this makes the orbital septum taut. It is better for the patient to look straight ahead or even up when palpating through the upper lid, and down when examining through the lower lid.

The trochlea and the adjacent portion of the superior oblique muscle, at the orbital

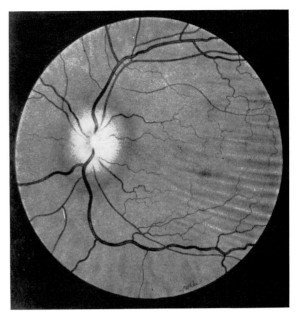

FIG. 17–1. Papilledema and retinal striae resulting from an encapsulated orbital hemangioma. Pressure of the tumor on the optic nerve produced papilledema, and pressure on the sclera produced horizontal retinal striae.

FIG. 17–2. Retinal folds from pressure of an orbital tumor on the sclera. The internal limiting layer is also involved in the folding. (Wolter JR, Jampel RS: Klin Monatsbl Augenheilkd 131: 433–438, 1957)

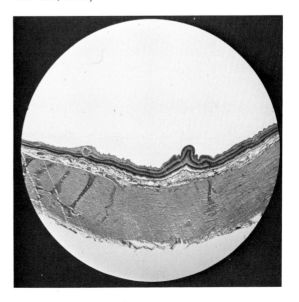

margin nasally and above, may be confused with an orbital mass. This is true to a lesser degree of the inferior oblique muscle at its origin along the orbital margin nasally and below.

The ratio of eye volume to orbital volume in infants and young children is approximately 4 to 5, as compared with approximately 1 to 4 in adults. Therefore, a relatively small expanding lesion produces exophthalmos in children. Because of the very small orbital space, a finger cannot be inserted between the globe and the external orbital margin to palpate the mass unless there is extreme proptosis. Orbital surgery in this age group consists primarily of obtaining biopsy tissue for diagnosis and, when indicated, performing an exenteration, the only means of completely excising the lesion.

Among the conditions that simulate a true exophthalmos are the following: a) asymmetry of the bony orbits, b) unilateral high myopia, c) early and mild hyperthyroidism, which produces a unilateral retraction of the upper lid, d) relaxation of one or more rectus muscles because of either paralysis or their undue recession at the time of a squint operation, and e) unilateral hydrophthalmos (buphthalmos).

Bony asymmetry, with the two orbital cavities having a different volume, may be congenital or acquired. The condition can be confirmed by x ray. Since irradiation around growth centers and not-yet-united epiphyses of bone tends to disturb growth, it may cause such a disparity in volume. Any type of radiation, even the implantation of radon seeds, may retard bony orbital growth in young patients and result in an orbit smaller than on the untreated side. This may cause some exophthalmos many years later. Since radiation is usually given because of an orbital tumor, the later appearance of exophthalmos may be mistaken for progression or recurrence of the tumor.

In two cases that have come to my attention, a unilateral high myopia of 18 to 25 diopters, with an emmetropic fellow eye, led to the belief that a proptosis, perhaps due to an orbital tumor, was present (Fig. 17–3).

Unilateral retraction of the upper lid in hyperthyroidism may simulate exophthalmos (Fig. 17–4). Without using an exophthalmometer, it may be impossible to distinguish between a unilateral wide palpebral aperture caused by retraction of the upper lid and a real exophthalmos.

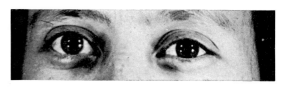

FIG. 17–3. Unilateral myopia of 25 diopters simulating exophthalmos. The right cornea protruded 4 mm more than the left, demonstrated by the exophthalmometer. The left eye was emmetropic.

FIG. 17–4. Retraction of the right upper lid in early hyperthyroidism, simulating unilateral exophthalmos.

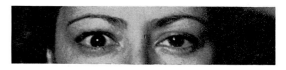

When one palpebral aperture is wider than the other, it may not be clear which one is normal. The inequality may be congenital or due to such conditions as Horner's syndrome, a mild congenital blepharoptosis, or any of the aforementioned causes of slight exophthalmos or simulating conditions.

The exophthalmometer, while useful, is far from being a precision instrument. This is readily apparent when one compares his own successive readings, or compares his readings with those of others. It must be kept in mind, when gauging the progression of a proptosis, that the readings are merely estimates. The Hertel, Luede, and Mutch exophthalmometers are all in general use. Although the Hertel instrument has an intrinsic error of 1–2 mm, it seems to be the best. To be properly secured, it must be fixed along the lateral orbital margin above or below the external canthal ligament. Faulty fixation, directly over the insertion of the external canthal ligament, results in incorrect readings.

Relative exophthalmos has been measured by the combined use of x ray and contact lenses with a small central lead dot.[39] Accurate measurement of the degree of exophthalmos has been facilitated by a combined radiograph and photograph.[93] Stereophotogrammetric exophthalmometry[5] seems to be impractical for routine systematic study of exophthalmos.

Some orbital lesions, particularly neoplasms, are known to increase the orbital pressure. In many instances the effects of this increased intraorbital pressure can be demonstrated by x ray. Instruments have been devised in an attempt to determine whether the orbital pressure is normal or elevated. The authors of a review of orbitonometric findings in 36 patients with unilateral exophthalmos concluded that such findings could not be solely relied on for diagnosis.[32]

EXPANDING LESIONS OF THE ORBIT

True tumors of the orbit are discussed in the appropriate chapters. The remainder, classified as simulating lesions rather than tumors, will be described briefly (in order of their frequency). Belonging in this group are granuloma, dermoid cyst, mucocele, retinocele (coloboma cyst), encephalocele, carotid-cavernous sinus fistula, fibrous dysplasia of bone, amyloid, and congenital orbital varix. The neoplasms and simulating lesions may be primary in the orbit or secondary to pathology at adjacent sites (cranium, sinuses, nasopharynx, lids), or result from metastasis or a systemic disease.

Our series of 504 expanding lesions of the orbit[82] (Table 17–1), treated and followed by one group, includes only cases diagnosed by biopsy or exploration; those with unconfirmed diagnoses were omitted. Cases were eliminated which weight some comparable series toward a particular specialty such as radiology or pathology. Also omitted were 59 cases of retinoblastoma in the orbit and 23 cases of postradiation sarcoma in or around the orbit, all seen in our retinoblastoma clinic and not considered routine cases.

In this series of consecutive cases studied clinically, the orbital manifestation of thyroid disease was the most common cause of unilateral proptosis. In an earlier series of 877 consecutive cases of orbital neoplasms and simulating lesions studied histologically in our pathology laboratory, granuloma was the most frequent cause of exophthalmos. In a series of exophthalmos cases studied in our x-ray laboratory, mucocele was the most common diagnosis, although it was not even listed in the histologic series because no tissue biopsy was taken. The low incidence of mucocele in the clinical series seems to be due to successful treatment of sinusitis by antibiotics.

CHRONIC GRANULOMA (PSEUDOTUMOR)

Virtually all granulomatous processes may manifest themselves in the orbit and simulate an orbital neoplasm. The term *granuloma* is used here in the older sense, to designate any tumorlike mass of chronic inflammatory tissue. This usage contrasts with the current tendency to reserve the term for lesions composed predominantly of large mononuclear cells and their modified forms, epithelioid and giant cells.

Some orbital granulomas can be identified as belonging to a specific category while others—unfortunately the larger group—cannot be so diagnosed and are referred to as pseudotumors. Before the lesion was well recognized, unnecessary radical surgery was often carried out in the belief that a tumor was present. In 1934 I reviewed the literature on pseudotumor of the orbit and found that unnecessary exenteration had been done without biopsy in 15 of 30 cases.[81]

Follow-up of the 140 patients in one study of pseudotumors of the orbit[11] revealed that 8.4% developed such lethal diseases as Wegener's granulomatosis, midline granuloma, malignant lymphoma, or leukemia, yet even retrospective examination of the original orbital biopsy tissue did not point to the correct diagnosis. Five of 13 patients with bilateral involvement subsequently developed a systemic disease, an incidence of almost 40% compared with 5.5% for unilateral cases. Five of the nine patients with histopathologic features in the "miscellaneous" category were later found to have Wegener's granulomatosis; biopsy specimens in all instances showed polymorphonuclear leukocytes as well as the usual chronic inflammatory cells.

Two cases of orbital granuloma were reported with occlusion of the retinal artery; the lesion in one case histologically resembled Wegener's granuloma.[43]

In Waldenström's macroglobulinemia affecting the lacrimal gland, clues to look for histologically are lymphocytes with PAS-positive intranuclear inclusions and the plasmacytoid differentiation of lymphocytes and reticulum cells.[60]

Since the pathologist's diagnosis of inflammatory pseudotumor does not eliminate the possible development of a serious or even lethal disease later, any progressive lesion should be biopsied repeatedly. The types of biopsy obtained in our series of orbital pseudotumors are shown in Figure 17–5.

TABLE 17–1. 504 Consecutive Cases of Expanding Lesions of the Orbit§

	No. of cases	Percentage (approx.)
Granuloma*	91	18
Hemangioma	61	12
Infantile 37		
Adult 24		
Lymphoma	48	10
Lymphangioma	39	8
Rhabdomyosarcoma	37	7
Epithelial tumors of lacrimal gland	25	5
(mixed and carcinomatous)		
Neurofibroma, neurilemoma and neuroma†	23	5
Dermoid	21	4
Mucocele	20	4
Carcinoma	20	4
Metastatic 10		
Extension 10		
Malignant melanoma	19	4
Conjunctiva to orbit 10		
Choroid to orbit 9		
Meningioma†	17	3
Glioma of optic nerve†	12	2
Hemangiosarcoma	8	2
Hemangiopericytoma 5		
Hemangioendothelioma 3		
Carcinoma—lid to orbit	7	2
Basal cell 4		
Meibomian gland 2		
Squamous cell 1		
Leiomyosarcoma	6	1
Neuroblastoma	6	1
Malignant melanoma–primary	5	1
Retinocele (coloboma cyst)	5	1
Carotid-cavernous sinus fistula	4	< 1
Mesenchymoma	4	< 1
Dermolipoma	4	< 1
Fibrous dysplasia	4	< 1
Osteoma	3	< 1
Amyloid	2	< 1
Ectopic lacrimal gland	2	< 1
Myxoma	2	< 1
Miscellaneous single cases‡	9	2

* The term *granuloma* is used in the older sense, to designate any tumor-like mass of chronic inflammatory tissue. This contrasts with the current tendency to reserve the term for lesions composed predominantly of large mononuclear cells and their modified forms, epithelioid and giant cells.

† When varying combinations of neurofibroma, meningioma or glioma were present in a single case, only the dominant component has been listed.

‡ Teratoma, myeloma, granular-cell myoblastoma, congenital orbital varix, mixed neurogenic tumor (encephalocele), osteosarcoma, chondrosarcoma, liposarcoma, and malignant schwannoma.

§ From Reese AB[82]

FIG. 17–5. Biopsy specimens of orbital granulomas from different histologic groups. **A.** An orbital granuloma featuring lymph follicles (group 1). **B.** An orbital granuloma showing focal and perivascular lymphocytes in an extraocular muscle (group 2). **C.** An orbital granuloma showing a diffuse chronic inflammation and some fat necrosis with giant cells (group 3a). The giant cells result from fat necrosis incidental to the inflammation and do not indicate that the lesion belongs to the giant-cell granuloma complex (e.g., tuberculosis, sarcoid or syphilis). **D.** An orbital granuloma showing a diffuse chronic inflammation with old fibrous scarring (group 3b). **E.** An orbital granuloma showing chronic inflammation and a significant number of polymorphonuclear leukocytes (group 3c), seen under higher power magnification in the inset. **F.** An orbital granuloma showing dense fibrous scarring (group 4). **G.** An orbital granuloma showing evidence of a preexisting vascular lesion—large vascular channels filled with blood and diffuse as well as focal chronic inflammation (group 5). In the inset, cholesterin spaces and, on the left, a dense area of phagocytized and free hematogenous pigment are seen under higher magnification. (Courtesy of A. W. Forrest.)

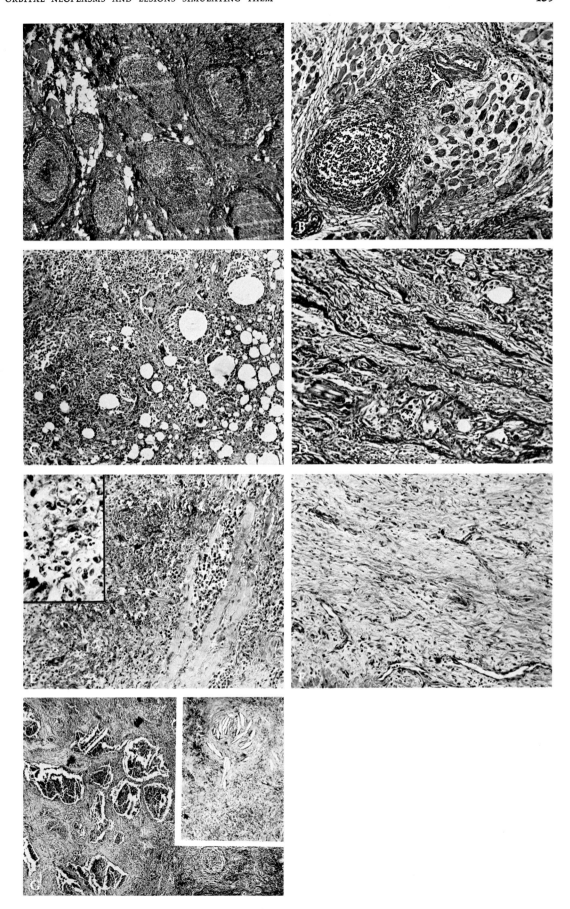

In my opinion, shared by others,[2,11] an appreciable number of so-called pseudo-tumors of the orbit are manifestations of collagen disease.

In a biopsy study of nonspecific orbital granulomas from our pathology laboratory,[37] the lesions were divided into five morphologic groups:

1. Lesions with formation of lymph follicles a prominent feature (Fig. 17–5A)
2. Lesions with focal and perivascular lymphocytic accumulations a prominent feature, usually with muscle involvement (Fig. 17–5B)
3. Lesions with chronic, widely diffused inflammation: with minimal tissue reaction (Fig. 17–5C), with old fibrous scarring (Fig. 17–5D), and with a significant number of polymorphonuclear leukocytes (Fig. 17–5E)
4. Lesions characterized essentially by an early fibrous scar and little inflammation (Fig. 17–5F)
5. Lesions with evidence of inflammation from a preexisting hemangioma or vascular anomaly (Fig. 17–5G)

Regarding lesions with focal and perivascular lymphocytic accumulations (group 2), chronic granuloma in some instances appears to originate in one or more of the extraocular muscles. Diplopia, the first symptom in about 25% of cases reported in the literature, often appears before the exophthalmos. Striated muscle is commonly found in the biopsy specimen. Cases of endocrine ophthalmopathy may fall into this group, as well as cases of chronic orbital myositis.

Regarding lesions interpreted as inflammation from a preexisting vascular lesion (group 5), three cases of this type require elucidation. Microscopic examination revealed endothelium-lined spaces associated with an extensive inflammatory reaction. Erythrocytes as well as phagocytosed hematogenous pigment and cholesterol slits indicated that the hemorrhagic aspect was prominent. A pathologic report on one patient showed that a cavernous hemangioma had been excised years earlier. Another patient had a long history of dilated and varicosed vessels of the lid, associated with repeated conjunctival hemorrhages. More varices, which could have caused frequent hemorrhage, were noted in the orbit after enucleation.

In a review of 16 cases of orbital granuloma that did not fit into a specific etiologic group,[52] the author found that the patients had exophthalmos associated with external ophthalmoplegia. Rapid visual loss was sometimes noted after an orbital exploration (the trigeminal nerve was affected in half the patients). He believed that these cases represented mild to fatal forms of collagen vascular disease. Because of possible visual loss following biopsy, he advised initial treatment by corticosteroids, reserving biopsy for cases where this treatment failed. While agreeing that orbital pseudotumors do not respond well to surgery, I feel that biopsy is required, especially if a neoplasm is suspected.

Necrotizing and Occlusive Angiitis

This disease group, characterized by a fibrinoid necrosis affecting the arteries, is often associated with a granulomatous tumefaction containing polymorphonuclear epithelioid and giant cells as well as eosinophils. Some features suggest an allergic diathesis triggered by many types of allergen. Included in this group of collagen diseases are Wegener's granulomatosis, midline lethal granuloma, dermatomyositis, temporal arteritis, and periarteritis nodosa. In an unusual case of pseudotumor, the only initial symptom was severe involvement of the left orbit in a 61-year-old man. When enucleation was performed 14 years later, the final diagnosis was periarteritis nodosa with a superimposed hypersensitivity angiitis.[94] An ocular or orbital lesion may be the first or only manifestation of the disease.[13,34,95] In a review of 100 cases of midline lethal granuloma,[26] there was ocular or orbital involvement in 42%.

ENDOCRINE OPHTHALMOPATHY

Endocrine ophthalmopathy, which is thought to be caused by a derangement of the pituitary-thyroid axis, is the commonest cause of unilateral proptosis. The most satisfactory explanation of the pathogenesis seems to be the presence in orbital tissues of autoimmune globulin, which promotes the synthesis of mucopolysaccharides, leading to edema and increased orbital pressure through osmosis.[58]

Lid retraction and lid lag are orbital manifestations of the mildest form of thyroid disease; lid fullness and conjunctival congestion represent a more advanced stage, while the very severe form is characterized by chemosis, proptosis, and disturbances of motility.[31] There is no consistent relationship between the severity of ocular symptoms and the stage of thyroid activity. However, the mild form of thyroid ophthalmopathy (thyrotoxic or noninfiltrative) almost invariably occurs with some degree of hyperthyroidism, whereas in the severe form (thyrotropic or infiltrative), thyroid activity may be increased, normal, or decreased. If the imbalance is brought under control too rapidly, thyrotoxicosis may result, followed by development or progression of the infiltrative ophthalmopathy. Eye manifestations of this disease are frequently associated with an emotional crisis. I believe that perseverance in questioning the patient may reveal something in his emotional background that preceded the onset.

When conventional tests (total thyroxine, radioactive iodine uptake, and serum cholesterol level) fail to reveal a dysfunction of the thyroid gland, the more sensitive Werner test is useful to determine suppression of radioactive iodine uptake after one week of oral triiodothyronine administration.[96]

Endocrine ophthalmopathy is always bilateral, although its exophthalmic component in the early stages is often unilateral. It has been pointed out[46] that the globe in all normal subjects sinks back when they are recumbent, resulting in exophthalmometric readings 1 to 3 mm lower than in the upright position. This author described four cases in which a postural difference was absent in the unaffected eye in patients with unilateral exophthalmos due to endocrine disturbance but present in patients with unilateral orbital tumor, and suggested that the method may be useful in differential diagnosis, to avoid unnecessary surgery in cases of endocrine exophthalmos. An increase in intraocular pressure during the upward gaze is also characteristic of endocrine ophthalmopathy because of the tethering effect of the inferior rectus muscle.

Intermittent exophthalmos due to an orbital varix has been reported in a 21-year-old woman after labor.[1] Intermittent exophthalmos and persistent headache in a 15-year-old girl with a congenital varix of the forehead and inferior orbital vein subsided after excision of the varix.[80]

When the differential diagnosis between an orbital tumor and unilateral endocrine ophthalmopathy proves difficult and an immediate decision must be made, the diagnosis can usually be confirmed by exploration through an external canthotomy. The orbit is first palpated to rule out a tumor, and then the extraocular muscles are palpated. If one or more muscles are enlarged, biopsy tissue can be taken. If the lacrimal gland is enlarged, a biopsy should be obtained because it may have the same pathology as the muscle.

Thyroid antibody tests may help to screen dysthyroid patients.[35] If the results are positive, further studies of thyroid function can be carried out; if negative, the patients can have an additional work-up for expanding lesions of the orbit. On the premise that we are dealing with an autoimmune disease, prednisone in immunosuppressive doses of 120–140 mg daily has been recommended.[97]

Orbital decompression, which may be indicated when the cornea is threatened from exposure, can be achieved by resecting the lateral wall of the orbit (temporal fossa), the orbital roof (anterior cranial cavity), the orbital floor (antrum), or the nasal wall of the orbit (ethmoids).[38] If secondary glaucoma from myopathy of the extraocular muscles becomes a real concern, it can usually be controlled by orbital decompression.

Endocrine ophthalmopathy seems to be associated with an elevated titer of long-acting thyroid stimulator (LATS), also known as thyroid-stimulating antibody (TSA).

Of the 37 cases of endocrine ophthalmopathy mentioned in the last edition of this book, a definite diagnosis was made in 28 by clinical evaluation. Only 8 of these patients had detectable abnormal thyroid function, of whom 3 had undergone thyroid surgery. In the other 20 cases, a presumptive diagnosis was made on the basis of eye findings only. Orbital surgery was carried out in 9 patients, as the possibility of an orbital tumor could not be ignored. Three of them had papilledema or a significant visual loss or both, 2 were thought to have retinal striae, and a palpable mass in one turned out to be a thyrotropic dacryoadenitis. Biopsy of an extraocular muscle revealed the diagnosis in 5 of the 9 cases, and markedly thickened extraocular muscles indicated the diagnosis without biopsy in the other 4.

EXOPHTHALMOS FROM A LESION IN A SINUS OR THE NASOPHARYNX

Exophthalmos may be due to tumor, inflammation, or granuloma primary in the sinuses. In our series, the antrum was the most common primary site for tumors because this sinus is most commonly affected by cancer. Involvement of the ethmoids leads to the highest incidence of exophthalmos because only the thin bony lamina papyracea separates the ethmoid from the orbit, and ethmoidal cancer is frequently associated with an infection that at times produces an orbital cellulitis.

Tumors of the frontal sinus sometimes reach the orbit, but more often mucoceles stemming from the frontal sinus cause a tumor mass that may be confused with a neoplasm. This is especially likely if the periosteum over the mucocele produces a layer of bone and simulates a solid tumor such as an osteoma, which occurred in over one-third of the cases in one series.[15] Mucoceles seldom produce a pronounced exophthalmos.

Tumors of the nasopharynx may also reach the orbit and produce exophthalmos. The primary site is usually the posterior wall—near the nasopharyngeal tonsil and its lateral extension into the pharyngeal recess—or, less frequently, the lateral wall. Nasopharyngeal tumors may reach the orbit by extension through the foramen lacerum and thence via the carotid groove along the internal carotid artery to the superior orbital fissure.[65]

In the early stages there may be no clinical sign of the tumor's presence. Because of difficulties in examining the primary site adequately, the first indication may be an eye symptom. When the primary site is still quite small, even small enough to be overlooked (especially when in the fossa of Rosenmüller), the tumor may already have reached the orbit and produced ocular symptoms. The patient therefore may first consult an ophthalmologist, who should keep in mind the possibility of latent tumors of the nose and throat. The juvenile nasopharyngeal angiofibroma mentioned in our series reached the orbit, caused a pronounced exophthalmos, and reduced the vision markedly.

In a combined Scandinavian–British series of 673 patients with malignant nasopharyngeal tumors,[44] over one third showed neuro-ophthalmic signs and symptoms, usually in the nature of ophthalmoplegia of the third, fourth, and sixth cranial nerves and a trigeminal neuralgia (cavernous sinus or superior orbital fissure syndrome). The majority of these patients were between 40 and 60 years of age, and twice as many males were affected. Tumor extension through the superior orbital fissure to the orbit may cause dysfunction of the optic nerve from toxic or pressure effects.

SPECIFIC INFLAMMATIONS OF THE ORBIT

Sarcoidosis of the orbit, which affects especially the lacrimal gland, may manifest itself as a palpable unilateral mass, producing some degree of proptosis as well as ptosis. Other inflammatory conditions of the orbit at times confused with a neoplasm are syphilitic gummas and tuberculomas. A tuberculous cold abscess in the orbit of a 4-year-old boy has been reported.[66] In one instance a localized orbital granuloma was caused by impregnation of talc in the wound during a squint operation 14 years earlier.[64] Also, granulomas may develop from foreign bodies such as wood, stubble, or metal that become embedded in the orbit unsuspected by the patient. An orbital granuloma resulted from injection of a lipid-based contrast medium for orbitography instead of a water-soluble medium.[33]

Infesting Agents

Larval granulomas due to *Toxocara canis* and also to *Cysticercus cellulosae* are discussed in the differential diagnosis of retinoblastoma (Ch. 3). Although no cases of *Toxocara canis* with orbital involvement have been found in the literature, I feel that they do occur. Three cases believed to belong in this group have not been added to our series because the diagnosis was presumptive. Among the infesting agents reported to cause orbital granuloma are *Cysticercus, Echinococcus,* and *Pasteurella tularensis.*

The orbit, including the eye muscles, and the eyeball may be affected by cysticercosis, resulting from ingestion of the ova of *Taenia solium.* The larva of this organism was found in a reddish-brown cystic mass in the lower fornix; serial sections showed the scolex with its suckers and hooklets.[4] The orbit is fairly often affected by *Taenia granulosa,* especially in countries where sheep-raising is extensive and there are many dogs.

The larva of *Hypoderma bovis* deposited in the orbit in a 13-year-old girl led to cellulitis.[83] In three reported cases of hydatid cyst of the orbit, the laboratory tests for hydatid disease were negative.[6] The authors suggested that orbital echinococcosis should be considered in cases of proptosis especially in countries where the disease is endemic. Since the enactment of strict laws governing meat inspection, this disease, common in the nineteenth century, is rarely seen. One such case was reported in Belgium.[18]

VASCULAR LESIONS

In a review of 67 patients with vascular anomalies of the orbit, 31 were considered to be congenital primary varices.[102] Contrast radiology was helpful in the diagnosis. The anomalies were of two main types: primary, due to a congenital venous malformation, and secondary, due to an arteriovenous shunt either intracranially or within the orbit.

An arteriovenous aneurysm between the internal carotid artery and the cavernous sinus may produce a pulsating exophthalmos. This usually results from trauma but may be idiopathic, particularly in elderly women. An orbital pulsation and a bruit are often present; when neither is found the condition may be confused with a neoplasm, usually a hemangioma. In a report on the ocular findings in 17 cases of carotid–cavernous sinus fistula,[48] the preferred treatment was combined cervical and intracranial internal carotid artery ligation with clipping of the ophthalmic artery. In rare cases, carotid-cavernous sinus fistula is associated with contralateral exophthalmos. The absence of ipsilateral exophthalmos may be due to a thrombus in the superior ophthalmic vein blocking the flow to orbital veins.[22]

A possible aneurysm of the ophthalmic artery or the internal carotid artery must be considered. In addition to exophthalmos, pain and oculomotor paralysis are common symptoms. Such lesions occur from the second to the sixth decade of life. In older patients, the aneurysm may be due to arteriosclerosis, but in younger people a congenital condition or an inflammatory process may be responsible. X rays may show early erosion of the sides of the sphenoid bone and sella turcica; pressure atrophy of the bone under the optic canal; enlargement of the superior orbital fissure; and, later, erosion and destruction of the bone of the optic canal. The clinical course progresses steadily with gradual and extensive destruction of the bone of the lateral orbital wall and increasing exophthalmos.

An idiopathic thrombophlebitis of the orbital veins may give a clinical picture suggesting an expanding neoplastic process.[103]

A patient with exophthalmos consulted me and after the usual tests my diagnosis was probable vascular abnormalities. A year later she had a subarachnoid hemorrhage from which she recovered with minimal hemiparesis. A neurosurgeon[79] successfully removed a congenital intracerebral arteriovenous malformation.

Hemorrhage

Unilateral exophthalmos may develop from hemorrhage in the orbit; in infants the hemorrhage may be caused by scurvy and in adults be either spontaneous or caused by trauma. When observed immediately after the injury the cause is usually obvious, but the hematoma formation may be delayed in the orbit as well as in the brain. Since the resulting exophthalmos is not directly related to the trauma, these delayed hematomas are often difficult to distinguish from neoplasms. When the trauma is primarily to the thorax instead of the head, strong compression of the thorax from this cause, as well as from coughing, vomiting or asphyxiation, may increase the pressure in the jugular veins. As these have no valves, the unobstructed pressure is transmitted to vessels of the skull where an orbital hemorrhage may ensue.

Orbital hematomas, so-called blood cysts, are most often sequelae of lymphangiomas, some of them previously unrecognized. Of two reported cases, one simulated a malignant tumor and the other extended into the cranium through the superior orbital fissure.[68] Also, orbital blood cysts may result from traumatic fat necrosis.

Subdural hematomas, encountered usually in neurologic practice, may cause unilateral exophthalmos. Among four reported cases of relapsing juvenile chronic subdural hematoma, three were of the middle fossa, of which two caused exophthalmos. The exophthalmos developed because of the orbit's decreased capacity, due to encroachment of the enlarged middle cranial fossa on the lateral orbital wall.[28] Demonstrable enlargement of the middle fossa in skull x rays is indicative of subtemporal subdural hematoma.[73]

MISCELLANEOUS ORBITAL LESIONS

Cholesteatomas

Cholesteatomas, or cholesterol-containing granulomas of the orbit, represent a heterogeneous group. The lesion cannot be specifically identified by the presence of cholesterol in a granuloma because this combination may occur in response to different processes. Some lesions represent dermoid or epidermoid cysts, so that biopsy from the wall of the lesion is imperative (see Ch. 15, Hamartomas, Progonomas, Choristomas, Miscellaneous Tumors and Tumefactions). Other lesions may represent eosinophilic granulomas or early Hand-Schüller-Christian disease. This was particularly true of cases in which the unilateral proptosis and diplopia were due to a process involving the frontoorbital bones.[71] The x rays showed characteristic osteolytic lesions of the lateral portion of the supraorbital ridge. Still other cholesterol-containing granulomas may result from orbital hematomas (blood cysts) caused basically by a lymphangioma or traumatic fat necrosis. A primary cholesteatoma of the orbit and cranial cavity producing exophthalmos has been described.[41]

Mixed Neurogenic Tumors

A mixed neurogenic tumor of the orbit may arise from a congenital rest or malformation such as an encephalocelelike protrusion of the brain which occurs during embryonic life, becomes partially or entirely separated, and develops independently in the orbit. These rests also occur at the base of the nose near the lacrimal fossa. Related lesions, encephalocele and meningocele, are discussed later.

Tumors from these ectopic brain rests contain bipotential cells. They may develop along the neuroblastic series, leading to neuroepitheliomatous tumors or even to malignant tumors such as neuroblastoma (retinoblastoma) and medulloblastoma. They more frequently develop along the spongioblastic series, however, in which case the majority resemble gliomas.

A number of primary mixed tumors of the orbit have appeared in the literature, and several have been seen here at the Eye Institute. They invariably affect children from 3 months to 6 years of age. A reported case in a 58-year-old woman is an exception.[14] Since ganglion cells were prominent in some of the tumors described, the question arises whether they could have originated in the ciliary ganglion. The tumor resembles a retinoblastoma if composed of anaplastic neuroblasts.[77]

Congenital Coloboma Cysts of the Orbit (Meningocele and Encephalocele)

At the 1957 meeting of the Verhoeff Society, I reported a case in which proptosis of the right eye since birth in a 14-month-old boy was believed to be due to a tumor of the optic nerve. Exploration through a Krönlein approach revealed that the large tumor was a congenital neurogenic rest (posterior encephalocele). It was generally agreed to have arisen from congenital ectopic brain tissue and to have reached the orbit through the sphenoidal fissure, shown by x rays to be enlarged.

Faulty closure of the fetal fissure may cause a wide range of ocular defects—from simple colobomas to craterlike holes of the disc (*Grubenbildung*), to cysts occurring anywhere from the posterior pole of the eye to the midbrain. The affected side often shows exophthalmos, microphthalmos, cryptophthalmos or anophthalmos, and other lesser congenital anomalies may be observed in the fellow eye. The basic developmental aberration, which manifests itself in various ways, has various designations, *e.g.*, coloboma cyst, meningocele, encephalocele, retinocele, and colobomatous orbitopalpebral cyst. The term *meningoencephalocystocele* implies ectopic brain and meninges in the apex of the orbit, which some investigators believe has no connection with the brain.[12] However, their cases seem to be related to a congenital neurogenic rest associated with a meningoencephalocele. In one reported case, a unilateral pulsating exophthalmos was due to a meningoencephalocele of the greater and lesser wings of the sphenoid and of the posterior portion of the orbital roof.[10]

It has been suggested that these lesions develop because the inner retinal layer of the optic cup grows more rapidly than the outer layer. The redundant retinal tissue becomes everted when normal fusion of the fetal fissure is delayed beyond the 11 mm stage. Virtually all coloboma cysts are associated with some degree of microphthalmos. In a review of 26 cases,[17] 5 were unilateral congenital orbital cysts with microphthalmos as the only associated defect. The only exception to my knowledge is a case in which the affected eye was of normal size, and a small coloboma was present only on the optic disc.[23]

In the embryonic formation of the bony orbit there may be gaps permitting cranioorbital herniations. Also, herniations may occur through natural openings and these defects may be anterior or posterior. The more common anterior type is located near the base of the nose. A sealed-off encephalocele presented as a mucocele of the ethmoid sinus in a 62-year-old woman; sequestered brain tissue was found in the sinus at operation.[59] The posterior type tends to occur in a natural opening such as the optic foramen or the superior orbital fissure. A bilateral anterior orbital meningoencephalocele in a 5-year-old girl has been described.[24]

The lesion usually appears in infants and children and very rarely in adults. It is frequently recognized because of a slowly progressive proptosis which sometimes pulsates. The diagnosis can usually be established by x ray.

A congenital meningoencephalocele must not be confused with orbital bone defects due to neurofibromas, which also may cause unilateral exophthalmos with pulsation. Some of these lesions are related to the primary orbital gliomas (see Ch. 4, Glioma of the Optic Nerve, Retina, and Orbit), which arise from partially or totally sequestered embryonic brain tissue persisting at the site of one of the several types of defects of the orbital wall previously mentioned. The lesions may involve structures outside of the orbit, in which case they should be treated by the neurosurgeon. Surgery is hazardous, however, and should be avoided if possible. A successfully treated case has been reported.[69]

Colobomatous cysts or retinoceles confined to the orbit are in the domain of the ophthalmic surgeon. These lesions at times fill the orbit, concealing the eye, which may be extremely small or rudimentary. They adhere closely to the optic nerve and should be dissected carefully, leaving the nerve and any eye present, no matter how microphthalmic.

A patient whom I treated had such a huge coloboma cyst of the orbit that the eye was almost unrecognizable. The cyst was dissected *in toto* from the small rudimentary eye and the optic nerve. The fellow eye was also microphthalmic but to a lesser degree. In later years the extremely small eye associated with the cyst proved to be the more useful one, permitting the patient to attend school with some visual aid. This case stresses the importance of saving any eye when the cyst is excised, however functionless or disfiguring it may seem.

The familial incidence of colobomatous orbitopalpebral cyst in natives of South Tunisia has been reported.[63] The authors, who cited four cases, had found several ocular anomalies in relatives of the probands and in their forebears up to the third generation.

Amyloid

In primary systemic amyloidosis involving the eye and adnexa, smooth, confluent, waxy yellow papules, nodules and masses as well as purpuric spots are found in the skin of the lids, the conjunctiva, and the orbit (Fig. 17–6). The ophthalmic lesions are often the

FIG. 17–6. Amyloid degeneration of the conjunctiva and orbit. A 38-year-old woman had noted redness of the right eye and a foreign-body sensation for two years. Several pathologists confirmed the clinical diagnosis of amyloid degeneration microscopically, with the aid of special staining. The translucent nodular appearance, particularly marked in the caruncle, is typical of this disease.

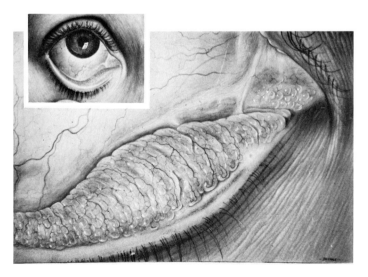

first clue to diagnosis of this systemic disease.[20] A unilateral primary subconjunctival amyloid tumor was found encircling the limbal and perilimbal area,[49] and a bilateral, secondary amyloid infiltration affected these same areas in an Indian woman with chronic trachoma.[7] A type of secondary amyloidosis is associated with chronic infectious processes and arthritis.

The waxy infiltrations consist of glycoproteins produced by cells of the reticuloendothelial system and are related to gamma globulins, Bence-Jones protein and other myeloma proteins.[78] As the blood vessel walls become infiltrated, systemic hemorrhagic vascular disease may develop almost anywhere in the body, including the retinal vessels. Amyloid may also infiltrate the vitreous, particularly in the familial form. In any case of amyloidosis the possibility of myeloma and perhaps a familial tendency must be considered, as well as association with systemic hemorrhagic vascular disease in the viscera or in the central nervous system.

Progressive exophthalmos results from an expanding lesion in the orbit. Usually some yellow infiltrate or waxy nodules in the skin or conjunctiva suggest the diagnosis. However, in some reported cases, progressive unilateral exophthalmos was present over a period of years before a biopsy revealed amyloidosis as the cause.[42,54,78]

There is no effective treatment for amyloidosis. When the tumefactions are removed surgically they gradually recur.

Necrosis of Uveal Melanomas

Necrotic malignant melanomas of the uvea may lead to exophthalmos by producing a severe inflammatory reaction with endophthalmitis and panophthalmitis. In these cases the diagnosis is presumptive, as the interior of the eye cannot be visualized. The condition is suggested in an eye that has been blind for some time prior to the inflammation. I saw one such case in which the intraocular melanoma had become completely necrotic and had set up a severe orbital inflammation associated with diffusion of tumor tissue throughout the orbit. Some of the tumor tissue was also recovered in the antrum.

Sclerosing Lipogranuloma

This lesion represents a granulomatous reaction to fat necrosis which sometimes follows trauma, although in many cases the cause is unknown.

One case in our series presented as a localized tumorlike mass in the lower lid which developed gradually over a one-year period in a 54-year-old man (Fig. 17–7). There was no history of trauma, and the cause of the spontaneous growth was unknown. Verhoeff concurred in the biopsy diagnosis of fat necrosis. Clinically, the mass was hard, freely movable, and not attached to the underlying structures or to the bone.

One case in a series of 14 was in the orbit and followed definite trauma;[88] there was no history of trauma in another case,[29] and in still another, the lesion developed after recurrent abscesses of the eyelids.[74]

Giant-Cell Tumor of the Tendon Sheath

Some authorities believe that a giant-cell tumor of the tendon sheath is a true neoplasm, whereas others consider it a granulomatous manifestation. I have encountered one such orbital lesion which was verified by Stout.

Giant-Cell Tumor of Bone

This controversial lesion is variously considered to be a true neoplasm, a granuloma, or a sequela of trauma. The lesion is usually located in the femur, tibia or radius, but about 10% are found in the head bones; the orbit may be involved secondarily.

Rare Intracranial Lesions

Hydrocephalus, some intracranial vascular lesions and, as previously mentioned, neurofibromatosis may produce changes in the bony orbital roof that lead to either herniation of the brain or sagging of the roof. Orbital volume is thus decreased, and exophthalmos may result. In these situations, the brain pulsations may be transmitted to the orbit.

NONNEOPLASTIC DISEASES OF BONE

Fibrous dysplasia (see Ch. 11, Connective Tissue and Other Mesenchymal Tumors) and its allied and simulating lesions may lead to osteosarcomas (Fig. 17–8). When the fibrous dysplasia is well localized (Fig. 17–9) (monostotic) and confined to the supraorbital plate, surgical excision may be indicated. In some instances orbital decompression and de-

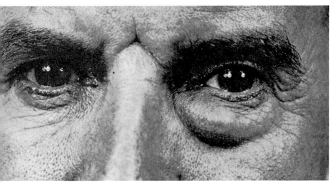
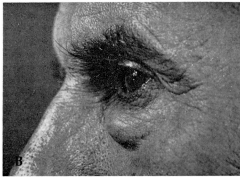

FIG. 17–7. Sclerosing lipogranuloma. **A.** Front view. **B.** Side view. **C.** Excised mass.

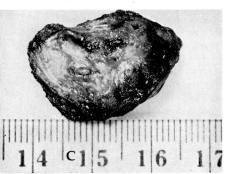

FIG. 17–9. Fibrous dysplasia of bone. Proptosis of the left eye had increased gradually over a three-month period in a 5-year-old girl. She had no symptoms and examination revealed no pathologic condition of either eye. Findings in a pediatric examination were normal except for the proptosis. X rays revealed an extensively thickened and sclerosed left side of the skull, with the upper maxilla, frontal squamosa, orbital plates, and sphenoid body and wings affected. Both maxillary sinuses, the left ethmoid, the frontal, and both sphenoid sinuses were opaque. One year later the clinical and x-ray findings were unchanged.

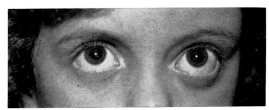

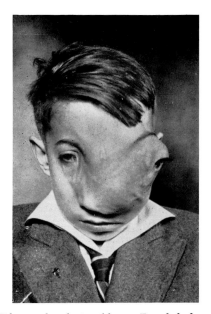

FIG. 17–8. Fibrous dysplasia of bone. Exophthalmos of the left eye was diagnosed as fibrous dysplasia when the patient was 3 years old. It progressed gradually until he died at age 16. Although not confirmed by biopsy, osteogenic sarcoma probably developed and proved fatal.

roofing of the optic foramen have proved beneficial.[55]

MISCELLANEOUS CONDITIONS

Some authorities have described an extremely rare serous orbital cyst originating in the bursa either between the tendon of the superior oblique muscle and the trochlea or between the levator muscle of the upper eyelid and the superior rectus muscle. Mesotheliomas or synoviomas which arise from serous surfaces could conceivably arise from Tenon's capsule in the orbit. Another extremely rare lesion, particularly in the United States, is a localized orbital lesion produced by a hydatid cyst.

Aneurysmal bone cysts of the orbital wall may cause exophthalmos.[36,56,86] They are painless, benign, and curable by incomplete excision. X-ray examination is noncontributory, and diagnosis rests upon biopsy.

DIAGNOSTIC AIDS

X RAYS

Various changes that occur in exophthalmos may be noted on x-ray films. They include calcium or bone formation, erosion or destruction of bony landmarks, hyperostosis, fossa formation, enlargement of the orbit, and changes in the optic canal.

Calcium or Bone Formation

When x rays are viewed in the stereoscope, any discrete area of increased density within the orbital cavity is apparent. Such densities may be due to an osteoma extending into the orbit from the paranasal sinuses, calcium in the wall of a mucocele in the orbit, or at times proliferation of fibrous dysplasia of bone.

Erosion or Destruction of Bony Landmarks

This finding should arouse suspicion. Carcinomas arising in the paranasal sinuses may involve the orbit after breaching the bony wall. Lacrimal gland tumors, as well as the granulomatous lesions of multiple myeloma and of the various histiocytoses, may cause destruction of adjacent bone. Sometimes it is impossible to determine whether a bone defect is due to invasion of the bone or to

pressure erosion. Other lesions that at times affect the bone in one of these ways are hemangiomas, lymphangiomas, malignant lymphomas, hemangiopericytomas, neurilemomas, rhabdomyosarcomas, and neuroblastomas.

Hyperostosis

Next to calcium or bone formation, increased density of an orbital bone is perhaps easiest to recognize, particularly if the two orbits can be compared. The mottled hyperostosis of meningioma is almost diagnostic, as is the hyperostosis in the lacrimal gland region associated with adenoid cystic carcinoma. Paget's disease of bone and other fibrous dys-

---

FIG. 17–10. X rays of orbits containing various ▶ types of neoplasms. **A.** Hemangioma of the right orbit which is markedly enlarged, evidently from increased intraorbital pressure. Soft-tissue density is also increased. Four concretions represent ossification or calcification in the hemangiomatous tissue. **B.** Mixed tumor of the lacrimal gland, with the right orbit showing increased density and porosity of the bony lacrimal gland fossa. The markings of the orbital roof are obscured in the outer half. **C.** Dermoid of the left orbit which caused a gross defect in the roof, characterized by loss of substance, increased radiolucency, clean-cut margins, and increased density of bone around the margin. The lesion is adjacent to, but does not communicate with, the frontal sinus. **D.** Metastatic sympathicoblastoma of the left orbit which is enlarged and shows characteristic erosion of the temporal line. **E.** Meningioma of the sphenoid ridge with orbital extension, and hyperostosis of the wings of the sphenoid bone and the lateral wall of the orbit. The optic canal and the superior orbital fissure are involved in the process. A benign osteoma of the left frontal sinus was unrelated to the meningioma. **F.** Neurofibromatosis of the right orbit from which the lateral wall and the posterior portion of the roof are absent. There are no normal shadows of the bone. These changes indicate a communication between the orbit and the cranial cavity; the cranial pulsations were transmitted directly to the orbital contents. **G.** Neurofibromatosis of the left orbit, in which the deformity and an increase in soft-tissue density were due to a mass of tumor tissue in the upper lid. **H.** In the left orbit, the optic canal is normal, and in the right it is markedly enlarged.

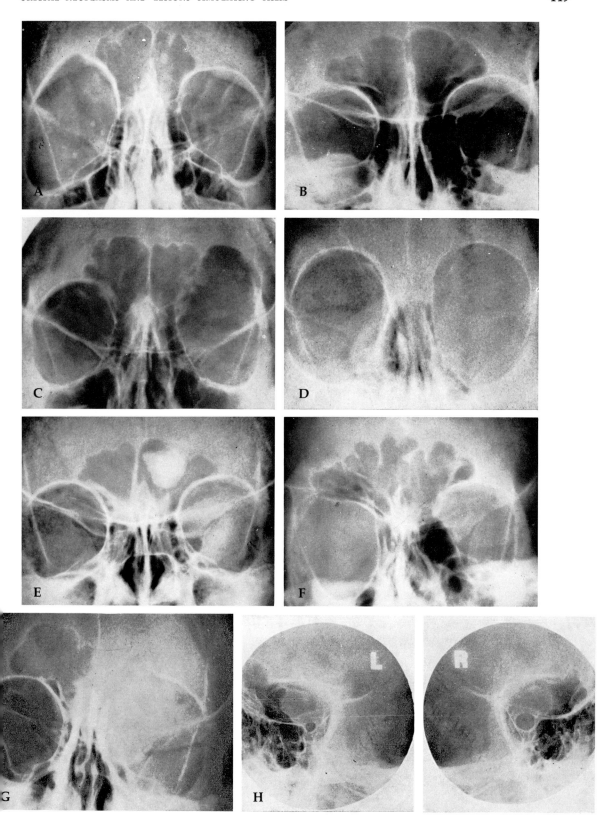

plasias often show hyperostosis, although a possible osteitis secondary to infection should not be overlooked in such cases. If the facial bones are involved, osteochondrosarcoma should be suspected.

Fossa Formation

This term usually refers to a smooth, rounded hollow lined with cortical bone, frequently produced by a dermoid cyst but sometimes by a benign mixed tumor of the lacrimal gland or a congenital rest that has long laid adjacent to bone.

Enlargement of the Orbit

In young patients an intraorbital mass often causes an increase in size of the orbit. The clinical history, considered with the patient's age and the x-ray findings, may suggest how long the process has been present. Any tumor can cause enlargement of the orbit, but the most common are hemangiomas and lymphangiomas. Soft-tissue infiltration, as in thyroid disease or chronic orbital granuloma, may also cause enlargement. Sometimes, e.g., in a case of mucocele from the paranasal sinuses or a neurofibromatosis, a large dehiscence in the orbital wall is associated with orbital enlargement. In the event of a communication between the orbit and the cranial cavity, there is often a pulsating exophthalmos. An aneurysm of the internal carotid artery may cause a posterior dehiscence, with or without enlargement of the orbit.

Optic Canal

Unilateral enlargement of the optic canal with associated clinical findings can confirm the diagnosis of glioma of the optic nerve. If both canals are enlarged, the glioma is probably continuous across the chiasm. The optic canal may be enlarged in neurofibromatosis with or without a glioma being present. The canal may be eroded if there is an aneurysm of the internal carotid artery.

Illustrations typifying these x-ray changes appear in Figure 17–10.

OTHER DIAGNOSTIC AIDS

Orbital pneumography, opaque contrast media, and angiography may be helpful adjuncts in diagnosis. Thermographic examina-

tion of 300 ophthalmic patients was reported to aid in identification of various conditions, particularly in eyes with opaque media.[45]

While electron microscopy has proved helpful in identifying orbital tumors otherwise difficult to classify,[51] it does not distinguish between benign and malignant lesions. See section Electron Microscopy of Tumors of the Eye and Ocular Adnexa, by Ramon L. Font, in Chapter 12. See also sections Ultrasonic Evaluation of Ocular and Orbital Tumors, by D. Jackson Coleman; Radiotherapy of Ocular and Orbital Tumors, by Patricia Tretter; and Special Radiodiagnostic Studies of the Orbit, Including Computerized Tomography, by Stephen L. Trokel, in Chapter 12.

TREATMENT OF ORBITAL NEOPLASMS AND SIMULATING LESIONS

In cases where an orbital mass is palpable, a Krönlein operation is usually indicated. However, it may be advisable to explore the orbit before this decision is made. Satisfactory appraisal is facilitated by a wide canthotomy and severing of the external canthal ligament. The index finger can then gain access to the orbit for palpation. In most instances a simple canthotomy is inadequate, and a resection of the lateral orbital wall is indicated. To proceed with the Krönlein operation requires extension of the canthotomy incision. Such an exploration helps the surgeon decide whether to try to remove the entire mass or obtain biopsy tissue.

In some instances of unilateral exophthalmos there are no positive findings. The innumerable nonneoplastic lesions that can cause this condition must be considered. When x rays show an increase in soft-tissue density or indicate increased orbital pressure, or both, some type of neoplasm must be seriously suspected even though patients with nonneoplastic disease can have similar findings.

It must be borne in mind that paralysis of one of the rectus muscles can itself produce an exophthalmos of as much as 2 mm. If an expanding lesion is associated with dysfunction of a rectus muscle, the ensuing proptosis is out of proportion to the size and extent of the offending lesion. In cases with no positive findings, or even with indeterminate findings, watchful waiting is often advisable.

CATEGORIES OF EXPANDING ORBITAL LESIONS

Table 17–1 shows that the large majority of primary expanding orbital lesions come under relatively few headings. Treatment of most of them is described in the respective separate chapters; granuloma (pseudotumor) and endocrine ophthalmopathy will be discussed here.

It is obvious that the diagnosis in each instance must be established before the treatment can be outlined and the prognosis considered. In most cases biopsy tissue must be removed; many experts in cancer treatment believe that taking a biopsy does not affect the prognosis adversely. The one exception is potentially malignant encapsulated tumors, as exemplified by epithelial tumors of the lacrimal gland. Well-encapsulated, accessible lesions may be excised without a preliminary biopsy.

Granuloma (Pseudotumor)

The most important step in management of such a lesion is to establish the correct diagnosis, preventing unnecessary and sometimes radical surgery when it is mistaken for a neoplasm. Without treatment the lesion may regress in time, even to the point of enophthalmos. In some instances regression seems to be hastened by corticosteroids. Also, irradiation may be effective, probably by dissipating the lymphocytic elements of the lesion and producing atresia of the vascular elements.

If a biopsy is performed it should be done with adequate surgical exposure, to avoid the possibility of hemorrhage becoming locked into the orbit and pushing the eye forward between the lids, thus leading to corneal ulceration and perforation with loss of the eye. Suturing the lid margins together and applying a firm pressure dressing may be additional safeguards.

If the vision is threatened through involvement of the optic nerve (due to pressure or some toxic effect), decompression by resection of the lateral wall of the orbit may be indicated.

Endocrine Ophthalmopathy

The management of endocrine ophthalmopathy falls mainly into the internist's province. Oral thyroid extract may be prescribed for patients with normal or low thyroid activity, but there is no definite evidence that this is helpful in treating the eye lesion. Regardless of therapy, the ophthalmopathy follows a fluctuating and unpredictable course, and generally tends to subside within 6 to 18 months.

It may be advisable to palpate the orbit through an external canthotomy when tests cannot confirm the diagnosis adequately; unilateral cases sometimes closely resemble expanding neoplastic lesions. If no tumor is present and the extraocular muscles are enlarged, the diagnosis can be established. Biopsy of an enlarged muscle may be advisable. If vision is jeopardized from corneal exposure or optic nerve damage, exploration can be carried out by resecting the lateral orbital wall (Krönlein) and removing the bone flap. This type of orbital decompression is effective only if the entire lateral wall is removed. Therefore, all of the wall posterior to the bone flap must be excised with a rongeur.

The author of a report on six cases of malignant exophthalmos operated upon by transantral orbital decompression considered the method "effective, simple and safe," though more successful in relieving proptosis than ocular muscle palsies.[91] In a follow-up study of 54 cases 1 to 20 years after decompression by this approach,[72] the author concluded that cosmetic restoration was facilitated without visual loss, corneal ulceration, or muscle paresis. The technique proved effective in a case of idiopathic malignant exophthalmos.[21]

The transmaxillary approach to the orbit, developed for decompression of malignant exophthalmos,[50] has been also advocated for removal of orbital tumors.[19]

Secondary glaucoma, which probably results from pressure of the enlarged extraocular muscles on the globe in Graves's disease, may be another indication for decompression of the orbit. Vision and appearance were improved in the majority of 17 patients treated for orbital decompression via the pterion.[4a]

The residual blemish of exophthalmos may be improved by a lateral tarsorrhaphy or by resecting the lateral wall of the orbit. The diplopia caused by limited upward movement of the eye, from splinting by the inferior rectus muscle, may be corrected in the static stage of the disease by recession of the inferior rectus muscle.

A procedure has been suggested for advancing lower eyelids to correct drooping in cases of exophthalmos.[76]

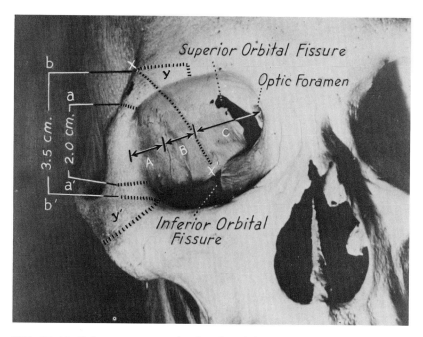

FIG. 17–11. Relevant anatomic landmarks of the bony orbit. *b-b'*—full resection of the lateral wall of the right orbit. *a-a'*—average resection of the orbital wall. *y*—extended lateral orbitotomy of Wright and of Stallard. *y'*—extended lateral orbitotomy of Barrie Jones. *x-x'*—junction of the orbital and cranial cavities. Arrow at *A*—site where the lateral wall breaks during performance of the Krönlein operation. Arrow at *B*—lateral wall that must be removed by rongeurs. Arrow at *C*—area including the superior orbital fissure traversed by important structures which must be crossed to reach a tumor at the apex of the orbit. This requires operation by palpation without direct exposure. (A. B. Reese.[82])

It must be reemphasized that the decision regarding therapy of all orbital lesions should be made only after the diagnosis has been established. The many different lesions encountered call for widely varying treatment.

SURGICAL PROCEDURES

Anatomic landmarks of the bony orbit are shown in Figure 17–11.

BIOPSY

Orbital lesions frequently lie deep beneath normal tissue. Therefore, some blunt dissec-

tion in important structures may be required to obtain biopsy material. After an external canthotomy with severance of all fibers of the external canthal ligament, the orbit is palpated. If the lesion proves to be widespread, biopsy material can be removed. But if it seems to be localized and encapsulated, the skin incision can be extended to permit a resection of the lateral bony wall (Krönlein operation) in the hope of achieving total excision.

Great care should be taken in removing biopsy tissue in cases where chronic granulomas (pseudotumors) are suspected. Because of possible brisk bleeding, tissue should not be excised deep in the orbit through a small incision. If the hemorrhage is locked in the orbit, the eye can be lost from exposure of the cornea or from sudden and marked elevation of the intraorbital pressure. Therefore, the surgical exposure should be ample to prevent a hematoma. Orbital granulomas as a group do not respond well to surgery. The basic process, of whatever nature, may be aggravated, leading to complications. These seem to stem mainly from vascular changes leading to occlusion of blood vessels which may cause macular pathology.

Biopsy of epithelial tumors of the lacrimal gland may also be hazardous. Potentially malignant tumors, such as benign mixed tumors, are usually encapsulated, and opening the capsule may cause seeding of the tumor cells into normal tissue.

EXTERNAL CANTHOTOMY (TRANSCONJUNCTIVAL APPROACH)

Orbital lesions located temporal to or in the muscle funnel are sometimes successfully approached by the transconjunctival route. A wide canthotomy is performed, and the upper and lower lids are freed from their fascial attachments to the orbital margins and periosteum for some distance above and below. The external canthal ligament and orbital septa are severed along the orbital margin. The external rectus muscle can usually be reflected without being severed from its insertion in order to give ample access to the muscle cone.

The orbit can be thoroughly palpated and a small anteriorly located lesion excised, although the exploration is not as satisfactory if there is little or no exophthalmos. The orbit cannot be palpated in an infant or a child unless there is marked exophthalmos because of the small orbital volume.

EXCISION THROUGH THE LIDS

A small, well-localized lesion in the anterior part of the orbit can be approached through the skin or the conjunctiva of the upper or lower lid. Since the approach through the upper lid may jeopardize the levator muscle, causing some degree of ptosis, it is reserved for small superficial lesions.

An anterior approach to some tumors in the upper part of the orbit has been reported to minimize the risk of damaging the levator muscle.[8] The skin incision is concentric with the upper margin of the orbit. Along the orbital rim the periosteum is incised and separated from the bone over the anterior roof of the orbit. The cut edge of the periosteum is grasped with strong-toothed forceps and pulled forward along with the adherent tumor.

Another anterior approach has been advocated principally for removing tumors of the optic nerve.[30] An incision is made through the skin along the lower margin of the orbit. The section is carried through the orbicularis muscle and the orbital septum deep into the orbit. The eye is rotated sharply upward by inserting a traction suture through the episclera at a point corresponding to 6 o'clock. A

tumor of the optic nerve is thus everted forward and excised. The inferior rectus muscle may be detached and resutured but this procedure is not always necessary. Severance of the optic nerve is followed by marked fundal changes (Fig. 17–12).

LATERAL ORBITOTOMY

The majority of orbital lesions can be approached by resecting the lateral wall of the orbit. This is particularly true of those in the muscle cone and temporal to the globe. There is very little orbital space in which tumors can arise nasal to the muscle cone, which is fortunate as the space is virtually inaccessible for surgery.

Krönlein Operation

The anatomy concerned in the Krönlein operation is shown in Figure 17–13 and the steps

FIG. 17–12. Fundus three months after excision of a meningioma arising from the optic nerve sheaths. The optic nerve, posterior ciliary arteries, and nerves were severed during surgery and the globe was left *in situ*. Diffuse pigment changes had occurred particularly around and over the site of the disc; in this same area were two sites of retinitis proliferans. The blood vessels in some places appeared as white lines; white atrophic areas were noted in the periphery below. (Courtesy of T. H. Johnson.)

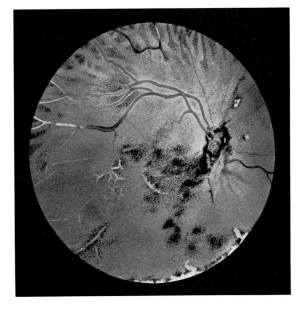

in the operation in Figure 17–14. A suture placed through the insertion of the external rectus muscle over the conjunctiva facilitates quick and easy identification of the muscle during surgery. The Berke incision extends horizontally from the external canthus for 5 cm or more, toward the upper level of the ear. It provides adequate exposure, and spectacles will conceal any visible operative incision. The upper and lower lids are freed from their fascial attachments, exposing the outer third of the orbital margin and the deep fascia covering the temporalis muscle. The external canthal ligament is severed. Its extensive attachments to the periosteum—for some distance above, below, and posteriorly—can be located and severed by putting the lids on a stretch. The lids can then be retracted completely, giving a wide exposure. The orbital septum is incised to provide sufficient space for palpation.

The surface of the aponeurosis of the temporalis muscle is a good cleavage plane, and the overlying skin and fascia are readily separated by blunt dissection except at the margin of the orbit, where scissors are needed. The lateral third of the margin is thus exposed.

The periosteum is incised with a knife along the lateral margin of the orbit and reflected from the lateral wall. A horizontal incision is then made in the periosteum. The upper and lower horizontal incisions are made in the bone with an oscillating saw. If this saw is not available, the bone can be incised through the thick orbital margin with

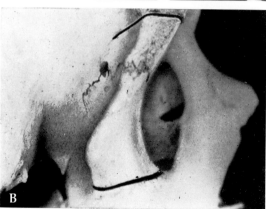

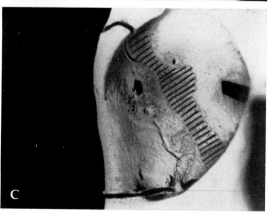

FIG. 17–13. Anatomy involved in the Krönlein operation. **A.** Horizontal section through orbits: (1) anterior thick part of the lateral orbital wall. (2) Anterior thin part of the lateral orbital wall adjacent to the temporal fossa. (3) Posterior thick part of the lateral orbital wall, formed by its junction with the lateral wall of the middle cranial fossa. (4) Posterior thin part of the lateral orbital wall, showing the orbital cavity in front and the cranial cavity behind. (5) Dehiscence in roof of the right orbit. (6) Roof of the right optic canal. (7) Temporal fossa (containing the temporal muscle in life). (8) Middle fossa of the cranial cavity (containing the temporal lobe of brain in life).

B. Right orbit viewed from the temporal side, showing position of the upper and lower bone cuts through lateral orbital wall.

C. Right orbit viewed from the nasal side, showing position of the upper and lower bone cuts through the lateral orbital wall. Shaded area represents cancellous bone between the lateral orbital wall and the lateral cranial wall, behind which lie the middle fossa of the cranial cavity and superior orbital fissure. Bone between the upper and lower cuts is easily broken and retracted laterally; the remaining bone posterior to the break is then rongeured as far as the shaded area. (Courtesy of R. N. Berke.)

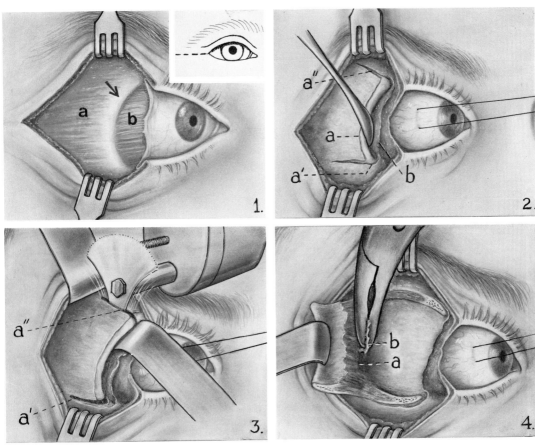

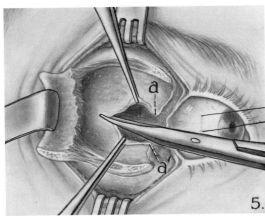

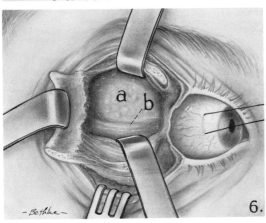

FIG. 17–14. Resection of the lateral wall of the orbit (Krönlein operation). *Step 1.* A horizontal skin incision (*inset*) is extended 5 cm or more from the external canthus, and a wide canthotomy exposes the lateral bony orbital wall (*arrow*). The fascia over the temporalis muscle is shown at *a* and the orbital fascia at *b*. *Step 2.* A traction suture previously placed in the lateral rectus muscle readily identifies it during surgery. The periosteum is incised along the orbital margin (*a*), and horizontal incisions are made at *a'* and *a''*. The periosteum is then reflected (*b*) from the inner aspect of the lateral orbital wall. *Step 3.* A retractor reflects the periosteum while the Stryker saw cuts the lateral bony orbital wall at *a'* and *a''*. *Step 4.* The lateral wall is broken with a rongeur and reflected, hinged to the temporalis muscle (*a*). The thin remaining posterior part of the wall (*b*) is removed with a rongeur. *Step 5.* The orbital fascia (*a-a'*) is cut horizontally with scissors. *Step 6.* The tumor (*a*) is lying in the muscle cone; *b* indicates the lateral rectus muscle.

a hammer and chisel. The thick margin is then broken, and the thin posterior wall is removed with a rongeur, or the anterior thick orbital margin can be partly incised by either a revolving saw or an ordinary·hand saw, after which the incision is completed with a chisel. The technique employing the hammer and chisel is adequate, particularly for children. A lower bone incision tangential to the margin of the orbit may extend into the zygomatic process; if so the bony flap will not break.

A similar incision is made below in the bone. The plane of the saw blade is slanted slightly backward, instead of being perpendicular, so that the incision is directed away from the anterior cranial fossa. The bony lateral wall of the orbit is then grasped with a rongeur and broken outward, with the temporalis muscle acting as a hinge. There is considerable variation as to how far back the wall breaks in different individuals; the thinnest portion may be just back of the margin or much deeper. The thin posterior edge of the wall is then rongeured down to the thick cancellous bone, where the lateral orbital and lateral cranial walls meet.

The periosteum is incised horizontally as far back as possible, and identifying sutures are placed in the two anterior edges of the periosteum so that the edges can be recognized for resuturing when the operation is finished. Only blunt dissection should be carried out in the orbit except when fibrous bands must be severed, which should be done under direct inspection if possible. It is seldom necessary to sever the external rectus muscle at its insertion for better exposure, as it can be retracted easily from the operative field. When the operation is over, the periosteum is resutured beginning at the anterior edge where the two identifying sutures were placed. The bony flap is next sutured in place and the lateral canthal ligament is reattached. The temporal fascia and the skin edges are closed. A double-arm suture on a rubber peg is placed in the center of the upper and lower lid margins to protect the cornea if proptosis should result from the surgery.

Even with the best possible exposure, one-third of the orbit posteriorly still remains inaccessible because it is sandwiched between the sinuses nasally and the anterior cranial fossa laterally. The lateral wall breaks about 12 mm posteriorly; another 12 mm portion still remains that must be removed with a rongeur. This leaves 20 mm of the posterior

lateral wall unexposed. Therefore, removal of a tumor in the posterior part of the orbit through a lateral orbitotomy would necessitate operating blindly across the superior orbital fissure, jeopardizing the important structures that traverse it.

Inadequate resection of the lateral wall is a common fault. The average resection in an adult is only about 2 cm, whereas a full resection should be about 3.4 cm.

The various extended lateral orbitotomies that have been proposed[53, 90, 101] give a wider base to the funnel in which the surgery is performed. However, the apex of the orbit still remains directly unapproachable from the lateral wall. If the orbital mass is diffuse with no cleavage planes, an attempt at total excision is usually contraindicated.

Complications

No tumor located mostly in the apex of the orbit can be completely excised without damaging important structures. These structures converge toward the apex of the orbit, and deep sharp dissection of this poorly exposed area carries the risk of damaging one or more of the extraocular muscles, the optic nerve, the blood supply to the optic nerve and eyeball, the levator muscle, and the ciliary ganglion. For these reasons, most of the untoward consequences in removing lesions involving the apex are probably due to attempts at surgical intervention beyond the point of diminishing returns.

In general, it is surprising that so few complications can be attributed unequivocally to surgery. The Krönlein procedure itself is not disfiguring. Blemishes and untoward sequelae usually result from manipulation in the orbit. The most frequently encountered sequelae of orbitotomy are limitations in abduction, ptosis, keratoconjunctivitis, sicca, diplopia, enophthalmos, occlusion of the central retinal artery or vein, optic atrophy, and macular pathology.

The limitation in abduction that often occurs after a lateral orbitotomy is seldom manifested as a tropia or a diplopia.

Some degree of ptosis is inevitable after complete excision of a lesion located in the upper part of the orbit. It is most often encountered following surgery around the lacrimal gland fossa; many lesions develop in this area and the levator muscle is closely related to, and integrated with, the lacrimal gland. If the tumor is malignant, excision must be complete and some degree of ptosis is likely to be the price.

Keratoconjunctivitis sicca may accompany lacrimal gland lesions and be aggravated by the surgery.

Enophthalmos stems from the decrease in orbital volume at the time of surgery. It seldom constitutes a blemish.

Occlusion of the central retinal artery and vein, optic atrophy, and macular changes are sometimes noted preoperatively, especially in the case of granulomas; surgery may exacerbate the underlying basic pathology. In two reported cases, occlusion of the central retinal artery was a complication of orbital granuloma.[43] Total unilateral visual loss following orbital surgery has been attributed to application of a pressure dressing tight enough to overcome the retinal arterial pressure.[61] The central retinal vessels are more likely to be injured during surgery in the inferior portion of the orbit where they emerge from the optic nerve, about 10 mm back of the globe. Macular pathology sometimes appears postoperatively from damage to the short posterior ciliary arteries.

In deep orbital dissections, where retraction is necessary for adequate exposure, care should be taken to prevent the retractor from pressing too hard on the eyeball, since very little pressure may occlude the central vessels.

Corneal anesthesia with neuroparalytic keratitis has also been reported as a sequela of orbitotomy.[9,92]

CRANIOTOMY

Ophthalmology shares the orbit with other specialities: neurology, rhinology, and maxillofacial pathology. Over the years, each has staked out its "orbital rights." Decompression of the orbit via the cranium has been advocated for cases of advanced exophthalmos in Graves's disease.[70] In a series of 123 orbital tumors, of which 108 were operated on by the transfrontal route, complications were reported to be rare and the results satisfactory.[16] Seven patients in another series were operated on by this routine for retrobulbar tumors.[84] However, I strongly disagree with the assertion that transfrontal craniotomy is indicated for virtually all expanding lesions of the orbit.[27]

Some neurosurgeons feel that many expanding orbital lesions extend to the cranium, but this seems to occur very seldom. The normal communication between the orbit and the cranium is by way of the superior orbital fissure and the optic nerve foramen. The superior orbital fissure syndrome is most unusual. An extension to the cranium through the optic nerve canal in cases of glioma, meningioma, and retinoblastoma is seldom demonstrated by x ray. A cranial extension directly through bone is extremely rare.

Our series of 504 expanding lesions of the orbit (Table 17–1) indicates that some patients with the following conditions may require craniotomy: neurofibroma, neurilemoma, neuroma, meningioma, glioma of the optic nerve, carotid–cavernous sinus fistula, mesenchymoma, fibrous dysplasia, congenital orbital varix, and mixed neurogenic tumor (encephalocele).

Perhaps only 2% of patients with neurofibroma, neurilemoma, or neuroma and the same percentage of those with mesenchymoma require craniotomy, whereas it is preferred for almost all patients in the other categories just listed. Thus, only about 8% of all patients with expanding lesions of the orbit seem to be candidates for neurosurgery.

The least accessible area by the Krönlein approach is the upper nasal part of the orbit. This quadrant, which is rarely affected, may possibly be better approached by way of the cranium.

If a tumor involves both the orbit and the adjacent intracranial cavity, it is preferable to do the intracranial surgery first to avoid opening that space to a potentially contaminated field. The neurosurgeon should place an easily identified barrier such as a plastic or metal plate at the site of the craniotomy so that if the orbit is later exenterated, the surgeon will have a chance for a clean excision of the orbital portion of the tumor. If a subtotal exenteration or a temporalis muscle transplant to the orbit is contemplated, there is no contraindication to performing the orbital surgery first.

It has been suggested that since osteomas involving the sinuses lie extradurally and in a potentially infected field, they should not be approached by way of the cranium.[62]

NASAL ORBITOTOMY

The medial bony wall of the orbit goes directly back to the optic foramen with no intervening structures. Therefore, a lesion is occasionally encountered at the apex of the orbit which is more accessible along the nasal wall than through the lateral wall. This approach is facilitated by resecting the lateral wall, mobilizing and retracting the temporalis muscle so that the globe can be pulled forward out of the apex. Lifting the globe forward with traction sutures on the four rectus muscles helps to increase the operating space and improve the exposure.[89] I believe that the nasal approach through the ethmoids is very seldom indicated for orbital neoplasms.

EXENTERATION

Until recently the ophthalmologist's surgical choice in treating orbital tumors lay between an orbitotomy and a total exenteration. The wide gap between these two extremes can be bridged considerably by a subtotal exenteration in the interest of a better cosmetic result. The objective after an exenteration is to produce a socket that will accommodate a prosthesis, or at least to leave a full orbit with the appearance of closed lids. The large cavity remaining after a total exenteration is humiliating to the patient, and any effort to improve his plight is worthwhile. The surgeon should decide what normal orbital tissues can be saved without jeopardizing the prognosis. The conjunctiva is the most indispensable tissue for socket restoration and the wearing of a prosthesis; and some or all of it can usually be salvaged.

The following are possibilities for subtotal exenteration:

1. When only the skin of the lids is left, it can be inverted to partially cover the bony orbit, the remainder of the denuded area being allowed to granulate. Alternatively, a temporalis muscle may be transplanted, with later restoration of the socket.
2. When the skin of the lids and the periosteum are left, the periosteum may be dissected from the bone until it thins out about halfway back; this free periosteum can be used to secure an implant.[25]
3. When the skin of the lids, the periosteum, the apical fat, and the posterior muscle cone are left, these tissues can be used to secure an implant in the apex of the orbit. The socket can later be restored and the patient fitted with a prosthesis.
4. When the skin of the lids, the periosteum, the apical fat, the posterior muscle cone,

and the conjunctiva are left, these tissues may secure an implant in the apex covered with conjunctiva, with the prosthesis fitted later.
5. When the contents of the upper and lower halves of the orbit can be spared, as is sometimes possible in cases of extensive epithelioma of the upper or the lower lid, the repair may be done by a Hughes operation in the case of a demiexenteration of the lower orbit and a reverse Hughes in the case of a demiexenteration of the upper orbit.

The tumor characteristics that determine the choice of operation are cohesiveness, encapsulation, and potential for metastasis.

Indications

1. Tumors that infiltrate, are not encapsulated, not cohesive, and nonmetastasizing may be excised extensively with some sacrifice of normal orbital tissue. If the tumor recurs, exenteration may then be performed. In this category are hemangiopericytoma, hemangioendothelioma, neurofibroma, mesenchymoma, fibrosarcoma, myxosarcoma, leiomyosarcoma, basal-cell carcinoma, meningioma, residual malignant melanoma, residual retinoblastoma, and some epithelial tumors of the lacrimal gland.
2. Tumors that infiltrate, are not encapsulated, and metastasize through the lymphatics. A subtotal exenteration with in-continuity resection of the lymphatics may be indicated in cases of malignant congenital melanoma, and total exenteration with in-continuity resection in late and recurrent cases. Tumors in this category are cancerous melanosis of the conjunctiva and malignant melanocytoma. Such in-continuity resection refers to removal of a block of tissue between the primary site of the tumor and the regional nodes. The purpose is to remove tumor cells lodged in the lymphatics, a phenomenon referred to as obstructed in-transit metastases.
3. Tumors that infiltrate and metastasize through the bloodstream. In these cases total exenteration is indicated. Tumors in this category are rhabdomyosarcoma, carcinoma of the lacrimal gland, and malignant melanoma extending to the uvea or elsewhere.

Technique

1. Simple, total exenteration. Two double-arm silk sutures are passed through the lid margins and tied in order to close the palpebral aperture. The suture ends should not be cut because they can provide traction to manipulate the lids. Incisions are made with a scalpel through the skin along the upper and lower lid margins just back of the cilia line. Both incisions are carried from one canthus to the other. The skin of the upper and lower lids is then reflected—above, below, nasally, and temporally—so that the bony orbital margin will be readily accessible. The dissection can be facilitated by a lateral extension of the skin incision beyond the external canthus. There is a considerable amount of bleeding, but it is not necessary to stop bleeding as it appears at each point. Proceeding quickly with reflection of the skin, the operator can control the bleeding after obtaining adequate exposure.

Once the bony orbital margin has been exposed, an incision should be made with a scalpel through the periosteum along the upper margin. At some point along this margin the periosteal elevator is inserted between the periosteum and the bone, and the periosteum is reflected as far back as possible from the orbital roof. Since resistance will be encountered in the regions of the superior oblique pulley and the external and internal canthal ligaments, a scalpel or scissors must be used. The bone in the roof of the orbit is quite thin and, even under normal circumstances, may have dehiscences. Therefore, in manipulating the periosteal elevator or other instrument, care should be taken to avoid entering the anterior cranial fossa.

Separation of the periosteum from the bone can be started again at the lower orbital margin, or the dissection that was started above can be continued around the lower half of the orbit. Resistance will be met at the origin of the inferior oblique muscle, which must be severed with scissors. After the periosteum has been separated as far posteriorly as possible with the elevator, blunt dissection should be carried out with the finger to the apex of the orbit. At certain sites the periosteum adheres so firmly to the bone that it cannot be completely separated, *e.g.*, over the areas of both the superior and inferior orbital fissures. Usually the supraorbital and infraorbital nerves are encountered at or near their course around the orbital margin. These nerves must be severed even though a postoperative anesthesia may result.

After the periosteum has been dissected as close as possible to the apex of the orbit, the orbital contents (surrounded for the most part by the periosteum) are removed *en masse* by severing the structures at the apex with heavy scissors. The moderate bleeding that usually ensues can be controlled satisfactorily by pressure. The skin of the upper and lower lids is tucked backward along the bony roof and floor of the orbit, and a pressure dressing is applied.

2. Simple exenteration with graft. A split-thickness skin graft cut from the abdomen is inserted into the orbital cavity on a gauze tampon. An appropriate amount of fluffed gauze is covered with a thin rubber tissue fixed by a rubber band. This round soft tampon, of a size to fit snugly in the orbit, is covered with a thin layer of petroleum jelly, which is in turn covered by the graft and plugged into the orbital cavity. The redundant graft around the base of the tampon is spread out over the margin of the orbit; the remaining skin of the lids is tucked around the roof and floor of the orbit. A pressure dressing is applied. The tampon is left *in situ* for six or seven days. After it is removed, petrolatum gauze is inserted at each dressing after the orbit has been cleaned. It is surprising that the graft always takes on this bare bone deprived of its periosteum. After six weeks or more the orbital cavity will be covered with epithelium (Fig. 17–15).

3. Exenteration with temporalis muscle implant (Fig. 17–16). In cases where it is unsafe to preserve the conjunctiva (*e.g.*, malignant melanoma of the conjunctiva, some basal-cell

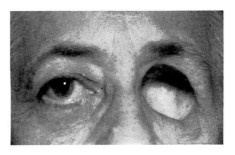

FIG. 17–15. Exenteration of the orbit with half-thickness skin graft.

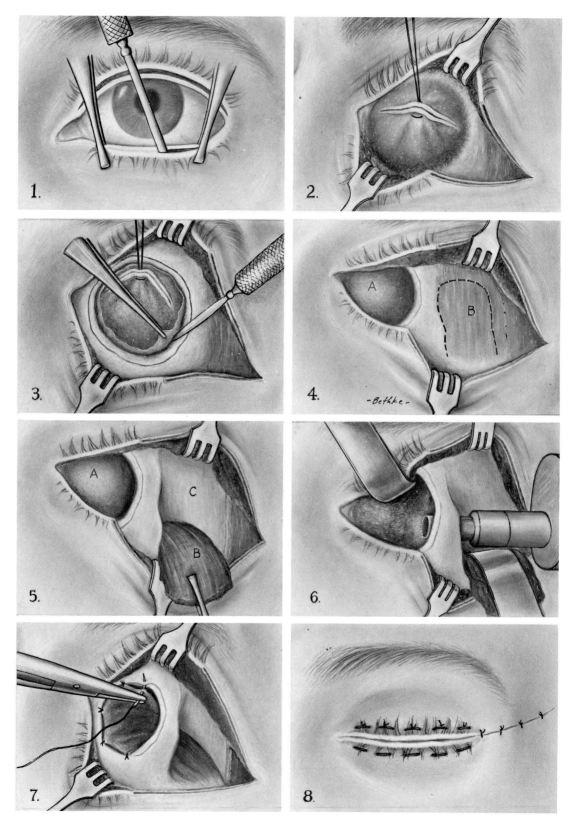

FIG. 17–16. Technique for exenteration of the orbit with a temporalis muscle transplant when the conjunctiva is sacrificed. *Step 1.* The upper and lower lids are split, leaving the cilia and skin anteriorly, and the tarsus, orbicularis, conjunctiva, palpebral muscle, and fascial planes posteriorly. *Step 2.* The margins of the posterior half of the lid are joined by a double-arm suture for easier manipulation during the exenteration. A horizontal skin incision extending temporally from the external canthus exposes the lateral bony wall and the temporalis muscle. *Step 3.* The periosteum is incised around the orbital margin and reflected from the bony orbit; the orbital contents along with the periosteum are removed. *Step 4.* The exenterated orbit is seen at *A,* and *B* shows the outlined portion of the temporalis muscle, with its fascia, which is to be transplanted. *Step 5.* The outlined portion (half or less of the muscle) is mobilized (*B*) from its fossa (*C*) after its fascia is freed from the zygoma. *Step 6.* With the temporalis muscle retracted from the field, a trephine opening is made through the lateral wall of the orbit with an oscillating saw. The opening is enlarged with a rongeur. *Step 7.* The temporalis muscle and its fascia are passed through the hole in the lateral wall and sutured to the cut edges of the periosteum after a plastic implant has been placed in the fossa behind the muscle. *Step 8.* The remaining anterior leaf of each lid is sutured with the borders everted, and the skin of the ◀ temple is sutured.

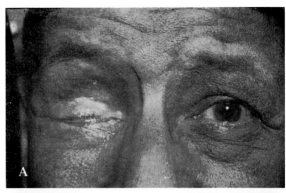

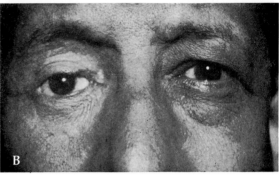

FIG. 17–17. Exenteration of the orbit with temporalis muscle transplant and restoration of the socket with a split-thickness skin graft. **A.** Appearance 6 months after exenteration of the orbit. **B.** Appearance 17 months later and 7 months after restoration of the socket.

or squamous-cell carcinomas), the socket is restored by a half-thickness skin graft either at the time of the original operation or later. It has been my practice to restore it later when a cure seems likely.

The upper and lower lids are each halved with a scalpel through the gray line that extends from one end of the lid to the other. At the extremities this incision may be completed with scissors. Anteriorly, halving of the lids leaves the cilia and skin intact; posteriorly, it leaves the tarsus, orbicularis, conjunctiva, palpebral muscle, and fascial planes intact. Division of the upper and lower lids is extended as far as the orbital margin above and below.

A 2 to 3 cm skin incision is made horizontally from the external canthus. Dissection of this skin, continuous with dissection of the skin of the upper and lower lids, is carried out above and below to expose the entire area over the temporalis muscle. Reflection of these upper and lower flaps (including the skin of both lids and of the temporal region) exposes the entire orbital cavity as well as a wide area in the temporal region.

The periosteum is then incised around the entire orbital circumference, and a total exenteration of the orbit, including the periosteum, is performed.

Next, an incision is made in the deep fascia of the temporalis muscle along the lateral wall of the orbit. The fascia is particularly adherent along the upper margin of the zygomatic process where it must be incised to release the temporalis muscle sufficiently. This muscle, with its fascia, must be freed from the temporal fossa and from under the zygomatic process to the site of its insertion into the coronoid process of the mandible, so that the muscle and its fascia are mobile enough to reach the orbit through the opening in the lateral wall. It is estimated that about two-thirds of the muscle is transplanted.

A round opening is made with the Stryker

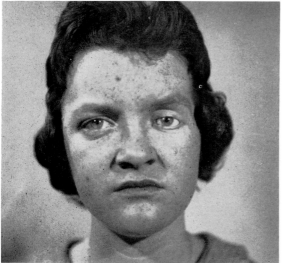

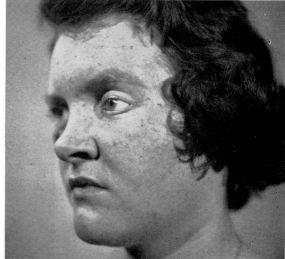

FIG. 17–18. Exenteration of the left orbit with temporalis muscle transplant and reconstruction of the socket with a split-thickness skin graft from the abdomen three years and four months later.

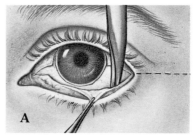

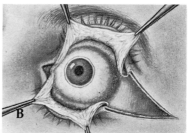

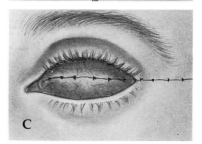

saw in the lateral wall of the orbit. This is enlarged with a rongeur, particularly below, but the anterior margin is left intact. A 20 mm plastic sphere is placed in the apex of the orbit (plastic is recommended instead of gold as it will not interfere with radiotherapy should that become necessary for a suspected or anticipated recurrence). The temporalis muscle and its fascia are passed through the opening into the orbit and sutured to the remaining periosteum in such a way that the muscle and fascia are fanned out to fill uniformly as much of the orbit as possible. The lid margins are approximated with two double-arm catgut sutures, and a pressure dressing is applied.

Restoration of the socket following a temporalis muscle implant with graft (Fig. 17–17). When enough time has elapsed after exenteration to make a recurrence seem unlikely, the socket may be restored. A knife cut is made between the two rows of cilia to a depth of 2 mm. The length of the incision and placement of the lateral and medial ends are determined with the palpebral fissure of the fellow eye in view, to ensure a good match. At the 2 mm depth, the surface of the underlying graft fascia is located, and the lids can be separated from it by combined sharp and blunt dissection which is carried above and below to the orbital rim.

FIG. 17–19. Exenteration of the orbit with a temporalis muscle transplant, followed by restoration of the socket with preserved conjunctiva. **A.** The conjunctiva is incised horizontally, nasally, and temporally and reflected from the globe. **B.** The reflected conjunctiva above and below is shown to be continuous with the horizontal Berke incision. **C.** Closure after routine exenteration and transplantation; the socket is lined with the preserved conjunctiva.

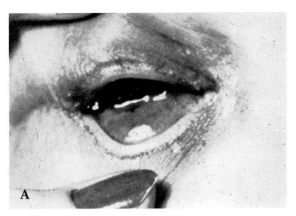

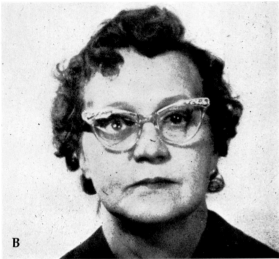

Two large plastic conformers are sutured back to back. A split-thickness skin graft about 5 × 8 cm, taken from the abdomen with a dermatome, is placed around the hand-molded conformers with the cut surface out. The edges of the skin graft should come together on the front surface of the plastic form, which is then placed under the lids. The upper and lower lid edges are drawn firmly together to push the skin graft as deeply into the fornices as possible. Excess protruding skin may be trimmed. The conformers are removed in five to seven days; when any devitalized skin has been excised, a prothesis can be fitted.

The socket may be restored with a split-thickness graft at the time of exenteration or later (Fig. 17–18).

Restoration of the socket following a temporalis muscle transplant with conjunctiva (Fig. 17–19). If the conjunctiva is not involved in the condition leading to exenteration, the technique can be modified as follows: Instead of the lids being split in the gray line, the entire thickness of each lid is preserved. The conjunctiva is divided at the limbus and reflected to the fornices. The knife cuts to the orbital rim are then made beneath the conjunctiva, and exenteration is carried out in the usual manner. After the temporalis muscle graft is sutured in place, the conjunctival opening is closed, as after an enucleation. A conformer should be used, and

FIG. 17–20. Exenteration of the right orbit with temporalis muscle transplant and restoration of the socket with preserved conjunctiva. A temporary prosthesis was inserted nine days postoperatively. **A.** The socket lined with conjunctiva one month after exenteration. **B.** Appearance at this time with a prosthesis.

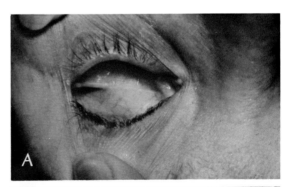

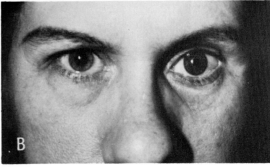

FIG. 17–21. Subtotal exenteration of right orbit and restoration of the socket with preserved conjunctiva. **A.** Socket four and a half months after exenteration. **B.** Patient with prosthesis three and a half months later. (Courtesy of I. S. Jones.)

a prosthesis can be fitted in two weeks (Fig. 17–20).

Improved cosmetic appearance after an orbital exenteration has been reported with use of a methyl methacrylate implant[40] or a conoidal acrylic implant especially fashioned to accommodate a facial prosthesis.[3]

Subtotal exenteration, leaving some amounts of skin, lid margin, conjunctiva, periosteum, orbital fat, and posterior muscle cone, or even the upper or lower nasal or temporal half of the orbit, is sometimes possible.

It is impractical to attempt to describe the many modifications and variations in technique. A competent surgeon will use the salvaged tissue to good advantage without relying on set rules. The value of saving tissues, especially the conjunctiva, cannot be overemphasized because it ensures a cosmetic result far superior to that obtained in the usual complete exenteration (Fig. 17–21).

REFERENCES

1. ABBOUD IA, HANNA LS: Intermittent exophthalmos. Br J Ophthalmol 55:628–632, 1971
2. AGRAWAL PK, DAYAL Y, AGARWAL LP: Pseudotumor of orbit; as a collagen disease manifestation. Orient Arch Ophthalmol 5:178–183, 1967
3. ALLEN L, BLODI FC: A conoidal exenteration implant. Trans Am Acad Ophthalmol Otolaryngol 78:617–621, 1974
4. AYOUB M, KAMEL I: Ocular cysticercosis. Bull Ophthalmol Soc Egypt 60:231–235, 1967
4a. BACKLUND EO: Pterional approach for orbital decompression. Acta Ophthalmol 46:535–540, 1968
5. BACKLUND EO, TORLEGARD K: Stereophotogrammetric exophthalmometry. Acta Ophthalmol (Kbh) 46:575–579, 1968
6. BAGHDASSARIAN SA, ZAKHARIA H: Report of three cases of hydatid cyst of the orbit. Am J Ophthalmol 71:1081–1084, 1971
7. BEHAL ML: Secondary amyloid infiltration around the limbus. Br J Ophthalmol 48:622–623, 1964
8. BENEDICT WL: Surgical treatment of tumors and cysts of the orbit. Am J Ophthalmol 32:763–773, 1949
9. BERKE RN: A modified Krönlein operation. Arch Ophthalmol 51:609–632, 1954
10. BERNASCONI V, GIOVANELLI M, PERRIA C: Meningo-encephalocele of posterior part of orbit. Neurochirurgia (Stuttg) 11:19–29, 1968
11. BLODI FC, GASS JD: Inflammatory pseudotumor of the orbit. Trans Am Acad Ophthalmol Otolaryngol 71:303–322, 1967
12. BÖKE W, MOHR HJ: Contribution to the knowledge of congenital orbital cysts. Klin Monatsbl Augenheilkd 151:225–230, 1967
13. BÖKE W, REICH H: Ocular involvement in Wegener's granulomatosis. Klin Monatsbl Augenheilkd 151:802–822, 1968
14. BOURQUET J, MAWAS J: Gliome encapsule de l'orbite. Bull Soc Ophtalmol Paris, 1931, pp 224–246
15. BOYCE DC, BOLKER N: Ocular manifestations of primary nasopharyngeal tumors. Am J Ophthalmol 32:1354–1358, 1949
16. BRENNER H, OSSOINIG K, VALENCAK E: Surgical treatment of orbital tumours. Wien Med Wochenschr 119:383–384, 1969
17. BRIGGS RM, CHASE RA, DELLÁPORTA A: Unilateral congenital orbital cyst with microphthalmos. Plast Reconstr Surg 41:376–380, 1968
18. BRIHAYE M, BASTIN J-P, DETILLEUX JM, HALET W: Hydatid cyst of the orbit. Bull Soc Belge Ophtalmol 146:317–328, 1967
19. BRIHAYE J, HOFFMANN GR, FRANÇOIS J, BRIHAYE-VAN GEERTRUYDEN M: Neurosurgical exophthalmos. Neurochirurgie 14:187–487, 1968
20. BROWNSTEIN MH, ELLIOTT R, HELWIG EB: Ophthalmologic aspects of amyloidosis. Am J Ophthalmol 69:423–430, 1970
21. BULTEAU V, CONSTABLE I: Transantral decompression of the orbit. Med J Aust 1:62–63, 1970
22. BYNKE HG, EFSING HO: Carotid-cavernous fistula with contralateral exophthalmos. Acta Ophthalmol (Kbh) 48:971–978, 1970
23. CALHOUN FP: Bilateral coloboma of the optic nerve associated with holes in the disc and a cyst of the optic sheath. Arch Ophthalmol 3:71–79, 1930
24. CHOLAN BS, PARMAR IPS, BHATIA JN: Anterior orbital meningoencephalocele. Am J Ophthalmol 68:144–146, 1969
25. COOPER WC: Personal communication
26. CUTLER WM, BLATT IM: Ocular manifestations of lethal midline granuloma (Wegener's granulomatosis). Am J Ophthalmol 42:21–35, 1956
27. DANDY WE: Orbital Tumors; Results Following the Transcranial Operative Attack. New York, Oskar Piest, 1941
28. DAVIDOFF LM, DYKE CG: Relapsing juvenile chronic subdural hematoma, clinical and roentgenographic study. Bull Neurol Inst NY 7:95–111, 1938
29. DAVIES GB, WONG PL: Sclerosing lipogranuloma in the orbit. Br J Ophthalmol 42:697–701, 1958
30. DAVIS FA: Primary tumors of the optic nerve (a phenomenon of Recklinghausen's disease); a clinical and pathologic study with a report of five cases and a review of the literature. Arch Ophthalmol 23:735–821; 957–1022, 1940
31. DAY RM: Ocular manifestations of thyroid disease; current concepts. Trans Am Ophthalmol Soc 57:572–601, 1959
32. DYER JA, HENDERSON JW: Orbitonometry in unilateral exophthalmos. Am J Ophthalmol 45:208–221, 1958
33. EIFRIG DE: Lipid granuloma of the orbit. Arch Ophthalmol 79:163–165, 1968
34. FAULDS JS, WEAR AR: Pseudotumour of the orbit and Wegener's granuloma. Lancet 2:955–977, 1960

35. Fells P, Koniach D, Kabir DJ: Diagnosis of dysthyroid exophthalmos. Trans Ophthalmol Soc UK 90:251–260, 1970

36. Fite JD, Schwartz JF, Calhoun FP: Aneurysmal bone cyst of the orbit (a clinicopathologic case report). Trans Am Acad Ophthalmol Otolaryngol 72:614–618, 1968

37. Forrest AW: Personal communication

38. Freedman A, Jones BR: Surgical problems in dysthyroid eye disease. Trans Ophthalmol Soc UK 87:431–445, 1967

39. Friedman B: Measurement of relative exophthalmos by roentgenography. US Navy Med Bull 45:482–487, 1945

40. Gass JD: Technique of orbital exenteration using methyl methacrylate implant. Arch Ophthalmol 82:789–791, 1969

41. Gigglberger H: Ueber das Cholesteatom der Orbita. Klin Monatsbl Augenheilkd 114:206–211, 1949

42. Goder G, Velhagen KH: Amyloid in the conjunctiva and orbit. Arch Klin Exp Ophthalmol 176:183–194, 1968

43. Godfrey RC: Occlusion of the retinal artery in two cases of orbital granuloma. Br J Ophthalmol 53:703–706, 1969

44. Godtfredsen E, Lederman M: Diagnostic and prognostic roles of ophthalmoneurologic signs and symptoms in malignant nasopharyngeal tumors. Am J Ophthalmol 59:1063–1069, 1965

45. Guibor P, Keeney AH: Thermography and ophthalmology. Trans Am Acad Ophthalmol Otolaryngol 74:1032–1043, 1970

46. Hauer J: Additional clinical sign of "unilateral" endocrine exophthalmos. Br J Ophthalmol 53:210–211, 1969

47. Hedges TR Jr, Leopold IH: Parallel retinal folds; their significance in orbital space-taking lesions. Arch Ophthalmol 62:353–355, 1959

48. Henderson JW, Schneider RC: The ocular findings in carotid-cavernous fistula in a series of 17 cases. Trans Am Ophthalmol Soc 56:123–144, 1958

49. Herndon BW: Perilimbal amyloid tumor. Am J Ophthalmol 66:515–520, 1968

50. Hirsch O: Surgical decompression of malignant exophthalmos. Arch Otolaryngol 51:325–335, 1950

51. Jakobiec FA, Tannenbaum M: Classification of orbital tumors based on electron microscopy. Proc. 2nd Int. Symp. on Orbital Disorders, Amsterdam 1973. Mod Probl Ophthalmol (Karger, Basel) 14:330–343, 1975

52. Jellinek EH: The orbital pseudotumor syndrome and its differentiation from endocrine exophthalmos. Brain 92:35–58, 1969

53. Jones BR: Surgical approaches to the orbit. Trans Ophthalmol Soc UK 40:368–381, 1970

54. Kassman T, Sundmark E: Orbital pseudo-tumors with amyloid. Acta Ophthalmol (Kbh) 45:220–228, 1967

55. King RB, Hayes GJ: Unilateral proptosis due to fibrous dysplasia of bone. Arch Ophthalmol 46:553–559, 1951

56. Kubicz S, Sobieszczanska-Radoszewska L: A case of aneurysmal cyst of the ethmoid and frontal bone in an 8-year-old boy. Otolaryngol Pol 16:665–669, 1962

57. Kubik J: Die Folgen der Bulbuskompression bei Raumbeengung in der Orbita. Klin Monatsbl Augenheilkd 80:513–518, 1928

58. Lavergne G, Winand R: Modern concepts on the pathogenesis and medical treatment of endocrine exophthalmos. Bull Soc Belge Ophtalmol 152:434–549, 1969

59. Leone CR Jr, Marlowe JF: Orbital presentation of an ethmoid encephalocele; report of a case in a 62-year-old woman. Arch Ophthalmol 83:445–447, 1970

60. Little JM: Waldenström's macroglobulinemia in the lacrimal gland. Trans Am Acad Ophthalmol Otolaryngol 71:875–879, 1967

61. Long JC, Ellis PP: Total unilateral visual loss following orbital surgery. Am J Ophthalmol 71:218–220, 1971

62. Love JG, Benedict WL: Transcranial removal of intraorbital tumors. JAMA 129:777–784, 1945

63. Mabrouk R, Chadli A, Djedidi H, Cheikh T-B: Four cases of colobomatous orbito-palpebral cysts; clinical, anatomopathological, and genetic study. Bull Mem Soc Fr Ophtalmol 81:173–194, 1968

64. McCormick JL, Macauley WL, Miller GE: Talc granulomas of the eye. Am J Ophthalmol 32:1252–1254, 1949

65. Martin HE: Personal communication

66. Mehra KS, Khanna NN, Nema HV, Mathur JS, Nagarajachar J, Tandon HD: Cold abscess in the orbit. Acta Ophthalmol (Kbh) 46:1067–1072, 1968

67. Morgan DC, Mason AS: Exophthalmos in Cushing's syndrome. Br Med J 2:481–483, 1958

68. Mortada A: Origin of orbital blood cysts. Br J Ophthalmol 53:398–402, 1969

69. Mortada A, El-Torach I: Orbital meningo-encephalocele and exophthalmos. Br J Ophthalmol 44:309–314, 1960

70. Naffziger HC: Progressive exophthalmos following thyroidectomy; its pathology and treatment. Ann Surg 94:582–586, 1931

71. Nicholls JVV: Cholesterol-containing granuloma of the orbital wall. Am J Ophthalmol 41:234–247, 1956

72. Ogura JH: Transantral orbital decompression for progressive exophthalmos; a follow-up of 54 cases. Med Clin North Am 52:399–407, 1968

73. Pfeiffer RL: Infratemporal subdural hematomas, a cause of exophthalmos. Trans Am Ophthalmol Soc 56:187–202, 1958

74. Pincus L: Primäre Rettnekrose (Lipogranulomatosis) der Orbita. Klin Monatsbl Augenheilkd 94:369–372, 1935

75. Plotz CM, Knowlton AI, Ragan C: The natural history of Cushing's syndrome. Am J Med 13:597–614, 1952

76. Quickert MH: Personal communication

77. Quinandeau P: Retinoblastome de l'orbite. Bull Soc Franc Ophtalmol 64:4–6, 1951

78. Raab EL: Intraorbital amyloid. Br J Ophthalmol 54:445–449, 1970

79. Ransohoff J: Personal communication

80. Rathbun JE, Hoyt WF, Beard C: Surgical management of orbitofrontal varix in Klippel-Trénaunay-Weber syndrome. Am J Ophthalmol 70:109–112, 1970

81. Reese AB: The etiology of exophthalmos (symposium). Complications; causes from primary

lesions in the orbit; surgery. Trans Am Acad Ophthalmol Otolaryngol 39:65–80, 1934–1935

82. REESE AB: Expanding lesions of the orbit (Bowman Lecture). Trans Ophthalmol Soc UK 91:85–104, 1971

83. SAKIC D: Parasites as a cause of exophthalmos in children. Ber Dtsch Ophthalmol Ges 69:111, 1968

84. SCHURMANN K, OPPEL O: Transfrontal orbitotomy as a method of operation in retrobulbar tumors. Klin Monatsbl Augenheilkd 139:130–159, 1961

85. SCHWARZ F, DER KINDEREN PJ, HOUTSTRA-LANZ M: Exophthalmos-producing activity in the serum and in the pituitary of patients with Cushing's syndrome and acromegaly. J Clin Endocrinol 22:718–725, 1962

86. SIEDENBIEDEL H: Brauner Tumor der Orbita: Gutartiger Riesenzellentumor. Klin Monatsbl Augenheilkd 122:86–90, 1953

87. SLANSKY HH, KOLBERT G, GARTNER S: Exophthalmos induced by steroids. Arch Ophthalmol 77:579–581, 1967

88. SMETANA HF, BERNHARD W: Sclerosing lipogranuloma. Arch Pathol 50:296–325, 1950

89. SMITH JL: Anterolateral approach to the orbit. Trans Am Acad Ophthalmol Otolaryngol 75:1059–1064, 1971

90. STALLARD HB: A plea for lateral orbitotomy with certain modifications. Br J Ophthalmol 44:718–723, 1960

91. STELL PM: Transantral orbital decompression in malignant exophthalmos. J Laryngol 82:613–621, 1968

92. TAKATS G: Surgery of the orbit. Arch Ophthalmol 8:259–268, 1932

93. TENGROTH B, BOGREN H, ZACKRISSON U: Human exophthalmometry. Acta Ophthalmol (Kbh) 42:864–874, 1964

94. VAN WIEN S, MERZ EH: Exophthalmos secondary to periarteritis nodosa. Am J Ophthalmol 56:204–208, 1963

95. WALTON EW: Pseudotumour of the orbit and polyarteritis nodosa. J Clin Pathol 12:419–426, 1959

96. WERNER SC: The Thyroid. New York, Harper & Row, 1955

97. WERNER SC: Management of the active severe eye changes of Graves' disease. Trans Am Acad Ophthalmol Otolaryngol 71:631–637, 1967

98. WILLIAMS AW: Exophthalmos in cortisone-treated experimental animals. Br J Exp Pathol 34:621–624, 1953

99. WOLTER JR: Parallel horizontal retinal folding. Am J Ophthalmol 53:26–29, 1962

100. WOLTER JR, JAMPEL RS: Retinal folds due to external pressure on the globe from tumors. Klin Monatsbl Augenheilkd 131:433–438, 1957

101. WRIGHT AD: Approach to orbital tumours. Trans Ophthalmol Soc UK 68:367–375, 1948

102. WRIGHT JE: Orbital vascular anomalies. Trans Am Acad Ophthalmol Otolaryngol 78:606–616, 1974

103. ZIMMERMAN LE, ROGERS JB: Idiopathic thrombophlebitis of orbital veins simulating primary tumor of orbit. Trans Am Acad Ophthalmol Otolaryngol 61:609–613, 1957

INDEX